# Bone and Joint Infections

Pietro Ruggieri • Rohan Parwani •
Khaled M. Emara • Andrea Angelini
Editors

# Bone and Joint Infections

Springer

*Editors*
Pietro Ruggieri
Department of Orthopedics &
Orthopedic Oncology
University of Padova
Padova, Italy

Khaled M. Emara
Department of Orthopedic Surgery
Ain Shams University Hospital
Cairo, Egypt

Rohan Parwani
Department of Orthopedics
PDU Medical College
Rajkot, Gujarat, India

Andrea Angelini
Department of Orthopedics &
Orthopedic Oncology
University of Padova
Padova, Italy

ISBN 978-3-031-96382-7 ISBN 978-3-031-96383-4 (eBook)
https://doi.org/10.1007/978-3-031-96383-4



This Springer imprint is published by the registered company Springer Nature Switzerland AG
The registered company address is: Gewerbestrasse 11, 6330 Cham, Switzerland

# Foreword

This project began as the vision of Professor Pietro Ruggieri, then Chair of the SICOT Infection Committee. The committee had the ambitious goal of creating a comprehensive textbook dedicated to infections, particularly those affecting the musculoskeletal system. The editors—Pietro Ruggieri, Andrea Angelini, Rohan Parwani, and Khaled Emara—were all inspired by their collective work on this committee and sought to share their expertise in this crucial field.

Infections related to bone and prostheses present unique challenges for orthopedic surgeons. Not only must they navigate complex medical issues, but they also need a deep understanding of infectious lesions, which can be as difficult to treat as tumors. In some cases, the approach to managing an infection, mirrors that of treating tumors, demanding a blend of knowledge for surgical intervention. While recent meta-analyses and reviews provide valuable information, nothing surpasses the insight gained from personal experience, which this book seeks to offer.

The authors, drawing on their work with the SICOT committee, have compiled their collective experience and knowledge into this volume. Each chapter serves as an update, addressing specific problems faced by orthopedic surgeons in the diagnosis and treatment of infections. The book covers not only surgical techniques but also diagnostic methods and tailored antibiotics treatments. Special attention is given to imaging, from traditional X-rays to advanced techniques like CT scans, MRIs, cytology, and bacterial cultures.

Current knowledge is supported by important references, providing a thorough guide to diagnosis, pathology, and treatment. Richly illustrated, the chapters include detailed pictures and tables to enhance understanding. This volume represents the collective work of the SICOT committee and will be an important educational resource within the field of orthopedic surgery. The four editors deserve both admiration and gratitude for their commitment to this significant work.

Finally, this book covers the tenure of three SICOT Presidents: Ashok Johari, Philippe Hernigou, and Vikas Khanduja.

Children's Orthopaedic Centre, Mahim (West) Ashok Johari
Mumbai, India
Henri Mondor Hospital, University Paris Philippe Hernigou
Créteil, France
Department of Trauma and Orthopedics Vikas Khanduja
Addenbrooke's-Cambridge University Hospital
NHS Foundation Trust, Cambridge, UK

# Preface

It is a great pleasure to present this volume on bone and joint infections published by Springer Nature.

This idea originated by a proposal of one of us (PR) to the other editors. We were all happy to work on this topic for several reasons. First of all, infections are becoming more and more a social and medical issue that raises concern for the future and implies the role and use of antibiotics. In fact, antibiotics are generally losing their efficacy for infectious diseases, this also due to the wide—maybe too wide—use that has been and is currently done.

The second reason is more specifically related to the field of orthopedics. As a matter of fact, the problem of periprosthetic infections in primary prosthetic reconstructions and complex revision surgeries in orthopedic oncology is increasing: it represents a true "emergency" for all us surgeons. Moreover, infections on bone and joint not related with primary surgery is an issue and it cannot always find a proper treatment in all orthopedic hospitals. One reason for that is that the treatment of orthopedic infections is becoming more and more a multidisciplinary task.

This book cannot have the ambition of completeness, as the topic of bone and joint infections is really an ocean; rather it tries to summarize in 28 chapters the crucial problems, in order to help orthopedic surgeons to refresh their knowledge and provide them with the most relevant references for each reported topic.

We wish to thank first of all the members of the SICOT Committee of Infections involved in authoring this book. Besides to them, other prominent members of SICOT contributed as authors: they all worked very hard, and we appreciate their tremendous effort and commitment.

We are sincerely thankful to Springer Nature for accepting our proposal and taking care of this publication with their usual precision and high-standard level.

Last, but not least: this volume could have never been possible without the strong approval and support of SICOT Presidential Line. Since it required a fair amount of time, we wish to make our acknowledgments to three consecutive Society Presidents for trusting us: Vikas Khanduja, Philippe Hernigou, Ashok Johari. To them, our sincerest gratitude.

We hope that this book can be useful to all orthopedic surgeons: the young ones for their education and progress, to the old ones for an update on the subject.

We wish all of you a pleasant, productive reading.

Padova, Italy Pietro Ruggieri
Padova, Italy Andrea Angelini
Rajkot, Gujarat, India Rohan Parwani
Cairo, Egypt Khaled Emara

# Contents

# 1 Bone and Joint Infections: Introduction and Epidemiology

Andrea Angelini and Pietro Ruggieri

## 1.1 Historical Background

Osteomyelitis, the infection and inflammation of long bones or bone marrow, has been documented in medical literature throughout history, from ancient Egypt and Greece to modern times. Various terms have been used to describe this condition, such as "cold of bones," "necrosis," "typhus," "carbuncle of the bone," "osteitis," "periostitis," "osteoperiostitis," and "periosteomyelitis." These terms all convey the notion of an inflammatory process affecting the bone [1]. The historical understanding of osteomyelitis has evolved significantly from ancient times, as evidenced by the descriptions found in early human remains and medical texts from Europe, Asia, and Northern Africa. Ancient Egyptian papyri, such as the Edwin Smith Surgical Papyrus, detailed bone involvement in open fractures with pus formation. Hippocrates later described osteomyelitis of the skull and long bones following wounds, noting that sequestra could depress scar tissue and underlying bone. Roman physicians Celsus and Galen emphasized the importance of suppuration for healing postfracture infections [2]. In the Medieval period, injuries sustained in battles and accidents were common causes of infections, often leading to chronic osteomyelitis. Moreover, poor sanitation and lack of aseptic surgical techniques contributed to the high incidence of infections.

By the late eighteenth and early nineteenth centuries, Hunter and Dorsey elucidated the mechanisms of sequestrum formation and bone necrosis, advocating for early incision to maintain periosteal blood supply and prevent abscesses. The discovery of microorganisms causing osteomyelitis by Pasteur in 1860 and Koch's isolation of the tubercle bacillus in 1882 marked significant advancements in understanding the disease's etiology [3]. At the same time, the introduction of antiseptic techniques by Joseph Lister significantly reduced postsurgical infections [4].

Throughout the 19th and 20th centuries, further insights were gained into osteomyelitis' pathophysiology and clinical manifestations, and in the past decades, new concepts were introduced, which include the immune system activation by osteocytes, cortical bone involvement, and *Staphylococcus aureus* is to be the main pathogen responsible for osteomyelitis [5]. The discovery of penicillin and the subsequent development of other antibiotics revolutionized the treatment of BJIs, dramatically reducing morbidity and mortality [6]. With the advent of advanced imaging techniques, including scintig-

A. Angelini · P. Ruggieri (✉)
Department of Orthopedics and Orthopedic Oncology, University of Padova, Padova, Italy
e-mail: andrea.angelini@unipd.it; pietro.ruggieri@unipd.it



P. Ruggieri et al. (eds.), *Bone and Joint Infections*, https://doi.org/10.1007/978-3-031-96383-4_1

raphy, ultrasonography, CT, MRI, and PET-FDG, the diagnosis and understanding of the early phases of osteomyelitis have markedly improved [7]. These modalities enable precise detection and detailed characterization of the infection, allowing for earlier and more accurate diagnosis and thereby enhancing the effectiveness of subsequent management strategies [8].

## 1.2 Epidemiology

The overall incidence of osteomyelitis in adults is 21.8 cases per 100,000 persons annually in the United States, with approximately 20% of these cases attributed to hematogenous spread [9]. The condition shows a higher prevalence in males and increases with age, although the reasons for this gender disparity remain unclear. In pediatric populations, the incidence of osteomyelitis varies, often influenced by different etiological factors compared to adults. *Staphylococcus aureus* is the most common pathogen implicated in both acute and chronic osteomyelitis, along with coagulase-negative staphylococci, aerobic gram-negative bacilli, Enterococcus, and various Streptococcal species [5]. The clinical presentation of osteomyelitis is heterogeneous, affecting individuals across all age groups and patient types (Table 1.1). High-risk and life-threatening conditions that predispose individuals to osteomyelitis and systemic infections include immunosuppression, diabetes with peripheral neuropathy, sickle cell anaemia, microangiopathies such as cardiovascular disorders and smoking, and intravenous drug use. These conditions significantly increase the risk of severe systemic infections. In immunocompromised patients, a broader spectrum of pathogens is observed, including *Mycobacterium tuberculosis* and Bacillus Calmette-Guérin in patients with bladder carcinoma, and fungal pathogens such as Candida species, Blastomyces, Cryptococcus, and Aspergillus. *Bartonella henselae* is associated with HIV-positive patients, and Pseudomonas and Enterococcal infections are frequently seen in intravenous drug users, whereas *Eikenella corrodens* and *Pasteurella multocida* are common following dog or human bites, respectively [10–13].

**Table 1.1** Pathogens and correlated population and conditions

| Pathogen | Population |
|---|---|
| *Staphylococcus aureus* | Children and adults, including posttrauma or prosthetic joint infections. |
| Bacile calmatte-Guerin | Bladder carcinoma patients |
| Streptococcal species, *Kingella kingae* | In children and newborns. |
| Blastomyces | Immune-suppressed patients |
| *Eikenella corrodens*, *Pasteurella multocida* | Dog bite/human bite |
| Salmonella | Children with Sickle Cell Anemia |
| Pseudomonas, Enterococcus | IV drug users |
| *Bartonella henselae* | HIV patients |
| Fungal species: Blastomyces, Cryptococcus, Aspergillus | Immune suppressed patients, long-term IV medications, parenteral nutrition patients |
| Mycobacterium Tuberculosis | Pott's disease after TB manifestation |

On the other hand, with the advent of joint replacement surgeries, prosthetic joint infections became a significant clinical issue in the modern age [14, 15]. The other two fields of interest on BJIs are the Healthcare-Associated Infections due to the increased use of invasive procedures and devices in hospitals led to a rise in nosocomial infections, and the emergence of antibiotic-resistant bacteria, such as methicillin-resistant *Staphylococcus aureus* (MRSA), that has complicated the management [16–18].

## 1.3 Classification, Pathogenesis, and Biofilm

Osteomyelitis is classified based on timing, staging, mechanism, and host status. Acute osteomyelitis occurs within the first 2 weeks of onset, subacute between one and several months, and chronic when the condition persists for months to years [19]. The Cierny-Mader classification system is a widely used method for classifying osteomyelitis based on the anatomic involvement (I: medullary, II: superficial, III: localized, IV: diffused), the involved bone, and host status (A host: normal, B host: systemic or local compromise, C host: where therapy is worse than the disease itself) (Figs. 1.1 and 1.2) [20]. Osteomyelitis can be divided into primary and secondary types: primary osteomyelitis results from a distant source of infection with hematogenous spread of microorganisms to the long bones, predominantly affecting children, while in adults, it primarily affects the vertebrae [21]. Secondary osteomyelitis arises due to trauma, surgery, oncologic conditions, or sepsis of various etiologies [22]. This form is often contiguous, occurring in young adults, whereas in older patients, it typically manifests with pressure ulcers [5, 23]. Biofilm formation, a crucial factor in osteomyelitis, begins when bacteria in the planktonic phase attach to a surface such as bone, implants, plates, polyethylene, or polymethylmethacrylate (PMMA) cement. Following adhesion, the bacteria enter a silent phase characterized by the formation of an extracellular polymeric substance (EPS) matrix that surrounds them. This matrix renders the bacteria more resistant to antibiotics due to the difficulty in penetrating the biofilm [24].

Osteomyelitis, due it its diverse etiologies, presents a diagnostic challenge requiring a high index of suspicion [25]. Acute osteomyelitis may manifest with localized symptoms such as swelling, erythema, warmth at the infection site, dull pain, fever, and potentially septic arthritis if the metaphysis is intracapsular. Special attention is warranted for new-onset back or neck pain accompanied by fever, bacteremia, endocarditis, and elevated C-reactive protein (CRP) and erythrocyte sedimentation rate (ESR) to diagnose vertebral osteomyelitis. Chronic osteomyelitis presents similarly but with symptoms persisting over a prolonged period, often with less pronounced fever [26] (Figs. 1.3 and 1.4).

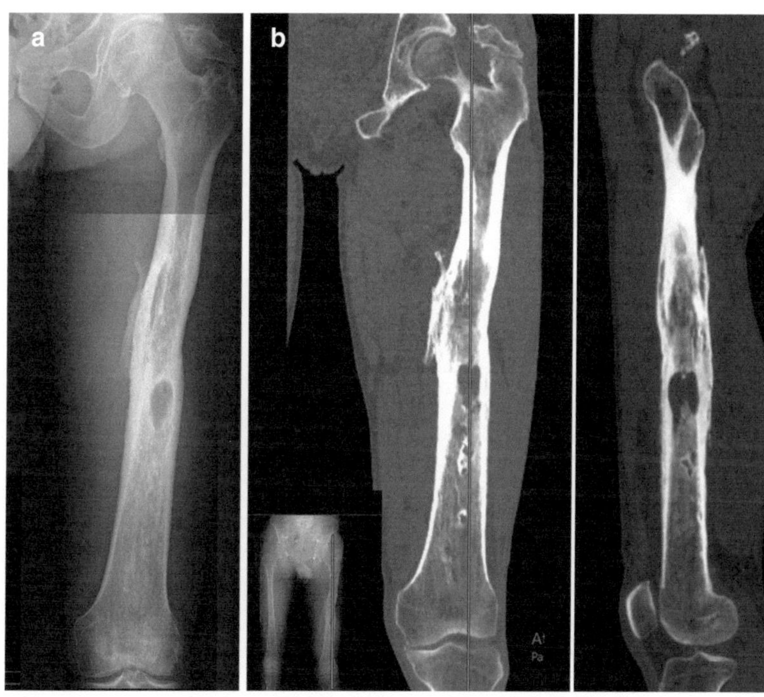


**Fig. 1.1** Stage 4 (diffuse osteomyelitis): an infection that involves the entire thickness of the bone and may result in structural instability. A 58-year-old woman with a history of a compound fracture of the femur. (**a**) Radiograph and (**b**) coronal and sagittal CT scans show a diffuse infection compromising the structural integrity of the bone

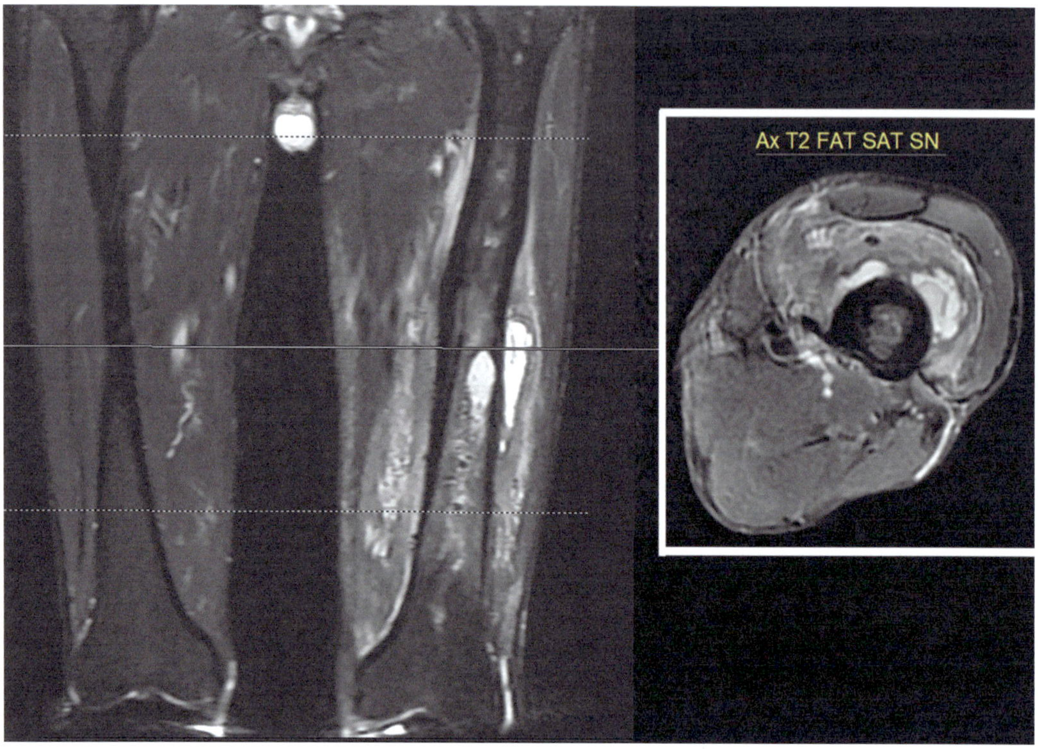


**Fig. 1.2** Same patient. MRI (STIR and T2-weighted FAT-SAT) clearly shows the involvement of soft tissues by the infectious process

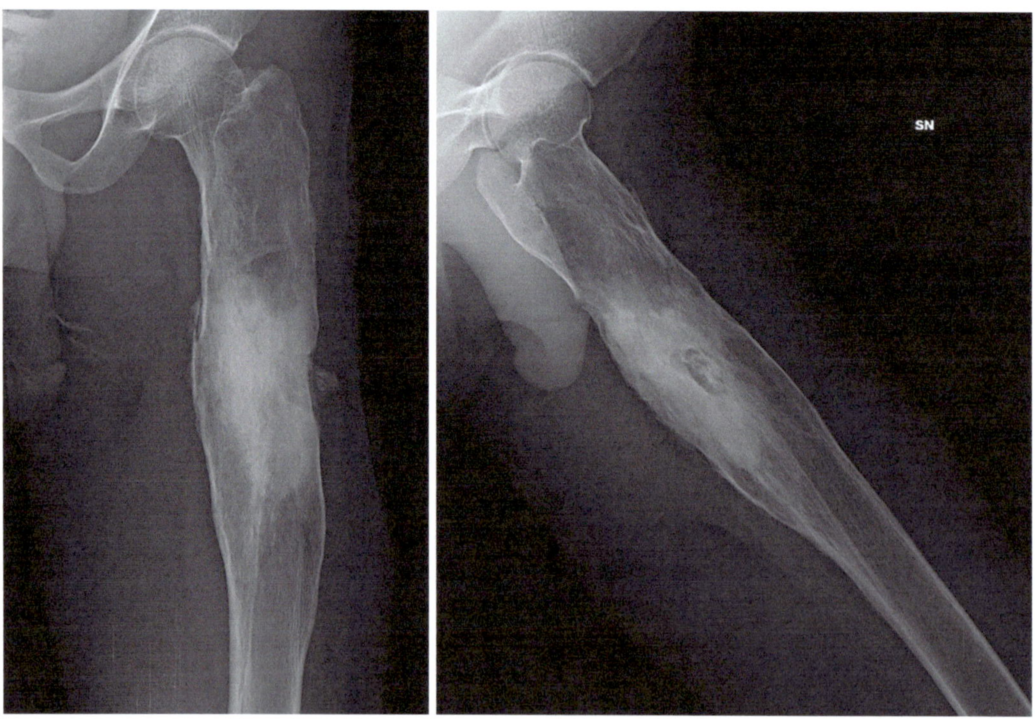


**Fig. 1.3** Chronic Osteomyelitis in a 21-year-old man with persistent pain in the thigh, swelling, and intermittent drainage from a sinus tract. Radiographs show periosteal reaction, cortical irregularities, and possible sequestrum (dead bone fragment)

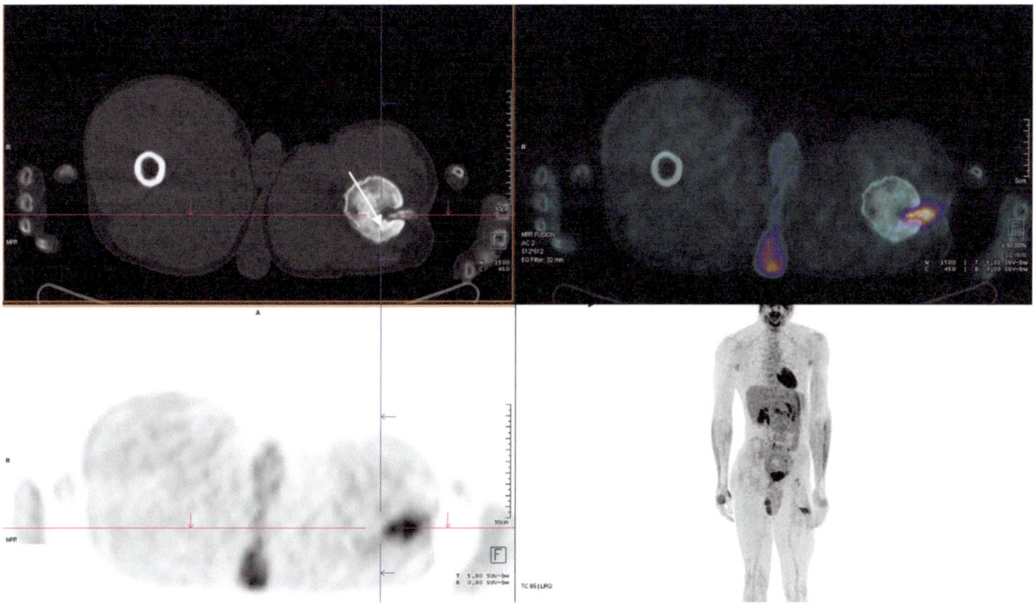

**Fig. 1.4** PET/CT Findings in chronic osteomyelitis. The midshaft of the femur shows significantly increased FDG uptake, indicating active infection and inflammation. The hot spots correlate with the areas of sinus tract extending from the bone to the surrounding soft tissue. The corresponding CT images reveal cortical irregularities and destruction, indicative of chronic osteomyelitis. Sequestra (white arrow) are visible as dense, sclerotic bone fragments within the medullary canal

## 1.4 Management

Before the discovery of penicillin, osteomyelitis management was primarily surgical, involving debridement, saucerization, and wound packing to facilitate secondary healing. This approach carried a high mortality rate due to sepsis. The introduction of antibiotics is considered a "game-changer" as they significantly reduced the mortality from staphylococcal osteomyelitis. However, with the emergence of antibiotic-resistant strains such as methicillin-resistant *Staphylococcus aureus* (MRSA), which account for approximately one-third of all staphylococcal infections [27], put the dealing physicians are faced with less effective treatments that necessitate more aggressive approaches [28]. Recent studies have validated a multidisciplinary treatment approach involving orthopedic surgeons, infectious disease specialists, radiologists, nurses, pediatricians, and social workers [29–31]. Evidence-based guidelines emphasize tailoring antibiotic regimens to the specific microorganism and patient host factors, along with various surgical interventions—such as curettage, Masquelet technique, osteotomy, Ilizarov bone handling, or negative pressure wound therapy—to address biofilm production and enhance recovery [6, 32, 33]. The management of BJIs has changed over time in relation to the evolution of epidemiological aspects. Improved sanitation, advances in trauma care and orthopedic surgery, and public health measures have reduced the overall incidence of infections, including BJIs. Moreover, vaccination programs (such as those against tuberculosis and other infectious diseases) have decreased the incidence of related bone and joint infections.

## 1.5 Conclusion

In summary, osteomyelitis is a complex condition to treat due to multiple factors and heterogeneity of the disease, requiring consideration of microorganisms, host factors, infection site, and clinical presentation. Clinicians must maintain a high level of suspicion and carefully tailor the best treatment to prevent severe complications such as sepsis, pathologic fractures, neurologic deficits, and even malignant transformation in long-standing infections. The epidemiology of BJIs reflects broader trends in medical and public health advancements, with significant improvements in prevention, diagnosis, and treatment over time. However, challenges remain, particularly with antibiotic resistance and healthcare-associated infections.

**Author Contributions** Conceptualization, project administration: AA, PR; data curation and formal analysis: AA, PR; supervision: PR; writing-original draft: AA; writing-review and editing: AA, PR; All authors have read and agreed to the published version of the manuscript.

**Institutional Review Board Statement** Not applicable.

**Informed Consent Statement** Written informed consent was obtained from patients at the time of admission to our Institute. However, all pictures have been reported anonymized.

**Consent for Publication (Include Appropriate Statements)** We confirm that this chapter, including related data, figures and tables, has not been published previously, it is not under consideration for publication elsewhere, and, if accepted, it will not be published elsewhere in the same form, in English or in any other language, without the written consent of the publisher.

**Conflicts of Interest/Competing Interests (Include Appropriate Disclosures)** Ruggieri P is a consultant for Stryker and Exactech (not relevant to the present manuscript). The other Authors declare that there are no relationships/conditions/circumstances that present a potential conflict of interest with the present manuscript.

**Availability of Data and Material (Data Transparency)** Manuscript data are embedded in the text and fully available on specific request.

**Funding** There was no external funding source in support of this study.

## References

1. Gross SD. The anatomy, physiology, and diseases of the bones and joints. John Grigg; 1830.
2. Broughton G 2nd, Janis JE, Attinger CE. A brief history of wound care. Plast Reconstr Surg. 2006;117(7 Suppl):6S–11S. https://doi.org/10.1097/01.prs.0000225429.76355.dd.
3. Breasted JH. The Edwin-Smith surgical papyrus. The Chicago University Press; 1930.
4. Toledo-Pereyra LH. Joseph Lister's surgical revolution. J Investig Surg. 2010;23(5):241–3. https://doi.org/10.3109/08941939.2010.520574.
5. Hofstee MI, Muthukrishnan G, Atkins GJ, Riool M, Thompson K, Morgenstern M, Stoddart MJ, Richards RG, Zaat SAJ, Moriarty TF. Current concepts of osteomyelitis: from pathologic mechanisms to advanced research methods. Am J Pathol. 2020;190(6):1151–63. https://doi.org/10.1016/j.ajpath.2020.02.007.
6. Cortés-Penfield NW, Kulkarni PA. The history of antibiotic treatment of osteomyelitis. Open Forum Infect Dis. 2019;6(5):ofz181. https://doi.org/10.1093/ofid/ofz181.
7. Hatzenbuehler J, Pulling TJ. Diagnosis and management of osteomyelitis. Am Fam Physician. 2011;84(9):1027–33.
8. Andre L, Clark MD, Accardo SI. Nuclear medicine musculoskeletal assessment, protocols, and interpretation, in StatPearls. Treasure Island: StatPearls PublishingCopyright © 2024, StatPearls Publishing LLC; 2024.
9. Kremers HM, Nwojo ME, Ransom JE, Wood-Wentz CM, Melton LJ 3rd, Huddleston PM 3rd. Trends in the epidemiology of osteomyelitis: a population-based study, 1969 to 2009. J Bone Joint Surg Am. 2015;97(10):837–45. https://doi.org/10.2106/JBJS.N.01350.
10. Burnett MW, Bass JW, Cook BA. Etiology of osteomyelitis complicating sickle cell disease. Pediatrics. 1998;101(2):296–7. https://doi.org/10.1542/peds.101.2.296.
11. Holt RIG, Cockram CS, Ma RCW, Luk AOY. Diabetes and infection: review of the epidemiology, mechanisms and principles of treatment. Diabetologia. 2024;67(7):1168–80. https://doi.org/10.1007/s00125-024-06102-x. Epub 2024 Feb 20.
12. Rehman S, Arif S, Ushakumari LG, Amreen J, Nagelli A, Moonnumackel SJ, Nair A. Assessment of bacterial infections and antibiotic regimens in intravenous drug users. Cureus. 2023;15(9):e45716. https://doi.org/10.7759/cureus.45716.
13. Secamilli EN, Drummond MR, Serrano JYM, Stelini RF, Cintra ML, Velho PENF. Is Bartonella sp. infec-

tion relevant in hematological malignancies in HIV-negative patients? A literature review. Leuk Res Rep. 2023;21:100402. https://doi.org/10.1016/j.lrr.2023.100402.
14. Anis HK, Ramanathan D, Sodhi N, Klika AK, Piuzzi NS, Mont MA, Higuera CA, Molloy RM. Postoperative infection in cementless and cemented total knee arthroplasty: a propensity score matched analysis. J Knee Surg. 2019;32(11):1058–62. https://doi.org/10.1055/s-0039-1678678.
15. Lemaignen A, Bernard L, Marmor S, Ferry T, Grammatico-Guillon L, Astagneau P. Scientific Committee for Complex Bone and Joint Infections Reference Centers (CRIOAc), on behalf of the CRIOAc network. Epidemiology of complex bone and joint infections in France using a national registry: the CRIOAc network. J Infect. 2021;82(2):199–206. https://doi.org/10.1016/j.jinf.2020.12.010.
16. Tsantes AG, Altsitzioglou P, Papadopoulos DV, Lorenzo D, Romanò CL, Benzakour T, Tsukamoto S, Errani C, Angelini A, Mavrogenis AF. Infections of tumor prostheses: an updated review on risk factors, microbiology, diagnosis, and treatment strategies. Biology (Basel). 2023;12(2):314. https://doi.org/10.3390/biology12020314.
17. Turner NA, Sharma-Kuinkel BK, Maskarinec SA, Eichenberger EM, Shah PP, Carugati M, Holland TL, Fowler VG Jr. Methicillin-resistant Staphylococcus aureus: an overview of basic and clinical research. Nat Rev Microbiol. 2019;17(4):203–18. https://doi.org/10.1038/s41579-018-0147-4.
18. Liu C, Bayer A, Cosgrove SE, Daum RS, Fridkin SK, Gorwitz RJ, Kaplan SL, Karchmer AW, Levine DP, Murray BE, Rybak JM, Talan DA, Chambers HF, Infectious Diseases Society of America. Clinical practice guidelines by the infectious diseases society of america for the treatment of methicillin-resistant Staphylococcus aureus infections in adults and children. Clin Infect Dis. 2011;52(3):e18–55. https://doi.org/10.1093/cid/ciq146.
19. He M, Arthur Vithran DT, Pan L, Zeng H, Yang G, Lu B, Zhang F. An update on recent progress of the epidemiology, etiology, diagnosis, and treatment of acute septic arthritis: a review. Front Cell Infect Microbiol. 2023;13:1193645. https://doi.org/10.3389/fcimb.2023.1193645.
20. Conway JD, Hambardzumyan V, Patel NG, Giacobbe SD, Gesheff MG. Immunological evaluation of patients with orthopedic infections: taking the Cierny-Mader classification to the next level. J Bone Jt Infect. 2021;6(9):433–41. https://doi.org/10.5194/jbji-6-433-2021.
21. Tsantes AG, Papadopoulos DV, Vrioni G, Sioutis S, Sapkas G, Benzakour A, Benzakour T, Angelini A, Ruggieri P, Mavrogenis AF. World association against infection in orthopedics and trauma W A I O T study group on bone and joint infection definitions. Spinal infections: an update. Microorganisms. 2020;8(4):476. https://doi.org/10.3390/microorganisms8040476.
22. Trovarelli G, Angelini A, Pala E, Cappellari A, Breda A, Ruggieri P. Infection in orthopaedic oncology: crucial problem in modern reconstructive techniques. Eur Rev Med Pharmacol Sci. 2019;23(2 Suppl):271–8. https://doi.org/10.26355/eurrev_201904_17501.
23. Bettale C, Chisari E, Parvizi J. 8.1 Osteomyelitis 8.1. 1 highlights (table 8.1) definition—infection of the bone or bone marrow epidemiology. In: Textbook of musculoskeletal disorders. Springer; 2023. p. 67.
24. Rather MA, Gupta K, Mandal M. Microbial biofilm: formation, architecture, antibiotic resistance, and control strategies. Braz J Microbiol. 2021;52(4):1701–18. https://doi.org/10.1007/s42770-021-00624-x. Epub 2021 Sep 23.
25. Forsberg JA, Potter BK, Cierny G 3rd, Webb L. Diagnosis and management of chronic infection. J Am Acad Orthop Surg. 2011;19(Suppl 1):S8–S19. https://doi.org/10.5435/00124635-201102001-00003.
26. Schmitt SK. Osteomyelitis. Infect Dis Clin N Am. 2017;31(2):325–38.
27. Al-Nammari SS, Bobak P, Venkatesh R. Methicillin resistant Staphylococcus aureus versus methicillin sensitive Staphylococcus aureus adult haematogenous septic arthritis. Arch Orthop Trauma Surg. 2007;127(7):537–42. https://doi.org/10.1007/s00402-007-0285-z.
28. Wang J, Wang L. Novel therapeutic interventions towards improved management of septic arthritis. BMC Musculoskelet Disord. 2021;22(1):530. https://doi.org/10.1186/s12891-021-04383-6.
29. Angelini A, Tiengo C, Sonda R, Berizzi A, Bassetto F, Ruggieri P. One-stage soft tissue reconstruction following sarcoma excision: a personalized multidisciplinary approach called "Orthoplasty". J Pers Med. 2020;10(4):278. https://doi.org/10.3390/jpm10040278.
30. Muller Q, Gerber F, Papadimitriou Olivgeris M, Di Summa P, Boillat Blanco N, Steinmetz S. Prise en charge multidisciplinaire des infections de fracture [Multidisciplinary approach to fracture-related infection]. Rev Med Suisse. 2022;18(808):2363–70. French. https://doi.org/10.53738/REVMED.2022.18.808.2363.
31. Trimaille A, Kerfant N, Henry AS, Ta P, Rouanet M, Le Nen D, Stindel E, Ansart S, Hu W. Multidisciplinary management of the bone and joint infection complicating treatment of an open fracture of the lower limb. Ann Chir Plast Esthet. 2020;65(5–6):380–93. https://doi.org/10.1016/j.anplas.2020.05.012.
32. Panteli M, Giannoudis PV. Chronic osteomyelitis: what the surgeon needs to know. EFORT Open Rev. 2017;1(5):128–35. https://doi.org/10.1302/2058-5241.1.000017.
33. Copley LA, Kinsler MA, Gheen T, Shar A, Sun D, Browne R. The impact of evidence-based clinical practice guidelines applied by a multidisciplinary team for the care of children with osteomyelitis. J Bone Joint Surg Am. 2013;95(8):686–93. https://doi.org/10.2106/JBJS.L.00037.

# Antibiotic Stewardship in Orthopedic Surgery

# 2

Khaled M. Emara, Ramy A. Diab, and Kyrillos Rashid

## 2.1 Introduction

Addressing different types of musculoskeletal infections necessitates a skilled hand from an orthopedic surgeon. These infections originate from surgical interventions, blood flow dispersal, immediate trauma, and other sources. Timely care is necessary to forestall catastrophic outcomes, including bone infection, joint inflammation, and implant failure. The strategic application of antibiotics, guided by scientific research, is critical to achieving optimal patient outcomes while counteracting the growing threat of drug resistance [1]. Additionally, controlling infections is a vital component of orthopedic surgery since, if neglected, they may have disastrous effects. In orthopedic procedures, antibiotics are essential for preventing and treating infections, and new developments in antibiotic regimes have completely changed how these infections are handled. This chapter investigates the current understanding and suggestions for effectively treating bone and joint infections, stressing the essential role of antibiotic sensitivity in orthopedic medical procedures. Moreover, it highlights their significance in assuring the best possible patient outcomes and the new procedures for antibiotic usage in various orthopedic surgery instances.

K. M. Emara · R. A. Diab · K. Rashid (✉)
Department of Orthopedic Surgery, Ain Shams University, Cairo, Egypt

## 2.2 Pathogenesis and Microbiology of Bone and Joint Infections

Effective treatment techniques are based on understanding the pathophysiology and microbiological origin of bone and joint infections, which is crucial [5]. *Staphylococcus aureus* holds the leading role in these instances, significantly affecting the unfolding of the related ailments. The struggle with methicillin-resistant strains originates from their innate defense systems [2]. It is essential to recognize that multiple factors contribute to these diseases. Various possible pathogens, including Streptococcus species, gram-negative bacilli, and anaerobes, contribute to the complex ecology of bone and joint diseases. Recent scientific research has shown that biofilm development on implant surfaces is crucial in encouraging persistent infections [9]. This discovery has broad repercussions since biofilms allow pathogens to resist host immune responses and common antibiotic treatments.

The formation of biofilms protects the microbial population from immune monitoring and forms a barrier that hinders the effectiveness of antimicrobial drugs [1]. This complex interaction between infections and biofilms highlights the urgent need for precisely planned treatment approaches that may successfully penetrate these biofilm barriers [4]. The conclusions drawn from these disclosures push for substituting precision-



P. Ruggieri et al. (eds.), *Bone and Joint Infections*, https://doi.org/10.1007/978-3-031-96383-4_2

guided interventions for broad-spectrum empirical therapies [2]. Identifying the microorganisms implicated and the distinctive features of their biofilm forms significantly impacts the effectiveness of antibiotic regimens [7]. In order to improve patient outcomes in orthopedic surgery, the next frontier in the therapy of bone and joint infections depends on focused, therapeutic methods that negotiate the complexity of microbial etiology and biofilm dynamics.

## 2.3 Diagnostic Modalities

Effective therapy of bone and joint infections depends heavily on accurate and prompt diagnosis, which directs the choice of suitable treatment approaches. We are now able to quickly and precisely detect these illnesses because of considerable improvements in diagnostic techniques. Modern imaging methods have become essential components of the diagnostic toolkit [6]. With its unmatched soft tissue contrast and multiplanar capabilities, magnetic resonance imaging (MRI) has completely changed how bone and joint infections may be seen. MRI enables the early diagnosis of infections even before radiographic abnormalities become obvious because it makes it easier to see small changes in the bone marrow and nearby soft tissues [17]. Nuclear scintigraphy, such as Technetium-99 m bone scans and Gallium-67 scans, also provides extraordinary sensitivity in identifying infection spots that are actively spreading, helping to localize the regions that need more research and treatment.

Molecular diagnostic equipment has become more popular in the age of individualized treatment. Microorganisms that cause disease may now be quickly and precisely identified thanks to polymerase chain reaction (PCR), which amplifies certain DNA sequences. It includes slow-moving or picky diseases that may be uncommon in traditional civilizations [7]. Additionally, the capability of PCR to provide profiles of antibiotic susceptibility enables doctors to customize medication early in the course of treatment, thereby improving patient outcomes [12]. In the diagnostic landscape, integration is crucial [9]. The infection's breadth, severity, and etiology may all be fully understood by integrating clinical, radiographic, and molecular results [8]. Orthopedic surgeons may create specialized treatment plans that focus on the distinctive traits of each illness, thanks to this multidimensional approach, which also improves diagnostic accuracy.

## 2.4 Antibiotic Stewardship Principles

Personalized Treatment: Antibiotic therapy's paradigm is changing from a one-size-fits-all strategy to customized treatment programs that consider unique patient traits, microbiological information, and bone and joint infection severity [9]. With this change, it is acknowledged that patient responses to medicines might vary and that different infecting bacteria have different susceptibilities [17]. Clinicians may maximize therapeutic results while lowering the risk of needless antibiotic usage by customizing therapy to unique patient characteristics, such as age, comorbidities, and prior antibiotic exposure. By preventing indiscriminate medication exposure, this strategy not only lowers the chance of negative effects but also prevents the development of antibiotic resistance [10]. Additionally, by using cutting-edge diagnostic technologies like molecular methods and genomic sequencing, doctors may quickly and correctly identify the causal organisms, allowing tailored antibiotic selection. With targeted and evidence-based therapy techniques, personalized treatment ushers in a new age of precision medicine in orthopedic surgery.

De-escalation and Duration: De-escalation tactics are critical in the therapy of bone and joint infections, according to recent recommendations. Clinicians should switch from broad-spectrum empiric antibiotics to narrower, more focused medications once microbiological culture data are available [11]. Since narrower-spectrum medicines successfully target the specific pathogen while sparing nonpathogenic bacteria, this method is consistent with optimizing antibiotic usage [11]. Additionally, shorter antibiotic courses may reduce side effects such as drug-related toxicity and secondary infections like *Clostridioides difficile* colitis. Additionally, the prudent use of antibiotics for a shorter period lessens the selection pressure on microbes, reducing the possibility of resistance emerging [5]. This strategy supports responsible antibiotic use in the context of bone and joint infections while aligning with the larger antimicrobial stewardship agenda, protecting antibiotic effectiveness for coming generations.

Combination Therapy: Treatment for complex bone and joint infections, often characterized by biofilm development or the presence of multidrug-resistant organisms, presents special difficulties. Combination antibiotic treatment, which involves giving two or more antibiotics simultaneously with various modes of action, may be the answer [9]. Combination treatment may improve microbiological eradication and stop the establishment of resistance by treating the infection from many perspectives [12]. Combination treatment has several advantages, but these must be carefully evaluated against any negative effects it can have, such as higher toxicity or the possibility of medication interactions [23]. A thorough knowledge of the relevant organisms, their resistance profiles, and their synergistic interactions should be the basis for selecting antibiotics. Meticulous clinical surveillance is necessary to evaluate the effectiveness and side effects of combination regimens [13]. As a result, although combination treatment has promise in treating complex infections, it must be used carefully and based on evidence if patient safety and therapeutic effectiveness are to be guaranteed.

Optimal Dosing and Route of Administration: Therapeutic antibiotic levels must be reached at the injection site for bone and joint infections to be successfully treated. Pharmacokinetic and bioavailability factors have a significant influence on dosing regimens [14]. Clinicians may adjust doses to reach effective concentrations at the infection site while reducing systemic toxicity by being aware of the drug's distribution, metabolism, and elimination characteristics. Additionally, new administration techniques have increased the range of available treatments [15]. The focused release of antibiotics at the infection site is made possible by local antibiotic delivery systems, such as antibiotic-impregnated bone cement or implant coatings, which encourage greater drug concentrations and minimize systemic exposure [5]. This targeted strategy reduces the possibility of systemic adverse effects while simultaneously improving antibacterial effectiveness [16]. The best delivery method, whether oral, intravenous, or local, depends on a thorough comprehension of the illness' features and the selected antibiotics' pharmacokinetics. In order to maximize therapeutic efficacy while limiting possible damage, it is important to achieve appropriate dose and administration procedures [17]. It ensures that antibiotics are delivered exactly where they are required.

An example of a "Comparative Antibiotic Protocols" table

| Orthopedic surgery type | Recommended antibiotics | Dosage and administration | Duration of prophylaxis | Additional considerations |
|---|---|---|---|---|
| Joint replacement | Cefazolin | 2 g IV within 1 h prior to incision | Single dose, up to 24 h post-op | Consider patient allergies, MRSA colonization |
| Fracture fixation | Ceftriaxone | 1 g IV pre-op, repeat if surgery >3 h | Single dose, up to 24 h post-op | Tailor for open fractures, patient's immune status |
| Spinal fusion | Vancomycin and cefazolin | 15–20 mg/kg IV within 1 h prior to incision, plus cefazolin 2 g IV | Single dose, up to 24 h post-op | Address MRSA risk, patient allergies |
| Revision surgery | Vancomycin and ciprofloxacin | Vancomycin 15–20 mg/kg IV within 1 h prior to incision, plus ciprofloxacin 400 mg IV | Multiple doses as per procedure duration | Tailor for implant-related infections, microbial culture results |

## 2.5 Surgical Management

The complete care of bone and joint infections includes surgery, a reliable ally that enhances the effectiveness of antibiotic therapy. Recent improvements in surgical methods have brought forth a new age of accuracy and inventiveness, enhancing the toolkit against these difficult illnesses [18]. The use of minimally invasive techniques and biofilm-targeted strategies is highlighted in this section, which also examines the changing landscape of surgical interventions. It also emphasizes the critical value of surgical debridement, the removal of infected hardware, and careful soft tissue management [19]. The surgical treatment of bone and joint infections has been transformed by the development of less invasive procedures. These procedures provide patients with quicker recoveries and lower postoperative morbidity since they have fewer incisions and less tissue damage. In order to precisely debride and remove infected tissue while limiting collateral damage, arthroscopy, for instance, offers a clear view into joint areas [20]. Additionally, the development of biofilm-targeted therapies intends to address the ongoing problem presented by bacteria entrenched in biofilms. These tenacious populations may be eliminated, recurring infections prevented, and more effective treatment made possible by methods utilizing antimicrobial coatings on implants or targeted drug delivery systems [21]. The precise surgical debridement procedure is essential to successfully managing bone and joint infections.

In order to stop the spread of the infection and provide an environment favorable for healing, this operation entails the excision of diseased tissue, necrotic bone, and surfaces coated with biofilm. It is often essential to remove contaminated hardware simultaneously as the germs, such as prosthetic joints or fixation devices [22]. To prevent recurrence and ensure that the future stages of therapy go as smoothly as possible, these niduses of infection must be carefully removed. Surgical procedures that include tissue preservation, reconstruction, or flap covering are essential to restore the integrity of the injured region. Surgeons strengthen the basis for later interventions and assist in eliminating infection by establishing a healthy environment for wound healing [23]. The idea of single-stage treatments has attracted interest in certain circumstances because it can simplify therapy. In one surgical procedure, this method involves the removal of contaminated implants, complete debridement, and prompt implant exchange [24].

Additionally, single-stage treatments seek to manage infection while limiting the patient's exposure to many operations using well-thought-out guidelines and patient selection criteria [25]. In addition to maximizing patient comfort, this strategy may save healthcare expenditures and cut the length of antibiotic medication.

## 2.6 Antibiotics' Importance in Orthopedic Surgery

Each orthopedic surgical approach is intended to address a specific musculoskeletal issue. No matter how complicated fracture fixations or subtle joint replacements are, lowering infection risks is a problem that affects all of them. Within this spectrum of surgical therapies, antibiotics stand out as crucial allies in the fight against infection-related issues [26]. Orthopedic surgeons can effectively stop the potential damage from post-surgical infections by harnessing their strength. It is not easy to overstate how crucial it is to use antibiotics sensibly in this situation. It significantly influences how quickly wounds heal, how long patients must stay in the hospital, and how well they will eventually recover from surgery [27]. The deliberate use of antibiotics by the orthopedic profession enhances its dedication to enhancing patient outcomes and ensuring that the promise of successful surgical treatments is upheld without exception.

## 2.7 Preventing Antibiotic Resistance

Stewardship of antibiotics is an essential part of the worldwide response to the growing danger of antimicrobial resistance. Orthopedic doctors significantly impact preventing the spread of microorganisms resistant to antibiotics in orthopedic surgery, where bone and joint infections are common [28]. This crucial function encompasses a range of tactics intended to maintain the effectiveness of antibiotics for both the present and future generations, in addition to clinical judgments.

***Infection Prevention Measures*** The key to infection control is still prevention. By applying strict infection prevention methods, orthopedic surgeons may significantly reduce the prevalence of infections in the bones and joints [29]. It calls for using sterile methods while performing surgery, appropriate wound care techniques, and fostering aseptic conditions in healthcare settings. The need for antibiotics may be decreased by avoiding infections altogether, lowering the selection pressure that feeds antibiotic resistance.

***Adhering to Evidence-Based Guidelines*** Orthopedic surgeons have access to a multitude of clinical advice and guidelines. Adopting evidence-based recommendations guarantees that the newest research and industry standards influence antibiotic treatment [30]. This method decreases the empirical use of antibiotics while maximizing treatment choice, dosage, and duration. Orthopedic surgeons may achieve positive patient outcomes while minimizing the probability of antibiotic resistance development by making treatment choices based on the best available data.

***Promoting Awareness among Healthcare Providers*** Fostering an awareness and education culture among medical professionals is essential in bone and joint infections. By participating in educational activities that stress the significance of sensible antibiotic use and the effects of antibiotic resistance, orthopedic surgeons may assume a leadership position in the medical community [31]. Surgeons may encourage a community commitment to antibiotic stewardship by facilitating multidisciplinary teamwork and disseminating information about emergent resistance trends. To ensure the healthcare team is informed and in sync with the most recent developments, they should also promote ongoing education on new diagnostic techniques, therapeutic modalities, and infection control techniques.

## 2.8 VI. Future Directions

With the persistent advancement of research and the introduction of cutting-edge technology, treating bone and joint infections is about to undergo significant changes. The use of pharmacogenomics in treatment plans is one possible route [31]. Clinicians can maximize treatment effectiveness while limiting adverse responses by customizing antibiotic selections depending on a patient's genetic profile [32]. This precise strategy has the potential to completely change the way we treat infections by guaranteeing that patients get the best care with the fewest risks. The subject of immunotherapy, which is quickly developing, provides a fascinating complement or alternative to conventional antibiotic treatment. A potential approach to preventing bone and joint infections is using the body's immune responses to pinpoint and eliminate invading organisms [18]. Monoclonal antibodies, vaccinations, and immune-modulating drugs all have the potential to strengthen the host's defenses, thereby improving outcomes and reducing the need for antibiotics.

Moreover, nanomedicine, which can control materials at the nanoscale, opens up new possibilities for treating infections and delivering drugs [3]. Antibiotic concentrations may be increased while systemic exposure is decreased by using nanoparticles to deliver the drugs directly to the sites of infection. By limiting the use of antibiotics widely, this focused strategy improves treatment effectiveness and slows the development of resistance [11]. While these developments provide promising futures, the core idea of antibiotic stewardship must remain unwavering. Responsible antibiotic usage guarantees that the limited supply of powerful antibiotics is preserved for the next generations in the face of developing therapies. Maintaining a balance between implementing new tactics and preserving the effectiveness of current antibiotics becomes more important when breakthrough medicines are developed.

In conclusion, a multidisciplinary approach to diagnosis and treatment is required for bone and joint infections, a serious concern in orthopedic surgery. Orthopedic surgeons may improve patient care while ensuring the continued effectiveness of antibiotics by practicing antibiotic stewardship, which is supported by current research and recommendations. Orthopedic surgeons may make a significant and scientifically sound contribution to the fight against musculoskeletal infections by adopting customized therapy, surgical innovation, and techniques to overcome resistance [12]. Additionally, the explosive expansion of antibiotic usage in orthopedic surgery is evidence of recent medical advances. Thanks to the adoption of cutting-edge techniques, like preoperative prophylaxis, intraoperative redosing, and precisely devised postoperative care, orthopedic surgeons are now at the forefront of infection management [20]. These cutting-edge techniques show a strong commitment to evidence-based approaches, ensuring patient welfare is always prioritized in orthopedic therapy. These recommendations improve patient outcomes, which is a testament to the dedication and expertise of medical professionals.

## Bibliography


1. Cheng S, Pan M, Hu D, Han R, Li L, Bei Z, et al. Adhesive chitosan-based hydrogel assisted with photothermal antibacterial property to prompt mice infected skin wound healing. Chin Chem Lett [Internet]. 2023 Mar 2 [cited 2023 Aug 10]; 34 108276. Available from: https://www.sciencedirect.com/science/article/pii/S1001841723001390
2. Corona A, De Santis V, Agarossi A, Prete A, Cattaneo D, Tomasini G, et al. Antibiotic therapy strategies for treating gram-negative severe infections in the critically Ill: a narrative review. Antibiotics [Internet]. 2023 Aug 1 [cited 2023 Aug 10];12(8):1262. Available from: https://www.mdpi.com/2079-6382/12/8/1262
3. Sanchez JA, Higgins RSD, Kent PS. Handbook of perioperative and procedural patient safety [internet]. Google books. Elsevier Health Sciences; 2023 [cited 2023 Aug 10]. Available from: https://books.google.com/books?hl=en&lr=&id=D0mzEAAAQBAJ&oi=fnd&pg=PA245&dq=Intraoperative+antibiotic+redosing+is+a+proactive+method+to+address+this+problem.&ots=NbxOxnmmsF&sig=PwNgAOSd9-6knnqe2Wr9attrj6g
4. Darwish RM, Matar SG, Snaineh AAA, Alsharif MR, Yahia AB, Mustafa HN, et al. Impact of antimicrobial stewardship on antibiogram, consumption and incidence of multi drug resistance. BMC Infect Dis. 2022;22(1):916.
5. Su Y, Yrastorza JT, Matis M, Cusick J, Zhao S, Wang G, et al. Biofilms: formation, research models, potential targets, and methods for prevention and treatment. Adv Sci. 2022 Aug 28;9(29):2203291.
6. Verhey JT, Haglin JM, Verhey EM, Hartigan DE. Virtual, augmented, and mixed reality applications in orthopedic surgery. Int J Med Robot Comput Assist Surg. 2020 Apr;16(2):e2067.
7. Day MA, Owens JM, Caldwell LS. Breaking barriers: a brief overview of diversity in orthopedic surgery. Iowa Orthop J [Internet]. 2019;39(1):1–5. Available from: https://www.ncbi.nlm.nih.gov/pmc/articles/PMC6604536/
8. Jud L, Fotouhi J, Andronic O, Aichmair A, Osgood G, Navab N, et al. Applicability of augmented reality in orthopedic surgery—a systematic review. BMC Musculoskelet Disord. 2020 Feb 15;21(1):103.
9. Anderson PA, Morgan SL, Krueger D, Zapalowski C, Tanner B, Jeray KJ, et al. Use of bone health evaluation in orthopedic surgery: 2019 ISCD official position. J Clin Densitom [Internet] 2019 Oct 1 [cited 2023 Aug 10];22(4):517–543. Available from: https://www.sciencedirect.com/science/article/pii/S1094695019301301
10. Li HK, Rombach I, Zambellas R, Walker AS, McNally MA, Atkins BL, et al. Oral versus intravenous antibiotics for bone and joint infection. N Eng J Med [Internet]. 2019;380(5):425–36. Available from: https://www.nejm.org/doi/full/10.1056/NEJMoa1710926.
11. McNally M, Sousa R, Wouthuyzen-Bakker M, Chen AF, Soriano A, Vogely HC, et al. The EBJIS definition of periprosthetic joint infection. Bone Joint J. 2021 Jan 1;103-B(1):18–25.
12. Sambri A, Spinnato P, Tedeschi S, Zamparini E, Fiore M, Zucchini R, et al. Bone and joint infections: the role of imaging in tailoring diagnosis to improve patients' care. J Pers Med [Internet] 2021 Dec 1 [cited 2023 Aug 11];11(12):1317. Available from: https://www.mdpi.com/2075-4426/11/12/1317
13. Ferry T, Boucher F, Fevre C, Perpoint T, Chateau J, Petitjean C, et al. Innovations for the treatment of a complex bone and joint infection due to XDR Pseudomonas aeruginosa including local application of a selected cocktail of bacteriophages. J Antimicrob Chemother. 2018 Jul 27;73(10):2901–3.
14. Thabit AK, Fatani DF, Bamakhrama MS, Barnawi OA, Basudan LO, Alhejaili SF. Antibiotic penetration into bone and joints: an updated review. Int J Infect Dis. 2019 Apr;81:128–36.

15. Ahmed SS, Haddad FS. Prosthetic joint infection. Bone Joint Res. 2019 Nov;8(11):570–2.
16. Tobudic S, Forstner C, Burgmann H, Lagler H, Steininger C, Traby L, et al. Real-world experience with dalbavancin therapy in gram-positive skin and soft tissue infection, bone and joint infection. Infection. 2019 Sep 13;47(6):1013–20.
17. Morata L, Cobo J, Fernández-Sampedro M, Guisado Vasco P, Ruano E, Lora-Tamayo J, et al. Safety and efficacy of prolonged use of Dalbavancin in bone and joint infections. Antimicrob Agents Chemother. 2019 May;63(5):e02280-18.
18. Izakovicova P, Borens O, Trampuz A. Periprosthetic joint infection: current concepts and outlook. EFORT Open Rev. 2019 Jul;4(7):482–94.
19. Broderick C, Hopkins S, Mack DJF, Aston W, Pollock R, Skinner JA, et al. Delays in the diagnosis and treatment of bone and joint tuberculosis in the United Kingdom. Bone Joint J. 2018 Jan;100-B(1):119–24.
20. Davido B, Saleh-Mghir A, Rottman M, Jaffal K, Salomon E, Bouchand F, et al. Native bone and joint infections caused by extended-spectrum β-lactamase-producing Enterobacterales: experience of a reference centre in the Greater Paris area. Int J Antimicrob Agents [Internet] 2022 Jan 1 [cited 2023 Aug 11];59(1):106497. Available from: https://www.sciencedirect.com/science/article/pii/S0924857921013388
21. Fang X, Cai Y, Mei J, Huang Z, Zhang C, Yang B, et al. Optimizing culture methods according to preoperative mNGS results can improve joint infection diagnosis. Bone Joint J. 2021 Jan 1;103-B(1):39–45.
22. Thakrar RR, Horriat S, Kayani B, Haddad FS. Indications for a single-stage exchange arthroplasty for chronic prosthetic joint infection. Bone Joint J. 2019 Jan;101-B(1_Supple_A):19–24.
23. Huang Z, Li W, Lee GC, Fang X, Xing L, Yang B, et al. Metagenomic next-generation sequencing of synovial fluid demonstrates high accuracy in prosthetic joint infection diagnostics. Bone Joint Res. 2020 Jul;9(7):440–9.
24. Marson BA, Deshmukh SR, Grindlay DJC, Scammell BE. Alpha-defensin and the Synovasure lateral flow device for the diagnosis of prosthetic joint infection. Bone Joint J. 2018 Jun;100-B(6):703–11.
25. Karczewski D, Winkler T, Renz N, Trampuz A, Lieb E, Perka C, et al. A standardized interdisciplinary algorithm for the treatment of prosthetic joint infections. Bone Joint J. 2019 Feb 1;101-B(2):132–9.
26. Abosala A, Ali M. The use of calcium Sulphate beads in Periprosthetic joint infection, a systematic review. J Bone Joint Infect. 2020;5(1):43–9.
27. Zeller V, Kerroumi Y, Meyssonnier V, Heym B, Metten MA, Desplaces N, et al. Analysis of postoperative and hematogenous prosthetic joint-infection microbiological patterns in a large cohort. J Infect. 2018 Apr;76(4):328–34.
28. Aggarwal VK, Weintraub S, Klock J, Stachel A, Phillips M, Schwarzkopf R, et al. 2019 Frank Stinchfield award: a comparison of prosthetic joint infection rates between direct anterior and non-anterior approach total hip arthroplasty. Bone Joint J. 2019 Jun 1;101-B(6_Supple_B):2–8.
29. Alamanda VK, Springer BD. The prevention of infection. Bone Joint J. 2019 Jan;101-B(1_Supple_A):3–9.
30. Wyles CC, Hevesi M, Osmon DR, Park MA, Habermann EB, Lewallen DG, et al. 2019 John Charnley Award: increased risk of prosthetic joint infection following primary total knee and hip arthroplasty with the use of alternative antibiotics to cefazolin. Bone Joint J. 2019 Jun;101-B(6_Supple_B):9–15.
31. Renz N, Yermak K, Perka C, Trampuz A. Alpha Defensin lateral flow test for diagnosis of Periprosthetic joint infection. J Bone Joint Surg. 2018 May;100(9):742–50.
32. Palan J, Nolan C, Sarantos K, Westerman R, King R, Foguet P. Culture-negative periprosthetic joint infections. EFORT Open Rev. 2019 Oct;4(10):585–94.

# Optimizing Antibiotic Treatment of Bone and Joint Infections: Pharmacokinetics and Pharmacodynamics

3

Marco Trevenzoli, Vincenzo Scaglione, and Annamaria Cattelan

## 3.1 Introduction

As a general rule, in bone and joint infections (BJIs) clinical success is obtained through the combination of antimicrobial and surgical approaches [1, 2] (Fig. 3.1).

Whenever possible, starting antibiotic therapy should be delayed until bone or synovial cultures are obtained, although blood cultures, if significant, can be reliable for aetiological in situ diagnosis. Patients treated with antibiotics recently, who do not require surgical intervention immediately, should discontinue antibiotics for at least 2 weeks before debridement to optimize microbiologic diagnosis [2].

The length of the clinical course before clinical approach is important since chronic BJIs are associated with avascular necrosis, determining bone sequestra (dead bone), and surgical debridement is necessary to restore optimal bone vascularization. Conversely, acute BJIs may be treated with antibiotic therapy alone because pathophysiological alterations should have only a small effect on drug exposure.

The choice of the adequate antibiotic therapy should take into account by presence of orthopedic hardware since bacteria may produce biofilm, determining a greater risk of clinical failure. Therefore, the therapeutic strategy must include the removal of prosthetic materials, which is an "overture" to an effective antibiotic therapy, determining source control, starting the real cure effectiveness.

As empiric antibiotic treatment, we recommend molecules highly penetrating bone and joint tissues with adequate coverage spectrum against Gram-positive bacteria (i.e., *Staphylococcus* spp.).

In a setting with high rates of methicillin-resistant *Staphylococcus aureus* (MRSA) or patients with risk factors for MRSA infections, adequate coverage should be included empirically, while extensive Gram-negative coverage should be tailored to patient characteristics.

M. Trevenzoli · V. Scaglione
Infectious and Tropical Diseases Unit, Department of Medicine-DIMED, Padua University Hospital, Padova, Italy

A. Cattelan (✉)
Infectious and Tropical Diseases Unit, Department of Medicine-DIMED, Padua University Hospital, Padova, Italy

Department of Molecular Medicine-DMM, University of Padua School of Medicine, Padova, Italy
e-mail: annamaria.cattelan@unipd.it



P. Ruggieri et al. (eds.), *Bone and Joint Infections*, https://doi.org/10.1007/978-3-031-96383-4_3

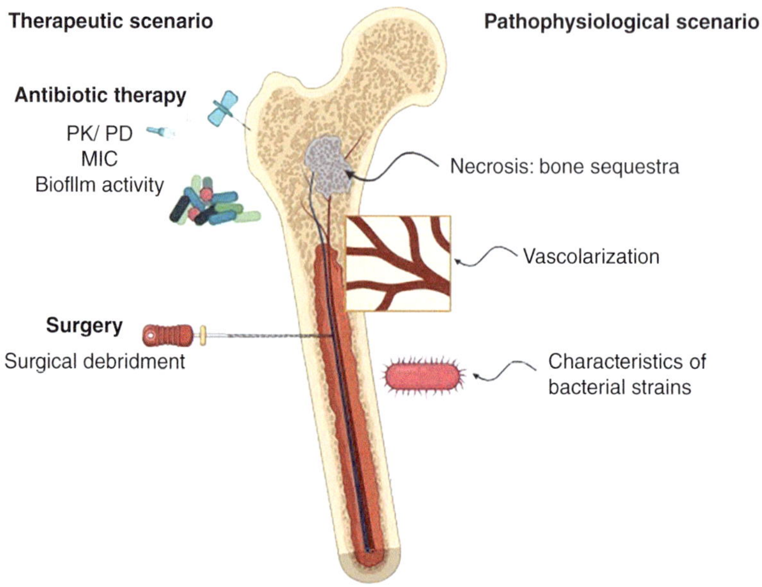


**Fig. 3.1** Key elements characterizing osteoarticular infections

## 3.2 Pharmacokinetics

Most pharmacokinetics (PK) studies are based on drug concentrations measured in plasma or serum, but this may not be the best measure of drug exposure at the action site, such as in bone.

Bone is a complex tissue composed of both organic and inorganic materials. Representing around 30–35% of bone mass, the organic matrix is made up of extracellular fluid, collagen fibrils, glycoproteins, and proteoglycans. Bone blood vessels pass through Havers' and Volkmann's canals, which are channels that run through the matrix of the bone. Bone cells (osteocytes in the mature form) are enclosed in the matrix and represents only 1–2% of bone mass, are enclosed in the matrix in their most mature form, osteocytes. The inorganic matrix, which makes up 65–70% of bone mass, is made up of hydroxyapatite (calcium-phosphate) crystals deposited within the organic matrix [3].

Bacteria and antibiotics are unlikely to be evenly distributed in bone tissue due to its heterogeneous composition. The precise localization of pathogens within bone remains a topic requiring further exploration. Considering bacterial size, for instance, the approximate diameter of *Staphylococcus aureus* (~1 μm), it is anticipated that these bacteria may disseminate through the Haversian canals and Volkmann canals, each with a diameter of around (~70 μm), yet not penetrate calcium-phosphate crystals. *S. aureus* demonstrates the ability to invade and persist within osteoblasts, potentially contributing to instances of relapse. Additionally, this pathogen is able to adhere to bone matrix components like collagen [4].

It is difficult to isolate and measure the concentrations of different components of bone. Therefore, most published studies rely on homogenized samples of bone, reporting total concentrations of the drug in these samples. It is worth noting that only the unbound drug is known to be active microbiologically, and this should be borne in mind when interpreting bone penetration findings. Total drug concentrations in the bone homogenate, however, if determined reliably and analyzed using Monte Carlo simulations and population pharmacokinetic (PK) modeling, might provide a better prediction of therapeutic success compared to serum concentrations, as serum concentrations are less representative of what is happening in the bone matrix [5].

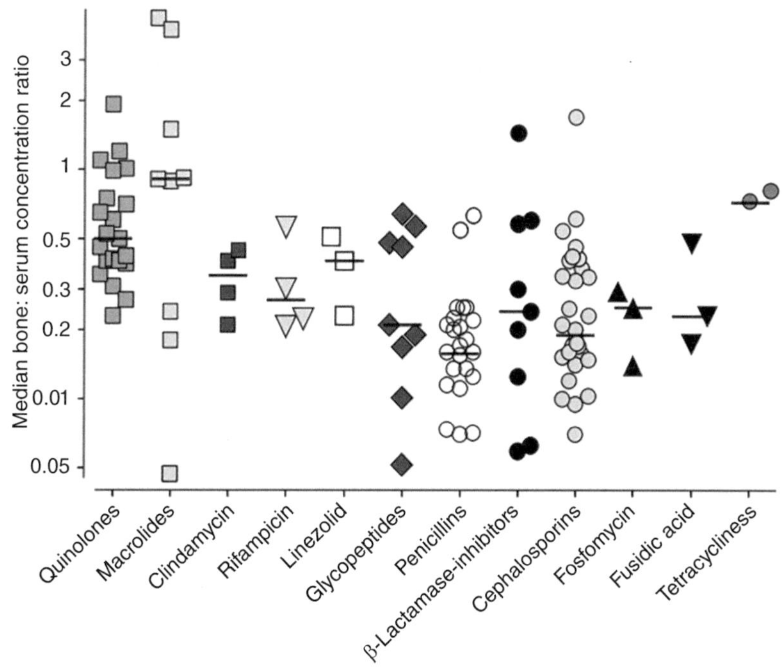


**Fig. 3.2** Different antibiotic groups' bone penetration. The lines indicate the medians of the groups, and each symbol indicates the median concentration ratio of one study. (Reproduced with permission of Springer from [5])

## 3.3 Fluoroquinolones

Fluoroquinolones are commonly used to treat bone infections due to their exceptional ability to penetrate bone tissue [5]. Compared to other antibiotic groups, fluoroquinolones exhibit some of the greatest median bone:serum concentration ratios, typically ranging from 0.3 to 1.2 (Fig. 3.2). This remarkable penetration might be attributed to the interaction between quinolones and calcium present in bone. However, it is important to note that only unbound or "free" antibiotic molecules are regarded as microbiologically active. Therefore, the actual concentrations of quinolones that are available for antimicrobial action are probably less than the overall concentrations in bone.

Interestingly, the bone:serum concentration ratios of the majority of quinolones tend to rise with time since the last dose, as recently observed for ciprofloxacin. This suggests a slow redistribution of quinolones from bone back into the blood circulation [6].

Additionally, quinolones generally exhibit good cellular penetration, which could be beneficial in treating osteomyelitis caused by *S. aureus*, as *S. aureus* has been shown to invade and persist within in vitro osteoblasts [4].

## 3.4 Macrolides and Clindamycin

Macrolides seem to be a heterogeneous group with respect to their pharmacokinetics in bone, with probably low bone penetration being reported for erythromycin and very high bone penetration being reported for azithromycin.

Indeed, concentrations in cortical bone of erythromycin were detected only in two of eight patients [7] while better data are reported for azithromycin in two recent studies in which patients were treated with 500 mg of azithromycin once a day for 3 days before periodontal surgery [8, 9]. In both studies, the average concentration of azithromycin in bone increased slightly from 12 h to 2.5 days, reached a peak of over 6, and then slowly decreased to about 2.5 at 6.5 days [8, 9]. However, it is not known how quickly azithromycin penetrates bone because the first samples were taken at 12 h.

Clindamycin is frequently said to have good bone penetration. However, the median bone:serum concentration ratio of 0.35 obtained from four clindamycin investigations is lower than that of fluoroquinolones (0.50) and linezolid (0.48) [5]. The majority of clindamycin research was carried out in the 70 s, before azithromycin, linezolid, and fluoroquinolones became available. So, at the time, clindamycin had better bone penetration than other antibiotics. All clindamycin investigations utilized bioassays, which may be affected by clindamycin's active metabolites. The findings of several investigations indicate that clindamycin has a bone penetration extent of 0.21–0.45, which is comparable to or somewhat greater than that of cephalosporins [5].

## 3.5 Tigecycline and Tetracyclines

Scant research is available regarding tetracyclines, and findings differ despite the high calcium-binding affinity of tetracyclines. Regarding tigecycline, initial bone sample analysis from 25 uninfected surgical patients revealed relatively low concentrations [10]. When the same samples were reanalyzed using a new liquid chromatography–tandem mass spectrometry (LC-MS/MS) assay, with a stabilizing agent, bone concentrations were found to be on average 9.5 times greater than with the previous approach [11]. This highlights how important it is to validate all facets of analytical approaches. Extensive penetration of tigecycline into bone has been reported in a more recent study in 33 uninfected surgical patients. Using a validated LC-MS/MS assay, the authors reported a bone:serum concentration ratio of 4.77 based on the ratio of appropriate use criteria (AUCs) in the matrices [12].

## 3.6 Cephalosporins

Many studies have been done on how well cephalosporins penetrate bone. For cefuroxime, the average ratio of bone concentration to serum concentration was 0.32 (range 0.09–0.55, 10 min to 6.5 h after a dose) in five investigations in which serum and uninfected bone concentrations were reported, with most samples above the limit of detection [5]. A recent study looked at the bone penetration of cefuroxime in uninfected surgery patients undergoing knee replacement [13]. In 9 patients who received the drug by short-term infusion and 9 patients who received it by continuous infusion, the respective bone:plasma concentration ratios on the basis of unbound AUCs after population PK modeling were 1.03 for cancellous bone and 0.35 for cortical bone; the corresponding ratios for continuous infusion were 1.15 and 0.65.

Ceftriaxone and cefamandole were tested in the same study on patients having hip replacement surgery. At 10–30 min after the dose, the average ratio of bone concentration to serum concentration was 0.156 (0.123–0.190) for ceftriaxone. At 8 h after the dose, the ratio of bone concentration to serum concentration for ceftriaxone was 0.142 (0.073–0.210), which is very similar to the ratio at 10–30 min. This suggests that ceftriaxone reaches equilibrium between serum and bone quickly [14]. However, a more recent study suggested that equilibrium is reached more slowly [15]. In 11 patients who were having surgery to remove dead bone from a broken leg that had become infected, the average ratio of bone concentration to plasma AUC for ceftriaxone was 0.093 in the outer bone (cortical bone) and 0.241 in the inner bone (cancellous bone) [16]. For cefazolin, the median ratio of bone concentration to serum concentration in eight patients with infected bones was 0.25 (range 0.06–0.41) over the course of a continuous infusion, with concentrations assessed using bioassay [17]. A more recent investigation performed using 24-h plasma sampling and bone microdialysis, and quantified cefazolin by high-performance liquid chromatography (HPLC), showed mean AUC-based bone:plasma concentration ratios of 0.74 ± 0.36 and 0.99 ± 0.59 for the left and right sternum of coronary artery bypass graft (CABG) patients [18].

## 3.7 Ceftobiprole

Ceftobiprole has been shown to penetrate bone tissue, with a cortical and cancellous bone-to-serum penetration ratio of 0.22 and 0.06, respectively, in patients undergoing elective total hip replacement [19]. However, there is no data on trough concentrations in bone, so it is not possible to assess whether PK/PD targets are achieved at the infection site [20].

## 3.8 Penicillins, Carbapenems, and β-Lactamase Inhibitors

Two studies by different groups in 1994 and 2001 looked at how well piperacillin/tazobactam penetrates uninfected hip bone in 12 patients each. The studies used the same methods to prepare and analyze the samples and found similar results. The ratio of bone concentration to plasma concentration was 0.2–0.3 for both piperacillin and tazobactam in both the outer bone (cortical bone) and the inner bone (cancellous bone) 1–1.5 h after the dose [21, 22]. More recently, a study looked at how well piperacillin/tazobactam penetrates uninfected jaw (7 patients) and hip (2 patients) bone [23]. The samples were prepared in a similar way to the previous studies, and the concentrations were assessed using a different method called LC-MS/MS. On average, 3 h (range 1–7 h) after the start of the infusion, the ratio of bone concentration to plasma concentration was 0.13 for tazobactam and 0.15 for piperacillin. These findings were somewhat lower and more varied than the results from the previous studies, which may be because different types of bone were studied and the samples were taken at different times. Studies using a different method, the bioassay, have reported a broad range of mean amoxicillin bone:serum concentration ratios. A study of 20 patients undergoing hip replacement surgery found that the ratio of bone AUC to serum AUC was 0.18 (0.11–0.29) for cancellous bone and 0.20 (10–90th percentile for inter-patient variability 0.16–0.25) for cortical bone [24]. The ratio of bone AUC to serum AUC for clavulanic acid in the same study was 0.10 (0.051–0.21) for cancellous bone and 0.15 (0.11–0.21) for cortical bone. Recently, a report reported bone-serum flucloxacillin concentration ratios, using HPLC analysis, of 0.07–0.08 and 0.05–0.06 for hip and knee bone, respectively, in the first hour and a half following administration of the drug [25]. Carbapenems have been the subject of only a few investigations, and the results are difficult to interpret because of problems with the methods used [5]. However, a recent study on ertapenem that involved taking samples over 2–28 h and analyzing them using liquid chromatography–mass spectrometry (LC-MS) and population PK modeling reported a bone:plasma concentration ratio of 0.025 in 10 patients [26].

## 3.9 Linezolid

Linezolid is more stable than many β-lactams, and all linezolid bone penetration studies have used HPLC to assess the drug concentrations. In 12 hip replacement patients, the average bone:serum concentration ratio at 30–50 mins following infusion initiation was 0.51 (95% confidence interval: 0.43–0.75) [27]. Similar penetration (0.40 ± 0.24) was found at 1.5 h in 12 elderly patients during knee replacement [28]. However, in 11 patients with infections associated with implants, the mean bone:plasma concentration ratio was lower (approximately 0.23) at the same dose as the two joint replacement studies and 0.5–1.5 h after the dose [29].

Two investigations have used microdialysis to measure linezolid concentrations in bone [18, 30]. In three patients with severe diabetic foot infections, the unbound AUC (fAUC) ratio in cancellous bone to plasma over 12 h was 1.09 ± 0.11 [30]. The 24-h sternal bone ratio in nine uninfected subjects undergoing coronary artery bypass grafting was 1.02 ± 0.47 for the right sternum and 0.82 ± 0.28 for the left sternum [18]. Ratios close to unity in the two investigations indicate that exposure to microbiologically active linezolid is comparable in bone interstitial fluid and plasma. The greater AUC ratio obtained from microdialysis, when contrasted with concentration ratios obtained from bone homogenate, aligns with linezolid's limited tendency to form chelate complexes with the bone inorganic matrix.

In other words, linezolid penetrates bone well, and the quantity of linezolid in bone is similar to the amount in blood plasma, meaning that linezolid can be effective in treating bone infections.

## 3.10 Trimetoprim/Sulfametoxazole

Cotrimoxazole also penetrates bone tissue, with a bone-to-serum ratio that is higher in cancellous bone (0.30) than in cortical bone (0.20) [31]. Interestingly, the synovial fluid-to-serum ratio for cotrimoxazole is even higher, at 0.61 for sulfamethoxazole and 0.74 for trimethoprim [32].

## 3.11 Daptomycin

Daptomycin penetrates well into bone in diabetic foot infections [33]. In one study, researchers measured daptomycin concentrations in the interstitial fluid of metatarsal bone and plasma in patients with diabetic foot infections. They determined that the average ratio of daptomycin concentrations in bone to plasma was 1.08, suggesting that daptomycin penetrates well into the bone tissue where infection is most likely to occur. This is remarkable given that daptomycin is highly bound to plasma proteins (about 90%) and has a high molecular weight.

Another study that measured the total area under the curve (AUC) of daptomycin in bone and plasma found much lower concentration ratios (0.095 for thigh bone and 0.082 for shin bone) [34]. This difference in results is likely because the first study measured unbound daptomycin concentrations, while the second study measured total daptomycin concentrations. Since daptomycin is highly bound to plasma proteins, the total daptomycin concentration in bone will be lower than the unbound plasma daptomycin concentration.

Overall, the evidence indicates that daptomycin penetrates well into bone in diabetic foot infections.

## 3.12 Fosfomycin

Fosfomycin penetrates bone tissue well. In a study of chronic osteomyelitis patients, the bone:serum ratio of fosfomycin was determined to be 0.43 [35]. This means that the fosfomycin concentration in bone is about 43% of the concentration in serum.

A single dose of 100 mg/kg of fosfomycin resulted in a mean $AUC_{0-12}$ of 511.0 ± 100.7 mg•h/kg in bone in patients with diabetic foot infections [35]. The $AUC_{0-12}$ measures the cumulative drug exposure over 12 h.

The optimal PK/PD target for fosfomycin against MRSA/methicillin-resistant *Staphylococcus epidermidis* (MRSE) is an $AUC_{0-24}$ h/minimum inhibitory concentration (MIC) ratio > 250. This means that the total amount of drug exposure over 24 h should be at least 250 times the MIC of the bacteria.

A dosing regimen of fosfomycin 200 mg/kg q24h (16 g/day in a 70 kg patient) should achieve optimal PK/PD target attainment at the infection site against MRSA/MRSE with an MIC value up to 4 mg/L. This is well below the clinical breakpoint of 32 mg/L, which means that the bacteria are still susceptible to the antibiotic at this concentration. Therefore, fosfomycin should not be utilized as a monotherapy [20].

## 3.13 Glycopeptides and Lipoglycopeptides

Glycopeptides, such as vancomycin and dalbavancin, penetrate bone tissue to some extent, but the degree of penetration varies according to the bone type and the specific glycopeptide.

A recent study determined that the ratio of vancomycin concentrations in cancellous bone to plasma was 0.45, while the ratio for cortical bone was 0.17. This indicates that vancomycin penetrates cancellous bone better than cortical bone.

A single dose of 1000 mg of dalbavancin resulted in a mean bone concentration of 4.1 ± 1.6 mg/kg at 14 days in subjects undergoing elective orthopedic interventions.

A dosing regimen of 1500 mg + 1500 mg 1 week apart is anticipated to result in a $C_{min}$ (minimum concentration) of >8.04 mg/L for around 5–6 weeks. This is considered to be the optimal PK/PD target attainment (fAUC/MIC >111.1) against MRSA and/or MRSE isolates with a MIC value up to the clinical breakpoint of 0.125 mg/L [36–38]. Therefore, dalbavancin can reach high enough concentrations in bone and synovial fluid to be effective against MRSA and MRSE infections. A dosing regimen of 1500 mg + 1500 mg 1 week apart is anticipated to maintain these high concentrations for around 5–6 weeks [20].

Overall, the evidence indicates that glycopeptides do penetrate bone tissue, but the degree of penetration varies according to the bone type and the specific glycopeptide. More research is needed to better understand the bone penetration of glycopeptides and to identify the optimal dosage and schedule for treating bone infections.

## 3.14 Pharmacodynamics and Monte Carlo Simulations

Pharmacodynamics (PD) studies how drugs impact biological systems. In the context of antibiotic therapy, PD involves studying the link between drug concentrations and the desired therapeutic effect [5].

For beta-lactam antibiotics, the key PD parameter is the T > MIC (time above the minimum inhibitory concentration). The T > MIC is the time during which the drug concentration surpasses the MIC of the bacteria being treated. In the case of other antibiotics, like fluoroquinolones, the key PD parameter is the area under the concentration-time curve above the MIC (fAUC/MIC). The fAUC/MIC is the total amount of drug exposure above the MIC over a given time period [5].

In bone penetration studies, it is not always possible to perform a PD analysis since bone penetration data is often sparse, with a small number of samples collected from each patient. Additionally, bone penetration data is often collected simultaneously for all patients. This complicates the comparison between the drug's bone concentration and the MIC of the bacteria being treated.

Overall, PD analysis of bone penetration data can be challenging, but it is important to report the approaches and assumptions used in bone penetration studies. This allows other researchers to understand the study's limitations and interpret the results carefully. Population PK modeling is a more sophisticated approach to analyzing bone penetration data and can provide estimates of the average and individual bone penetration parameters.

Population modeling is à powerful instrument for analyzing bone penetration data. It can account for both the average penetration and its variability between subjects. This information can be used for predicting the expected concentration-time profiles for different dosage regimens and to estimate the probability of achieving a PK/PD target.

One example of how population modeling has been utilized to study bone penetration is the work of Landersdorfer CB et al [39]. These researchers developed a population PK model for moxifloxacin in bone and serum. They then used the model for predicting the probability of achieving PK/PD targets for positive microbiological and clinical outcomes in osteomyelitis patients. Simulation results suggested that a dose of 400 mg moxifloxacin administered one time a day would achieve a ≥ 90% probability of target attainment for MICs up to 0.375 mg/L in cancellous bone and serum and 0.5 mg/L in cortical bone [39].

This is a promising result, but it is worth noting that the model relied on data from a small number of patients and that clinical trials are needed to validate the results. Additionally, the

PK/PD targets used in the simulation were derived from data on ciprofloxacin, not moxifloxacin. Therefore, it is important to interpret the findings with caution.

Although population modeling is a valuable tool for studying bone penetration and for predicting the probability of achieving PK/PD targets, it is important to conduct well-designed clinical studies to collect high-quality bone penetration data that herald clinical outcomes.

## 3.15 Conclusion

In the context of BJIs, the PK/PD antimicrobial profile is particularly important to get clinical success.

(a) One of the key challenges in treating BJIs is that antibiotics can have difficulty penetrating bone and joint tissue. This is due to several factors, including the dense bone matrix, the existence of biofilms, and the limited blood supply to some areas of bone. As a result, it is important to choose antibiotics that have good bone and joint penetration and ask for an orthopedic consultation to get surgical toilette to optimize the action of the antimicrobial therapy.

(b) Another important PK/PD consideration for BJIs is the time-dependent or dose-dependent elimination of bacteria. This implies that some antibiotics, such as beta-lactams, are more effective at killing bacteria when they are maintained at an elevated concentration for a long period. Conversely, dose-dependent molecules like fluoroquinolones or aminoglycosides require more attention to the appropriateness of the individual dosage than to the maintenance of an adequate plasma level. Anyway, whatever the mechanism of action, it is important to achieve and maintain adequate concentrations of the molecule at the infection site.

(c) Lastly, the spectrum of activity of antibiotics when choosing treatment for BJIs must be considered. The spectrum of activity refers to the range of bacteria that an antibiotic is effective against. For BJIs, it is important to choose, at least initially, an antibiotic that has a spectrum of activity against the most prevalent pathogens, taking into account that Gram-positive bacteria are the most frequently involved.

(d) In addition to the PK/PD considerations listed above, it is also important to individualize antibiotic treatment for BJIs according to the patient's clinical condition, clinical compliance, the possibility of an allergic response, or the concomitant therapies with their relative interactions.

Treating an infection means treating the patient globally; the use of knowledge relating to the metabolism of the antibiotic must not make us forget the empathy that must be sought with the patient to establish a strong therapeutic alliance.

## References

1. Lew DP, Waldvogel FA. Osteomyelitis. Lancet. 2004;364(9431):369–79. https://doi.org/10.1016/S0140-6736(04)16727-5.
2. Zimmerli W, Ochsner PE. Management of infection associated with prosthetic joints. Infection. 2003;31(2):99–108. https://doi.org/10.1007/s15010-002-3079-9.
3. Florencio-Silva R, Sasso GR, Sasso-Cerri E, Simoes MJ, Cerri PS. Biology of bone tissue: structure, function, and factors that influence bone cells. Biomed Res Int. 2015;2015:421746. https://doi.org/10.1155/2015/421746.
4. Jevon M, Guo C, Ma B, Mordan N, Nair SP, Harris M, et al. Mechanisms of internalization of Staphylococcus aureus by cultured human osteoblasts. Infect Immun. 1999;67(5):2677–81. https://doi.org/10.1128/IAI.67.5.2677-2681.1999.
5. Landersdorfer CB, Bulitta JB, Kinzig M, Holzgrabe U, Sorgel F. Penetration of antibacterials into bone: pharmacokinetic, pharmacodynamic and bioanalytical considerations. Clin Pharmacokinet. 2009;48(2):89–124. https://doi.org/10.2165/00003088-200948020-00002.
6. Landersdorfer CB, Kinzig M, Hohl R, Kempf P, Nation RL, Sorgel F. Physiologically based population pharmacokinetic modeling approach for ciprofloxacin in bone of patients undergoing orthopedic surgery. ACS Pharmacol Transl Sci. 2020;3(3):444–54. https://doi.org/10.1021/acsptsci.0c00045.
7. Sorensen TS, Colding H, Schroeder E, Rosdahl VT. The penetration of cefazolin, erythromy-

cin and methicillin into human bone tissue. Acta Orthop Scand. 1978;49(6):549–53. https://doi.org/10.3109/17453677808993236.

8. Malizia T, Batoni G, Ghelardi E, Baschiera F, Graziani F, Blandizzi C, et al. Interaction between piroxicam and azithromycin during distribution to human periodontal tissues. J Periodontol. 2001;72(9):1151–6. https://doi.org/10.1902/jop.2000.72.9.1151.
9. Malizia T, Tejada MR, Ghelardi E, Senesi S, Gabriele M, Giuca MR, et al. Periodontal tissue disposition of azithromycin. J Periodontol. 1997;68(12):1206–9. https://doi.org/10.1902/jop.1997.68.12.1206.
10. Rodvold KA, Gotfried MH, Cwik M, Korth-Bradley JM, Dukart G, Ellis-Grosse EJ. Serum, tissue and body fluid concentrations of tigecycline after a single 100 mg dose. J Antimicrob Chemother. 2006;58(6):1221–9. https://doi.org/10.1093/jac/dkl403.
11. Ji AJ, Saunders JP, Amorusi P, Wadgaonkar ND, O'Leary K, Leal M, et al. A sensitive human bone assay for quantitation of tigecycline using LC/MS/MS. J Pharm Biomed Anal. 2008;48(3):866–75. https://doi.org/10.1016/j.jpba.2008.06.020.
12. Bhattacharya I, Gotfried MH, Ji AJ, Saunders JP, Gourley I, Diehl A, et al. Reassessment of tigecycline bone concentrations in volunteers undergoing elective orthopedic procedures. J Clin Pharmacol. 2014;54(1):70–4. https://doi.org/10.1002/jcph.201.
13. Tottrup M, Soballe K, Bibby BM, Hardlei TF, Hansen P, Fuursted K, et al. Bone, subcutaneous tissue and plasma pharmacokinetics of cefuroxime in total knee replacement patients – a randomized controlled trial comparing continuous and short-term infusion. APMIS. 2019;127(12):779–88. https://doi.org/10.1111/apm.12996.
14. Lovering AM, Walsh TR, Bannister GC, MacGowan AP. The penetration of ceftriaxone and cefamandole into bone, fat and haematoma and relevance of serum protein binding to their penetration into bone. J Antimicrob Chemother. 2001;47(4):483–6. https://doi.org/10.1093/jac/47.4.483.
15. Gergs U, Clauss T, Ihlefeld D, Weiss M, Ponicke K, Hofmann GO, et al. Pharmacokinetics of ceftriaxone in plasma and bone of patients undergoing hip or knee surgery. J Pharm Pharmacol. 2014;66(11):1552–8. https://doi.org/10.1111/jphp.12282.
16. Garazzino S, Aprato A, Baietto L, D'Avolio A, Maiello A, De Rosa FG, et al. Ceftriaxone bone penetration in patients with septic non-union of the tibia. Int J Infect Dis. 2011;15(6):e415–21. https://doi.org/10.1016/j.ijid.2011.03.003.
17. Zeller V, Durand F, Kitzis MD, Lhotellier L, Ziza JM, Mamoudy P, et al. Continuous cefazolin infusion to treat bone and joint infections: clinical efficacy, feasibility, safety, and serum and bone concentrations. Antimicrob Agents Chemother. 2009;53(3):883–7. https://doi.org/10.1128/AAC.00389-08.
18. Andreas M, Zeitlinger M, Wisser W, Jaeger W, Maier-Salamon A, Thalhammer F, et al. Cefazolin and linezolid penetration into sternal cancellous bone during coronary artery bypass grafting. Eur J Cardiothorac Surg. 2015;48(5):758–64. https://doi.org/10.1093/ejcts/ezu491.
19. Azanza Perea JR, Sadaba Diaz de Rada B. Ceftobiprole: pharmacokinetics and PK/PD profile. Rev Esp Quimioter. 2019;32(Suppl 3):11–6.
20. Gatti M, Tedeschi S, Zamparini E, Pea F, Viale P. Pharmacokinetic and pharmacodynamic considerations for optimizing antimicrobial therapy used to treat bone and joint infections: an evidence-based algorithmic approach. Expert Opin Drug Metab Toxicol. 2023;19(8):511–35. https://doi.org/10.1080/17425255.2023.2255525.
21. Incavo SJ, Ronchetti PJ, Choi JH, Wu H, Kinzig M, Sorgel F. Penetration of piperacillin-tazobactam into cancellous and cortical bone tissues. Antimicrob Agents Chemother. 1994;38(4):905–7. https://doi.org/10.1128/AAC.38.4.905.
22. Boselli E, Breilh D, Debon R, Duflo F, Bel JC, Saux MC, et al. Penetration of piperacillin/tazobactam (4 g/500 mg) into synovial tissue. J Chemother. 2002;14(1):54–8. https://doi.org/10.1179/joc.2002.14.1.54.
23. Al-Nawas B, Kinzig-Schippers M, Soergel F, Shah PM. Concentrations of piperacillin-tazobactam in human jaw and hip bone. J Craniomaxillofac Surg. 2008;36(8):468–72. https://doi.org/10.1016/j.jcms.2008.06.003.
24. Landersdorfer CB, Kinzig M, Bulitta JB, Hennig FF, Holzgrabe U, Sorgel F, et al. Bone penetration of amoxicillin and clavulanic acid evaluated by population pharmacokinetics and Monte Carlo simulation. Antimicrob Agents Chemother. 2009;53(6):2569–78. https://doi.org/10.1128/AAC.01119-08.
25. Torkington MS, Davison MJ, Wheelwright EF, Jenkins PJ, Anthony I, Lovering AM, et al. Bone penetration of intravenous flucloxacillin and gentamicin as antibiotic prophylaxis during total hip and knee arthroplasty. Bone Joint J. 2017;99-B(3):358–64. https://doi.org/10.1302/0301-620X.99B3.BJJ-2016-0328.R1.
26. Chambers J, Page-Sharp M, Salman S, Dyer J, Davis TME, Batty KT, et al. Ertapenem for osteoarticular infections in obese patients: a pharmacokinetic study of plasma and bone concentrations. Eur J Clin Pharmacol. 2019;75(4):511–7. https://doi.org/10.1007/s00228-018-2597-z.
27. Lovering AM, Zhang J, Bannister GC, Lankester BJ, Brown JH, Narendra G, et al. Penetration of linezolid into bone, fat, muscle and haematoma of patients undergoing routine hip replacement. J Antimicrob Chemother. 2002;50(1):73–7. https://doi.org/10.1093/jac/dkf066.
28. Rana B, Butcher I, Grigoris P, Murnaghan C, Seaton RA, Tobin CM. Linezolid penetration into osteo-articular tissues. J Antimicrob Chemother. 2002;50(5):747–50. https://doi.org/10.1093/jac/dkf207.
29. Kutscha-Lissberg F, Hebler U, Muhr G, Koller M. Linezolid penetration into bone and joint tissues

infected with methicillin-resistant staphylococci. Antimicrob Agents Chemother. 2003;47(12):3964–6. https://doi.org/10.1128/AAC.47.12.3964-3966.2003.
30. Traunmuller F, Schintler MV, Spendel S, Popovic M, Mauric O, Scharnagl E, et al. Linezolid concentrations in infected soft tissue and bone following repetitive doses in diabetic patients with bacterial foot infections. Int J Antimicrob Agents. 2010;36(1):84–6. https://doi.org/10.1016/j.ijantimicag.2010.03.007.
31. Saux MC, Le Rebeller A, Leng B, Mintrosse J. Bone diffusion of trimethoprim and sulfamethoxazole high pressure liquid chromatography (HPLC) (author's transl). Pathol Biol (Paris). 1982;30(6):385–8.
32. Sattar MA, Cawley MI, Holt JE, Sankey MG, Kaye CM. The penetration of trimethoprim and sulphamethoxazole into synovial fluid. J Antimicrob Chemother. 1983;12(3):229–33. https://doi.org/10.1093/jac/12.3.229.
33. Traunmuller F, Schintler MV, Metzler J, Spendel S, Mauric O, Popovic M, et al. Soft tissue and bone penetration abilities of daptomycin in diabetic patients with bacterial foot infections. J Antimicrob Chemother. 2010;65(6):1252–7. https://doi.org/10.1093/jac/dkq109.
34. Montange D, Berthier F, Leclerc G, Serre A, Jeunet L, Berard M, et al. Penetration of daptomycin into bone and synovial fluid in joint replacement. Antimicrob Agents Chemother. 2014;58(7):3991–6. https://doi.org/10.1128/AAC.02344-14.
35. Schintler MV, Traunmuller F, Metzler J, Kreuzwirt G, Spendel S, Mauric O, et al. High fosfomycin concentrations in bone and peripheral soft tissue in diabetic patients presenting with bacterial foot infection. J Antimicrob Chemother. 2009;64(3):574–8. https://doi.org/10.1093/jac/dkp230.
36. Dunne MW, Puttagunta S, Sprenger CR, Rubino C, Van Wart S, Baldassarre J. Extended-duration dosing and distribution of dalbavancin into bone and articular tissue. Antimicrob Agents Chemother. 2015;59(4):1849–55. https://doi.org/10.1128/AAC.04550-14.
37. Cojutti PG, Rinaldi M, Zamparini E, Rossi N, Tedeschi S, Conti M, et al. Population pharmacokinetics of dalbavancin and dosing consideration for optimal treatment of adult patients with staphylococcal osteoarticular infections. Antimicrob Agents Chemother. 2023;65(5):e02260-20. https://doi.org/10.1128/AAC.02260-20.
38. Cojutti PG, Tedeschi S, Gatti M, Zamparini E, Meschiari M, Siega PD, et al. Population pharmacokinetic and Pharmacodynamic analysis of Dalbavancin for long-term treatment of subacute and/or chronic infectious diseases: the major role of therapeutic drug monitoring. Antibiotics (Basel). 2022;11(8):996. https://doi.org/10.3390/antibiotics11080996.
39. Landersdorfer CB, Kinzig M, Hennig FF, Bulitta JB, Holzgrabe U, Drusano GL, et al. Penetration of moxifloxacin into bone evaluated by Monte Carlo simulation. Antimicrob Agents Chemother. 2009;53(5):2074–81. https://doi.org/10.1128/AAC.01056-08.

# 4 Aetiology and Pathogenesis: Causative Agents

Franziska Ziegenhain and Gerrolt Nico Jukema

Bone, joint and soft tissue infections in orthopaedic and trauma infections are a devastating incident in the treatment of patients, generating significant disease burden and a high financial impact [1, 2]. Understanding the aetiology and pathogenesis is critical for prevention and reducing patients' threats as well as improving treatment of these infections. The different factors contributing to the occurrence of bone and joint infections are complex and impact one another significantly. Patient's general and local (soft) tissue factors, as well as the pathogens, influence the outcome and the course of treatment. This chapter concentrates on outlining the aetiology and pathogenesis of bone and joint infections, and will give some considerations about their treatment in trauma surgery.

## 4.1 Aetiology

### 4.1.1 Definition

The Centers for Disease Control and Prevention (CDC) define a surgical site infection (SSI) as an infection that occurs in a part of the body that has undergone surgery. Infections can be divided into superficial wound infections and deep infections that involve organs and or bones and joints. Infection following and involving implanted hardware forms a separate subgroup [3].

F. Ziegenhain · G. N. Jukema (✉)
Department of Trauma Surgery, University Hospital Zurich, Zurich, Switzerland
e-mail: Franziska.ziegenhain@usz.ch; GerroltNico.Jukema@usz.ch

### 4.1.2 Risk Factors

#### 4.1.2.1 Patient-Specific Risk Factors

Different risk factors of the patient that influence the occurrence of bone and joint infections have been described over the years [4, 5]. Systemic as well as local conditions have a tremendous impact. Patients with systemic diseases that influence the immune system are at a significantly higher risk of developing osteomyelitis and or septic arthritis. These diseases include metabolic conditions like diabetes, arteriosclerosis and obesity, as well as immunodeficiencies like HIV, immunosuppressant medications and malignancies. Diabetes mellitus is hereby of special interest, as up to 20% of these patients suffer from diabetic foot syndrome with osteomyelitis [6]. Substance abuse, especially smoking and alcoholism, are known risk factors as well [7, 8]. These patients tend to have impaired wound healing. Depending on the degree of the abuse, noncompliance is also a patient factor to take into consideration. Some of these conditions are accessible for optimising preoperatively, if time allows [9]. Prior to elective surgery, these at-risk patients should be treated by an interdisciplinary


P. Ruggieri et al. (eds.), *Bone and Joint Infections*, https://doi.org/10.1007/978-3-031-96383-4_4

team. Elective surgery should, when possible, be postponed until the pre-existing conditions are improved. Medication of patients with known diabetes and suboptimal glucose sugar levels should be adjusted preoperatively whenever possible to reach normal glucose levels, and therefore reduce the risk of infection.

Local status, i.e. reduced blood circulation (e.g. in patients with arteriosclerosis), closed damaged soft tissue (classification according to Tscherne-Oestern [10]) and open fractures (classification according to Gustilo-Anderson [11, 12]) are related to the occurrence of infections of the bone and joints. The importance of acknowledging the local soft tissues and treating fractures with extensive soft tissue accordingly is reflected in the multitude of scores and definitions. The Tscherne-Oestern and Gustilo-Anderson classifications are widely used to describe the soft tissue injury in combination with a fracture. They provide the surgeon with a tool to estimate the level of tissue damage and treat the patient accordingly. This is especially important as open fractures have a significantly higher rate of infections.

The initial management, meaning a carefully carried out debridement by the most skilled surgeon available and initial (perioperative) antibiotic therapy where needed, determines the course of the healing process. In general, in case of an open fracture, every wound should have a surgical debridement with lavage in the operating room under sterile conditions as soon as possible after admission [13]. In cases with extended soft tissue damage, negative pressure wound therapy can support a favorable outcome in the treatment of extensive soft tissue damage, especially as it benefits the local circulation and the reduction of bacterial growth. The number of patients who are initially more in need of (free) flap plastic surgery can be successfully reduced by staged application of negative pressure wound therapy.

The complex interaction between host factors and local infection for the course of the disease is reflected in the classification that was proposed in 1985 by Cierny and Mader [4, 14]. Factors that are taken into account to determine the host class are systemic factors like malnutrition, renal failure, diabetes mellitus, immunodeficiency, alcohol or tobacco abuse, extreme age and hypoxia, among others. For local factors, compromising conditions such as lymphedema, vascular disease, scarring, nerve damage, radiation disease and major vessel compromise are recognised to have a major influence on outcome.

#### 4.1.2.2 Bacteria

***Staphylococcus aureus***

*Staphylococcus aureus* is the most commonly found pathogen in bone and joint infections. This is due to its high virulence and ubiquitous occurrence. Several cell-associated and extracellular factors contribute to this. *Staphylococcus aureus* produces several adhesions that allow it to attach to tissue as well as foreign body surfaces [15]. After adhesion, the bacteria produces factors like protein A, coagulase and other capsular polysaccharides that shield the pathogen from the human immune system [16–18]. This biofilm forms an almost impossible to penetrate wall for the human immune system and antibiotic treatment, and thus protects the embedded bacteria. It also protects the bacteria from mechanical disruption during surgical debridement. With various exotoxins and hydrolases, *S. aureus* causes damage and ultimately (necrotic) destruction of the infected tissue [19, 20] and is uniquely adapted to survive in the skeletal structure. Next to biofilm formation, the bacteria can infiltrate cells. Studies have shown infiltration of osteoclasts and osteocytes by bacterial species [21, 22]. The activation of osteoclasts leads to further bone loss, and the survival of the cells might support long-term colonisation. With its high virulence and ability to form colonies, *S. aureus* promotes the formation of abscesses in bone infections. The forming necrotic tissue protects the bacteria further from clearance by antibiotic agents and neutrophil cells [23, 24]. The combination of these various mechanisms to spread and survive in the skeletal system explains the predominance of *S. aureus* in bone and joint infections.

#### 4.1.2.3 Other Causative Agents

While *S.aureus* is the most prevalent bacteria in bone and joint infections, other commonly found bacteria include *strepto-* and *pneumococcus* species. Depending on the location and cause of the infection, different bacterial species will be involved.

Especially in nosocomial infections, multiresistant bacteria like methicillin-resistant *Staphylococcus aureus* (MRSA), *Pseudomonas* and *Enterobacteria* can be found [25]. These pathogens present their own unique challenges, as antibiotic treatment is often complicated for treatment of these particular infections. Preferably, these patients should be treated in specialised centres by an experienced, multidisciplinary team.

Implant-associated bone and joint infections become particularly challenging if biofilm-generating bacteria are involved. Next to *Staphylococcus aureus*, *Pseudomonas aeruginosa* and *Staphylococcus epididermidis* are able to form biofilms and hence expand their virulence [26–28].

Different body regions also play a role in the different microbiomes that are found. Mixed infections are predominantly prevalent in the face, oral region and pelvis due to the common local skin flora. *M. tuberculosis* is more frequently found in infections of the spine [29].

If a pre-existing infection of an organ system is the cause of bone or joint infections, bacteria are typically the same as primarily found in those infections. Antibiotic treatment should be adapted accordingly if there is suspicion of (ongoing) systemic spread of the primary infection like bacteremia or sepsis.

As bacteria and antibiotic resistance profiles vary in between countries and even between hospitals in a country, it is highly recommended to follow the local anti-infective guidelines for initial treatment and to adapt antibiotic therapy as soon as the causative agents are identified according to their resistance pattern.

Properly carrying out of sampling is of essence to provide adequate antibiotic treatment (Table 4.1).

#### 4.1.2.4 Path of Infection

In general, two different pathways of infection are distinguished. Endogen infections, mostly caused by haematogenous and septic spreading, are frequently showing monobacterial colonisation. The origin is usually a bacterial infection like tonsillitis, a soft tissue infection or, for example a visceral organ infection like an appendicitis. They are more regularly found in children and

**Table 4.1** Overview of the most common bacteria found in different types of bone and joint infections [6, 29–34]

| Type of infection | Commonly found bacteria | Polymicrobial infections | Gram-negative infections |
|---|---|---|---|
| Post-traumatic/fracture related | *Staphylococcus aureus*<br>*Staphyloccocus epididermidis*<br>*Streptococcus* spp.<br>*Pseudomonas* spp.<br>*Enterobacteria* spp. | >20% | app. 20% |
| Haematogenous infections | *Staphylococcus aureus*<br>*Streptococcus* spp.<br>*Pseudomonas* spp. | app. 20% | >10% |
| Vertebral infections | *Staphylococcus aureus*<br>*Staphylococcus epididermidis*<br>*Streptococcus* spp.<br>*Enterococccus* spp.<br>*Diphtheroids*<br>*Pseudomonas* spp.<br>*Enterobacteriaceae* spp. | >15% | >10% |
| Implant-related infections | *Staphylococcus aureus*<br>*Staphylococcus epididermidis* | >10% | >5% |

young adolescents [35]. Metaphyseal bone with its extensive blood supply and low blood flow rate is especially susceptible for bacterial attachment and growth of the germs. Depending on the age of the individual, spreading of the infection to the joint is possible. It is less likely in children over the age of 2 years with open epiphyseal plates and normally no shared blood supply of the meta- and epiphysis [36]. Children under the age of approximately two and adults can suffer from a spreading per continuitatem towards the joint, resulting in septic arthritis [37].

In contrast, exogen osteitis and septic arthritis are often multibacterial infections after trauma as well as iatrogenic after surgeries (e.g. surgical site infection). For that reason, treatment is often challenging and requires a different approach [38].

In post-traumatic infections, details about patient's injury are critical for prevention and successful treatment of infection. For example, injuries in the farming environment with contaminated wounds need different antibiotic therapy [39]. Knowledge of these exceptions and where to expect different bacterial species are essential for clinical management. International and local antibiotic guidelines should be considered. Patients with pre-existing conditions are at higher risk of developing bone and joint infections after trauma due to their compromised immune system [5]. Close surveillance and early intervention are key to successful treatment.

Iatrogenic infections after surgical intervention (so-called surgical site infections) were reduced significantly over the last years by the implementation of several preventive measures (for example, the perioperative administration of an antibiotic drug [40, 41]. Similar to post-traumatic infections, in elective surgery pathogens are introduced to the bone and or joint from the skin/outside. Therefore, skin-related species like *Staphylococcus aureus* are frequently found in these infections. Normally, in an acute surgical site infection, local symptoms like swelling, redness and painful tenderness are present, sometimes with generalised symptoms like fever. Laboratory examination shows elevated inflammatory markers correlating to the response of the immune system. If an infection after orthopaedic and trauma surgery cannot be treated successfully in the acute and early phase, it eventually becomes a chronic infection, with formation of infected (granulation) tissue, osteonecrosis and fistulae at the surgical site [34, 42, 43].

### 4.1.3 Acute Osteomyelitis and Septic Arthritis

By definition of the CDC acute bone and joint infections after surgery are limited to a time period of 30 (acute onset) to up to 90 days within 1 year if an implant is in place (late onset [3]). In the early stage, patients normally complain of local symptoms like redness, swelling, pain at the operation site and systemic reactions like fever, fatigue and general sickness. The onset is typically within a short time period. Wounds might present with secretion and possibly pus. As already stated, the critical incident in bone infection is the development of a biofilm, especially if osteosynthesis hardware or prosthesis with plastic components are in situ [27]. Biofilm prevents an effective antibiotic treatment and builds a hard-to-penetrate layer for the human (cellular) immune system and antibiotic drugs to destroy bacteria. The definitive formation of this biofilm occurs early after the start of infection, over the time of days to weeks, so the timeframe is essential in the successful treatment of these infections. An acute infection leads to a quick and strong immune response. Histologic findings include erosions and destruction of bone and neutrophils [44]. Underlying conditions such as diabetes benefit the rapid expansion of the infection due to lack of adequate perfusion and reduced immune response [5]. In fracture-related infections, inadequate fixation and/or soft tissue damage favor the occurrence of an acute or ongoing persistent infection like osteomyelitis. This is aggravated in patients with extensive soft tissue damage and according to Gustilo Anderson's Classification in Grade II and III open fractures. To reduce the risk of an acute or an ongoing infection, adequate wound and soft tissue management from the early start in open fracture treatment, for example with negative pressure wound therapy, is mandatory [45].

### 4.1.4 Chronic Osteomyelitis and Septic Arthritis

Chronic infections of the bone and/or joint are defined by an onset of more than 30 days after a surgery [3]. A chronic infection can occur after an insufficiently treated acute infection. The residual bacteria eventually causes the formation of granulation tissue, sequesters and osteonecrosis. Persistent secretion often results in the formation of chronic fistulas [42]. If the infection is fracture and/or implant-related, non-union of the fracture can occur [46]. In some cases, the only clinical and radiological sign of a chronic osseous infection can be a non-union at the fracture site. The clinician treating the patient should always be alerted by the absence of fracture union, especially in patients with underlying diseases and or history of extensive soft tissue damage at the fracture site. Histopathological findings include formation of granulation tissue, periosteal reaction and fibroplasia [38, 47].

## 4.2 Negative Pressure Wound Therapy

Especially in Grade II and III open fractures according to Gustilo Anderson, the risk of an acute or later, a chronic infection is higher and related to the extent of damage and loss of soft tissues.

Chronic infection will develop more easily if the local vascularisation of soft tissue and bone is compromised. To reduce the initial bacterial burden in an open trauma wound and/or fracture and to reduce the risk of an ongoing infection, modern techniques like negative pressure wound therapy can support a faster and better clinical outcome [48–51]. By use of two different types of reticulated foam with different physical and mechanical properties (polyurethane or polyvinylalcohol foam) in the wound, the wound, together with the foams, is covered with an occlusive semipermeable wound drape and connected with a negative pressure machine. This negative wound pressure system at the wound site stimulates the local blood perfusion and will reduce soft tissue edema [52]. The local blood flow is stimulated and the immune system of the injured patient can be more effective in its action against a local infection and consequently can reduce the systemic sequelae of a local infection. Especially, the negative wound pressure therapy with instillation technique has proven to be strongly effective in reducing the risk of recurrent infections in trauma and orthopaedic patients with (recurrent) soft tissue and bone infections [48, 53]. Even in cases with implanted hip and knee prosthesis with acute infection, the installation technique with an antiseptic polyhexanide solution (0.04%) was favorable in retaining the prosthesis in acute infections [52].

**Case Report**
A 17-year-old man suffered a grade IIIB open comminuted patella fracture during holidays abroad in a motorbike accident (Fig. 4.1), with severe putrid arthritis of the knee joint. Initial

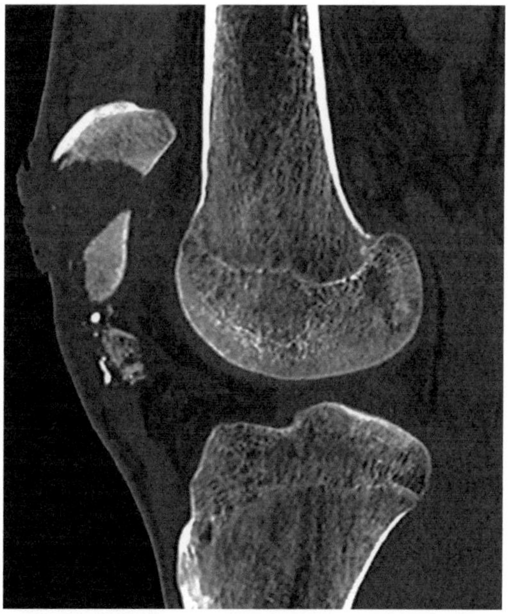

**Fig. 4.1** Comminuted and dislocated patella fracture

limited wound exploration followed by primary closure of the wound was performed. The patient was repatriated on day nine by airplane to our hospital. An extended wound revision with debridement, removal of multiple foreign bodies (small stones, grass) and synovectomy of the knee joint and lavage was performed (Fig. 4.2), followed by negative wound pressure therapy. Intravenous antibiotic therapy according to the resistance pattern of the isolated bacterial species was administered. Multiple intraoperative swabs and soft tissue probes showed cultures of *Enterobacter cloacae, Enterococcus* species *and Corynebacterium* species. Two weeks later, a definitive osteosynthesis of the patella (Fig. 4.3) with tension wire was performed, associated with a negative pressure wound therapy with instillation technique using polyhexanide solution (0.04%) was performed (Fig. 4.4). Four days after the Instillation technique, wound swabs became sterile. Seven days after the tension wire osteosynthesis, the wound was closed by secondary intention with uneventful healing (Fig. 4.5). Removal of the hardware after consolidation of the patella fracture was done 5 months later (Fig. 4.6) in com-

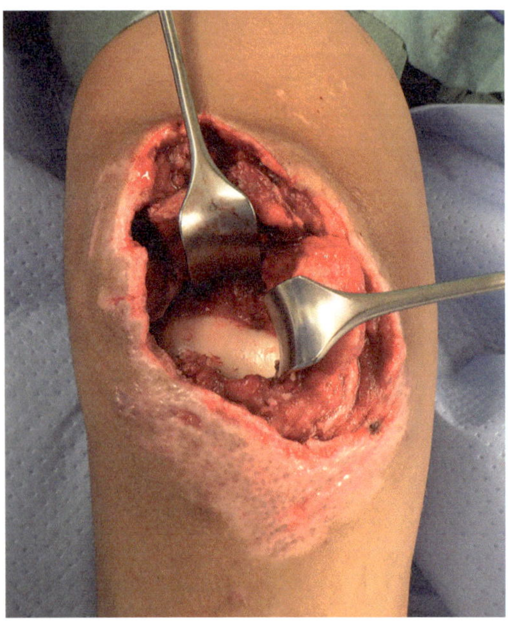

**Fig. 4.2** Intraoperative situs of the open knee joint: severe infection of the joint with granulation tissue

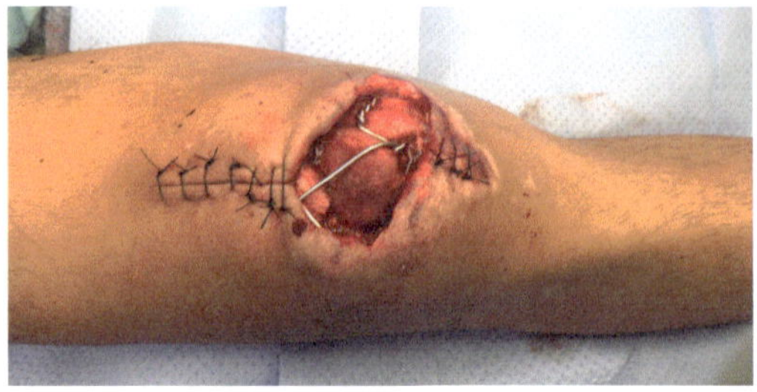

**Fig. 4.3** Tension wire osteosynthesis of the patella

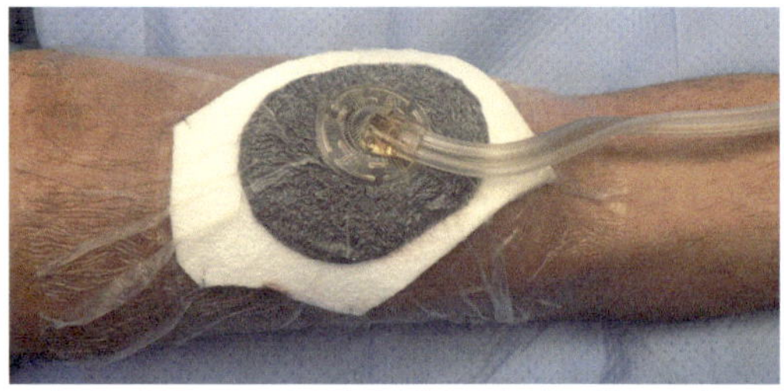

**Fig. 4.4** Negative Pressure Instillation Technique (note the double tubing: a suction and a smaller sized instillation tube) with polyvinylalcohol (white foam) and polyurethane foam (black foam)

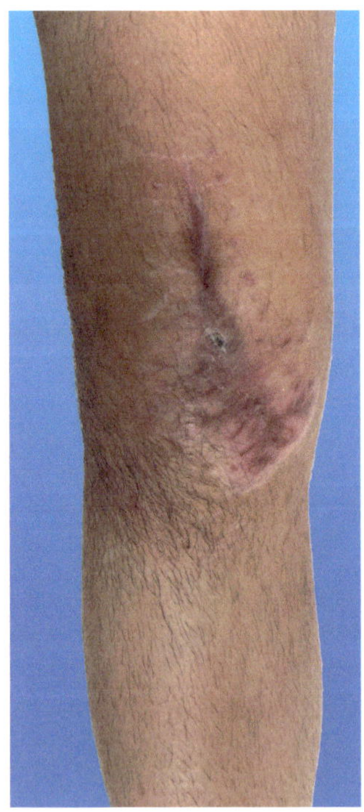

**Fig. 4.5** Soft tissues 4 months after trauma

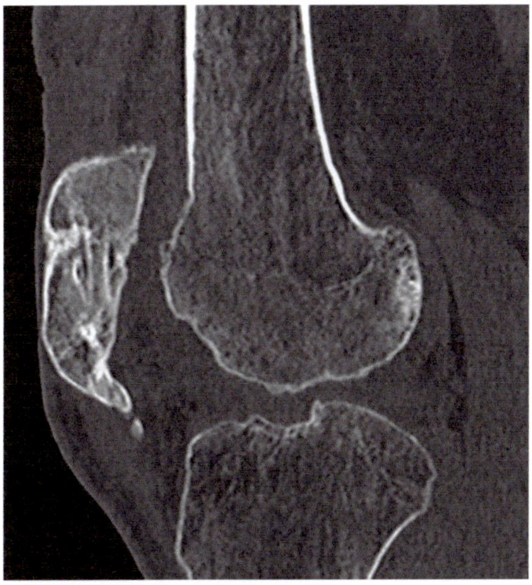

**Fig. 4.6** Radiological outcome (CT) 1 year after trauma

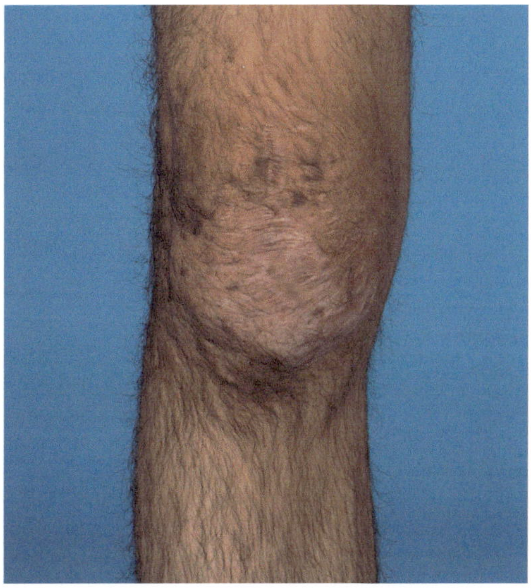

**Fig. 4.7** Soft tissues of the knee joint after 15 months

bination with an arthrolysis of the knee joint. Now, 2.5 years after the accident, the patient is doing well with a wide range of motion of the knee joint (Flexion 130 degrees, full extension) without any signs of infection (Figs. 4.7 and 4.8).

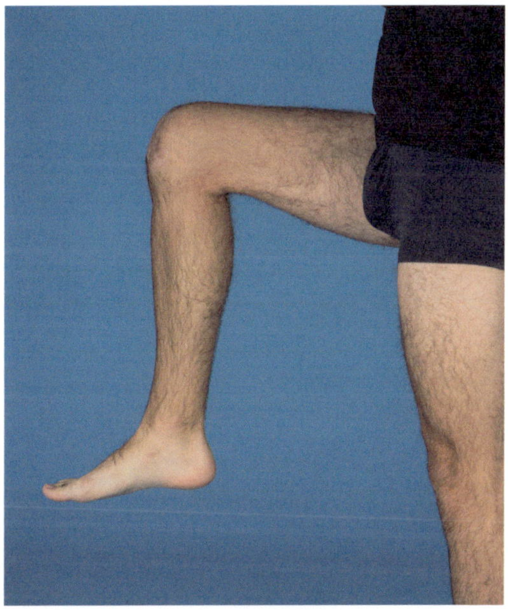

**Fig. 4.8** Clinical outcome after 15 months

### 4.2.1 Summary

Soft tissue and bone infections in orthopaedic and trauma surgery have a high risk for recurrence, especially if osteosynthesis hardware like plates, intramedullary nails and prosthesis are in situ. For that reason, from the very beginning, the care for soft tissues should have the highest priority to reduce the risk of an infection in emergency trauma situations, which can end up in chronic bone and joint infections. In case of closed fractures with soft tissue injury and even more in primary open fractures, from the very first start fracture treatment should be brought in line with the soft tissue damage ('do not further harm'). The experience of the orthopaedic and trauma surgeon plays an important role in the timing of the following procedures, aiming to reduce the risk of infection.

Debridement and lavage of soft tissue injuries are still the corner stone for future care, but modern wound treatment concepts like negative pressure wound pressure therapy with installation technique of polyhexanide solution, can guide us to an improved outcome for patients in combination with a shorter hospital stay and reduced number of operative procedures needed for patient's recovery and finally to achieve a better outcome.

## References


1. O'Connor O, Thahir A, Krkovic M. How much does an infected fracture cost? Arch Bone Jt Surg. 2022;10(2):135–40.
2. Hogan A, Heppert VG, Suda AJ. Osteomyelitis. Arch Orthop Trauma Surg. 2013;133(9):1183–96.
3. Prevention CCfDCa. Surgical Site Infection (SSI) (Available from: https://www.cdc.gov/hai/ssi/ssi.html).
4. Cierny GI. A clinical staging system for adult osteomyelitis. Contemp Orthop. 1985;10:17–37.
5. Kremers HM, Nwojo ME, Ransom JE, Wood-Wentz CM, Melton LJ 3rd, Huddleston PM 3rd. Trends in the epidemiology of osteomyelitis: a population-based study, 1969 to 2009. J Bone Joint Surg Am. 2015;97(10):837–45.
6. Goh TC, Bajuri MY, Nadarajah SC, Abdul Rashid AH, Baharuddin S, Zamri KS. Clinical and bacteriological profile of diabetic foot infections in a tertiary care. J Foot Ankle Res. 2020;13(1):36.
7. Schmidt BM, Keeney-Bonthrone TP, Hawes AM, Karmakar M, Frydrych LM, Cinti SK, et al. Comorbid status in patients with osteomyelitis is associated with long-term incidence of extremity amputation. BMJ Open Diabetes Res Care. 2023;11(6):e003611.
8. Chien HI, Yang KC, Liu WC, Ho YY, Tsai WH, Chen LW. Haematogenous Klebsiella pneumoniae osteomyelitis. Int Orthop. 2021;45(7):1693–8.
9. Truntzer J, Vopat B, Feldstein M, Matityahu A. Smoking cessation and bone healing: optimal cessation timing. Eur J Orthop Surg Traumatol. 2015;25(2):211–5.
10. Oestern HJ, Tscherne H. Pathophysiologie und Klassifizierung des Weichteilschadens bei Frakturen [Pathophysiology and classification of soft tissue damage in fractures]. Orthopade. 1983;12(1):2–8. German
11. Gustilo R, Anderson JT. Prevention of infection in the treatment of one thousand and twenty five open fractures of long bones. Retrospective and prospective analyses. Bone joint Surg Am. 1976;58:453.
12. Gustilo RB, Mendoza RM, Williams DN. Problems in the management of type III (severe) open fractures: a new classification of type III open fractures. J Trauma. 1984;24(8):742–6.
13. Gustilo RB, Anderson JT. Prevention of infection in the treatment of one thousand and twenty-five open fractures of long bones: retrospective and prospective analyses. J Bone Joint Surg Am. 1976;58(4):453–8.
14. Mader JT, Shirtliff M, Calhoun JH. Staging and staging application in osteomyelitis. Clin Infect Dis. 1997;25(6):1303–9.
15. Elasri MO, Thomas JR, Skinner RA, Blevins JS, Beenken KE, Nelson CL, Smeltzer MS. Staphylococcus aureus collagen adhesin contributes to the pathogenesis of osteomyelitis. Bone. 2002;30(1):275–80.
16. Smeltzer MS, Gillaspy AF. Molecular pathogenesis of staphylcoccal osteomyelitis. Poult Sci. 2000;79(7):1042–9.
17. Costerton JW, Lewandowski Z, Caldwell DE, Korber DR, Lappin-Scott HM. Microbial biofilms. Ann Rev Microbiol. 1995;49:711–45.
18. Costerton W, Veeh R, Shirtliff M, Pasmore M, Post C, Ehrlich G. The application of biofilm science to the study and control of chronic bacterial infections. J Clin Invest. 2003;112(10):1466–77.
19. Hussain M, Wilcox MH, White PJ. The slime of coagulase-negative staphylococci: biochemistry and relation to adherence. FEMS Microbiol Lett. 1993;104(3):191–207.
20. Arciola CR, Hansch GM, Visai L, Testoni F, Maurer S, Campoccia D, et al. Interactions of staphylococci with osteoblasts and phagocytes in the pathogenesis of implant-associated osteomyelitis. Int J Artif Organs. 2012;35(10):713–26.
21. Ellington JK, Harris M, Webb L, Smith B, Smith T, Tan K, Hudson M. Intracellular *Staphylococcus aureus*. A mechanism for the indolence of osteomyelitis. J Bone Joint Surg Br. 2003;85(6):918–21.
22. Yang D, Wijenayaka AR, Solomon LB, Pederson SM, Findlay DM, Kidd SP, Atkins GJ. Novel insights into Staphylococcus aureus deep bone infections: the involvement of osteocytes. MBio. 2018;9(2):e00415-18.
23. Hofstee MI, Riool M, Terjajevs I, Thompson K, Stoddart MJ, Richards RG, et al. Three-dimensional in vitro Staphylococcus aureus abscess communities display antibiotic tolerance and protection from neutrophil clearance. Infect Immun. 2020;88(11):e00293-20.
24. Cheng AG, DeDent AC, Schneewind O, Missiakas D. A play in four acts: Staphylococcus aureus abscess formation. Trends Microbiol. 2011;19(5):225–32.
25. Nohl A, Hamsen U, Jensen KO, Sprengel K, Ziegenhain F, Lefering R, et al. Incidence, impact and risk factors for multidrug-resistant organisms (MDRO) in patients with major trauma: a European multicenter cohort study. Eur J Trauma Emerg Surg. 2022;48(1):659–65.
26. Cazander G, van Veen KE, Bouwman LH, Bernards AT, Jukema GN. The influence of maggot excretions on PAO1 biofilm formation on different biomaterials. Clin Orthop Relat Res. 2009;467(2):536–45.
27. Morgenstern M, Post V, Erichsen C, Hungerer S, Bühren V, Militz M, et al. Biofilm formation increases treatment failure in Staphylococcus epidermidis device-related osteomyelitis of the lower extremity in human patients. J Orthop Res. 2016;34(11):1905–13.
28. Cazander G, van de Veerdonk MC, Vandenbroucke-Grauls CM, Schreurs MW, Jukema GN. Maggot excretions inhibit biofilm formation on biomaterials. Clin Orthop Relat Res. 2010;468:2789–96.
29. Park KH, Kim DY, Lee YM, Lee MS, Kang KC, Lee JH, et al. Selection of an appropriate empiric antibiotic regimen in hematogenous vertebral osteomyelitis. PLoS One. 2019;14(2):e0211888.

30. Gerometta A, Rodriguez Olaverri JC, Bitan F. Infections in spinal instrumentation. Int Orthop. 2012;36(2):457–64.
31. Rosteius T, Jansen O, Fehmer T, Baecker H, Citak M, Schildhauer TA, Geßmann J. Evaluating the microbial pattern of periprosthetic joint infections of the hip and knee. J Med Microbiol. 2018;67(11):1608–13.
32. Yu Y, Kong Y, Ye J, Wang A, Si W. Microbiological pattern of prosthetic hip and knee infections: a high-volume, single-centre experience in China. J Med Microbiol. 2021;70(3)
33. Kuehl R, Tschudin-Sutter S, Morgenstern M, Dangel M, Egli A, Nowakowski A, et al. Time-dependent differences in management and microbiology of orthopaedic internal fixation-associated infections: an observational prospective study with 229 patients. Clin Microbiol Infect. 2019;25(1):76–81.
34. Masters EA, Ricciardi BF, Bentley KLM, Moriarty TF, Schwarz EM, Muthukrishnan G. Skeletal infections: microbial pathogenesis, immunity and clinical management. Nat Rev Microbiol. 2022;20(7):385–400.
35. Funk SS, Copley LA. Acute Hematogenous osteomyelitis in children: pathogenesis, diagnosis, and treatment. Orthop Clin North Am. 2017;48(2):199–208.
36. Brown DW, Sheffer BW. Pediatric septic arthritis: an update. Orthop Clin North Am. 2019;50(4):461–70.
37. Ross JJ. Septic arthritis of native joints. Infect Dis Clin N Am. 2017;31(2):203–18.
38. Metsemakers WJ, Morgenstern M, McNally MA, Moriarty TF, McFadyen I, Scarborough M, et al. Fracture-related infection: a consensus on definition from an international expert group. Injury. 2018;49(3):505–10.
39. Wynn M, Kesler K, Morellato J, Higginbotham R, Robertson M, Marsh JL, Hogue M. Agricultural trauma causing open fractures: is antibiotic coverage against anaerobic organisms indicated? J Orthop Trauma. 2022;36(2):e51–e5.
40. Fuglestad MA, Tracey EL, Leinicke JA. Evidence-based prevention of surgical site infection. Surg Clin North Am. 2021;101(6):951–66.
41. Leaper DJ, Edmiston CE. World Health Organization: global guidelines for the prevention of surgical site infection. J Hosp Infect. 2017;95(2):135–6.
42. Beck-Broichsitter BE, Smeets R, Heiland M. Current concepts in pathogenesis of acute and chronic osteomyelitis. Curr Opin Infect Dis. 2015;28(3):240–5.
43. Hofmann SR, Kapplusch F, Girschick HJ, Morbach H, Pablik J, Ferguson PJ, Hedrich CM. Chronic Recurrent Multifocal Osteomyelitis (CRMO): presentation, pathogenesis, and treatment. Curr Osteoporos Rep. 2017;15(6):542–54.
44. Lew DP, Waldvogel FA. Osteomyelitis. Lancet. 2004;364(9431):369–79.
45. Timmers MS, Graafland N, Bernards AT, Nelissen RG, van Dissel JT, Jukema GN. Negative pressure wound treatment with polyvinyl alcohol foam and polyhexanide antiseptic solution instillation in posttraumatic osteomyelitis. Wound Repair Regen. 2009;17(2):278–86.
46. Nicholson JA, Makaram N, Simpson A, Keating JF. Fracture nonunion in long bones: a literature review of risk factors and surgical management. Injury. 2021;52(Suppl 2):S3–S11.
47. Mais DD, Hackman S, Ross J. Histopathologic findings in culture-positive secondary osteomyelitis. Ann Diagn Pathol. 2021;50:151661.
48. Argenta LC, Morykwas MJ. Vacuum-assisted closure: a new method for wound control and treatment: clinical experience. Ann Plast Surg. 1997;38(6):563–77.
49. Morykwas MJ, Argenta LC, Shelton-Brown EI, McGuirt W. Vacuum-assisted closure: a new method for wound control and treatment: animal studies and basic foundation. Ann Plast Surg. 1997;38(6):553–62.
50. Fleischmann W, Becker U, Bischoff M, Hoekstra H. Vacuum sealing: indication, technique, and results. Eur J Orthop Surg Traumatol. 1995;5(1):37–40.
51. Jukema GN, Bøhm HJ, HIerholzer G. Vakuumversiegelung: ein neues Konzept zur Behandlung von Wechteil-und Knocheninfektionen [Vacuum occlusion: a new concept in treatment of soft tissue and bone infections]. Langenbecks Arch Chir (Chir Suppl Kongressbericht). 1997;114:581–5.
52. Lehner B, Fleischmann W, Becker R, Jukema GN. First experiences with negative pressure wound therapy and instillation in the treatment of infected orthopaedic implants: a clinical observational study. Int Orthop. 2011;35(9):1415–20.
53. Webb LX. The impact of negative pressure wound therapy on orthopaedic infection. Orthop Clin N Am. 2017;48(2):167–79.

# 5 Bacterial Resistance

Marco Trevenzoli, Vincenzo Scaglione,
and Annamaria Cattelan

## 5.1 Introduction

Penicillin, the initial antibiotic employed historically, demonstrated remarkable efficacy in treating bacterial infections among soldiers during World War II. However, penicillin-resistant bacteria emerged just a few years later. In response, new antibiotics were developed, but bacteria quickly evolved resistance to these as well. By the 1980s, the discovery of new antibiotics had slowed to a crawl. As a result, bacterial infections caused by multidrug-resistant or extensively drug-resistant pathogens are now a major global health threat [1].

Antimicrobial resistance (AMR) occurs when microorganisms change their susceptibility to antimicrobial pattern over time, resulting in no longer responding to antibiotics, making infections harder to treat and increasing the risk of disease spreading, severe illness, and death.

In Europe, more than 670,000 infections occur every year, and 33,000 people die due to bacteria resistant to antibiotics, with billions of Euros in cost for healthcare systems [2].

Several factors are linked to AMR:

- The overuse and misuse of antimicrobials in humans and animals.
- The spread of antibiotic-resistant bacteria through healthcare settings.
- The emergence of new antibiotic resistance genes.

Antibiotic therapy may be considered a double-edged sword. On one hand, from the ecological impact, the best antimicrobial molecule is not the one given. On the other hand, antimicrobial therapy saves lives.

Several bacteria have been highlighted in recent years for the AMR issue [3]:

Methicillin-resistant *Staphylococcus aureus* (MRSA).
Vancomycin-resistant *Enterococcus* (VRE).
Carbapenem-resistant *Enterobacterales* (CRE).
Multidrug-resistant *Pseudomonas aeruginosa* (MDR PA).
Carbapenem-resistant *Acinetobacter baumannii* (CRAB).

M. Trevenzoli · V. Scaglione
Infectious and Tropical Diseases Unit, Department of Medicine-DIMED, Padua University Hospital, Padova, Italy
e-mail: marco.trevenzoli@aopd.veneto.it; vincenzo.scaglione@aopd.veneto.it

A. Cattelan (✉)
Infectious and Tropical Diseases Unit, Department of Medicine-DIMED, Padua University Hospital, Padova, Italy

Department of Molecular Medicine-DMM, University of Padua School of Medicine, Padova, Italy
e-mail: annamaria.cattelan@unipd.it



P. Ruggieri et al. (eds.), *Bone and Joint Infections*, https://doi.org/10.1007/978-3-031-96383-4_5

In addition, in bone and joint infections (BJIs), the complex anatomy of bones and joints can make it difficult for antibiotics to reach the site of infection.

Several measures can be implemented to reduce the risk of AMR, including: (i) antimicrobial stewardship (AS) programs in order to maximize clinical outcome avoiding unnecessary and ecological collateral damage due to antimicrobials [4]; (ii) practicing hand hygiene, both in and out of healthcare settings [5, 6]; (iii) vaccination campaigns for relevant contagious diseases [7]; (iv) development of new antibiotics and other treatments for infections [8].

## 5.2 Antimicrobial Resistance: Innate, Acquired, and Adaptive

- Innate resistance is the natural ability of a bacterium to resist an antibiotic. For example, all Gram-negative bacteria have an outer membrane that makes them resistant to many antibiotics such as glycopeptides.
- Acquired resistance develops when a bacterium gains the ability to resist an antibiotic to which it was previously sensitive. This can happen through mutation or horizontal gene transfer.
- Adaptive resistance is a temporary state of resistance that a bacterium can develop in response to exposure to an antibiotic. It is thought to be caused by changes in gene expression [9–11].

Horizontal gene transfer is the most typical way that bacteria acquire resistance genes. It can arise through three main mechanisms:

- Transformation: bacteria take up free DNA from the surrounding environment.
- Transduction: This is a process in which a bacteriophage, which is a virus that infects bacteria, transfers DNA from one bacterium to another.
- Conjugation: This is a process in which two bacteria exchange DNA directly [1].

## 5.3 Mechanisms of Antibiotic Resistance

Antibiotic resistance is typically caused by the destruction or modification of antibiotics, changes to the targets that antibiotics attack, or reduced accumulation of antibiotics in bacterial cells. This can happen through reduced permeability of the cell wall or increased efflux of antibiotics from the cell. Alternatively, antibiotic resistance can be the result of a global adaptation of the entire bacterial cell [1].

The following text describes the principal resistance mechanisms associated with the most frequently used antibiotics for the pathogens commonly encountered in clinical practice.

### 5.3.1 Antibiotic Destruction

The production of beta-lactamase enzymes, which break down beta-lactam antibiotics, is a major cause of penicillin resistance.

In 1940, the first β-lactamases were described [12], a year before penicillin entered clinical practice. Over 1000 β-lactamases since then has been reported from a variety of bacteria, and they represent the most frequent resistance mechanism leading to Gram-negative bacteria β-lactam resistance.

In the chromosome or in mobile genetic elements can be found genes encoding β-lactamases, which have facilitated their transmission among bacteria. In the 1960s, TEM-1, a plasmid-encoded β-lactamase, was discovered in Gram-negative bacteria. Since then, the introduction of new β-lactams has been followed by the identification of new β-lactamases that can break down the new compound.

For example, in the early 1980s, the introduction of third-generation cephalosporins was quickly followed by the identification of plasmid-encoded β-lactamases in 1983 that could possibly hydrolyze third-generation cephalosporins (Extended-Spectrum β-Lactamases-ESBLs) [13, 14].

Another beta-lactamase group of great clinical importance in Gram-negative bacteria includes:

Carbapenemases: These enzymes are able to hydrolyze carbapenems, which are the most potent beta-lactam antibiotics. Carbapenem-resistant bacteria are a major threat to public health, as there are very few antibiotics that are still effective against them.

Metallo-beta-lactamases (MBLs): MBLs are a class of beta-lactamases that are resistant to beta-lactamase inhibitors, such as clavulanic acid and tazobactam. In addition, all of these enzymes can efficiently hydrolyze carbapenems, while only monobactams are uniformly resistant to hydrolysis by these versatile enzymes. Consequently, bacteria producing metallo-beta-lactamases (MBLs) are challenging to treat, and their prevalence is steadily increasing [15].

The emergence of new beta-lactamase groups is a major challenge for public health. It is important to continue to develop new antibiotics and new strategies to prevent the spread of beta-lactamase-producing bacteria.

### 5.3.2 Antibiotic Modification

The primary mechanism responsible for clinically significant resistance to aminoglycosides and chloramphenicol is the enzymatic modification of the antibiotic molecule.

Aminoglycoside-modifying enzymes (AMEs) are a group of enzymes that can modify aminoglycoside antibiotics by adding various chemical groups to them. This modification might reduce the ability of the antibiotic to bind to its target and makes it less effective. AMEs are encoded by genes that are often located on mobile genetic elements (MGEs), such as plasmids and transposons, allowing genes to be easily transferred between different bacteria [16].

In parallel, chloramphenicol acetyltransferases (CATs) are a group of enzymes that can acetylate chloramphenicol, which is a specific type of antibiotic. Acetylation reduces the activity of chloramphenicol and makes it less effective at killing bacteria. Much like AMEs, CAT genes exhibit a propensity for residing on MGEs, enabling facile inter-bacterial transfer and thereby contributing to the widespread dissemination of antibiotic resistance. This intricate interplay of enzymatic modifications unveils the complex molecular dynamics that underscore the adaptability and persistence of antibiotic resistance mechanisms in bacterial populations [17].

### 5.3.3 Modifications of Antibiotic-Activating Enzymes

Nitrofurantoin is a prodrug that requires activation by bacterial reductases to become effective. The two main nitroreductases involved in nitrofurantoin activation are NfsA and NfsB. Mutations in the genes encoding these enzymes can lead to nitrofurantoin resistance [18].

### 5.3.4 Target Replacement or Target Bypass

Methicillin resistance in *Staphylococcus aureus* and the mechanism underlying β-lactam resistance in *Streptococcus pneumoniae* is a replacement of the bacterial penicillin-binding proteins (PBPs).

Penicillin-binding proteins (PBPs) are enzymes that are essential for cell wall synthesis in bacteria. β-lactam antibiotics work by inhibiting PBPs, which prevents the bacteria from building a strong cell wall.

For *Streptococcus pneumoniae*, β-lactam resistance can be caused by the replacement of native PBP genes with mosaic PBP genes, which are created by the recombination of foreign DNA and native DNA from β-lactam-resistant streptococci. This process is known as transformation [19].

For *Staphylococcus aureus*, methicillin resistance is caused by the acquisition of the mecA gene. The mecA gene encodes a unique PBP called PBP2a, which has a very low affinity for all β-lactam antibiotics. This allows *Staphylococcus aureus* to continue building a strong cell wall even in the presence of β-lactam antibiotics [20].

Other examples of antibiotic resistance mediated by the replacement of bacterial targets include:

Glycopeptide resistance in *Enterococci*: *Enterococci* can acquire resistance to glycopeptide by replacing the glycopeptide target (the terminal d-Alanine-d-Alanine moiety of peptidoglycan precursors) with a different molecule, reducing the binding affinity of the antibiotic molecule [21].

Trimethoprim resistance in bacteria: Trimethoprim inhibits dihydrofolate reductase (DHFR), an enzyme involved in folate metabolism. Bacteria can become resistant to trimethoprim by acquiring genes that encode trimethoprim-resistant DHFR enzymes.

Sulfonamide resistance in bacteria: Sulfonamides inhibit dihydropteroate synthase (DHPS), an enzyme involved in folate metabolism. Bacteria can become resistant to sulfonamides by acquiring genes that encode sulfonamide-resistant DHPS enzymes [22].

### 5.3.5 Target Site Alteration

Linezolid is an antibiotic that binds to the 23S rRNA and inhibits protein synthesis. Mutations in the 23S rRNA can prevent linezolid from binding, determining resistance to linezolid. Other mechanisms of linezolid resistance include: mutations in the ribosomal proteins L3 and L4; methylation of the 23S rRNA by the cfr enzyme [21, 23]. Other examples are mutations in genes encoding the gyrase and/or topoisomerase IV enzymes which represent the most common mechanism of quinolone resistance [24]. Rifampicin resistance is mostly the result of mutations in the RNA polymerase beta subunit gene [25].

### 5.3.6 Decreased Permeability of the Bacterial Outer Membrane

A permeability barrier that can restrict the entry of antibiotics is the outer membrane of Gram-negative bacteria [26]. Porins are the main route of entry for hydrophilic antibiotics into Gram-negative bacteria. They are small proteins that form channels in the outer membrane. The type and the number of porins expressed on the outer membrane could possibly affect the entry of hydrophilic antibiotics, and, hence, the susceptibility of the bacterial cell to them. Porin loss, conductance of modification of the size of porins, minimized expression of porins, and changes in porin expression, are all associated with resistance to several molecules [27].

Examples of porin-mediated antibiotic resistance in Gram-negative bacteria:

- Penicillin resistance in *Neisseria gonorrhoeae*: *N. gonorrhoeae* can develop penicillin resistance by reducing the expression of the porin OmpC [28].
- Cephalosporin resistance in *Enterobacterales*: *Enterobacterales* can develop cephalosporin resistance by reducing the expression of the porins OmpF and OmpC [29].
- Fluoroquinolone resistance in *Pseudomonas aeruginosa*: *P. aeruginosa* can develop fluoroquinolone resistance by reducing the expression of the porins OprD and OprF [30].

### 5.3.7 Efflux Pumps

Bacterial efflux pumps are molecular systems that use energy to transport toxic molecules out of the cell.

Efflux pumps can be classified into two main types:

1. Multidrug efflux pumps: These pumps are typically chromosomally encoded and can transport a wide range of antibiotics and other compounds out of the cell.
2. Substrate-specific efflux pumps: these pumps are often located on MGEs and are specific for a particular type of antibiotic or compound.

Efflux pumps contribute to antibiotic resistance decreasing antibiotic concentration inside the cell below the level needed to kill the bacteria [27, 31].

## 5.4 Biofilm

Biofilms are a major challenge in healthcare, as they can lead to persistent and difficult-to-treat infections [32]. They are often found on medical devices, such as implants and catheters, but can also form on natural surfaces, such as teeth and wounds, or dead bone.

Biofilms are made up of a variety of microorganisms, including bacteria, fungi, and algae, which are embedded in a sticky matrix of extracellular polysaccharides. This matrix provides the microorganisms with protection from the outside environment, including antibiotics [33].

Biofilms are also able to coordinate their behavior. This allows them to share nutrients, communicate with each other, resist antibiotics, and develop new ways to evade the immune system.

As a result of these factors, biofilm infections can be very hard to treat and, in several cases, the only way to cure a biofilm infection is to remove the infected device or tissue [32, 33].

## 5.5 Steps in Biofilm Formation

Genetic research reveals that biofilm formation is a multistep process that requires specialized cell signalling (quorum sensing) and transcription of a unique set of genes. Moreover, several factors can influence biofilm formation, such as temperature, nutrient availability, and pH [34–36].

Biofilms contain channels that separate microcolonies, and their mechanical stability is due to the viscoelastic properties of the extracellular polymeric substance (EPS) matrix.

Researchers have identified a few common steps in biofilm formation:

1. Initial attachment to the surface: Bacteria first attaches to a surface through a variety of mechanisms, such as electrostatic interactions, van der Waals forces, and specific adhesins.
2. Microcolony formation: Once attached, bacteria begin to multiply and form microcolonies. This process is mediated by quorum sensing, a cell-to-cell communication system that allows bacteria to coordinate their behavior.
3. Maturation and architecture formation: The biofilm continues to mature and develop a complex architecture. This process involves the production of the EPS matrix, which encases the bacteria and provides them with protection.
4. Detachment and dispersion: Once mature, the biofilm can detach from the surface and disperse the bacteria to new locations. This process is also mediated by quorum sensing.

Each step in the biofilm formation process is regulated by a different set of genes. For example, genes involved in initial attachment to the surface are different from genes involved in EPS production.

The viscoelastic properties of the EPS matrix play an important role in the mechanical stability of the biofilm, protecting bacteria from antibiotics and other environmental stressors.

Conversely, certain bacterial strains do not generate EPS and instead disperse directly into the environment through a process called sloughing. This detachment mechanism can be triggered by various factors, including mechanical stress induced by fluid flow or shear forces. Additionally, the production of enzymes that actively degrade the EPS matrix can contribute to the sloughing phenomenon, enabling these bacteria to efficiently release into their surroundings.

For example, *Escherichia coli* produces N-acetyl-heparosan lyase; *Pseudomonas aeruginosa* produces alginate lyase; or *Streptococcus equi* produces hyaluronidase.

Even bacteria that do produce EPS can detach from the biofilm and disperse. This process is known as active dispersal. Active dispersal is often triggered by environmental cues, such as nutrient limitation or overcrowding.

During active dispersal, also upregulate the expression of genes involved in flagella and increase enzymes production to degrade the EPS matrix. In this way, bacteria break free from the biofilm and are able to move to new locations [32–36].

## References


1. Christaki E, Marcou M, Tofarides A. Antimicrobial resistance in bacteria: mechanisms, evolution, and persistence. J Mol Evol. 2020;88(1):26–40. https://doi.org/10.1007/s00239-019-09914-3.
2. Control ECfDPa. Antimicrobial resistance in the EU/EEA (EARS-net) – annual epidemiological report 2019. Stockholm: ECDC; 2020.
3. Organization WH. WHO publishes list of bacteria for which new antibiotics are urgently needed. 2017.
4. Lanckohr C, Bracht H. Antimicrobial stewardship. Curr Opin Crit Care. 2022;28(5):551–6. https://doi.org/10.1097/MCC.0000000000000967.
5. Weinstein RA. Controlling antimicrobial resistance in hospitals: infection control and use of antibiotics. Emerg Infect Dis. 2001;7(2):188–92. https://doi.org/10.3201/eid0702.010206.
6. Allegranzi B, Pittet D. Role of hand hygiene in healthcare-associated infection prevention. J Hosp Infect. 2009;73(4):305–15. https://doi.org/10.1016/j.jhin.2009.04.019.
7. Rosini R, Nicchi S, Pizza M, Rappuoli R. Vaccines against antimicrobial resistance. Front Immunol. 2020;11:1048. https://doi.org/10.3389/fimmu.2020.01048.
8. Tarin-Pello A, Suay-Garcia B, Perez-Gracia MT. Antibiotic resistant bacteria: current situation and treatment options to accelerate the development of a new antimicrobial arsenal. Expert Rev Anti-Infect Ther. 2022;20(8):1095–108. https://doi.org/10.1080/14787210.2022.2078308.
9. Lee JH. Perspectives towards antibiotic resistance: from molecules to population. J Microbiol. 2019;57(3):181–4. https://doi.org/10.1007/s12275-019-0718-8.
10. Munita JM, Arias CA. Mechanisms of Antibiotic Resistance. Microbiol Spectr. 2016;4:2. https://doi.org/10.1128/microbiolspec.VMBF-0016-2015.
11. Holmes AH, Moore LS, Sundsfjord A, Steinbakk M, Regmi S, Karkey A, et al. Understanding the mechanisms and drivers of antimicrobial resistance. Lancet. 2016;387(10014):176–87. https://doi.org/10.1016/S0140-6736(15)00473-0.
12. Abraham EP, Chain E. An enzyme from bacteria able to destroy penicillin. 1940. Rev Infect Dis. 1988;10(4):677–8.
13. Knothe H, Shah P, Krcmery V, Antal M, Mitsuhashi S. Transferable resistance to cefotaxime, cefoxitin, cefamandole and cefuroxime in clinical isolates of Klebsiella pneumoniae and Serratia marcescens. Infection. 1983;11(6):315–7. https://doi.org/10.1007/BF01641355.
14. Paterson DL, Bonomo RA. Extended-spectrum beta-lactamases: a clinical update. Clin Microbiol Rev. 2005;18(4):657–86. https://doi.org/10.1128/CMR.18.4.657-686.2005.
15. Agarwal V, Tiwari A, Varadwaj P. An extensive review on beta-lactamase enzymes and their inhibitors. Curr Med Chem. 2023;30(7):783–808. https://doi.org/10.2174/0929867329666220620165429.
16. Ramirez MS, Tolmasky ME. Aminoglycoside modifying enzymes. Drug Resist Updat. 2010;13(6):151–71. https://doi.org/10.1016/j.drup.2010.08.003.
17. Schwarz S, Kehrenberg C, Doublet B, Cloeckaert A. Molecular basis of bacterial resistance to chloramphenicol and florfenicol. FEMS Microbiol Rev. 2004;28(5):519–42. https://doi.org/10.1016/j.femsre.2004.04.001.
18. Osei SJ. Genomic insights into nitrofurantoin resistance mechanisms and epidemiology in clinical Enterobacteriaceae. Future Sci OA. 2018;4(5):FSO293. https://doi.org/10.4155/fsoa-2017-0156.
19. Chambers HF. Penicillin-binding protein-mediated resistance in pneumococci and staphylococci. J Infect Dis. 1999;179(Suppl 2):S353–9. https://doi.org/10.1086/513854.
20. Moellering RC Jr. MRSA: the first half century. J Antimicrob Chemother. 2012;67(1):4–11. https://doi.org/10.1093/jac/dkr437.
21. Miller WR, Munita JM, Arias CA. Mechanisms of antibiotic resistance in enterococci. Expert Rev Anti-Infect Ther. 2014;12(10):1221–36. https://doi.org/10.1586/14787210.2014.956092.
22. Huovinen P. Resistance to trimethoprim-sulfamethoxazole. Clin Infect Dis. 2001;32(11):1608–14. https://doi.org/10.1086/320532.
23. Ma X, Zhang F, Bai B, Lin Z, Xu G, Chen Z, et al. Linezolid resistance in enterococcus faecalis associated with urinary tract infections of patients in a tertiary hospitals in China: resistance mechanisms, virulence, and risk factors. Front Public Health. 2021;9:570650. https://doi.org/10.3389/fpubh.2021.570650.
24. Aldred KJ, Kerns RJ, Osheroff N. Mechanism of quinolone action and resistance. Biochemistry. 2014;53(10):1565–74. https://doi.org/10.1021/bi5000564.
25. Alifano P, Palumbo C, Pasanisi D, Tala A. Rifampicin-resistance, rpoB polymorphism and RNA polymerase genetic engineering. J Biotechnol. 2015;202:60–77. https://doi.org/10.1016/j.jbiotec.2014.11.024.
26. Nikaido H. Outer membrane barrier as a mechanism of antimicrobial resistance. Antimicrob Agents Chemother. 1989;33(11):1831–6. https://doi.org/10.1128/AAC.33.11.1831.
27. Fernandez L, Hancock RE. Adaptive and mutational resistance: role of porins and efflux pumps in drug resistance. Clin Microbiol Rev. 2012;25(4):661–81. https://doi.org/10.1128/CMR.00043-12.
28. Lou H, Chen M, Black SS, Bushell SR, Ceccarelli M, Mach T, et al. Altered antibiotic transport in OmpC mutants isolated from a series of clinical strains of multi-drug resistant E. Coli. PLoS One. 2011;6(10):e25825. https://doi.org/10.1371/journal.pone.0025825.

29. Masi M, Vergalli J, Ghai I, Barba-Bon A, Schembri T, Nau WM, et al. Cephalosporin translocation across enterobacterial OmpF and OmpC channels, a filter across the outer membrane. Commun Biol. 2022;5(1):1059. https://doi.org/10.1038/s42003-022-04035-y.
30. Straatsma TP, Soares TA. Characterization of the outer membrane protein OprF of Pseudomonas aeruginosa in a lipopolysaccharide membrane by computer simulation. Proteins. 2009;74(2):475–88. https://doi.org/10.1002/prot.22165.
31. Poole K. Efflux-mediated antimicrobial resistance. J Antimicrob Chemother. 2005;56(1):20–51. https://doi.org/10.1093/jac/dki171.
32. Hurlow J, Couch K, Laforet K, Bolton L, Metcalf D, Bowler P. Clinical biofilms: a challenging frontier in wound care. Adv Wound Care (New Rochelle). 2015;4(5):295–301. https://doi.org/10.1089/wound.2014.0567.
33. Seth AK, Geringer MR, Hong SJ, Leung KP, Mustoe TA, Galiano RD. In vivo modeling of biofilm-infected wounds: a review. J Surg Res. 2012;178(1):330–8. https://doi.org/10.1016/j.jss.2012.06.048.
34. Donlan RM. Biofilms: microbial life on surfaces. Emerg Infect Dis. 2002;8(9):881–90. https://doi.org/10.3201/eid0809.020063.
35. Federle MJ, Bassler BL. Interspecies communication in bacteria. J Clin Invest. 2003;112(9):1291–9. https://doi.org/10.1172/JCI20195.
36. Shaw T, Winston M, Rupp CJ, Klapper I, Stoodley P. Commonality of elastic relaxation times in biofilms. Phys Rev Lett. 2004;93(9):098102. https://doi.org/10.1103/PhysRevLett.93.098102.

# 6 "Diagnosis of Bone and Joint Infections from Sample to Culture"

Ferdinando Da Rin de Lorenzo

The prevention of surgical site infections (SSI) is a priority within the objectives of the National Health System. The negative consequences that postoperative infections entail (morbidity, length of hospitalization, and mortality) represent particularly serious events both for the individual patient and for the community, in consideration of the healthcare resources necessary to treat them. Therefore, prevention is the watchword for these pathologies, but also the diagnosis, as early as possible. Before carrying out an evaluation of the tests to arrive at a diagnosis of periprosthetic joint infection (PJI), an answer must be given to what a periprosthetic infection is. There are many guidelines for identifying a PJI, such as that of the Infectious Diseases Society of America [1], that of the European BJIS [2], that of Musculoskeletal Infection Society (MSIS) [3], and that from WAIOT [4] [Fig. 6.1]. We will examine what was reported by the Philadelphia Consensus Conference [5–7] and that is, an infection occurs when:

- *two positive cultures are taken with phenotypically identical organisms,*
  *or*
- *the presence of a fistula in communication with the outside,*
  *or*
- *having three of the following minor criteria:*

(a) C-reactive protein (CRP-PCR) and erythrocyte sedimentation rate (ESR) in serum elevated;
(b) elevated white blood cell (WBC) count O++;
(c) change in the leukocyte esterase stripe in the sampled fluid;
(d) high percentage of polymorphonuclear neutrophils (PMN%) in the collected fluid;
(e) positive histological analysis of the tissue in the peri-lesional area; and.
(f) a single positive culture. (85%).

Based on what is stated above, it is easy to understand that the diagnosis is based on a set of factors and elements which combined can give us a definitive diagnosis. It is also clear that being faced with bone exposure leaves no doubt about a diagnosis of infection.

On the basis of what has been reported, we must take into consideration the various tests that we should do to arrive at a certain diagnosis, but before doing this we must do a *clinical examination*, but, alas, the clinical signs of pain, joint stiffness, fever [8], of the redness, swelling, and increase in temperature in the periprosthetic region, are to be considered signs and symptoms with low specificity for a PJI [9].

F. Da Rin de Lorenzo
Codivilla-Putti Institutes, National Reference Center for the diagnosis and treatment of bone infections, Cortina d'Ampezzo, Italy
e-mail: darin.ferdinando@iol.it



P. Ruggieri et al. (eds.), *Bone and Joint Infections*, https://doi.org/10.1007/978-3-031-96383-4_6

| Definition Source | MSIS 2011 [1] | IDSA 2013 [4] | ICM 2013 [5] | ICM 2018 [7] | Proposed EBJIS 2018 [8] |
|---|---|---|---|---|---|
| Scoring system | 1 of the 2 Major Criteria<br>OR<br>≥4 of 6 Minor Criteria* | ≥1 Positive Criteria* | 1 of the 2 Major Criteria<br>OR<br>≥3 of 5 Minor Criteria* | 1 of the 2 Major Criteria<br>OR<br>Minor criteria scoring ≥6 Infected<br>3–5 Possibly infected<br>("Consider further molecular diagnostics such as next-generation sequencing")<br><3 Not infected* | ≥1 Positive Criteria |
| | *"PJI may be present if fewer than four of these criteria are met" | *"The presence of PJI is possible even if the above criteria are not met ( .. .)" | *"PJI may be present without meeting these criteria,( ... )." | *"Proceed with caution in: adverse local tissue reaction, crystal deposition disease, slow growing oranisms*" | |
| Criteria | Major:<br>1. Sinus tract communicating with the prosthesis;<br>2. A pathogen is isolated by culture from at least two separate tissue or fluid samples obtained from the affected prosthetic joint<br><br>Minor:<br>(a) Elevated ESR (>30 mm/hr) and CRP (>10 mg/L) concentration<br>(b) Elevated synovial leukocyte COWlt<br>(c) Elevated PMN%<br>(d) Purulence in the affected joint<br>(e) Isolation of a microorganism in one culture of periprosthetic tissue or fluid<br>(f) Greater than five neutrophils per high-power field in five high-power fields observed from histologic analysis of periprosthetic tissue at ×400 magnification | 1. Sinus tract communicating with the prosthesis<br>2. Purulence without other etiology surrounding the prosthesis<br>3. Acute inflammation seen on histopathological examination of the periprosthetic tissue<br>4. ≥2 intraoperative cultures or combination of preoperative aspiration and intraoperative cultures yielding an indistinguishable organism (the growth of a virulent microorganism (e.g., Staphylococcus aureus) in a single specimen of a tissue biopsy or synovial fluid is also considered as indicative of a PJI] | Major<br>1. A sinus tract communicating with the joint<br>2. Two positive periprosthetic cultures with phenotypically identical organisms,<br><br>Minor:<br>(a) Elevated ESR (>30 mm/hr) and CRP (> 100 mg/L for acute infections; >10 mg/L.. for chronic infections)<br>(b) Elevated synovial fluid WBC count (>10,000 cells/mL for acute infections; >3,000 cells/mL for chronic infections) or ++ change on leukocyte esterase test strip<br>(c) Elevated PMN% (>90% for acute infections; >80% for chronic infections)<br>(d) Positive histological analysis of periprosthetic tissue (> 5 neutrophils per high-power field in five high-power fields observed on periprosthetic tissue at ×400 magnification)<br>(e) A single positive culture | Major:<br>1. Sinus tract with evidence of communication to the joint or visualization of the prosthesis<br>2. Two positive growths of the same organism using standard culture methods<br><br>Minor:<br>(a) Elevated CRP (>100 mg/L for acute infections; >10 mg/L.. for chronic infections) or D-Dimer (unknown threshold for acute infection; >860 ug/L for chronic infection) (score 2)<br>(b) Elevated ESR (no role for acute infections; >30 mm/hr for chronic infections) (score 1)<br>(c) Elevated synovial WBC count (>10,000 cells/mL for acute infections; >3,000 cells/mL for chronic infections) OR Leukocyte Esterase (++ for acute and chronic infections) OR Positive alphadefensin (score 3)<br>(d) Elevated synovial PMN% (>90% for acute infections; >70% for chronic infections) (score 2)<br>(e) Single positive culture (score 2)<br>(f) Positive histology (score 3)<br>(g) Positive intraoperative purulence (score 3) | 1. Purulence around the prosthesis or sinus tract<br>2. Increase synovial fluid leukocyte count (>2,000 cells/mL or >70 % granulocytes)<br>3. Positive histopathology<br>4. Confirmatory microbial growth in synovial flui<t periprosthetic tissue, or sonication culture<br><br>("Confirmatory microbial growth in periprosthetic tissue: if positive in ≥1 specimen in highly virulent organisms or ≥2 in low vilulent pathogens; sonication culture considered positive if >50 colony-forming units/mL of sonication fluid.") |

**Fig. 6.1** Comparison of the diagnostic criteria, adopted in five periprosthetic joint infection (PJI) definitions, published from 2011 to 2018. (Reproduced from [4] under the terms and conditions of the Creative Commons Attribution (CC BY) license (http://creativecommons.org/licenses/by/4.0/)). The table outlines major and minor criteria for each source, including factors like sinus tract communications, elevated inflammatory markers and positive cultures. Each column details specific diagnostic criteria and notes, highlighting differences and similarities across the guidelines

Before delving into the tests to be considered, it is good to make a distinction by giving the definitions of some terms used in the evaluation of tests, namely sensitivity, specificity, negative predictive value *(NPV)*, and positive predictive value *(PPV)*. *Sensitivity* = Probability that the test is positive if an individual is sick. Ability to correctly classify sick subjects. *Specificity* = Probability that the test will be negative if an individual is healthy. Ability to correctly classify healthy subjects. *PV* = probability of presence or absence of disease given the positive or negative test result and the likelihood ratios = measures of informativeness of the diagnostic test define by how much the probability of disease is changed to positive or negative given the test result [10–13]. It is not possible to identify an acceptable value for the predictive and negative value of a diagnostic test in the context of peri-prosthetic infection (PIJ) because the negative or positive probabilistic diagnosis is achieved through an ordered series of diagnostic tests starting from those with the least invasiveness or frequently through a minimal basis of diagnostic tests that modify the a priori probability of disease given by the clinical history, physical examination and risk factors for PPH. The only generic indication that we are allowed to give is to use less invasive tests with a high negative predictive value at the beginning of the diagnostic process which can more likely allow us to exclude the disease and interrupt the diagnostic process for the majority of patients tested. In the population testing positive for these tests, further investigations will be carried out to exclude false positives [14–16].

## 6.1 Blood Chemistry Tests

These are generally the first tests done when PJI is suspected as they are not very invasive and can already give us information, especially if associated with a clinic which, although not specific, can alarm us.

Let us start with the hematochemical dosage of polymerase chain reaction *(PCR)* and erythrocyte sedimentation rate *(ESR)*. Normal ESR values in humans are 1–10 mm, and 1–15 mm in women. Normal C-reactive protein (CRP) values are the same for men as for women 0–0.8 mg/dl. It should be considered that normal values of these two elements do not indicate the absence of infection, and this can happen [17–22]:

- In low virulence infections such as *Cutibacterium acnes* or *Propionibacterium acnes*.
- In fungal infections.
- In tuberculosis.
- In *Staphylococcal epidermidis* infections.
- In patients using anti-inflammatories, immunosuppressants, or antibiotics.
- In immunosuppressed patients.

It should be considered that the ESR and CRP values can remain high postoperatively for up to 6 weeks [23] after a prosthesis operation. It is useful to carry out a preoperative hematochemical evaluation of both ESR and CRP, which can be based on postoperatively because in patients with autoimmune rheumatic diseases, the values are already high without the presence of ongoing infections. In the postoperative period, the trend will therefore be followed based on the previous blood sample and noting the stability or decrease in values; an increase in the blood should lead to suspicion of an ongoing infection.

Another hematological test is *interleukin 6*, which is an inflammatory cytokine produced in response to infection or inflammation by monocytes and macrophages and is more elevated than in aseptic mobilizations and normalizes in the 6 h following surgery.

Also in the blood sample, other elements such as *D-dimer* can be evaluated. D-Dimer is assuming an interesting diagnostic value from a diagnostic point of view in PJI [24, 25].

When we talk about D-dimer, we are referring to a protein fragment (of fibrin), the result of the natural degradation of the clots present in our organism. It tends to be detectable in the blood if we are faced with a phenomenon of fibrinolysis, i.e., when the counterbalancing process of blood coagulation starts (vascular or tissue damage can trigger it). This process, therefore, allows the formation of the D-dimer: how? The body must block any hemorrhage (blood loss) with the formation of clots (composed of networks of fibrin and platelets). After repairing the damage, the networks are no longer necessary and the clots are slowly destroyed by plasmin (enzyme), giving rise to mini-fragments, the D-dimer. Usually, the doctor can request the measurement of the D-dimer when the patient shows symptoms linked to a possible deep vein thrombosis or pulmonary embolism. The D-dimer is not present in physiological conditions in human blood (or, more correctly, it is present in very low concentrations); the normal and reference values of the D-dimer are less than or equal to 500 ng/mL *Fibrinogen Equivalent Units* (FEU). The molecular weight of the D-dimer is around 180,000 daltons, and the half-life is equal to 4–6 h, in other words, this means that during this time interval, its plasma concentration is halved. Therefore, it does not have a specific biological function. Its measurement, however, provides very useful indirect information about the activation of the patient's coagulation system.

D-dimer can be increased in various physiological and pathological conditions:

**Physiological Causes**

- Advanced age (increase in elderly subjects >65 years, perhaps related to less mobility and atherosclerosis)
- Neonatal period
- Pregnancy (expression of the increased hypercoagulability inherent to the condition)
- Menstrual cycle
- Laboratory limitations (more frequent with the classic latex test: interference from plasma proteins, haemolysis, cross-reacting substances, and antibodies)

**Pathological Causes**

- Hospitalized and/or severely disabled subjects
- Current infections (sepsis due to Gram-negative bacteria)
- Major trauma
- Brain stroke
- Myocardial infarction
- Heart failure
- Tumors
- Disseminated intravascular coagulation (DIC)
- Surgical interventions
- Liver disease
- Nephropathies
- Chronic inflammatory diseases such as lupus erythematosus and rheumatoid arthritis)
- Venous thromboembolism
- Thrombolytic therapy

The test has a sensitivity between 93 and 95% and approximately 50% specificity in the diagnosis of thrombotic disease, while in a work by Qian Hu et al. [26] on a sample of 40 patients affected by PJI, 37 patients with aseptic loosening and 59 patients with extra-articular infection, the sensitivity of the D-dimer was 87.50% and a specificity of 78.38%, while for the sum of the CRP and ESR values the sensitivity was 75.00% and the specificity of 83.78%. Shahi and other authors [27] compared 245 patients; 23 with primary prosthesis, 56 with revision prosthesis for aseptic loosening, 57 revision prosthesis for PJI, and 29 reimplantations and evaluated CRP, ESR, and D-dimer and the result was very interesting: the median D-dimer level was significantly higher ($p < 0.0001$) for patients with PJI (1110 ng/ml [range, 243–8487 ng/ml]) compared to patients with aseptic failure (299 ng/mL [range, 106–2571 ng/mL]). Using the Youden index, 850 ng/mL was determined to be the optimal cut-off value for serum D-dimer for diagnosis of PJI. Serum D-dimer outperformed both ESR and serum CRP, with a sensitivity of 89% and specificity of 93%. ESR and CRP had a sensitivity of 73% and 79%, respectively, and a specificity of 78% and 80%. The sensitivity and specificity of the combined ESR and CRP were 84% (95% confidence interval [CI], from 76% to 90%) and 47% (95% CI, from 36% to 58%).

They concluded that it appears that serum D-dimer is a promising marker for the diagnosis of PJI. This test can also be of great use in determining the optimal time for replantation.

However, some factors must be considered:

- False positives: can be due to various causes such as liver disease, a high rheumatoid factor value, inflammation, malignant tumors, trauma, pregnancy, recent surgery, as well as advanced age.
- False negatives: occur in particular if the sample is collected too soon after the formation of thethrombus or if the test is performed with a serious delay (in the order of several days).
- Furthermore, ongoing anticoagulant treatment can make the test negative because it prevents the extension of the thrombus.
- False values can be obtained if the sample tube is not sufficiently filled (a falsely low value is recorded if it is underfilled and a falsely high value if overfilled). This is due to the dilution effect of the anticoagulant (the sample is collected correctly when the blood-anticoagulant ratio is equal to 9:1).
- In elderly patients, the D-dimer has a reduced specificity and is therefore less useful. However, it is possible to construct age-dependent cut-off values in order to adapt and make the execution of the test is useful even in elderly subjects.
- The evaluation laboratory testing is different between the various laboratories, and, furthermore, the evaluation is different whether on serum or on plasma, even if the latter data is not significant as demonstrated by Korte and Riesen [28]. Therefore, even if the cut-off was detected for the PJI of 850, it is thought that this is not a value identifying the PJI because it can also be detected in aseptic mobilizations.

The D-dimer has entered the evaluation parameters of a possible PJI, but neither the mechanism by which it is formed in a PJI nor what is the cut-off value that can give us a diagnosis is still clear certain of PJI. There will certainly be further studies that will provide these answers in the future.

Another easily identifiable blood element is *fibrinogen (Fbg)* [29–31], which is a protein present in the blood whose main role is linked to hemostasis, i.e., the set of physiological processes that allows blood loss (hemorrhage) to be stopped in any area of the body. Chemically, it is a glycosylated protein (glycoprotein) which is produced in the liver and endothelial cells in the form of dimers with a molecular weight of 340 kDa; the individual monomers that constitute it, in turn, are made up of simple amino acid chains. Its half-life in circulating plasma is between 3 and 5 days. High fibrinogen values are usually associated with prothrombotic conditions, while low values correlate with hemorrhagic conditions. *Fibrinogen values* can be detected through *normal blood tests* and normal parameters, which indicate correct functioning of the coagulation mechanism and are the following:

- Women: 200–430 mg/dl;
- Men: 200–375 mg/dl.
- Normal values 200–393 mg/dL (Source: Mayo).

The correlation between D-dimer, fibrinogen, and fibrin degradation products is an indicator of a septic condition as highlighted in various works [26, 32–34]. Plasma Fbg showed similar diagnostic performance compared to CRP and ESR in predicting positive culture results in PJI. Plasma D-dimer showed high specificity but low sensitivity. In the study by Xi Chen and AA, Fbg and D-dimer did not show better diagnostic performance with different pathogens and different types of PJI. Further studies are needed to investigate the difference between serum D-dimer and plasma D-dimer in the arthroplasty population [35].

If exposures and/or fistulas are present, a *culture examination and a superficial antibiogram* can be performed by taking a local sample. The superficial sampling must be done with accuracy because it could reveal germs that are not pathogenic ones, and therefore a sterile field must be created, and the performer must equip himself with all the equipment as if he were carrying out a simple surgical operation. Many authors discourage the performance of superficial swabs as in many cases it is polymicrobial or does not correspond to deep-seated pathogens, creating difficulties in antibiotic coverage [36, 37].

Another test, but in this case a little more invasive, is the *examination of the synovial fluid,* on which many tests can be performed:

- The white blood cell count with the percentage of polymorphonuclear cells (PMN).
- The dosage of PCR and ESR (blood).
- Leukocyte esterase.
- Alpha defensin.
- D-Dimer.
- Calprotectin.
- Culture examination with antibiogram.
- The search for the germ with molecular and other techniques.

*Arthrocentesis* [38] is indicated in the presence of an intra-articular effusion and increased blood inflammation indices, but also in the case of negative serological tests, if there is a strong clinical suspicion of PJI. In some cases, the technique makes use of ultrasound, especially in the hip, while for the knee it is recommended to do it with the knee flexed so that the liquid collects entirely in the intra-condylar space, even if normally the knee joint is entered in the subpatellar space. Hip arthrocentesis is more difficult and actually produces false positives from 3% to 16% [39]. If there is not enough fluid, some authors recommend the introduction of physiological saline in modest quantities [40–43]. In general there are no contraindications to arthrocentesis unless there is a skin infection in the area to be punctured, the use of anticoagulants that could create a hemarthrosis [44] or a systemic septic disease that could be the act of arthrocentesis to create a joint infection, but there are no studies that support these risk conditions, even if being an invasive gesture it can cause synovial irritation and pain. In this way, with a single sample, more data can be obtained [45]. This system is part of the Point-of-Care (POCT). They are widespread in many branches of medicine. Their name derives from their location (at the patient's bed) and not from the type of examination they allow to be performed. They are also sometimes called rapid, satellite, or remote tests; in general, however, the term POCT refers to all those tests that can be performed close to the patient or in the place where health care is provided. The results are ready in a short time and allow their immediate use. The first evaluation that is done after having performed the arthrocentesis is to evaluate *the physical aspect,* which can give us information, and thus the viscosity and color (Fig. 6.2).

From this clearly invasive test, multiple pieces of information can be obtained such as *the white blood cell count, with differential polymorphonuclear count*, an important test to evaluate a joint infection. In fact, it has an excellent specificity with a cut-off >3000 cells/μL and a percentage of neutrophils >80%, this value can be differentiated between knee and hip [45–47]. To be accurate, the white blood cell count should be performed within 2 h of arthrocentesis, as white blood cells may agglutinate over time. In particularly viscous synovial fluids, hyaluronidase can be used (15 U/ml for 15 min at 30 °C), which decreases the viscosity and allows greater handling.

***Leukocyte Esterase Test*** It is an enzyme present in neutrophils and granulocytes (white blood cells), whose main task is to degrade the proteins that support the connective matrix (molecules with the role of tissue support). It is carried out using a stick, normally used for urinalysis (Fig. 6.3).

An extemporaneous exam that can be evaluated directly even if for greater objectivity it can be evaluated by an optical reader (Fig. 6.4), therefore, is no longer a personal evaluation but given by an impartial and highly validated system.

*Alpha-defensin* (Fig. 6.5) is a peptide with antimicrobial action that is particularly abundant in neutrophils where it is produced in response to an infectious stimulus.

| ***Color*** | ***Aspect*** | ***Viscosity*** | ***Synovial fluid*** |
|---|---|---|---|
| light yellow | transparent | preserved | non-inflammatory |
| light yellow or citrine | slightly cloudy | moderately reduced | moderately inflammatory |
| dark yellow. | cloudy. | reduced | frankly inflammatory |
| greenish-yellow | purulent or milky | variable | septic |

**Fig. 6.2** Some macroscopic characteristics found in the various synovial fluids

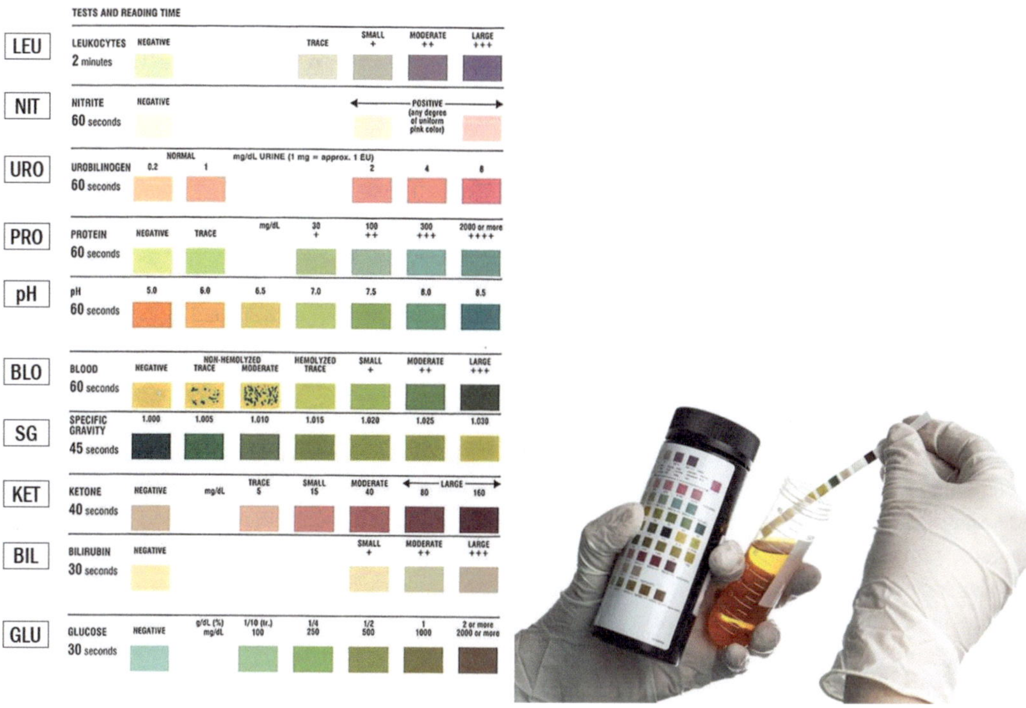


**Fig. 6.3** As can be seen from the following images. Each test has a corresponding color range indicating levels from negative to large, with specific reading times in minute and seconds

It presents some characteristics:

- It is not influenced by the preventive administration of antibiotics.
- It covers a wide spectrum of potential pathogens.
- It is not influenced by other inflammatory conditions.
- It does not give valid results in the presence of a high saline dilution of the sample.
- The aspiration of a hematoma not from a validation of the test.
- In metallosis from a false positive rate of 30%.

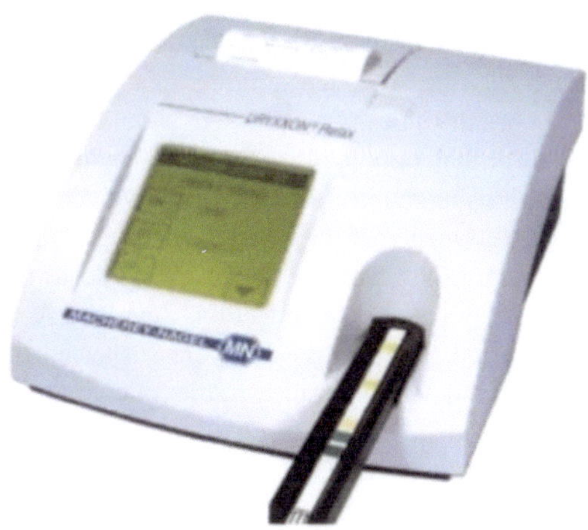

**Fig. 6.4** Optical reader

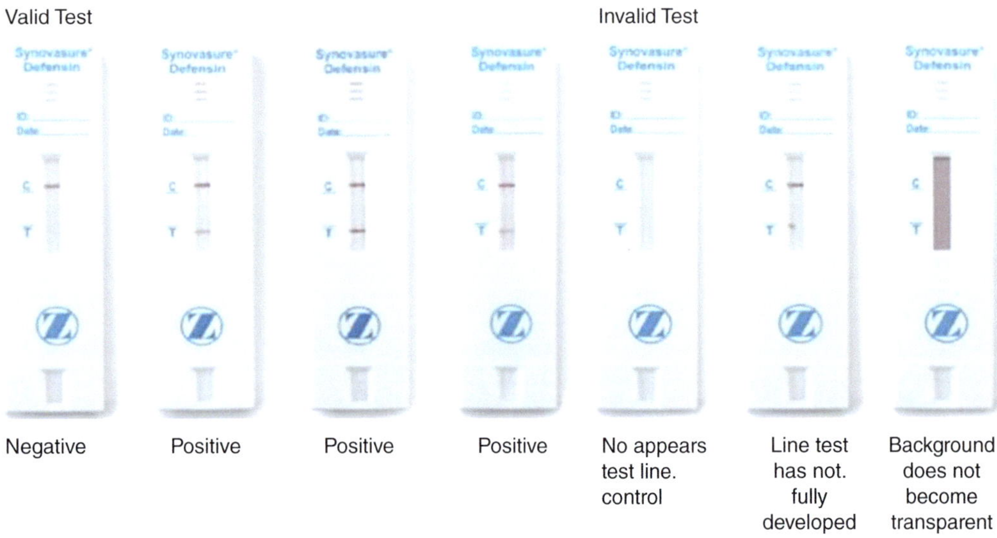


**Fig. 6.5** Some examples of Synovasure-defensin test results

Leukocyte esterase has a very low cost and has a specificity and sensitivity equal to alpha defensing, which has a higher cost [48]. There are many studies on alpha defensin but the comparison with esterase is similar [49].

*Calprotectin* is a very important substance for diagnosing numerous inflammatory diseases. Calprotectin is a peptide (protein) present throughout the body, but particularly concentrated especially in neutrophilic granulocytes and also in monocytes and macrophages. Capable of binding to oxygen and zinc, the main function of calprotectin consists in a counteracting action against the growth of bacteria and fungi within the body (the so-called antimicrobial activity). The normal values of this protein should always be lower than 500 mcg/g, while they begin to be suspicious or doubtful when they are between 50 0 and 120 mcg/g; if they were to be higher than 120 mcg/g, however, the test can be said to be completely positive for infection. Zeyu and A.A [50]. tested 63 patients who were suspected of having a PJI and the result was the following:

The median calprotectin level was 776 μg/ml (interquartile range [IQR] 536 5–1132) in the PJI group and 54.5 μg/ml (IQR, 38 75–78 0.25) in the aseptic failure (AF) group ($p < 0\ 05$). Using a threshold of 173 μg/ml, the sensitivity was 95 2%, with a 97 6% specificity, and the AUC was 0.993. The sensitivity of calprotectin of the antibiotic-treated PJI group was 100% versus 90 9% of the nonantibiotic-treated PJI group. Although 47.6% (ten cases) of the patients in the PJI group received antibiotics before aspiration, the diagnostic efficacy of calprotectin was not affected. The sensitivity and specificity of ESR, CRP, SF-WBCs, and SF-PMNs ranged from 76 (2%) to 90 (5%) and 64 (3%) to 85 (7%), respectively [50].

*It must be considered that the presence of blood inside the joint and the use of anticoagulants can alter the diagnostic tests.*

The culture test from synovial fluid has a high specificity (approximately 98%) but low sensitivity (approximately 68%). A negative culture test therefore does not exclude the presence of PJI. On the other hand, a false positivity rate of 13% was reported. Shmerling in 1994 claims that the "best reason" to perform an arthrocentesis is the diagnosis of an infection [51, 52]. A positive gram stain can in fact lead to a reasoned therapy in a very short time, the positivity of a culture allows a diagnosis, and a therapeutic choice makes it possible to monitor the therapy and the pathological course with a second blood sample

[53]. There are two methods for managing the withdrawal:

A) Immediately, after collection, inoculate an aliquot (≥ 1 ml per bottle) into blood culture bottles for aerobic and anaerobic microorganisms. Transfer the remaining aspirate into sterile containers with anticoagulant for subsequent culture analyzes and with EDTA (dithiothreitol) for the total leukocyte count and differential neutrophil polymorphonuclear count.
B) Transfer the aspirate into sterile containers with anticoagulant for subsequent culture and EDTA analyzes for the total leukocyte count and differential neutrophil polymorphonuclear count.

The samples must be kept at a temperature of 4 °C and should reach the laboratory within 2 h, keeping in mind that there is a significant loss of bacteria already 6 h after sampling due to the presence of killer bacteria. Antibiotics should be discontinued at least 2 weeks before arthrocentesis to ensure positive culture results; however, it is necessary to know that antibiotic therapy can inhibit the proliferation of some microorganisms even for months [54].

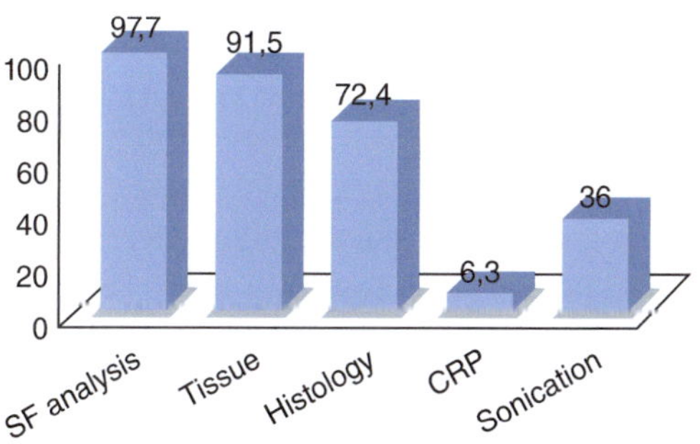


*The value of intra-articular tests has greater significance than blood chemistry tests. The examination of the synovial fluid is, to date, the most important examination in the diagnosis of PJI.* (*Based on data taken from Suflan S. Ahmad, Roland Becker, Antonia F Chen, Sandro Kohl EKA survey: diagnosis of prosthetic knee joint infection September 2016, Knee Surgery Sports Traumatology Arthroscopy 24(10) https://doi.org/10.1007/s00167-016-4303-y*)

The data set carries a score, as reported in the following scheme developed at the Philadelphia 2018 consensus conference (Fig. 6.6), differentiating the values between the acute form and the chronic form.

Other biomarkers from synovial fluid are being evaluated. In a recent work, 16 biomarkers were studied of which 5 gave a value of high specificity and sensitivity: alpha-defensin, the mutated ELA-2 gene, the Bactericial permeability-increasing (BPI) protein, neutrophil gelatinase-associated lipocalin (NGAL), and lactoferrin. Eight other biomarkers (IL-8, C-reactive protein, resistin, thrombospondin, IL-1, IL-6, IL-10, and IL-1) have showed AUC greater than 0.9 [55]. Results: Five biomarkers, including human α-defensin 1–3, neutrophil elastase 2,bactericidal/permeability-increasing protein, neutrophil gelatinase-associated lipocalin, and lactoferrin, correctly predicted the MSIS classification of all patients in this study, with 100% sensitivity and specificity for the diagnosis of PJI. Eight additional biomarkers demonstrated excellent diagnostic strength, with an area under the curve of greater than 0 9.

Another very recent test about which there are still some uncertainties and which can be performed when sampling synovial fluid is *molecular diagnostics for the identification of pathogens in septic arthritis and periprosthetic infections (PJI).*

*For this very recent topic, I availed myself of the collaboration of Prof. Pier Francesco Indelli and Doctor Emanuele Chisari whom I thank.*

Next-generation sequencing (NGS) is a molecular diagnostic method that offers a more efficient, cost-effective, and validated technique for identifying the pathogens responsible for periprosthetic joint infections (PJIs). NGS outperforms traditional culture and PCR methods in microbial detection, particularly in complex cases like polymicrobial infections or when traditional biomarkers fail. It is especially useful for identifying causative pathogens in culture-negative PJIs [56], which can occur due to previous antimicrobial therapy, user error, or limitations of current detection methods. Because of this, recent reports [57, 58] are recommending

| Major Criteria (at least on of the following) | Decision |
|---|---|
| Two positive growths of the same organism using standard culture methods. | Infected |
| Sinus tract with evidence of communication to the joint or visualization of the prosthesis | |

| Minor Criteria | Thershold | | Score | Decision |
|---|---|---|---|---|
| | Acute[€] | Chronic | | |
| CRP (mg/L)<br>D-D Dimer (μg/L) | 100<br>Unknown | 10<br>860 | 2 | Combined preoperative and postoperative score:<br>≥6 Infected<br>3 to 5 Inconclusive*<br><3 Not Infected |
| Elevated Serum ESR (mm/hr) | No rule | 30 | 1 | |
| Elevated Synovial WBC (cell/μL)<br>*or*<br>Leukocyte Esterase<br>*or*<br>Positive Alpha-defensin (signal/cutoff) | 10.000<br>++<br>1.0 | 3,000<br>++<br>1.0 | 3 | |
| Elevated Synovial PMN (%) | 90 | 70 | 2 | |
| Signle Positive Culture | | | 2 | |
| Positive Histology | | | 3 | |
| Positive Intraoperative Purulence[γ] | | | 3 | |

*This criteria were never validated on acute infection. [γ]No role in suspected adverse local tissue reaction.
*Consider further moleular diagnostics such as next-generation sequencing

**Fig. 6.6** Proposed 2018 ICM criteria for PJI

the use of molecular diagnostics for a prompt septic arthritis/PJI diagnosis. Nucleic acid amplification techniques, such as polymerase chain reaction (PCR) and Next Generation Sequencing (NGS), represent the most appealing for the scientific community because of the capability to accelerate the diagnosis, identify causative agents, and direct targeted antibiotic therapy [59, 60]. NGS provides comprehensive pathogen detection, supporting accurate and targeted treatment decisions in PJI management. Next-Generation Sequencing (NGS) for Periprosthetic Joint Infections (PJI) involves a detailed process to identify pathogens:

1. Sample Collection and Preparation: NGS begins with collecting a sample, typically synovial fluid or tissue, from the infected joint.
2. DNA Extraction: DNA is extracted from the collected sample. This DNA includes genetic material from the patient and any microbes present in the sample.
3. Library Preparation: The extracted DNA is processed to prepare a sequencing library. This involves fragmenting the DNA into smaller pieces and adding specialized adapters for sequencing.
4. Sequencing: The library is then sequenced. NGS allows for the simultaneous sequencing of millions of DNA fragments, producing a vast amount of genetic data in a single run.
5. Data Analysis: The sequenced data is analyzed using bioinformatics tools. This involves aligning the sequences against known microbial genomes to identify the specific pathogens present in the sample.
6. Pathogen Identification: By comparing the sequenced data to reference databases, the specific pathogens causing the infection are identified.
7. Report Generation: A report is generated that lists the identified pathogens, which helps in guiding the treatment plan.

This molecular diagnostic tool (Biofire Joint Infection panel, Biomerieux, Salt Lake City, USA) is capable to identify, in less than an hour, 39 microorganisms, including 14 Gram-negative bacteria and two yeasts and eight antimicrobial resistance (AMR) genes from synovial fluid specimens, allowing for rapid microbiological identification and subsequently targeted adequate antimicrobial therapy. In a recent multicenter study, this panel has shown a sensitivity of 90.9% and a specificity of 98.5% [61]: the major limitation of this diagnostic technology is the lack of coagulase-negative *staphylococci* (i.e., *S. Epidermidis*) and Gram-positive rods (i.e., *Cutibacterium Acnes*) in its diagnostic spectrum, but beyond these limitations, the molecular test appears to be the ideal diagnostic tool for acute joint infections, both in native joints as well as in PJI: in fact, acute joint infections are mainly caused by *S. aureus* and Gram-bacilli (*Escherichia coli, Enterobacter cloacae* complex, *Klebsiella, Pseudomonas aeruginosa)* which are included in the panel.

In chronic infections, where coagulase-negative *staphylococci* play a major role, next generation sequencing (NGS, which can quickly sequence DNA, represents a modern and innovative diagnostic methodology, especially in culture-negative scenarios. Recent reports have highlighted that the NGS technique, especially in its metagenomic variation (mNGS), had a 95.9% sensitivity and a 95.2% specificity [62]. The limitation of NGS stays in its very high sensitivity [63]: in a recent study, surgeons from the American Association of Hip and Knee Surgeons (AAHKS), using NGS in a study on culture negative PJI, reported pathogen identification in 65.9% of cases; more than 90% of those PJI were polymicrobial [64]. This last finding raised a major, still unanswered, question: does the threshold of reads for distinguishing real pathogens from background signals (knee microbioma?) [65] need to be established before the widespread use of NGS as the most emerging technology for microorganism identification in septic arthritis and PJI scenarios?

The diagnosis of septic arthritis and PJI in the setting of equivocal test results, negative cultures, or chronic, indolent infection can raise significant dilemmas, especially without a single, "gold standard" diagnostic test available. Molecular diagnostics represent revolutionary technologies that could disrupt the traditional diagnostic paradigm of musculoskeletal infections.

Another series of tests that can be requested consists of radiological ones, which range from the least demanding to those that have a greater impact on the patient.

**The X-ray (Figs. 6.7, 6.8 and 6.9)** Is perhaps the first test done when faced with the symptoms of a painful prosthesis and can give us some information, such as the relationship between the prosthesis and the bone structure. Lytic areas or periosteal reactions can be detected, but all these images are nonspecific because they can also concern, for example, aseptic loosening. It should be considered that lysis occurs when there is significant bone loss (at least 30%), so in the initial stages, it is difficult to establish a diagnosis.

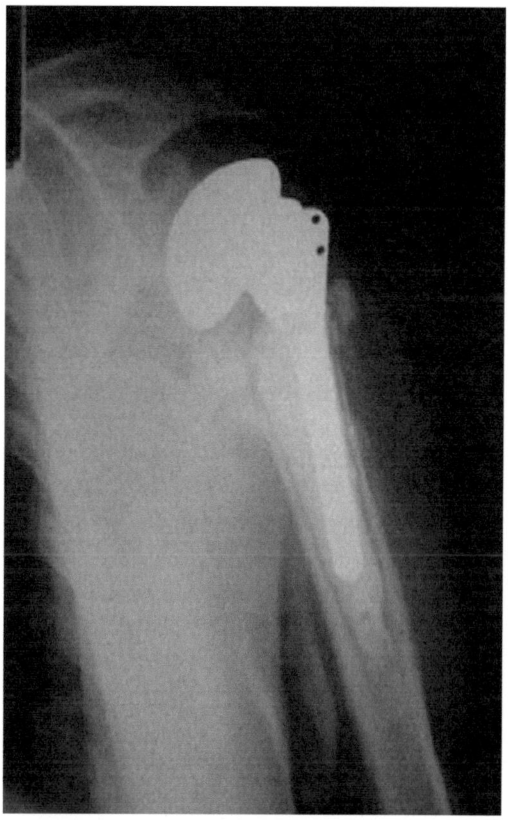

**Fig. 6.7** X-ray of a cemented anatomical shoulder prosthesis, where a separation between the cement and the bone is visible but without other signs and tests it is not possible to say whether it is an infection or an aseptic loosening

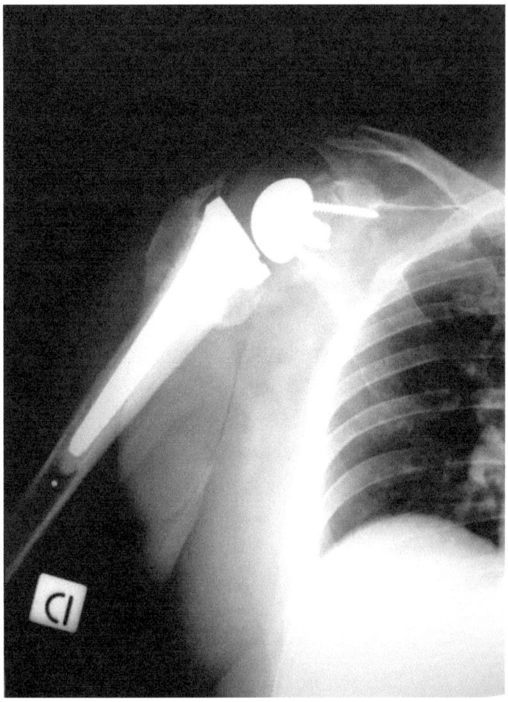


**Fig. 6.8** Another example of an X-ray of a cemented reverse shoulder replacement, where you can see a notch in the proximal humerus but without other signs and tests you can't tell if it's an infection or aseptic loosening

Therefore, if it were negative, it would not exclude that there is an ongoing PJI [66, 67].

In Figs. 6.7 , 6.8, and 6.9. There are two X-rays; an anatomical prosthesis and a reverse prosthesis, both infected and showing no radiographic sign of a septic diagnosis. Although in the case on the anatomical prosthesis we notice a gap between the cement and the prosthesis, nothing tells us whether it is a septic loosening or not septic. The situation is similar for the knee x-rays. It should be noted that they were all septic forms.

An associated exam is *fistulography* (Fig. 6.10) [68] if, obviously, there is a fistula as in the image below. It is an exam that is performed without anesthesia and uses a buttoned needle and a contrast medium, in our case lipiodol, which is made up of 1 ml of solution containing active ingredients: mixture of ethyl esters of iodinated fatty acids of plant origin equal to 480 mg of iodine.

Density: 1280 at 15 ° C.

Viscosity: 65 centipoises at 15 ° C.

Iodine content: 1 g contains 0. 38 g of iodine—1 ml contains 0.48 g of iodine Lipiodol Ultra Fluid does not contain excipients. In general, the dose administered varies from 1 to 20 ml, according to the needs of the different radiological investigations carried out. Administer Lipiodol Ultra Fluid using an adequate glass syringe and a cannula, by slow injection or cannulation.

*Lipiodol Ultra Fluid must not be administered intravenously and intra-arterial but only locally.*

Fistulography can give us indications on the main focus or on any abscess collections, useful for, possibly, under ultrasound control, to do an aspiration that can help us find the germ responsible for the infection and, consequently, the antibiogram.

Another test that can be easily carried out, with low invasiveness and low cost is *ultrasound* (Fig. 6.11) [69, 70], a test used in PJI to identify collections above or below the fascia which, always under ultrasound control, can be evacuated to perform, above all, the search for any pathogen. It has the advantage of being able to be done dynamically to evaluate any prosthetic and/or joint impingement and any existing relationships with the vascular system. Therefore, it does not have the diagnostic capabilities of a PJI or differentiation but guides in fine needle aspirates and biopsies without the use of ionizing radiation.

**MRI (Fig. 6.12) [71–73]** as in the case below, can help us highlight foci that would not have been highlighted on X-ray, having a sensitivity for the soft parts. The presence of metal has always been a contraindication, but the arrival of less ferromagnetic materials and the technical growth of equipment has made it possible to reduce artifacts. One fact is that this system does not use ionizing radiation and, therefore, in patients who need repeated tests this may be a possibility. The possibility of performing it in open environments should be considered, especially for those who suffer from claustrophobia.

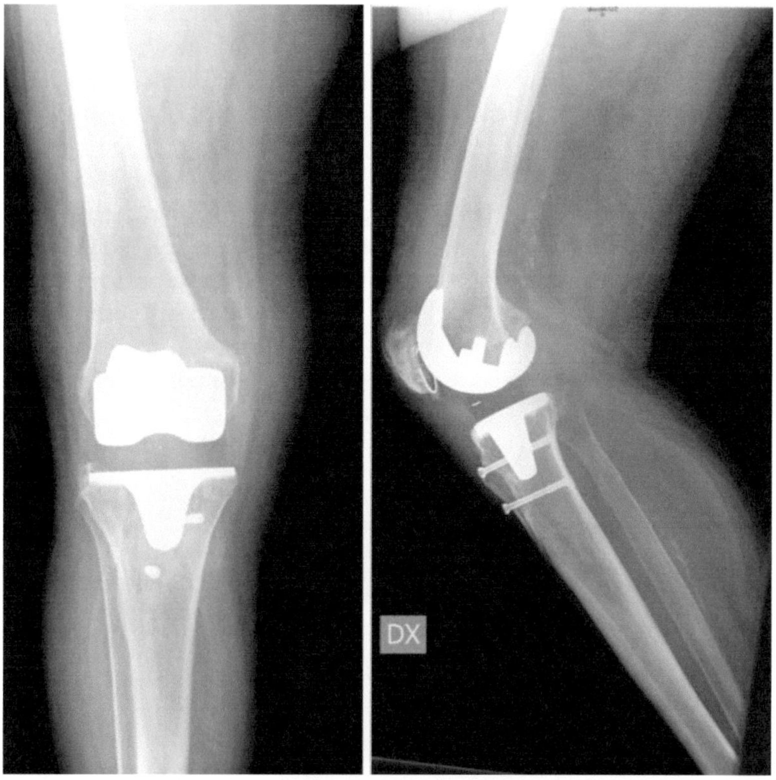


**Fig. 6.9** Another example where the X-ray does neither show any sign of apparent infection, nor other signs of loosening

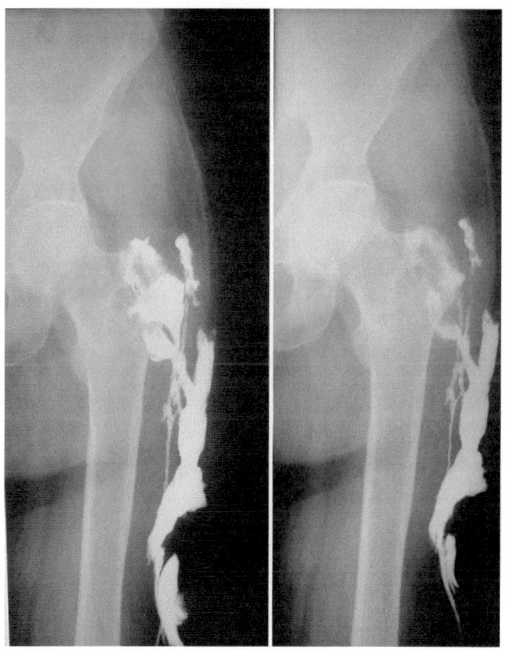

**Fig. 6.10** An example of fistolography of an infection of the greater trochanter which, thanks to the examination, made us understand that the joint had not been affected by the infection. It is a test whose importance has been lost but in some cases, it is useful and is not complicated to perform

**Computed Tomography (CT) [74, 75]** This exam allows us to better analyze the relationships between bone and prosthesis. It is a test that hardly helps us in making a diagnosis of PJI, as the manifestations of the infection are evident when the infection is already established, and, therefore, in the initial stages, it is of little help. The presence of the prosthesis, then, creates artefacts, even if today it is possible to perform image subtraction CT scans, which avoid artefacts.

**The Triphasic Bone Scan [76–78]** is a test that must be requested when at least 2 years have passed since the implantation of a hip prosthesis, while at least 4 years after the implantation of a knee and shoulder prosthesis, in how long the bone manipulation takes place and would certainly give false positives. It is a test that is performed by injecting a bisphosphonate analogue labeled with metastable Technetium-99 (99mTc) into the blood. Similarly, to unlabeled bisphosphonates, this radiopharmaceutical is incorporated into the crystals of hydroxyapatite of the newly affixed bone matrix, providing information relating to osteoblastic metabolism. In the suspicion of an infection, the most appropriate bone scan is the one acquired in triphasic mode, i.e., exploring three fundamental functional moments of the infectious process: vascularization, permeability vascular, and bone metabolism. In the presence of an infection, in fact, all three of these phases are enhanced and therefore positive on the triphasic bone scan. It should be considered that the increased metabolism is typical of other forms in addition to the infectious one, such as aseptic loosening, tumors, and osteometabolic pathologies. Therefore, its negativity (negative predictive value) indicates the non-presence of a septic pathology. Therefore, high sensitivity but low specificity.

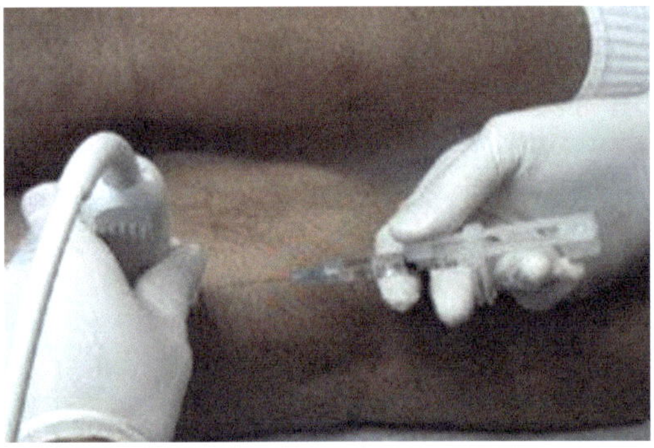

**Fig. 6.11** Aspiration of a septica area under ultrasound guidance

**Scintigraphy with Autologous Labeled Leukocytes (Fig. 6.13) [79–81]** Should be requested, possibly associated with SPECT/CT (Fig. 6.14) method or spinal cord scintigraphy, in cases in which serological tests and those on

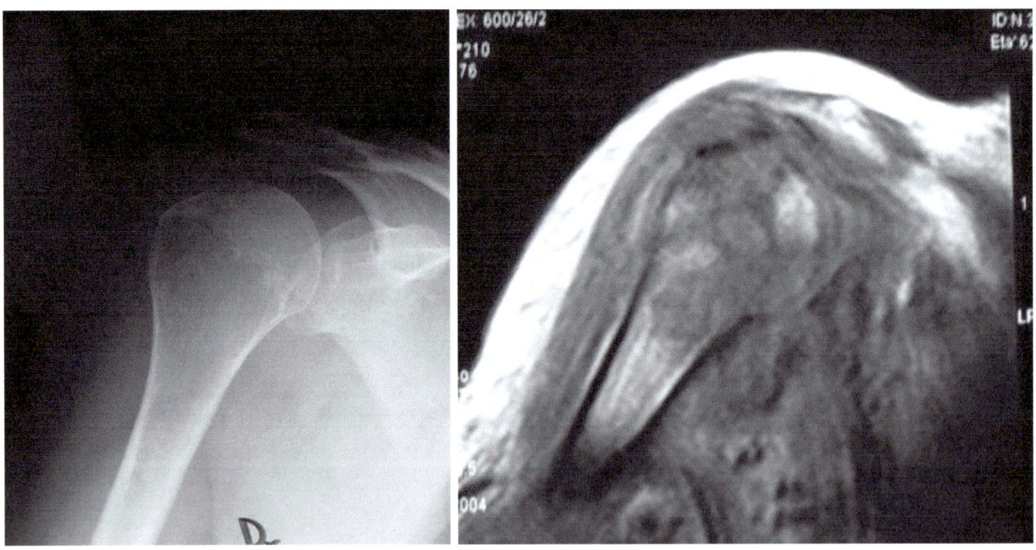

**Fig. 6.12** An example of MRI that highlights endo-epiphyseal foci of the humerus that cannot be seen on a simple X-ray

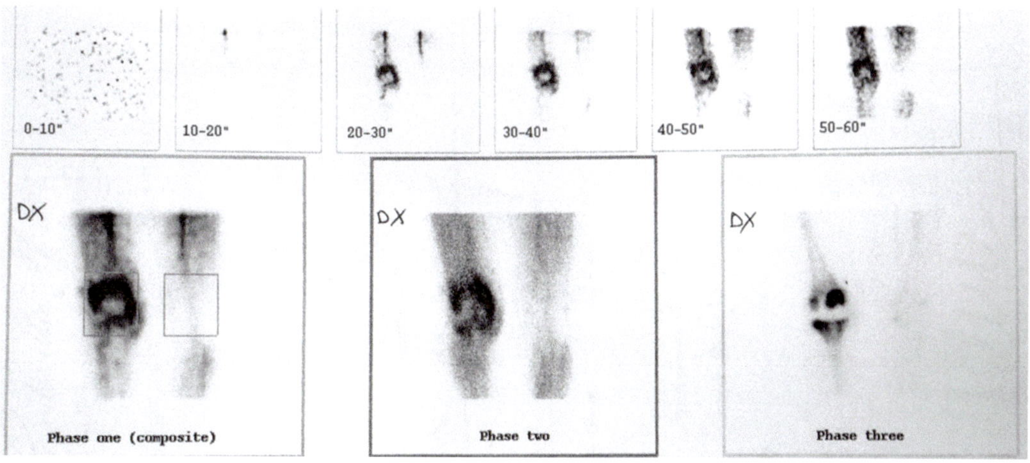


**Fig. 6.13** An example of a scan with autologous labeled leukocytes in a case of periprosthetic knee infection

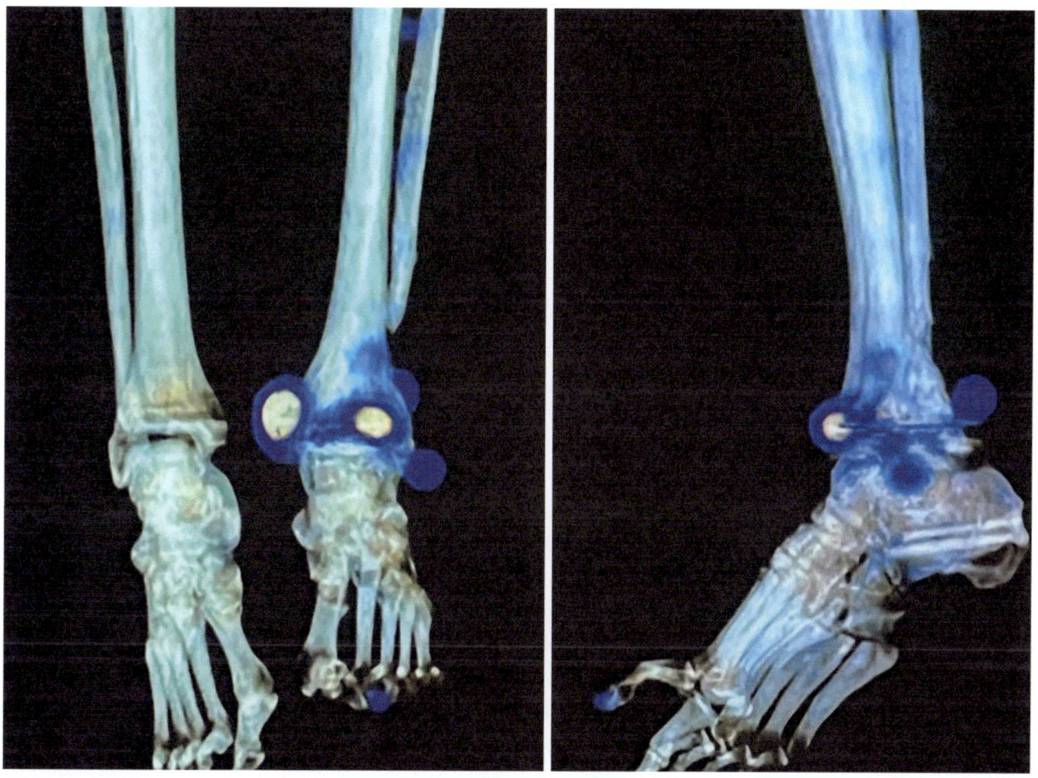

**Fig. 6.14** The SPECT/CT is considered the best technique that can contribute to the evaluation of the presence and extent of the infection both in the diagnostic phase, in the case of suspected infection, and as a control after appropriate medical and/or surgical treatment, to exclude the persistence of the infection

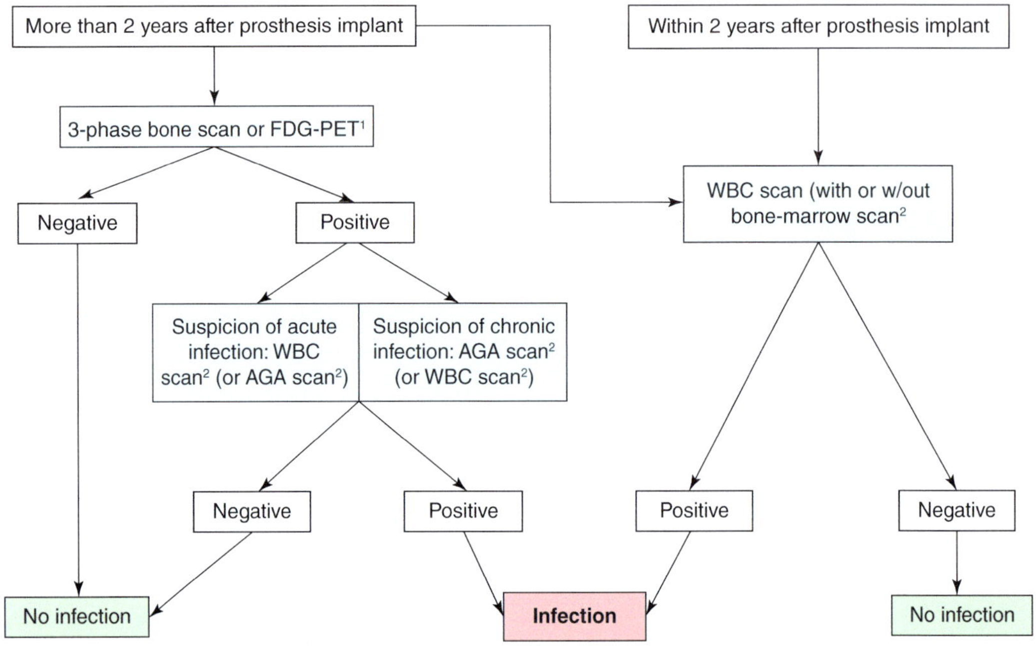


**Fig. 6.15** Nuclear Medicine Flow chart for diagnosing infection after prosthesis implant. Signore, LM Sconfienza, O. Borens, AW.J.M. Glaudemans, VC Pullicino, A Trampuz, H. Winkler, O. Gheysen, FM.H.M. VanhoenackerN Petrosillo, P C. Jutte "Consensus document for the diagnosis of prosthetic joint infections: a joint paper by the EANM, EBJIS, and ESR (with ESCMID endorsement)" A. Signore et Al. European Journal of Nuclear Medicine and Molecular Imaging https://doi.org/10.1007/s00259-019-4263-9

synovial fluid are not sufficient to confirm or exclude the diagnosis of infection. Scintigraphy with leukocytes labeled with 111-Indium (111In) or 99 m-Technetium (99mTc) is still the "gold standard" nuclear medical test for the diagnosis of infectious processes and is therefore indicated in the majority of infectious pathologies, if performed and interpreted according to the guidelines provided by the European Society of Nuclear Medicine (EANM) (Fig. 6.15). Therefore, in compliance with the pathophysiology of infections, it is necessary to acquire images at multiple times (30 min–1 h; 2–4 h; and 20–24 h after the administration of the labeled autologous leukocytes) in order to verify the trend of radioactivity. In case of increased uptake in extent and/or extent of uptake, we speak of infection, on the contrary, if the uptake shows a reduction/stability over time, it is a sterile inflammation. Adding SPECT/CT provides better localization of the septic process and its extension by differentiating between periprosthetic-bony localization and soft parts, with an accuracy that, in some cases, reaches 100%. This test is also valid in low infections where the bone tournover is not very high. Another fact, especially for the acute forms, both hematogenous and post-prosthesis surgery, is that the exam can be done approximately a month later and that it is not conditioned by the use of antibiotics even if some authors recommend their use. Suspension 10–15 days before the exam.

**PET (Positron Emission Tomography)/CT with F-FDG (fluorodeoxyglucose) [82–84]** Another, but invasive, test is *the biopsy* (Fig. 6.16), which is performed under amplioscopic control and under local anesthesia, but it must also be performed intraoperatively. It consists of taking at least in 6 samples from the bone-prosthesis or bone-cement-prosthesis space. Each withdrawal must be indicated for the headquarters made as the septic process is

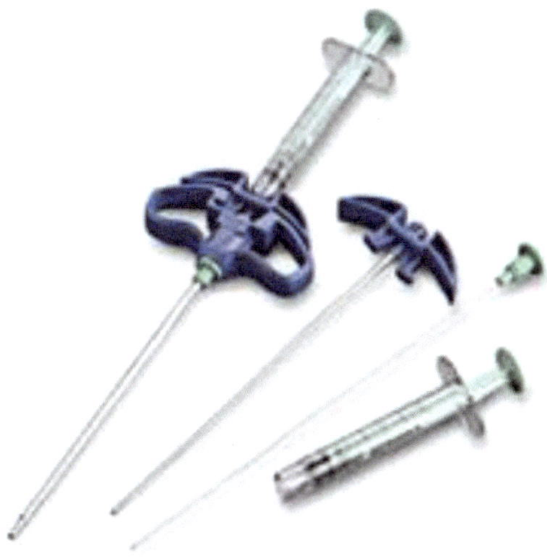

**Fig. 6.16** Material for biopsy sampling both under closed amplioscopic control and in the open surgical phase

not uniform in the whole articulation. Culture research on the germ and a histological examination can be carried out on the sample which should evaluate the presence of neutrophilic polymorphonuclear leukocytes indicative of infection which should be at least five neutrophils per field at high magnification (400x). As you can easily understand, it's evaluation of several tests that together contribute to the dignosis of infection. The experience and relationship with other specialists (radiologists, microbiologists, infectious disease of infection, anatomical pathologists, plastic surgeons) is crucial.

Another test that can be done in situations of high fever and/or sepsis is *the blood culture* which can give us information on the circulating germ. Some authors consider it of little significance as the isolation of the bacterium(s) is much more important batteries in the joint field. But the most important thing is that if we are faced with septicemia it is very important to treat, regardless of the germ found in the joint, also the blood culture germ, even if the positivity of the blood culture in the context of a PJI varies from 4% to 25% [85]. Some works have shown that the isolated germs in blood culture and from intraoperative sampling coincided in 86% and 100% of cases [86, 87]. At this point, we have made the diagnosis of PJI or we still have doubts but we have decided that we must operate on the patient by removing the prosthesis. We may not even have a positive culture test or we may find ourselves faced with the doubt that it is an aseptic loosening. I will not go into the merits of the various surgical techniques of removal and/or reimplantation with passage through an antibiotic spacer but I will focus on the diagnostic part of this surgical act which involves some gestures that can help us identify, in a safer way, the responsible germ of the pathology or give certainty about the diagnosis of PJI:*The microbiological examination* must be done regardless of the preoperative diagnosis and consists of 3–5 samples in the areas of doubtful appearance due to infection. Each sample must be done by changing the sample material and must be placed in a sterile test tube describing the site of the sample itself. Material must be subjected to aerobic and anaerobic culture for at least 15 days. The number of samples is also given by the clinical situation. In the suspicion of a low infection, samples should be more than 5. The material collected may consist of synovial tissue, the membrane that surrounds the prosthesis, in the bone and, if necessary, cement always close to the prosthesis and the bone. The samples must be taken to the laboratory as soon as possible to prevent the killer bacteria from attacking the pathogenic bacteria, lysing them. The sample must be stored at −4 °C. The removed prosthesis can follow two paths, both perfectly similar in terms of results and both use a system to break the biofilm [88–90] which is not only present on the prostheses but also in the periprosthetic tissues, and, therefore, all the material taken must be sent for analysis with the following methods, and thus allow the identification of the pathogenic germ and the subsequent sensitivity to the antibiotics tested and are:

- *Sonication (physical method)* [91]; this consists of subjecting both cellular suspensions to the action of ultrasound, to cause the rupture of biological membranes and recover the intracellular contents, and proteins or DNA, to obtain fragments of uniform molecular mass. In our case it serves to break the biofilm of the germs that are positioned on the prosthesis but also in the periprosthetic tissues.

*Dithiothreitol (DTT) (chemical method)* [92] is chemically classified as a thiol. It is a solid, white compound, very soluble in water, with a typical "rotten egg" odor, an odor that is accentuated when the compound passes into solution, especially if concentrated. It belongs to the family of reducing chemical compounds. It is one of the strongest reducing agents known in the biological and laboratory fields, capable of breaking disulfide bridges of both most proteins and organic compounds, even at room temperature. It was used in the past to break up the sputum in the search for mycobacterium in pulmonary tuberculosis and this ability is used today to break up the biofilm both on the prosthesis and on the tissues.The only clinical finding of *purulent material* (Fig. 6.17) on intra-operative examination, although highly suggestive of PPI, cannot be considered in itself a certain sign of periprosthetic infection, therefore it is still recommended to complete the diagnosis with a microbiological and anatomical-pathological examination. "Pus" is a dense fluid with a creamy appearance and a yellowish-white color, which forms during particular types of inflammation. It is made up of decaying white blood cells, which can be mixed with bacteria (live and/or dead), in this case representing a sign of infection. However, the accumulation of white blood cells and the formation of purulent material can also be caused by "aseptic" inflammation therefore in the absence of infecting microorganisms; on the basis of this observation, authoritative experts have highlighted the limits of clinical evaluation both regarding the subjectivity of the definition of "purulent material" and regarding the impossibility of clinically appreciating the true cause of a purulent collection; in fact, only the microscopic examination and the possible isolation of the pathogenic agent can allow us to unequivocally establish the septic or aseptic nature of a purulent collection [93]. Purulent material can also be found in the presence of metallosis [94, 95], pseudotumors due to wear of biomaterials [96], some rheumatic diseases such as gout [97] or other crystal deposition diseases [98], aseptic loosening or other bone pathologies such as, for example, osteonecrosis [98].

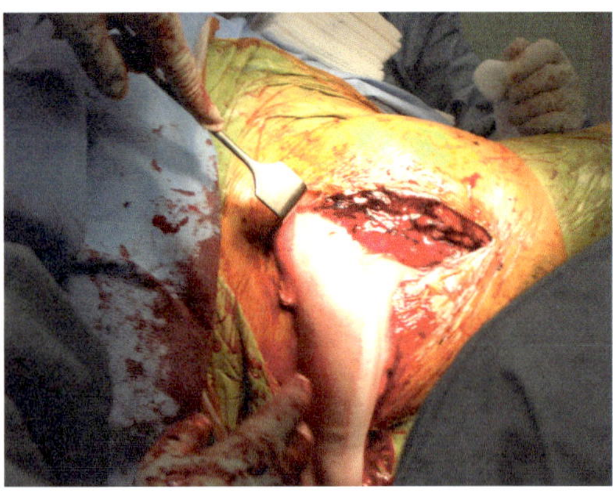

**Fig. 6.17** Pus leakage during PJI surgery

As the conclusion of this chapter, I would like to draw attention to what EBJIS has proposed with a new definition of PJI, trying to give a new value to infections given that there is not yet, to date, a valid test to define the presence of an infection and therefore a further differentiation was made by dividing them into unlikely infections, probable infections, and confirmed infections [99]. Based on the above, Shohat and A.A [100]. Combined a stepwise clinical algorithm that could collect all the characteristics we have described. Patients who had a low-virulence infection and patients who were culture-negative were considered. Developed a stepwise clinical algorithm based on the revised 2018 MSIS definition. They applied the algorithm to a multicentered cohort of patients and demonstrated high sensitivity (96.6%) and specificity (99.5%) (Fig. 6.18).

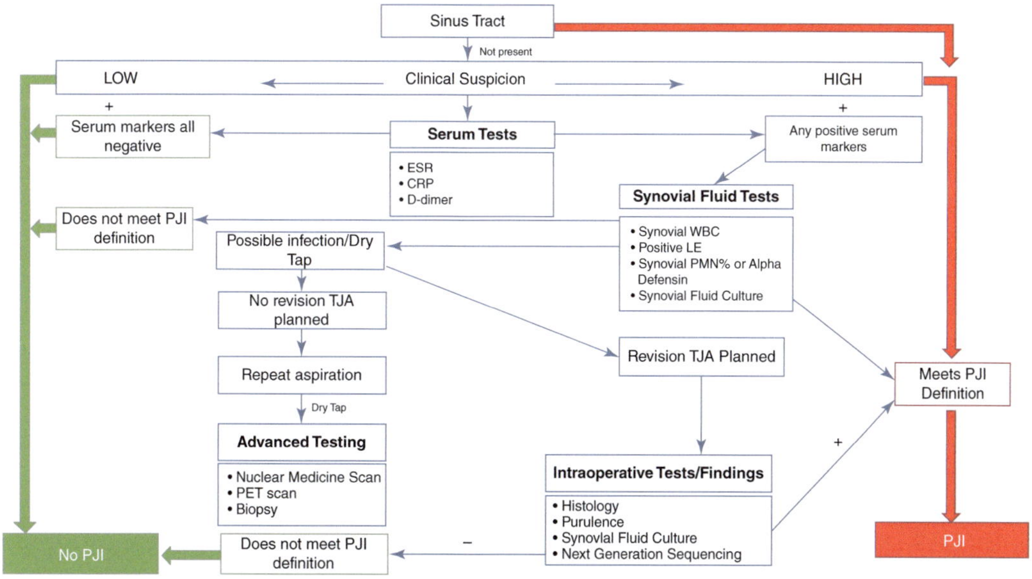


**Fig. 6.18** Like all algorithms, this one can also have some negativity but it is an indication that the whole world is taking action to fight this terrible pathology. (Stepwise clinical algorithm adapted from Shohat et al. (2019) [100] based on the revised 2018 MSIS criteria proposed by Parvizi et al. (2018) [6]

## References


1. Osmon DR, Berbari EF, Berendt AR, et al.; Infectious Diseases Society of America. Diagnosis and management of prosthetic joint infection: Clinical practice guidelines by the Infectious Diseases Society of America. Clin Infect Dism2013;56:e1-e25. https://doi.org/10.1093/cid/cis803.
2. Martin McNally, Ricardo Sousa, Marjan Wouthuyzen-Bakker, Antonia F Chen, Alex Soriano, H Charles Vogely, Martin Clauss, Carlos A Higuera, Rihard Trebše The EBJIS definition of periprosthetic joint infection. Bone Joint J. 2021;103-B(1):18–25.
3. Parvizi J, Zmistowski B, Berbari EF, et al. New definition for periprosthetic joint infection: From the workgroup of the Musculoskeletal infection Society. Clin Orthop Relat Res 2011;469:2992e4. https://doi.org/10.1007/s11999-011-2102-9.
4. Romano CL, Khawashki HA; Benzakour T, et al. The W.A.I.O.T. definition of high- grade and low-grade peri-prosthetic joint infection. J Clin Med 2019;8(5). https://doi.org/10.3390/jcm8050650.
5. Parvizi J, Gehrke T; International Consensus Group on Periprosthetic Joint Infection. Definition of periprosthetic joint infection. J Arthroplast 2014;29:1331. https://doi.org/10.1016/j.arth.2014.03.009.
6. Parvizi J, Tan TL, Goswami K, et al. The 2018 definition ofperiprosthetic hip and knee infection: an evidence-based and validated criteria. J Arthroplast 2018;33:1309-14.e2. https://doi.org/10.1016/j.arth.2018.02.078.
7. Parvizi J, Gehrke, T. Proceedings of the Second International Consensus Meeting on Musculoskeletal Infection. Hip and Knee Section Data Trace Publishing Company: Brooklandville, MD, USA, 2018.
8. Zeng Y, Feng W, Qi X, et al. Differential knee skin temperature following total knee arthroplasty and its relationship with serum indices and outcome: a prospective study. J Int Med Res 2016;44:1023–33. https://doi.org/10.1177/0300060516655237.
9. Allami MK. Superficial incisional infection in arthroplasty of the lower limb: interobserver reliability of the current diagnostic criteria. J Bone Joint Surg Br 2005;87-B:1267-71. https://doi.org/10.1302/0301-620X.87B9.16672.
10. Pepe MS. The statistical evaluation of medical tests for classification and prediction. Oxford Statistical Science Series- 28. Oxford University Press 2003.
11. Alijanipour P, Bakhshi H, Parvizi J. Diagnosis of periprosthetic joint infection. The threshold for serological markers. Clin Orthop Relat Res 2013;3186–95.
12. McGee S. Simplifying likelihood ratios. J Gen Intern Med 2002;17:647–50.
13. Mol BW, Lijmer JG, Evers JLH, et al. Characteristics of good diagnostic studies. Sem Reprod Med 2003; 21:17–25. https://doi.org/10.1055/s-2003-39991.
14. Djulbegovic B, Hozo I, Schwartz A, et al. Acceptable regrein medical decision making. Medical Hypotheses 1999;53:253–9. https://doi.org/10.1054/mehy.1998.0020.

15. Trevethan R. Sensitivity, specificity, and predictive values: foundations, pliabilities, and pitfalls in research and practice. Front Public Health 2017;5:1–7.
16. Zeman DH. The "best" diagnostic test. Sw Health and Production 1997;5:159–60.
17. Assasi N, Blackhouse G, Campbell K, et al. Comparative value of erythrocyte sedimentation rate (ESR) and C-reactive protein (CRP) testing in combination versus individuallyb for the diagnosis of undifferentiated patients with suspected inflammatory disease or serious infection: a systematic review and economic analysis. Ottawa: CADTH; 2015 Nov. (CADTH health technology assessment; no.140)
18. Bray C, Bell LN, Liang H, et al. Erythrocyte sedimentation rate and C-reactive protein measurements and their relevance in clinical medicine. WMJ2016;115: 317–21
19. Brigden M. The erythrocyte sedimentation rate. Postgrad Med 1998;103:257–74.
20. Deirmengian CA, Citrano PA, Gulati S, et al. The C-reactive protein may not detect infections caused by less-virulent organisms. J Arthroplasty 2016;31:S152-5. https://doi.org/10.1016/j.arth.2016.01.060.
21. Harrison M. Erythrocyte sedimentation rate and C-reactive protein. Aust Presc 2015;38:93–4. https://doi.org/10.18773/austprescr.2015.034.
22. McArthur BA, Abdel MP, Taunton MJ, Osmon DR, Hanssen AD. Seronegative infections in hip and knee arthroplasty: periprosthetic infections with normal erythrocyte sedimentation rate and C–reactive protein level. Bone Joint J. 2015;97–B:939–944. https://doi.org/10.1302/0301-620X.97B7.35500.
23. Parvizi J, Della Valle CJ. AAOS clinical practice guideline: diagnosis and treatment of periprosthetic joint infections of the hip and knee. J Am Acad Orthop Surg. 2010;18:771–772.
24. Balato G, De Franco C, Balboni F, De Matteo V, Ascione T,Baldini A. Lippi G. The role of D-dimer in periprosthetic joint infection: a systematic review and meta-analysis.
25. Li C, Margaryan D, Ojeda-Thies C, Perka C, Trampuz A. Meta-analysis of serum and/or plasma D-dimer in the diagnosis of periprosthetic joint infection. J Orthop Surg Res 2020;15:298. https://doi.org/10.1186/s13018-020-01808-1.
26. Qian Hu , Yaoyang Fu , Lingli Tang . Serum D-dimer as a diagnostic index of PJI and retrospective analysis of etiology in patients with PJI. Clin Chim Acta 2020:506:67–71. https://doi.org/10.1016/j.cca.2020.03.023. Epub 2020 Mar 13
27. Shahi A, Kheir MM, Tarabichi M, Hosseinzadeh HRS, Tan TL, Parvizi J. Serum D-dimer test is promising for the diagnosis of periprosthetic joint infection and timing of reimplantation. J Bone Joint Surg. 2017;99(17):1419–1427. https://doi.org/10.2106/JBJS.16.01395.
28. Korte W, Riesen W. Latex-enhanced immunoturbidimetry allows D-dimer determination in plasma and serum samples. Clin Chem 2000;46:871–2.
29. Yang F., Zhao C., Huang R. , Ma H. , Wang X. , Wang G. , Zhao X. Plasma fibrinogen in the diagnosis of periprosthetic joint infection. Sci Rep. 2021 Jan 12;11(1):677. https://doi.org/10.1038/s41598-020-80547-z.
30. Li R, Shao HY, Hao LB, Yu BZ, Qu PF, Zhou YX, Chen JY. Plasma fibrinogen exhibits better performance than plasma d-dimer in the diagnosis of periprosthetic joint infection: a multicenter retrospective study. J Bone Joint Surg Am. 2019;101(7):613–9. https://doi.org/10.2106/JBJS.18.00624.
31. Miao RQ, Cao L, Nueraijiang Y, Zhang XG, Wuhuzi W, Ren JD, Jiang RD, Wang Q. Diagnostic value of D-dimer for chronic periprosthetic infection after hip and knee joint replacement.
32. Qian Hu , Yaoyang Fu , Lingli Tang . Serum D-dimer as a diagnostic index of PJI and retrospective analysis of etiology in patients with PJI. Clin Chim Acta 2020:506:67–71. https://doi.org/10.1016/j.cca.2020.03.023. Epub 2020 Mar 13.
33. Li Xue, Li Tao, Xueyi Li, Yan Wang, Biao Wang, Yanping Zhang, Ning Gao, Yanying Dong, Nan Xu, Chaoliang Xiong, Ting Zhou, Zeshi Liu, Hailong Liu, Juntao He, Ke Li. Plasma fibrinogen, d-dimer, and fibrin degradation product as biomarkers of rheumatoid arthritis. Scientific Reports volume 11, Article number: 16903 (2021).
34. Burzynski, L. C. et al. The coagulation and immune systems are directly linked through the activation of interleukin-1alpha by thrombin. Immunity 50, 1033-1042 e1036. https://doi.org/10.1016/j.immuni.2019.03.003.
35. Chen X, Wenwei Qian, Xisheng Weng, Jin Lin, Jin Jin, Yiou Wang & Shibai Zhu Different diagnostic performance of plasma fibrinogen and D-dimer in periprosthetic joint infection: a propensity score matched study. BMC Musculoskeletal Disorders volume 22, Article number: 422 (2021).
36. Cuñé J, Soriano A, Mart.nez JC, Garc.a S, Mensa J. A superficial swab culture is useful for microbiologic diagnosis in acute prosthetic joint infections. Clin Orthop Relat Res. 2009;467:531–535. https://doi.org/10.1007/s11999-008-0553-4.
37. Aggarwal VK, Higuera C, Deirmengian G, Parvizi J, Austin MS. Swab cultures are not as eff ective as tissue cultures for diagnosis of periprosthetic joint infection. Clin Orthop Relat Res. 2013;471:3196–3203. https://doi.org/10.1007/s11999-013-2974-y.
38. Yee DK, Chiu KY, Yan CH, et al. Review article: joint aspiration for diagnosis of periprosthetic infection. J Orthop Surg (Hong Kong) 2013;21:236–40. https://doi.org/10.1177/230949901302100225.
39. Phillips WC, Kattapuram SV. Efficacy of preoperative hip aspiration performed in the radiology department. Clin Orthop Relat Res 1983:141–6.
40. Ross JJ. Septic Arthritis of Native Joints. Infect Dis Clin North Am. 2017;31(2):203–218. [PubMed].
41. Cooper CA. Centesis studies in critical care. Crit Care Nurs Clin North Am. 2010;22(1):95–108. [PubMed].
42. Partridge DG, Winnard C, Townsend R, et al. Joint aspiration, including culture of reaspirated saline after a 'dry tap', is sensitive and specific for the diagnosis

of hip and knee prosthetic joint infection. Bone Joint J 2018;100B:749–54. https://doi.org/10.1302/0301-620X.100B6.BJJ-2017-0970.R2.
43. Li R, Lu Q, Chai W, et al. Saline solution lavage and reaspiration for culture with a blood culture system is a feasible method for diagnosing periprosthetic joint infection in patients with insufficient synovial fluid. J Bone Joint Surg 2019;101:1004–9. https://doi.org/10.2106/JBJS.18.01052.
44. Yui JC, Preskill C, Greenlund LS. Arthrocentesis and joint injection in patients receiving direct oral anticoagulants. Mayo Clin Proc 2017;92:1223–6. https://doi.org/10.1016/j.mayocp.2017.04.007.
45. Parvizi J, Delia Valle CJ. AAOS clinical practice guideline: Diagnosis and treatment of periprosthetic joint infections of the hip and knee. J Am Acad Orthop Surg 2010;18:771–2. https://doi.org/10.5435/00124635-201012000-00007
46. Trampuz A, Hanssen AD, Osmon DR, et al. Synovial fluid leukocyte count and differential for the diagnosis of prosthetic knee infection. Am J Med 2004; 117:556-62. https://doi.org/10.1016/j.amjmed.2004.06.022.
47. Sendi P, Müller AM, Berbari E. Are all joints equal? Synovial fluid analysis in periprosthetic joint infection. J Bone Joint Infect 2018;3:258–9. https://doi.org/10.7150/jbji.30491.
48. De Vecchi E, Romanò CL, De Grandi R, et al. Alpha defensin, leukocyte esterase, C-reactive protein, and leukocyte count in synovial fluid for pre-operative diagnosis of periprosthetic infection. Int J Immunopathol Pharmacol 2018;32:2058738418806072. https://doi.org/10.1177/2058738418806072.
49. Marson BA, Deshmukh SR, Grindlay DJC, et al. Alpha-defensin and the Synovasure lateral flow device for the diagnosis of prosthetic joint infection: a systematic review and meta-analysis. Bone Joint J 2018;100-B(6):703–11. https://doi.org/10.1302/0301620X.100B6.BJJ-2017-1563.R1.
50. Zhang Z, Cai Y, Bai G, Zhang C, Li W, Yang B, Zhang W. The value of calprotectin in synovial fluid for the diagnosis of chronic prosthetic joint infection Bone Joint Res. 2020;9(8):450–457. https://doi.org/10.1302/2046-375898BJR-2019-0329.R2 eCollection 2020 Aug.
51. Shmerling RH, Synovial fluid analysis. A Critical Reappraisal. Rheumatic disease clinics of North America 1994;20:503–12.
52. Shmerling RH, Delbanco TL. Synovial fluid test. What should be ordered? JAMA 1990; 264:1009-14.
53. Shirtliff ME, Mader JT. Acute Septic Arthritis. Clinical Microbiology Reviews 2002;15:527–44.
54. Barrack RL, Harris WH. The value of aspiration of the hip joint before revision total hip arthroplasty. J Bone Joint Surg Am 1993;75:66–76 https://doi.org/10.2106/00004623-199301000-00010.
55. Deirmengian C, Kardos K, Kilmartin P, Cameron A, Schiller K, Parvizi J. Diagnosing periprosthetic joint infection: has the era of the biomarker arrived? Clin Orthop Relat Res. 2014;472(11):3254–62.
56. Yoon H-K, Cho S-H, Lee D-Y, Kang B-H, Lee S-H, Moon D-G, et al. A review of the literature on culture-negative periprosthetic joint infection: epidemiology, diagnosis and treatment. Knee Surg Relat Res 2017;29:155–64.
57. Indelli PF, Ghirardelli S, Violante B, Amanatullah DF. "Next-Generation Sequencing for Pathogen Detection in Periprosthetic Joint Infections". EFORT Open Reviews. EOR. 6(4):2001. https://doi.org/10.1302/2058-5241.6.200099.
58. Saeed K (2014) Diagnostics in prosthetic joint infections. J Antimicrob Chemother 69(Suppl 1):i11–i19. https://doi.org/10.1093/jac/dku248.
59. Saeed K, Ahmad N, Pallett A, Guiver M, Marsh P (2010) Specific staphylococcal polymerase chain reaction can be a complementary tool for identifying causative organisms and guiding antibiotic management in orthopaedic infections. Curr Ortho Pract 21:628–631.
60. Saeed K, Ahmad-Saeed N (2015) The impact of PCR in the management of prosthetic joint infections. Expert Rev Mol Diagn 15(7):957–964. https://doi.org/10.1586/14737159. 2015. 10464 37
61. Esteban J, Salar-Vidal L, Schmitt BH, Waggoner A, et al (2023) Multicenter evaluation of the BIOFIRE Joint Infection Panel for the detection of bacteria, yeast, and AMR genes in synovial fluid samples. J Clin Microbiology.
62. Huang Z, Li W, Lee GC, et al. Metagenomic next-generation sequencing of synovial fluid demonstrates high accuracy in prosthetic joint infection diagnostics: mNGS for diagnosing PJI. Bone Joint Res 2020; 9:440–449.
63. Mei J, Hu H, Zhu S, Ding H, Huang Z, Li W, Yang B, Zhang W, Fang X. Diagnostic role of mNGS in polymicrobial periprosthetic joint infec-tion. J. Clin. Med. 2022, 10.
64. Goswami K, Clarkson S, Caleb DP, Dennis D, et al. An Enhanced Understanding of Culture-Negative Periprosthetic Joint Infection with Next Generation Sequencing. JBJS-AM, 2022, 104, 1523–1529.
65. Fernandez-Rodriguez D, Baker CM, Tarabichi Saad, Johnson EE et al. The Mark Coventry Award: Human Knee has a Distinct Microbiome. Implications for Periprosthetic Joint Infections. J Arthroplasty (2023) 38, S2-S6.
66. Lyons CW, Berquist TH, Lyons JC, et al. Evaluation of radiographic findings in painful hip arthroplasties. Clin Orthop Relat Res 1985;(195):239–51.
67. Math KR, Zaidi SF, Petchprapa C, et al. Imaging of total knee arthroplasty. Semin Musculoskelet Radiol 2006;10:47–63. https://doi.org/10.1055/s-2006-934216.
68. Berquist TH, Bender CE. Maus TP, Ward EM, Rand JA. Pseudobursae: a useful finding in patients with painful hip arthroplasty AJR Am J Roentgenol, 148 (1) (1987), pp. 103–106.
69. Soliman SB, Davis JJ., Muh SJ., Vohra ST., van Holsbeeck MT. Ultrasound evaluations and guided procedures of the painful joint arthroplasty. Skeletal radiology volume 51, pages 2105–2120 (2022)

70. Klauser AS, Tagliafico A, Allen GM, et al. Clinical indications for musculoskeletal ultrasound: a Delphi-based consensus paper of the European Society of Musculoskeletal Radiology. Eur Radiol. 2012;22:1140–8.
71. Plodkowski AJ, Hayter CL, Miller TT, et al. Lamellated hyper-intense synovitis: potential MR imaging sign of an infected knee arthroplasty. Radiology 2013;266:256–60. https://doi.org/10.1148/radiol.12120042.
72. Lee YH, Lim D, Kim E, et al. Usefulness of slice encoding for metal artifact correction (SEMAC) for reducing metallic artifacts in 3-T MRI. Magn Reson Imaging 2013;31:703–6. https://doi.org/10.1016/j.mri.2012.11.004.
73. Li AE, Sneag D, Greditzer HG 4th, et al. Total knee arthroplasty: diagnostic accuracy of patterns of synovitis at MR imaging. Radiology 2016;281:499–506. https://doi.org/10.1148/radiol.2016152828.
74. Cyteval C, Hamm V, Sarrabère MP, et al.Painful infection at the site of hip prosthesis: CT imaging. Radiology 2002;224:477–83. https://doi.org/10.1148/radiol.2242010989.
75. Cahir JG, Toms AP, Marshall TJ, et al. CT and MRI of hip arthroplasty. Clin Radiol 2007;62(12):1163–1171; discussion 1172–1173. https://doi.org/10.1016/j.crad.2007.04.018
76. Love C, Marwin SE, Palestro CJ. Nuclear medicine and the infected joint replacement. Semin Nucl Med 2009;39:66–78 https://doi.org/10.1053/j.semnuclmed.2008.08.007
77. Ouyang Z, Li H, Liu X, et al. Prosthesis infection: diagnosis after total joint arthroplasty with three-phase bone scintigraphy. Ann Nucl Med 2014;28:994–1003. https://doi.org/10.1007/s12149-014-0899-5.
78. Glaudemans AW, de Vries EF, Vermeulen LE, et al. A large retrospective single-centre study to define the best image acquisition protocols and interpretation criteria for white blood cell scintigraphy with 99mTc-HMPAO-labelled leucocytes in musculoskeletal infections. Eur J Nucl Med Mol Imaging 2013;40:1760–9 https://doi.org/10.1007/s00259-013-2481-0.
79. Signore A, Sconfienza LM, Borens O, et al. Consensus document for the diagnosis of prosthetic joint infections: a joint paper by the EANM, EBJIS, and ESR (with ESCMID endorsement). Eur J Nucl Med Mol Imaging 2019; 46:971-88. https://doi.org/10.1007/s00259-019-4263-9.
80. Roca M, de Vries EF, Jamar F, et al. Guidelines for the labelling of leucocytes with (111) In-oxine. Inflammation/Infection Taskgroup of the European Association of Nuclear Medicine.Eur J Nucl Med Mol Imaging 2010;37:835–41. https://doi.org/10.1007/s00259-010-1393-5.
81. De Vries EF, Roca M, Jamar F, et al. Guidelines for the labelling of leucocytes with (99m) Tc-HMPAO. Inflammation Infection Taskgroup of the European Association of Nuclear Medicine. Eur J Nucl Med Mol Imagin g 2010; 37:842-8. https://doi.org/10.1007/s00259-010-1394-4.
82. Love C, Tomas M B, Tronco G G, Palestro C J. FDG PET of infection and inflammation 1. Radiographics 2005;25(5):1357–68.
83. Manthey N, Reinhard P, Moog F, Knesewitsch P, Hahn K, Tatsch K. The use of [18 F] fluorodeoxyglucose positron emission tomography to differentiate between synovitis, loosening and infection of hip and knee prostheses. Nucl Med Commun 2002;23(7):645–53.
84. Palestro C J. Radionuclide imaging of osteomyelitis. Semin Nucl Med 2015;45(1):32–46.
85. Klement MR, Siddiqi A, Rock JM, et al. Positive blood cultures in periprosthetic joint infection decrease rate of treatment success. J Arthroplasty 2018;33:200-204.e1. https://doi.org/10.1016/j.arth.2017.08.034.
86. Kuo FC, Goswami K, Klement MR, Shohat N, Parvizi J. Positive blood cultures decrease the treatment success in acute hematogenous periprosthetic joint infection treated with debridement, antibiotics, and implant retention. J Arthroplast. 2019;34(12):3030–3034.e1. https://doi.org/10.1016/j.arth.2019.06.053. Epub 2019 Jul 1. PMID: 31376976
87. Zeller V. Kerroumi Y. Meyssonnier V. Heym B. Metten M.A. Desplaces N. et alAnalysis of postoperative and hematogenous prosthetic joint-infection microbiological patterns in a large cohort.J Infect. 2018;76:328–334.
88. Romanò CL, Romanò D, Morelli I, et al. The concept of biofilm-related implant malfunction and "low-grade infection". Adv Exp Med Biol 2017;971:1–13. https://doi.org/10.1007/5584_2016_158 https://doi.org/10.1007/5584_2016_158.
89. Sendi P. Banderet F. Graber P. Zimmerli W. Clinical comparison between exogenous and haematogenous periprosthetic joint infections caused by Staphylococcus aureus.Clin Microbiol Infect. 2011;17:1098–1100.
90. Romanò CL, Romanò D, Morelli I, et al. The concept of biofilm-related implant malfunction and "low-grade infection". Adv Exp Med Biol 2017;971:1–13. https://doi.org/10.1007/5584_2016_158.
91. Trampuz A, Piper KE, Jacobson MJ, et al. Sonication of removed hip and knee prostheses for diagnosis of infection. N Engl J Med 2007;357:654–63. https://doi.org/10.1056/NEJMoa061588
92. Drago L, Signori V, De Vecchi E, et al. Use of dithiothreitol to improve the diagnosis of prosthetic joint infections. J Orthop Res 2013;31:1694–9. https://doi.org/10.1002/jor.22423.
93. Alijanipour P, Adeli B, Hansen EN, et al. Intraoperative purulence is not reliable for diagnosing periprosthetic joint infection. J Arthroplasty 2015;30:1403–6. https://doi.org/10.1016/j.arth.2015.03.005.
94. Jacobs JJ, Gilbert JL, Urban RM. Corrosion of metal orthopaedic implants. J Bone Joint Surg Am 1998;80:268–82. https://doi.org/10.2106/00004623-199802000-00015.
95. Judd KT, Noiseux N. Concomitant infection and local metal reaction in patients undergoing revision of metal on metal total hip arthroplasty. Iowa Orthop J 2011;31:59–63.

96. Watters TS, Eward WC, Hallows RK, et al. Pseudotumor with superimposed periprosthetic infection following met-al-on-metal total hip arthroplasty: a case report. J Bone Joint Surg Am 2010;92:1666-9. https://doi.org/10.2106/JBJS.I.01208.
97. Malech HL, Deleo FR, Quinn MT. The role of neutrophils in the immune system: an overview. Methods Mol Biol 2014;1124:3–10. https://doi.org/10.1007/978-1-62703-845-401.
98. Kim TY, Kim SJ, Lee YK, et al. Accumulation of fatty marrow in the osteonecrotic hip mimicking joint infection. Clin Orthop Relat Res 2012;470:877–82. https://doi.org/10.1007/s11999-011-2048-y.
99. McNally M, Sousa R, Wouthuyzen-Bakker M, Chen AF, Soriano A, Vogely HC, et al. The EBJIS definition of periprosthetic joint infection: a practical guide for clinicians. Bone Joint J. 2021; 103:18–25 This paper represents a project of the European Bone and Joint Infection Society (EBJIS) and represents a novel treatment algorithm that was formed at the annual EBJIS meeting in 2018 with over 450 delegates.
100. Shohat N, Tan TL, Della Valle CJ, Calkins TE, George J, Higuera C, et al. Development and validation of an evidence-based algorithm for diagnosing periprosthetic joint infection. J Arthroplast. 2019; 34:2730–2736.e1

# 7 New Diagnostic Tools for the Diagnosis of Periprosthetic Joint Infection

Saad Tarabichi, Elizabeth A. Abe, Juan D. Lizcano, and Javad Parvizi

## 7.1 Introduction

Total joint arthroplasty (TJA) is one of the most common elective procedures worldwide [1]. Periprosthetic joint infection (PJI) is a devastating complication and a well-documented cause of implant failure following arthroplasty procedures [2]. Despite concerted international efforts, large arthroplasty registries have demonstrated that the incidence of PJI is on the rise [3]. Recent estimates have placed the incidence of PJI between 0.5 and 2% after total knee arthroplasty (TKA) and 0.5–1% after total hip arthroplasty (THA).

The diagnosis of PJI remains challenging as a single "gold standard" test with absolute accuracy has not yet been identified [4, 5]. Physicians often rely on a combination of serological tests, synovial markers, intraoperative findings, and clinical judgment in the workup of patients with a painful prosthetic joint [6]. In recent years, advancements in technology have provided surgeons with new modalities to improve diagnostic confidence in this setting [7]. However, the introduction of multiple novel tests that have not been robustly validated has led to confusion regarding appropriate test selection and questions surrounding their cost-effectiveness [8, 9].

In order to ensure that a diagnosis of PJI is not missed, physicians must employ a high index of suspicion in all patients presenting with a painful prosthesis. Regardless of the affected joint, the diagnosis of PJI typically involves two steps. Patients first undergo venipuncture for analysis of serological markers; if these markers are elevated, arthrocentesis is then performed, and synovial fluid is sent off for biomarker evaluation. The second step in the diagnosis of PJI involves the attempted identification of the infecting organism. In addition to biomarker testing, culture is routinely performed on synovial fluid obtained during arthrocentesis, as this may facilitate targeted antimicrobial therapy, which in turn greatly improves the chances of treatment success [10–12]. For over a century, culture has been the gold standard for identifying pathogens in this setting. However, it can still miss up to 45% of infecting organisms, emphasizing the need for improved diagnostic tests [13].

S. Tarabichi
Department of Orthopaedic Surgery, Mayo Clinic Arizona, Phoenix, USA

E. A. Abe
Department of Orthopaedic Surgery, Mayo Clinic Rochester, Rochester, USA
e-mail: abe.elizabeth@mayo.edu

J. D. Lizcano
Department of Orthopaedic Surgery, University of Florida, Gainesville, USA
e-mail: jlizcano78@gmail.com

J. Parvizi (✉)
International Joint Center, Acibadem University, Istanbul, Turkey


P. Ruggieri et al. (eds.), *Bone and Joint Infections*, https://doi.org/10.1007/978-3-031-96383-4_7

The purpose of this chapter is to provide an overview of new diagnostic tests that are currently being utilized to help identify PJI.

## 7.2 New Diagnostic Tools

### 7.2.1 Serological Tests

#### 7.2.1.1 D-dimer

D-dimer has garnered attention following reports of its ability to predict outcomes in patients with bacteremia and sepsis [14, 15]. Recently, there has been data in the orthopedic literature to suggest that D-dimer can be a useful marker for the diagnosis of PJI. In a study by Shahi et al., serum D-dimer (sensitivity 89%, specificity 93%) was found to have the best diagnostic utility for the diagnosis of PJI of the hip and knee, outperforming both C-reactive protein (CRP) (sensitivity 79%, specificity 80%) and erythrocyte sedimentation rate (ESR) (sensitivity 73%, specificity 78%) [16]. Furthermore, Tarabichi et al. found that plasma D-dimer demonstrated the highest sensitivity (94%) for the diagnosis of PJI caused by indolent organisms [17]. Despite this, several studies have also put into question the diagnostic utility of D-dimer for PJI. Li et al. found that at a threshold of 1250 ng/mL, plasma D-dimer yielded an AUC of 0.657, sensitivity of 64%, and specificity of 65% in the diagnosis of PJI [18]. Nevertheless, it is important to recognize that D-dimer levels may be falsely elevated in patients with certain medical conditions including systemic inflammatory diseases and cancer [19].

#### 7.2.1.2 Fibrinogen

While originally described as an important meditator of neutrophil adherence in patients with sepsis, fibrinogen has gained traction as a potential marker for the diagnosis of PJI [20]. In a study by Yang et al., fibrinogen was found to have an AUC of 0.916, sensitivity of 86.0%, and specificity of 90.0% [21]. In contrast, CRP had an AUC of 0.901, sensitivity of 91.2%, and specificity of 82.7%, while ESR had an AUC of 0.822, sensitivity of 70.2%, and specificity of 85.9%. Xu et al.. performed a meta-analysis of the literature and found that fibrinogen had a AUC, sensitivity, and specificity of 0.830, 79%, and 73%, respectively [22]. There has also been recent data to suggest that plasma fibrinogen may be useful in patients with a known history of coagulation-related abnormalities [23].

#### 7.2.1.3 Neutrophil-to-Lymphocyte Ratio

Serum neutrophil-to-lymphocyte ratio (NLR) was first identified as a predictor of adverse outcomes in patients with cardiovascular disease and cancer [24, 25]. In a study of 245 revision TKA patients, Yu et al. found that serum NLR (AUC 0.802, sensitivity 85.0%, specificity 68.3%) outperformed CRP (AUC 0.793, sensitivity 70.0%, specificity 79.2%), ESR (AUC 0.744, sensitivity 63.2%, specificity 74.0%), and WBC count (AUC 0.632, sensitivity 35.0%, specificity 94.1%) in the diagnosis of acute PJI [26]. Conversely, a separate study of 158 revision TJA patients by Ye et al. found poor overall accuracy with an AUC of 0.660, sensitivity of 57.4%, and specificity of 77.9% [27]. Additionally, a recent meta-analysis found that NLR had a pooled sensitivity and specificity of 72.0% and 74.0%, respectively, for hip and knee PJI [28].

#### 7.2.1.4 Procalcitonin

Procalcitonin (PCT) is primarily produced by parafollicular and neuroendocrine cells [29]. As such, a number of studies have attempted to determine the utility of PCT in the diagnosis of PJI. In a recent metanalysis that included 1835 patients, Yoon et al. found that serum PCT had a pooled AUC, sensitivity, and specificity of 0.830, 53%, and 92%, respectively [30]. Similarly, Busch et al. found that serum PCT, using a cutoff of 0.1 ng/mL, exhibited a sensitivity and specificity of 26% and 81%, respectively [31]. Given its low sensitivity, serum PCT is currently not utilized in the workup of patients with a painful prosthesis.

#### 7.2.1.5 Platelet Count to Mean Platelet Volume Ratio

It is now well-established that activated platelets possess antimicrobial properties [32]. In a study of 4938 revision TJA patients, Paziuk et al. found that when using a threshold of 31.7, serum PC/mPV ratio demonstrated an AUC of 0.690, sensitivity of 48.1%, and specificity of 80.9% for the diagnosis of PJI [33]. In contrast, CRP and ESR both demonstrated significantly higher accuracy, with a reported AUC of 0.872 and 0.851, respectively. Another study of 538 revision TKAs by Tirumala et al. found that PC/mPV ratio, at a cutoff of 30.8, exhibited an AUC of 0.850, sensitivity of 87.9%, and specificity of 75.9% [34].

### 7.2.2 Synovial Tests

#### 7.2.2.1 Mass Spectrometry

Mass spectrometry (MS) is best known for its superior accuracy in the identification of different microbial species [35]. More recently, MS has also demonstrated near perfect accuracy in the diagnosis of PJI, with one study reporting an AUC of 0.975 [36]. Notwithstanding, MS machines are expensive and require highly trained laboratory personnel to be able to perform analyses. As a result, spectro-analysis is often inaccessible and is therefore not routinely performed in patients with suspected PJI.

#### 7.2.2.2 Alpha Defensin

Over the last few years, many studies have attempted to determine the diagnostic value of alpha-defensin in the identification of PJI. Although most synovial markers have demonstrated high accuracy [37–39], Frangiamore et al. found that alpha-defensin outperformed other markers, yielding an AUC of 0.950, sensitivity of 100%, and specificity of 98% [40]. However, it is important to note that three recent studies have shown no additional benefit to the routine measurement of alpha-defensin as its diagnostic accuracy was comparable to other readily available synovial markers such as WBC count and PMN% [41–43]. While the utility of alpha-defensin as a routine screening test for all patients undergoing revision TJA may be limited, it can be a useful adjunct to aid in diagnosis of PJI for patients with equivocal laboratory findings.

#### 7.2.2.3 Synovial C-Reactive Protein

Synovial CRP first gained attention following reports on its diagnostic utility in the workup of patients with inflammatory arthritis [44]. Subsequently, in a study of 64 patients undergoing revision TKA, Parvizi et al. found that synovial CRP exhibited an AUC of 0.910, sensitivity of 84.0%, and specificity of 97.1% in the diagnosis of PJI [45]. In a more recent study of 612 revision TJAs, Baker et al. demonstrated that synovial CRP, at a cutoff of 6.9 mg/L, yielded an AUC of 0.951, sensitivity of 74.2%, and specificity of 98.0% [46]. Furthermore, they also found that although the correlation between serum and synovial CRP was strong ($r = 0.703$), it was not completely linear, leading them to hypothesize that synovial cells were also capable of local CRP production.

#### 7.2.2.4 Synovial Interlukin-6

Given the recent inclusion of serum IL-6 in the AAOS guidelines [47], several studies have also attempted to ascertain the diagnostic value of synovial IL-6 in patients with suspected PJI. In a study of 73 revision TJA patients, Jacovides et al. demonstrated an AUC of 0.950, sensitivity of 87.1%, and specificity of 100% using a synovial IL-6 threshold of 4270 pg/mL [48]. A recent meta-analysis by Xie et al. found a pooled AUC of 0.960, sensitivity of 91%, and specificity of 90% in the diagnosis of hip, knee, and shoulder PJI. However, due to the wide range of proposed diagnostic thresholds (359.3 pg/mL–13,350 pg/mL), the authors concluded that the utilization of a universal cut-off for synovial IL-6 may not yet be suitable.

#### 7.2.2.5 Calprotectin

Although calprotectin has been widely recognized as a marker for intestinal inflammation, recent studies in the orthopedic literature have evaluated its potential as a biomarker for PJI [49]. In a study by Warren et al., synovial calprotectin, at a threshold of 50 mg/L, was shown to have an AUC of 0.969, sensitivity of 98.1%, and specificity of 95.7% [50]. Furthermore, a meta-analysis by Peng et al. found that synovial calprotectin demonstrated a pooled AUC, sensitivity, and specificity of 0.980, 94.0%, and 93.0%, respectively [51]. However, the literature on calprotectin remains limited, and additional studies with larger sample sizes are required to ascertain its diagnostic utility in the workup of PJI.

### 7.2.3 Pathogen Identification

#### 7.2.3.1 Culture Sonication

Even with the advent of newer technologies, culture remains the most popular test for pathogen isolation in PJI [52]. In a recent meta-analysis, culture demonstrated a pooled sensitivity and specificity of 70% and 97%, respectively, in the diagnosis of PJI [53]. In order to maximize the diagnostic yield of culture, the ICM on musculoskeletal infection recommends that at least 3–5 "high-quality" intraoperative samples be obtained from patients undergoing revision TJA [54]. More recently, sonication of the implant has garnered attention in this setting following promising reports in the literature. This technique disrupts sessile bacteria that are present in biofilm in order to help improve the overall yield of culture. Furthermore, it has been suggested that sonication culture is not impacted by the administration of antibiotics. In one study, the authors found that implant sonication culture demonstrated a sensitivity and specificity of 97% and 90%, respectively, in the diagnosis of PJI [55].

#### 7.2.3.2 Polymerase Chain Reaction and Next-Generation Sequencing

Molecular techniques, such as multiplex polymerase chain reaction (PCR) and next-generation sequencing, can detect and identify bacterial and fungal DNA without the need for isolation on culture [56]. Hence, these techniques are highly sensitive and can significantly increase the chances of pathogen identification, compared to traditional culture [57]. Multiplex PCR, through the use of primers, can detect both microbial DNA and resistance genes. However, its diagnostic capabilities are dependent on the availability of gene-specific primers that only exist for a selection of microbes [58]. Next-generation sequencing (NGS) is another molecular technique that has recently gained traction in this setting following favorable reports in the literature [59, 60]. In contrast to multiplex PCR, NGS targets two specific regions of the rRNA gene: (1) 16S region to detect bacteria and (2) the internal transcribed spacer region to identify fungi. This results in the production of sequence reads that are then referenced against the GenBank database from the National Institute of Health. In a recent study, NGS was capable of identifying a pathogen in 65.9% of culture-negative patients [61]. Nevertheless, as molecular techniques become more readily available, their superior sensitivity and faster turnaround time may allow surgeons to administer more targeted antimicrobial therapy sooner, increasing the chances of treatment success in patients with PJI [62].

## 7.3 Conclusion

Despite significant efforts from the orthopedic community, we are yet to identify a single "gold standard" test for the diagnosis of PJI. Hence, the diagnosis of PJI can be extremely challenging. In this chapter, we highlight new tests that have garnered interest for their utility in the diagnosis of PJI.

## References

1. Sloan M, Premkumar A, Sheth NP. Projected volume of primary total joint arthroplasty in the U.S., 2014 to 2030. J Bone Joint Surg Am. 2018 Sep 5;100(17):1455–60.
2. Kurtz S, Ong K, Lau E, Mowat F, Halpern M. Projections of primary and revision hip and knee arthroplasty in the United States from 2005 to 2030. J Bone Joint Surg Am. 2007 Apr;89(4):780–5.

3. Springer BD, Cahue S, Etkin CD, Lewallen DG, McGrory BJ. Infection burden in total hip and knee arthroplasties: an international registry-based perspective. Arthroplast Today. 2017 Jun;3(2):137–40.
4. Wasterlain AS, Goswami K, Ghasemi SA, Parvizi J. Diagnosis of periprosthetic infection: recent developments. JBJS. 2020 Aug 5;102(15):1366–75.
5. Goh GS, Parvizi J. Diagnosis and treatment of culture-negative periprosthetic joint infection. J Arthroplasty [Internet]. 2022 Jan 31 [cited 2022 May 11]; Available from: https://www.sciencedirect.com/science/article/pii/S0883540322000778
6. Shahi A, Tan TL, Kheir MM, Tan DD, Parvizi J. Diagnosing periprosthetic joint infection: and the winner is? J Arthroplasty. 2017 Sep;32(9S):S232–5.
7. Patel R, Alijanipour P, Parvizi J. Advancements in diagnosing periprosthetic joint infections after total hip and knee arthroplasty. Open Orthop J. 2016;10:654–61.
8. Tarabichi S, Chen AF, Higuera CA, Parvizi J, Polkowski GG. 2022 American association of hip and knee surgeons symposium: periprosthetic joint infection. J Arthroplasty. 2023 Feb 2;S0883–5403(23):00065–7.
9. Diaz-Ledezma C, Lichstein PM, Dolan JG, Parvizi J. Diagnosis of periprosthetic joint infection in Medicare patients: multicriteria decision analysis. Clin Orthop Relat Res. 2014 Nov;472(11):3275–84.
10. Yang J, Parvizi J, Hansen EN, Culvern CN, Segreti JC, Tan T, et al. 2020 Mark Coventry Award: microorganism-directed oral antibiotics reduce the rate of failure due to further infection after two-stage revision hip or knee arthroplasty for chronic infection: a multicentre randomized controlled trial at a minimum of two years. Bone Joint J. 2020 Jun;102-B(6_Supple_A):3–9.
11. Patel R, Osmon DR, Hanssen AD. The diagnosis of prosthetic joint infection: current techniques and emerging technologies. Clin Orthop Relat Res. 2005 Aug;437:55–8.
12. Tarabichi S, Goh GS, Zanna L, Qadiri QS, Baker CM, Gehrke T, et al. Time to positivity of cultures obtained for periprosthetic joint infection. J Bone Joint Surg Am. 2023 Jan 18;105(2):107–12.
13. Palan J, Nolan C, Sarantos K, Westerman R, King R, Foguet P. Culture-negative periprosthetic joint infections. EFORT Open Rev. 2019 Oct 7;4(10):585–94.
14. Pulivarthi S, Gurram MK. Effectiveness of D-dimer as a screening test for venous thromboembolism: an update. N Am J Med Sci. 2014 Oct;6(10):491–9.
15. Han YQ, Yan L, Zhang L, Ouyang PH, Li P, Lippi G, et al. Performance of D-dimer for predicting sepsis mortality in the intensive care unit. Biochem Med (Zagreb). 2021 Jun 15;31(2):020709.
16. Shahi A, Kheir MM, Tarabichi M, Hosseinzadeh HRS, Tan TL, Parvizi J. Serum D-dimer test is promising for the diagnosis of periprosthetic joint infection and timing of reimplantation. J Bone Joint Surg Am. 2017 Sep 6;99(17):1419–27.
17. Tarabichi S, Goh GS, Baker CM, Chisari E, Shahi A, Parvizi J. Plasma D-dimer is noninferior to serum C-reactive protein in the diagnosis of periprosthetic joint infection. J Bone Joint Surg Am. 2023 Feb 9;105(7):501–8.
18. Li R, Shao HY, Hao LB, Yu BZ, Qu PF, Zhou YX, et al. Plasma fibrinogen exhibits better performance than plasma D-dimer in the diagnosis of periprosthetic joint infection: a multicenter retrospective study. J Bone Joint Surg Am. 2019 Apr 3;101(7):613–9.
19. ten Wolde M, Kraaijenhagen RA, Prins MH, Büller HR. The clinical usefulness of D-dimer testing in cancer patients with suspected deep venous thrombosis. Arch Intern Med. 2002 Sep 9;162(16):1880–4.
20. Kirschenbaum LA, McKevitt D, Rullan M, Reisbeck B, Fujii T, Astiz ME. Importance of platelets and fibrinogen in neutrophil-endothelial cell interactions in septic shock. Crit Care Med. 2004 Sep;32(9):1904–9.
21. Yang F, Zhao C, Huang R, Ma H, Wang X, Wang G, et al. Plasma fibrinogen in the diagnosis of periprosthetic joint infection. Sci Rep. 2021 Jan 12;11(1):677.
22. Xu H, Xie JW, Yang JL, Huang ZY, Pei FX. Role of D-dimer and fibrinogen in the diagnosis of periprosthetic joint infection: a systematic review and meta-analysis. Orthop Surg. 2021;13(3):692–700.
23. Xu H, Xie J, Yang J, Chen G, Huang Q, Pei F. Plasma fibrinogen and platelet count are referable tools for diagnosing periprosthetic joint infection: a single-center retrospective cohort study. J Arthroplasty. 2020 May 1;35(5):1361–7.
24. Angkananard T, Anothaisintawee T, McEvoy M, Attia J, Thakkinstian A. Neutrophil lymphocyte ratio and cardiovascular disease risk: a systematic review and meta-analysis. BioMed Res Int. 2018 Nov 11;2018:e2703518.
25. Boissier R, Campagna J, Branger N, Karsenty G, Lechevallier E. The prognostic value of the neutrophil-lymphocyte ratio in renal oncology: a review. Urol Oncol: Semin Orig Investig. 2017 Apr 1;35(4):135–41.
26. Yu BZ, Fu J, Chai W, Hao LB, Chen JY. Neutrophil to lymphocyte ratio as a predictor for diagnosis of early Periprosthetic joint infection. BMC Musculoskelet Disord. 2020 Dec;21(1):1–7.
27. Ye Y, Chen W, Gu M, Liu Q, Xian G, Pan B, et al. Limited value of serum neutrophil-to-lymphocyte ratio in the diagnosis of chronic periprosthetic joint infection. J Orthop Traumatol. 2021 Sep 18;22(1):37.
28. Festa E, Ascione T, Bernasconi A, Di Gennaro D, Basso MA, Guarino A, et al. Diagnostic performance of neutrophil to lymphocyte ratio, monocyte to lymphocyte ratio, platelet to lymphocyte ratio, and platelet to mean platelet volume ratio in periprosthetic hip and knee infections: a systematic review and meta-analysis. Diagnostics. 2022 Sep;12(9):2033.
29. Vijayan AL, Vanimaya RS, Saikant R, Lakshmi S, Kartik R, et al. Procalcitonin: a promising diagnostic marker for sepsis and antibiotic therapy. J Intensive Care. 2017 Aug 3;5(1):51.

30. Yoon JR, Yang SH, Shin YS. Diagnostic accuracy of interleukin-6 and procalcitonin in patients with periprosthetic joint infection: a systematic review and meta-analysis. Int Orthop. 2018 Jun;42(6):1213–26.
31. Busch A, Jäger M, Engler H, Haversath M, Bielefeld C, Landgraeber S, et al. Is Procalcitonin (PCT) a reliable biomarker for preoperative diagnosing of low grade periprosthetic joint infection? A prospective study. BMC Musculoskelet Disord. 2020 Apr;20(21):257.
32. Gaertner F, Ahmad Z, Rosenberger G, Fan S, Nicolai L, Busch B, et al. Migrating platelets are mechano-scavengers that collect and bundle bacteria. Cell. 2017 Nov 30;171(6):1368–1382.e23.
33. Paziuk T, Rondon AJ, Goswami K, Tan TL, Parvizi J. A novel adjunct indicator of periprosthetic joint infection: platelet count and mean platelet volume. J Arthroplasty. 2020 Mar 1;35(3):836–9.
34. Tirumala V, Klemt C, Xiong L, Chen W, van den Kieboom J, Kwon YM. Diagnostic utility of platelet count/lymphocyte count ratio and platelet count/mean platelet volume ratio in periprosthetic joint infection following total knee arthroplasty. J Arthroplasty. 2021 Jan;36(1):291–7.
35. Fox A. Mass spectrometry for species or strain identification after culture or without culture: past, present, and future. J Clin Microbiol. 2006 Aug;44(8):2677–80.
36. Li R, Song L, Quan Q, Liu MW, Chai W, Lu Q, et al. Detecting periprosthetic joint infection by using mass spectrometry. J Bone Joint Surg Am. 2021 Oct 20;103(20):1917–26.
37. Parvizi J, Jacovides C, Antoci V, Ghanem E. Diagnosis of periprosthetic joint infection: the utility of a simple yet unappreciated enzyme. JBJS. 2011 Dec 21;93(24):2242–8.
38. Lee YS, Koo KH, Kim HJ, Tian S, Kim TY, Maltenfort MG, et al. Synovial fluid biomarkers for the diagnosis of periprosthetic joint infection: a systematic review and meta-analysis. J Bone Joint Surg Am. 2017 Dec 20;99(24):2077–84.
39. Deirmengian C, Kardos K, Kilmartin P, Cameron A, Schiller K, Parvizi J. Diagnosing periprosthetic joint infection: has the era of the biomarker arrived? Clin Orthop Relat Res. 2014 Nov;472(11):3254–62.
40. Frangiamore SJ, Gajewski ND, Saleh A, Farias-Kovac M, Barsoum WK, Higuera CA. A-defensin accuracy to diagnose periprosthetic joint infection-best available test? J Arthroplasty. 2016 Feb;31(2):456–60.
41. Ivy MI, Sharma K, Greenwood-Quaintance KE, Tande AJ, Osmon DR, Berbari EF, et al. Synovial fluid α defensin has comparable accuracy to synovial fluid white blood cell count and polymorphonuclear percentage for periprosthetic joint infection diagnosis. Bone Joint J. 2021 Jun;103-B(6):1119–26.
42. Kleeman-Forsthuber LT, Johnson RM, Brady AC, Pollet AK, Dennis DA, Jennings JM. Alpha-defensin offers limited utility in routine workup of periprosthetic joint infection. J Arthroplasty. 2021 May;36(5):1746–52.
43. Heckmann ND, Wang JC, Liu KC, Won P, Chung BC, Mayer L, et al. Refining the role of routine synovial alpha-defensin in periprosthetic joint infection following total knee arthroplasty: an analysis of limitations. J Arthroplasty [Internet]. 2023 Jun 8 [cited 2023 Jun 12]; Available from: https://www.sciencedirect.com/science/article/pii/S088354032300637X
44. Zamani B, Jamali R, Ehteram H. Synovial fluid adenosine deaminase and high-sensitivity C-reactive protein activity in differentiating monoarthritis. Rheumatol Int. 2012 Jan 1;32(1):183–8.
45. Parvizi J, Jacovides C, Adeli B, Jung KA, Hozack WJ, Mark B. Coventry award: synovial c-reactive protein: a prospective evaluation of a molecular marker for periprosthetic knee joint infection. Clin Orthop Relat Res. 2012 Jan;470(1):54–60.
46. Baker CM, Goh GS, Tarabichi S, Shohat N, Parvizi J. Synovial C-reactive protein is a useful adjunct for diagnosis of periprosthetic joint infection. J Arthroplasty. 2022 Jun 22;S0883–5403(22):00678–7.
47. Tubb CC, Polkowksi GG, Krause B. Diagnosis and prevention of periprosthetic joint infections. J Am Acad Orthop Surg. 2020 Apr;28(8):e340–8.
48. Jacovides CL, Parvizi J, Adeli B, Jung KA. Molecular markers for diagnosis of periprosthetic joint infection. J Arthroplasty. 2011 Sep;26(6 Suppl):99–103.e1.
49. Summerton CB, Longlands MG, Wiener K, Shreeve DR. Faecal calprotectin: a marker of inflammation throughout the intestinal tract. Eur J Gastroenterol Hepatol. 2002 Aug;14(8):841–5.
50. Warren J, Anis HK, Bowers K, Pannu T, Villa J, Klika AK, et al. Diagnostic utility of a novel point-of-care test of calprotectin for periprosthetic joint infection after total knee arthroplasty: a prospective cohort study. J Bone Joint Surg Am. 2021 Jun 2;103(11):1009–15.
51. Peng X, Zhang H, Xin P, Bai G, Ge Y, Cai M, et al. Synovial calprotectin for the diagnosis of periprosthetic joint infection: a diagnostic meta-analysis. J Orthop Surg Res. 2022 Jan 4;17(1):2.
52. Kim SJ, Cho YJ. Current guideline for diagnosis of periprosthetic joint infection: a review article. Hip Pelvis. 2021 Mar;33(1):11–7.
53. Li C, Ojeda-Thies C, Trampuz A. Culture of periprosthetic tissue in blood culture bottles for diagnosing periprosthetic joint infection. BMC Musculoskelet Disord. 2019 Jun 22;20(1):299.
54. Zmistowski B, Della Valle C, Bauer TW, Malizos KN, Alavi A, Bedair H, et al. Diagnosis of periprosthetic joint infection. J Arthroplasty. 2014 Feb;29(2 Suppl):77–83.
55. Rothenberg AC, Wilson AE, Hayes JP, O'Malley MJ, Klatt BA. Sonication of arthroplasty implants improves accuracy of periprosthetic joint infection cultures. Clin Orthop Relat Res. 2017 Jul;475(7):1827.

56. Tsui CKM, Woodhall J, Chen W, Lévesque CA, Lau A, Schoen CD, et al. Molecular techniques for pathogen identification and fungus detection in the environment. IMA Fungus. 2011 Dec;2(2):177–89.
57. Sigmund IK, Holinka J, Sevelda F, Staats K, Heisinger S, Kubista B, et al. Performance of automated multiplex polymerase chain reaction (mPCR) using synovial fluid in the diagnosis of native joint septic arthritis in adults. Bone Joint J. 2019 Mar;101-B(3):288–96.
58. Fenollar F, Roux V, Stein A, Drancourt M, Raoult D. Analysis of 525 samples to determine the usefulness of PCR amplification and sequencing of the 16S rRNA gene for diagnosis of bone and joint infections. J Clin Microbiol. 2006 Mar;44(3):1018–28.
59. Tarabichi M, Alvand A, Shohat N, Goswami K, Parvizi J. Diagnosis of Streptococcus canis periprosthetic joint infection: the utility of next-generation sequencing. Arthroplast Today. 2018 Mar;4(1):20–3.
60. Tarabichi M, Shohat N, Goswami K, Parvizi J. Can next generation sequencing play a role in detecting pathogens in synovial fluid? Bone Joint J. 2018 Feb;100-B(2):127–33.
61. Goswami K, Clarkson S, Phillips CD, Dennis DA, Klatt BA, O'Malley MJ, et al. An enhanced understanding of culture-negative periprosthetic joint infection with next-generation sequencing: a multicenter study. J Bone Joint Surg Am. 2022 Jun 20;104(17):1523–9.
62. Tarabichi M, Shohat N, Goswami K, Alvand A, Silibovsky R, Belden K, et al. Diagnosis of periprosthetic joint infection: the potential of next-generation sequencing. J Bone Joint Surg Am. 2018 Jan 17;100(2):147–54.

# 8 Osteoarticular Infections in Children

Ashok N. Johari, Ashish S. Ranade, and Raashid Anjum

## 8.1 Introduction

Musculoskeletal infections in pediatric patients present a wide range of conditions, including osteomyelitis, septic arthritis, pyomyositis, abscess, or a combination of these. With the advent of newer investigative modalities, the diagnosis of unusual and subtle infections has increased. The advances in diagnosis and treatment of pediatric musculoskeletal infections have led to decreased morbidity and mortality, however, they still pose a significant risk of morbidity and mortality, especially in developing countries [1, 2]. The reported incidence of musculoskeletal infections in children is 2–13 per 100,000 of the population in developed nations and up to 200 cases/100000 of the population in developing countries with no clear sex predilection [3–5]. There are many studies that report a decrease in the incidence of pediatric musculoskeletal infection over a period of time, and many other studies report the opposite [6, 7]. The incidence of septic arthritis alone in the pediatric age group is reported to be 5.5–12/100000 children, and an increased propensity of males compared to females, up to three times, is seen. The most common joint to be affected in septic arthritis is the hip, followed by knee, and more than 20% of cases can have multiple joint involvement at the same time [8–10]. With the advances in diagnostics, the incidence of pediatric osteoarticular infection has increased. Early diagnosis and management are of pivotal significance for an optimum outcome. Delay in diagnosis is not infrequent, especially in developing countries, due to late presentation, lack of resources, variability in presentation, late or injudicious management, etc., and this is associated with potentially disabling morbidities like limb length discrepancies, angular deformities, and other growth disturbances. The optimum management of musculoskeletal infections in the pediatric age group warrants a coordinated approach between the orthopedic surgeon, radiologist, microbiologist, pediatrician, and allied services [11].

A. N. Johari (✉)
Children's Orthopaedic Centre, Mumbai, India

A. S. Ranade
Deenanath Mangeshkar Hospital, Pune, India

R. Anjum
All India Institute of Medical Sciences, Jammu, India


P. Ruggieri et al. (eds.), *Bone and Joint Infections*, https://doi.org/10.1007/978-3-031-96383-4_8

## 8.2 Etiology

The most common mode of infection is hematogenous spread from a symptomatic or asymptomatic bacteremia or secondary to the contiguous source of infection or a direct inoculation [12]. The commonest microorganism causing acute osteomyelitis or septic arthritis in children is *Staphylococcus aureus,* accounting for 60–90% of cases irrespective of the age group, followed by Streptococcus species and Gram-negative organisms in a small subset of patients (<5%). In neonates, the incidence of Group B Streptococcus sepsis is increased, whereas the incidence of cases with *H. influenzae* has significantly decreased due to the universal immunization for the same. Salmonella sp. should be considered in osteomyelitis of the diaphyseal region and in patients with sickle cell disease. Other commonly encountered bacteria causing infections in the pediatric age group include *Kingella kingae*, *Streptococcus pyogenes*, *Mycobacterium tuberculosis*, atypical mycobacteria, and *N. gonorrhea*; however, this is not an exhaustive list, and there are many reports of infection with uncommon microbial agents. In recent years, the incidence of methicillin-resistant *Staphylococcus aureus* (MRSA) has increased, and the incidence stands at 9–30% as per the published literature [13]. Panton–Valentin Leucocidin (PVL) producing strains of *Staphylococcus aureus* are responsible for extensive tissue necrosis. PVL is a cytotoxin that can be produced by different strains of both methicillin-sensitive *Staphylococcus aureus* (MSSA) and methicillin-resistant *S. aureus* (MRSA) [14]. In a study from Europe, the incidence of PVL-producing strains was found to be 18.6% [15]. The common microorganisms causing musculoskeletal infections at different ages are presented in Table 8.1. This is not an exhaustive list and shows only the common pathogens.

**Table 8.1** Shows commonly encountered microorganisms in different age groups

| Age of child | Microorganisms | Empirical antibiotics |
|---|---|---|
| Neonates (0–4 weeks) | Group A and B *Streptococcus* sp., *Staphylococcus aureus*, *Enterobacter* sp. | First/Second generation Cephalosporin or Oxacillin + Gentamicin |
| 1 month–4 months | *Staphylococcus aureus*, *Klebsiella pneumoniae*, *Streptococcus pyogenes*, *Kingella kingae*, *E. coli*, *Enterobacter* sp. | First/Second generation Cephalosporin Clindamycin |
| 4 months to 04 years | *Staphylococcus aureus*, Group A *Streptococcus* sp., *Kingella kingae*, *Enterobacter* sp. | First/Second generation Cephalosporin. Clindamycin |
| >04 years | *Staphylococcus aureus*, *H. influenzae*, *Enterobacter* sp. Group A B haemolytic Streptococcus | First/Second generation Cephalosporin or Ampicillin Clindamycin |
| Sickle cell patients | *Staphylococcus aureus*, *Salmonella* sp. (Pathognomonic) | First/Second generation Cephalosporin or Ampicillin or Chloramphenicol |

## 8.3 Investigative Modalities in Osteoarticular Infections in Children

The diagnosis of musculoskeletal infections in children is mainly clinical, based on the signs and symptoms as discussed in the subsequent section, and test parameters supplement the clinical diagnosis. However, taking an appropriate history and performing an accurate examination of the child is a challenging task, and the surgeon needs to be extremely perceptive to gather as much information as possible.

## 8.4 Clinical Diagnosis

The clinical presentation of a child with musculoskeletal infection depends upon the type of infection (osteomyelitis/septic arthritis/pyomyositis), the site of infection, virulence of the causative agent, immune status, and age of the child [16]. The common presenting symptoms and signs are pain, fever, inability to bear weight, local warmth, erythema, tenderness, reduced mobility of the affected part, and sick general condition. However, it is not necessary to have all the signs and symptoms in each patient, and there can be a variable presentation. An antecedent history of minor trauma is often present in many cases and should be enquired about. Neonates and infants do not have a fully developed immune system, and the presenting symptoms can be subtle in such cases. A high index of suspicion is required to avoid delays in diagnosis and treatment. A similar subtle presentation is seen in children with immunodeficiency syndromes, malnourishment, and concomitant comorbid conditions like HIV or Tuberculosis. Dartnell J et al. in a systematic review of more than 12,000 cases of pediatric musculoskeletal infections noted the most common clinical feature as localized pain (seen in 81%); local rise of temperature, swelling and tenderness in 70%, fever in 62%, and restricted mobility in 50% of cases [2].

## 8.5 Laboratory Investigations

The investigations that should be obtained in a suspected case of musculoskeletal infection include a complete blood count with erythrocyte sedimentation rate and a differential leucocyte count. The leucocyte count is generally elevated with increased neutrophil count; however, in subacute infections in neonates and children with immunodeficiency, the values can be within normal range. C-reactive protein (CRP), an acute phase reactant, is a sensitive marker of acute infection and should be obtained; it is the single most important independent predictor of infection. An attempt should be made to obtain a tissue/fluid sample wherever possible for culture, sensitivity, and Gram staining. The British Orthopaedic Association and British Society for Children's Orthopaedic Surgery recommend that microbiology samples should be taken prior to antibiotic therapy, but this should not delay treatment in sick children [17]. Dartnell J et al. in a systematic review on acute osteomyelitis noted an increased white blood cell (WBC) count in 36% of children on presentation, raised C-reactive protein (CRP) in 81%, and elevated erythrocyte sedimentation rate (ESR) in 91% of cases [2]. The laboratory markers supplement the clinical suspicion or diagnosis of infection and are not definitive per se. More recently, procalcitonin has emerged as a sensitive and specific indicator of infection; it has a normal range of <0.1 ng/ml and levels above 0.4 ng/ml are highly indicative of infection [18, 19].

Kocher (1999) laid down criteria for the diagnosis of septic arthritis of hip and to differentiate it from a benign transient synovitis of hip [20]. The original criteria included the following parameters

1. Inability to bear weight
2. Temperature > 38° C
3. WBC > 12,000/$mm^3$
4. ESR > 40 mm/hr

The probability of having septic arthritis of hip increased to more than 90% when three or more criteria were met. Caird et al. modified Kocher's criteria to include a CRP level of more than 20 mg/l. The addition of CRP level increased the positive predictability of infection to more than 97% when all the parameters were met. Moreover, the authors noted a CRP level of more than 20 mg/l to be the most significant independent predictor of infection [21]. Despite the relevance of this criteria, there are certain drawbacks too; it can be applied to the hip joint only and is unable to differentiate between osteomyelitis of acetabulum from septic arthritis of hip joint. In any case, it is serving the intended purpose very well. Copley et al. developed a severity of illness score for patients of acute hematogenous osteomyelitis based on clinical, laboratory, and radiographic parameters to help objectively assess the severity and stratify the patients [22]. It comprised of three categories, mild (0–3), moderate [4–6], and severe (>7). The authors further noted severity of illness scoring system to be accurate with respect to physician panel assessment in 88%, 60%, and 78% for mild, moderate, and severe categories, respectively. The detailed parameters of severity of illness scoring system are presented in Table 8.2. Mignemi et al. devised a three-tier classification system that can be applied to all pediatric musculoskeletal infections in the emergency department for stratification [23]. It is based on the severity of infection and degree of dissemination. The operational definitions of the three classes are shown in Table 8.3. There is a need for further research on predictive algorithms and scoring systems for their application at large in different ethnicities and geographic areas [24]. In a study by Hollmig ST et al., the authors noted that the children older than 8 years with an elevated CRP level at admission had a significantly increased risk of deep vein thrombosis (DVT) (40%) [25].

**Table 8.2** Copley's severity of illness score [22] for acute hematogenous osteomyelitis patients

| S. no | Parameter | Score |
|---|---|---|
| 1. | CRP initial | |
| | < 10<br>10–15<br>> 15 | 0<br>1<br>2 |
| 2. | CRP 48 h | |
| | < 5<br>5–10<br>>10 | 0<br>1<br>2 |
| 3. | CRP 96 h | |
| | < 5<br>5–10<br>>10 | 0<br>1<br>2 |
| 4. | Respiratory rate | |
| | > 125% of midrange normal<br>< 125% of midrange normal | 1<br>0 |
| 5. | Febrile days on antibiotics | |
| | < 2<br>> 2 | 0<br>1 |
| 6. | ICU admission | |
| | No<br>Yes | 0<br>1 |
| 7. | Disseminated disease | |
| | No<br>Yes | 0<br>1 |

Mild (0–3), Moderate (4–6), and Severe > 7

**Table 8.3** Three-tier stratification system for pediatric musculoskeletal infections by Mignemi et al. [23]

| Inflammation | Local Infection | Dissemination |
|---|---|---|
| All of the following must be true (if available)<br>1. Negative blood culture.<br>2. Negative local culture.<br>3. Not fulfilling the criteria for local and disseminated types. | One of the following must be true<br>1. Imaging diagnostic for single-site osteomyelitis or pyomyositis.<br>2. Local culture positive and/ or tissue/fluid consistent with infection[a].<br>3. Criteria for disseminated type are not met. | For two or more anatomic sites, at least one of the following must be true<br>1. Imaging diagnostic for osteomyelitis or pyomyositis.<br>2. Local culture positive and/ or tissue or fluid consistent with infection[a].<br>3. Two or more positive blood cultures.<br>4. Thromboembolic disease. |

[a]cell count >50,000, grossly purulent

## 8.6 Biopsy

In cases where definitive diagnosis remains elusive, a bone or tissue biopsy may be necessary. Biopsy allows for direct examination of affected tissues, facilitating identification of pathogens and guiding appropriate treatment strategies.

## 8.7 Radiological Investigations

**Radiographs** The X-rays show no findings for the initial 1 week or 10 days, except for possible changes or distortion in soft tissue planes. The radiologic changes of osteomyelitis like bone lysis, periosteal reaction, and increased joint space can be seen at 2 weeks.

**Ultrasonography** An ultrasonogram can be done to localize an abscess, to assess the extent of soft tissue involvement, and in aspiration of joint; however, it is a highly operator-dependent investigation modality and cannot detect changes in the bone.

**Magnetic Resonance Imaging (MRI)** MRI is the investigation of choice to assess the extent of bone changes and any soft tissue collection; it is a highly sensitive modality in the early course of infection. The MRI shows infection as a low signal intensity on T1-weighted images and increased signal intensity on T2-weighted and short tau inversion recovery (STIR) images [26–28]. The contrast-enhanced MRI is not routinely ordered for every case, but is useful for localizing an intramedullary or muscular abscess. In addition to the diagnosis of musculoskeletal conditions, MRI also helps in surgical planning, like approach and localizing any associated pyomyositis.

**Nuclear Scans** Another diagnostic modality which can be useful, especially in multisite infections or when the local signs are minimal, is bone scintigraphy or technetium 99-scan ($^{99m}Tc$), which can pick up the physiologically active bone areas as a hot spot. It is triphasic having an initial flow phase followed by blood pool phase and the final delayed phase after 2–4 h. Musculoskeletal infections cause a focal absorption in the delayed phase, which is attributed to the increased activity of osteoblasts; however, it can be tricky, especially if the hotspot localizes close to a physis. The disadvantages of bone scan are the lack of details on the size of collection, exposure to ionising radiation, and false-negative results that may occur in subperiosteal abscess [29].

**Computerised Tomograms (CT)** The use of CT in acute pediatric musculoskeletal infections is limited because of increased exposure of ionizing radiation to the child and its low sensitivity and specificity compared to magnetic resonance imaging. It has a role in chronic osteomyelitis to plan surgery and assess the sequestrum/involucrum status. Judicious use of investigations should be done to supplement the clinical diagnosis of musculoskeletal infection.

## 8.8 Medical Management

### 8.8.1 Acute Osteomyelitis

It is the most common infection of bone in the pediatric age group. The most common mode of infection is hematogenous spread, and it affects the metaphyseal region of bone owing to the hairpin bend arrangement of vessels, sluggish flow of blood, rich vascularity, and being a physiologically active site. Treatment of acute osteomyelitis involves general care of the child, selection and administration of an appropriate antibiotic, rest to the affected part, and surgery when indicated. An attempt should be made to obtain a tissue/fluid sample for culture and sensitivity prior to starting empirical treatment with broad-spectrum antibiotics. However, it should not delay the onset of treatment in sick cases, where antibiotics, as per the local hospital/institution policy, are started immediately without waiting for the culture and sensitivity tests. Obtaining a blood sample for culture at the time of intravenous cannula application is a safe practice without causing any delay in institution of treatment. An algorithmic approach to the management of acute osteomyelitis of the proximal tibia/distal femur is presented in Flowchart 8.1. The duration of the antibiotic course in acute osteomyelitis is generally 6 weeks, with initial 2 weeks of intravenous antibiotics followed by oral route. The time period for shifting to oral antibiotics is also not clearly defined and should be based on the recovery of patient manifested by clinical improvement of signs and symptoms and a decrease in laboratory parameter like CRP and ESR. There are many studies in the literature evaluating the outcome of a short course (<3 weeks) versus a traditional 6-week antibiotic regimen in acute osteomyelitis with no significant differences [30, 31]. However, the authors recommended to prolong the duration in vertebral osteomyelitis and severe infections caused by MRSA. The decision to intervene surgically should be based on the clinical condition of the patient. Surgery, which may include abscess drainage and debridement is indicated when there is a large abscess collection, subperiosteal abscess, failure of nonoperative treatment (IV antibiotics), and formation of abscess while on conservative treatment [32]. An algorithmic approach to management of acute osteomyelitis of distal femur/proximal tibia is presented in Flowchart 8.1.

### 8.8.2 Septic Arthritis

Septic arthritis is an acute inflammation of the joint which is mostly hematogenous in origin or secondary to transmission from an adjacent source of infection like osteomyelitis. The metaphyseal vessels in children younger than 2 years of age cross the physis and can cause septic arthritis early in the course of osteomyelitis especially in joints where metaphyseal part is intracapsular like hip and shoulder. Although septic arthritis can affect any joint, it most commonly affects the hip and knee joints. Unlike acute osteomyelitis, septic arthritis warrants an urgent decompression to prevent rapid joint destruction due to acute inflammatory response,

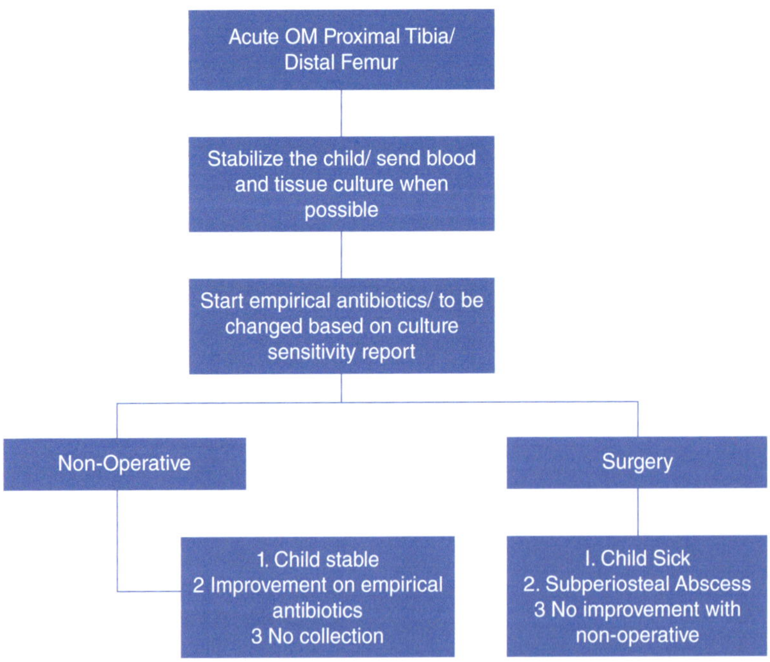


**Flowchart 8.1** An algorithmic approach to operative and nonoperative treatment of acute osteomyelitis of the proximal tibia/distal femur

bacterial toxins, and release of cartilage-degrading enzymes. Wherever possible, an attempt should be made to obtain joint fluid/pus for culture sensitivity testing before starting antibiotics; however, it should not delay the start of treatment. The choice of empirical antibiotic is mostly dependent upon local susceptibility pattern and institutional policy, generally, a third-generation cephalosporin or a broad-spectrum antibiotic covering the likely causative microbes should be started. Joint decompression should be done at the earliest to prevent joint destruction. Decompression can be done through an open arthrotomy or arthroscopically, although there are no significant differences in the outcome, an open arthrotomy is the preferred technique by most surgeons. The antibiotics are continued for 2–4 weeks with regular checks on clinical improvement, inflammatory markers, and cell counts. The transition from parenteral to oral antibiotics is a grey area with no well-defined guidelines; the decision depends upon improvement in symptoms and reducing markers and is taken on a case-to-case basis. If the symptoms persist, there should be a repeat decompression with debridement, and antibiotics should be started as per the culture report. A regular follow-up is needed to check the condition of the joint and any growth arrest in the long term.

## 8.9 Pyomyositis

Pyomyositis is an acute inflammation of the striated muscles, often associated with a history of minor trauma. The incidence was initially higher in the tropical regions, but now the incidence is increasing in the temperate regions as well. Most cases are secondary to hematogenous spread, but why a localized muscle is involved is still unclear. A likely mechanism can be a local trauma to the muscle, leading to the release of iron from the myoglobin, which can provide an opportunity for the bacteria to grow and cause a localized abscess in the muscle. The pyomyositis presents in a similar way like septic arthritis or osteomyelitis with fever, pain, inability to move the part, localized tenderness, local swelling, warmth, erythema, and often a history of trauma. The most common site of pyomyositis is the iliopsoas muscle, followed by the thigh muscles. In almost 30% of cases in the tropics, it can present at multiple sites at the same time. The investigations are done on the same lines, an X-ray is taken to rule out any bone involvement, ultrasonography is a reliable modality for the diagnosis of pyomyositis, but MRI is the gold standard for localizing the infection and simultaneously ruling out any bone or joint involvement, including neoplasms. The treatment of pyomyositis is based on the presence of abscess and associated systemic symptoms or sepsis. Prior to the formation of a collection, which is labelled as Stage I, it can be managed nonoperatively with broad-spectrum antibiotics, keeping in view the regional susceptibility pattern and institutional guidelines. In Stage II, there is a frank abscess collection which warrants an early decompression and antibiotics as per the hospital policy, which can be altered as per the culture and sensitivity. The Stage III has sepsis and systemic symptoms and is taken up as an orthopedic emergency warranting an urgent decompression, IV antibiotics, and intensive care unit (ICU) care of the patient [31, 33, 34].

The treatment or detailed review of each and every pediatric musculoskeletal infection, like vertebral osteomyelitis, diskitis, skeletal tuberculosis, and low-grade chronic infections like brucellosis, is extensive and beyond the scope of this chapter. We have tried to discuss the brief outline and approach toward musculoskeletal infections in children.

## 8.10 Surgical Management

The treatment of musculoskeletal infection is demanding, and often multidisciplinary care is required. Despite variability in treatment protocols, the treatment principles that remain ubiquitous are organism identification, correct antibiotic selection and delivery of the antibiotics, and prevention of ongoing tissue damage.

## 8.11 Acute Osteomyelitis

Although a vast majority of acute osteomyelitis is treated medically, surgical treatment is necessary for a select few. The indications for surgery are the presence of abscess (subperiosteal/soft tissue abscess/intramedullary abscess), acute osteomyelitis with concomitant septic arthritis and/or pyomyositis, complex infections as per the new classification, and for osteomyelitis cases that show no improvement despite 48–72 h of antibiotic treatment. [35, 36] In addition to clinical examination, imaging (USG and MRI) helps to determine the extent of the disease. Imaging is also useful in deciding on the site and extent of incision.

The surgical treatment entails removal of necrotic tissue that facilitates antibiotics reaching the site of infection, and washout to reduce the bacterial load to halt the infection spread, obtaining cultures and tissue for histopathological exam (Fig. 8.1a–d). This debridement and washout are many times combined with drilling a hole in the bone or making a bone window for draining the intramedullary abscess. The surgical approach depends on the bone involved. After surgical treatment, a drain may be used if the collection is large. After the surgical procedure, the affected extremity is protected with a splint, and medical management is continued. The clinical condition of the child and the inflammatory laboratory parameters are monitored. A repeat surgical procedure may be needed if there is a worsening in the condition of the child. Although the treatment is straightforward, there are several controversies regarding surgical procedures: the best approach to debride, the extent of debridement, the role of repeat surgery, and the use of drains. Also, the role of bone drilling has been debated. It remains unknown whether bone drilling should be done for every case of acute osteomyelitis or if it should be offered to a select few. In addition, the optimal way to create a bone window, its size, and its location in the bone (round or trough shape) remains unknown. [36, 37] The role of local drug delivery systems is emerging. The local drug delivery system offers the advantage of higher drug concentration at the site of infection and avoids systemic toxicity. In addition, it helps with dead space management. A recent study compared surgery along with antibiotic-loaded calcium sulphate to surgery without a local drug delivery system. The first group had a faster fall in CRP (4.8 ± 2.5 versus 13 +/−9.6 days. [38] Although promising early results, more evidence is needed to define the role of local drug delivery systems in treating acute osteomyelitis. Also, there are no clear evidence-based recommendations for postoperative care, including the duration of extremity immobilization, and when to return to sports from the viewpoint of pathological fracture prevention. After the index procedure, secondary procedures are often required. The reported rate of secondary procedures is 15–33% [39, 40]. Typically, the indications for secondary or repeat procedures are persistent pain, MRSA infection, and worsening clinical condition of the patient and lab parameters. The treatment principles for repeat surgical procedures remain the same.

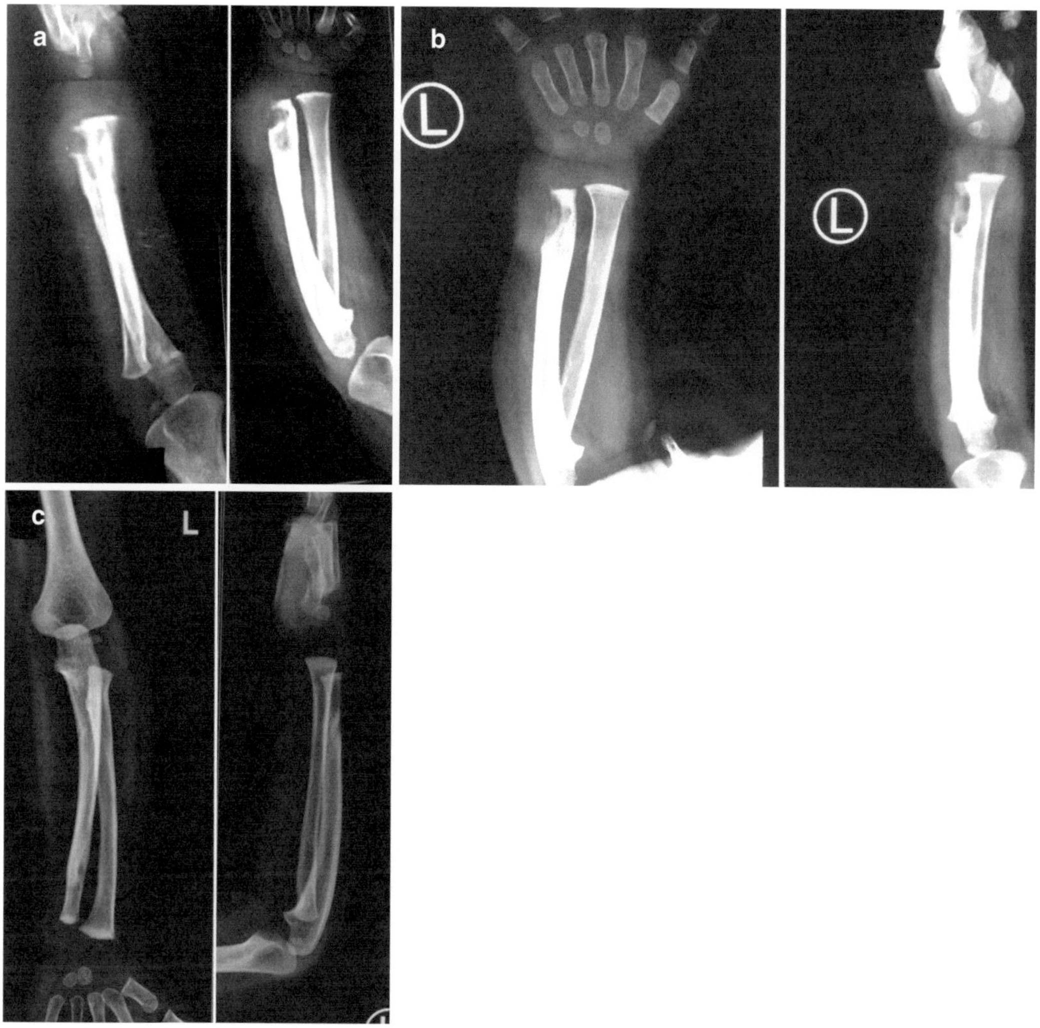


**Fig. 8.1** (**a**) An 1-year old with discharging sinus and abscess over the left forearm. His CRP and ESR were raised, and the total leucocyte count was 21,000/cmm. He was treated with debridement and washout. The cultures grew Methicillin-sensitive *Staphylococcus aureus*. The histopathology showed changes suggestive of tuberculous osteomyelitis. Diagnosis of tuberculous osteomyelitis with super-added staphylococcal osteomyelitis was made. (**b**) Radiograph at 6-month follow-up. The patient was on antituberculosis treatment and a removable forearm splint. (**c**) Radiographs at 18-month follow-up showing resolution of the lytic lesion. (**d**) Radiographs and clinical pictures at 6-year- follow-up showing slightly short ulna and completely healed bony lesion

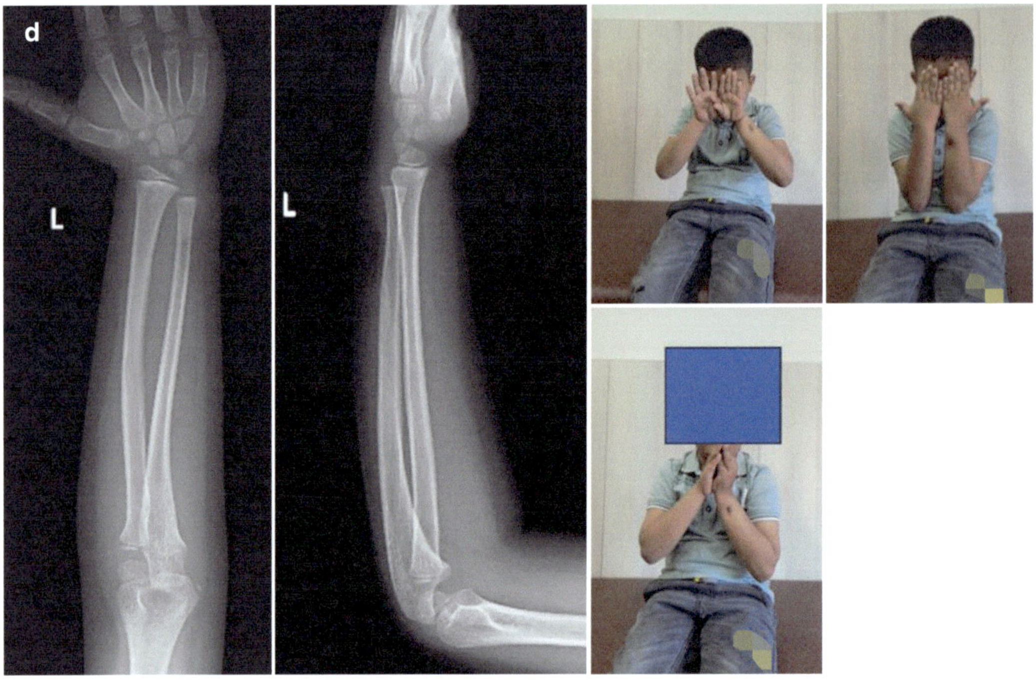


**Fig. 8.1** (continued)

## 8.12 Septic Arthritis

In contrast to acute hematogenous osteomyelitis, septic arthritis always necessitates surgical treatment. The treatment principles are decompression of the joint, washout of inflammatory fluid, and debridement to decrease the bacterial load. The indications for surgical treatment are confirmed or clinical diagnosis of septic arthritis. Joint aspiration and synovial fluid analysis remain an excellent tool for diagnosing septic arthritis. However, the facilities for joint aspiration and synovial fluid analysis may not be available universally. It is recommended to diagnose septic arthritis based on clinical and laboratory parameters. [41, 42] The diagnosis of septic arthritis warrants urgent surgical treatment. Delays give rise to sequelae (Fig. 8.2a–h).

When to do the surgery?

It is recommended to do the surgery at the earliest. [43] The duration between the onset of symptoms and the drainage procedure has a bearing on outcomes. Guidelines recommend doing the joint decompression on an emergent basis, but it remains unknown whether delaying it by a few hours makes any difference. It remains unknown whether doing the procedure in the middle of the night versus doing it in the morning makes any difference in the outcomes. A delay of more than 24 h has shown poor outcomes. The treatment of late-presenting septic arthritis remains problematic. It has been shown to have suboptimal outcomes and poor results. [44–47] This highlights the need for early diagnosis and appropriate referral. This is crucial for saving the joint and to achieve good results.

The arthrotomy and washout can be done by different means, although an open arthrotomy and washout remain the most commonly used approach. Surgical treatment of septic arthritis can be achieved via open arthrotomy, needle aspiration (one-time or repeated procedures), or arthroscopic washout. Various factors need to be taken into consideration while choosing the best option. These factors include the age of the patient, size of the joint involved, availability of instruments and personnel in addition to training, and comfort level of the surgeon performing the procedure. [48–51].

The hip joint is the most commonly involved joint for septic arthritis. Hip joint septic arthritis can be treated via open arthrotomy using an anterior or medial approach. With the anterior approach, an anterior incision is made and the interval between sartorius and tensor fascia lata is identified. Through this interval, the rectus femoris is split to expose the anterior hip capsule. A small window is made in the capsule to open the hip joint. The tissue is sent for culture and histopathology. Wash is given using normal saline. It is important to open the joint and identify the femoral head for complete decompression of the joint. A suction drain may be used for the hip joint and removed after it stops draining. However, there are other approaches, such as needle aspiration or hip arthroscopy, for treating septic arthritis of the hip. The European Society guidelines advocate surgeon preference depending on his/her experience. [52].

Needle aspiration, although a simple technique, carries the risk of inadequate drainage. However, needle aspiration remains a minimally invasive alternative, especially in neonates or if the child is medically unfit to undergo a longer procedure. Similarly, hip arthroscopy offers an alternative to open arthrotomy. It is possible to do debridement and also obtain tissue for histopathological examination. El Sayed prospectively compared arthroscopy versus open arthrotomy and showed that the results are similar in both procedures. The hospital duration was significantly shorter in the arthroscopy group compared to the open arthrotomy group (3.8 days versus

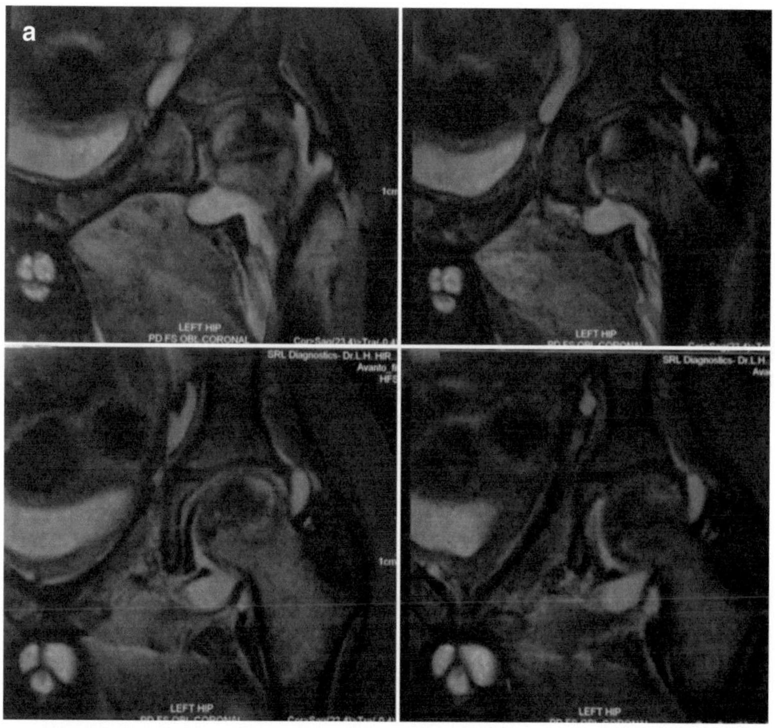


**Fig. 8.2** (**a** and **b**): An 8-year old had febrile illness and pain in the left hip which started on the sixth March 2020. He was diagnosed to have multiorgan sepsis, septic arthritis of left hip with left femoral vein thrombosis. Antibiotics and thrombolytics were started. He was operated 15 days later, on the 21st March 2020, for hip decompression. (**c**) 7 months from onset, avascular necrosis of the femoral epiphysis with hinged abduction is visible. No treatment was given. (**d**) A year since the onset of infection, the hinged abduction is very visible on the X-ray and MRI. An arthrogram was done along with an adductor tenotomy, and the hip was contained in a hip spica at another centre. (**e**) 3 months after the adductor tenotomy, the hip appears contained. (**f**) 1 year and 8 months since the adductor tenotomy, the hip remains contained. (**g**) Functionally, the child is doing well and is able to sit cross-legged and can also do the split. (**h**) Status of the hip on X-ray nearly 3 years and 11 months since the onset

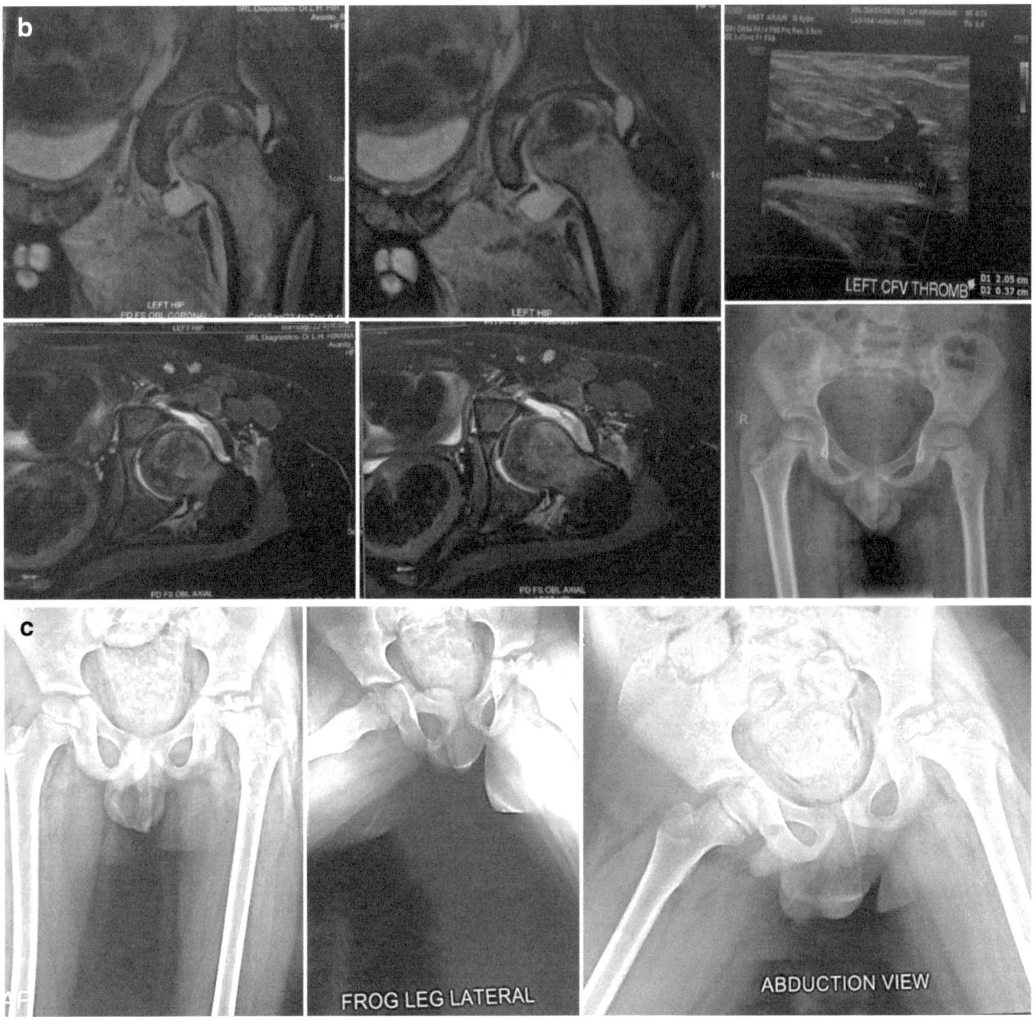


**Fig. 8.2** (continued)

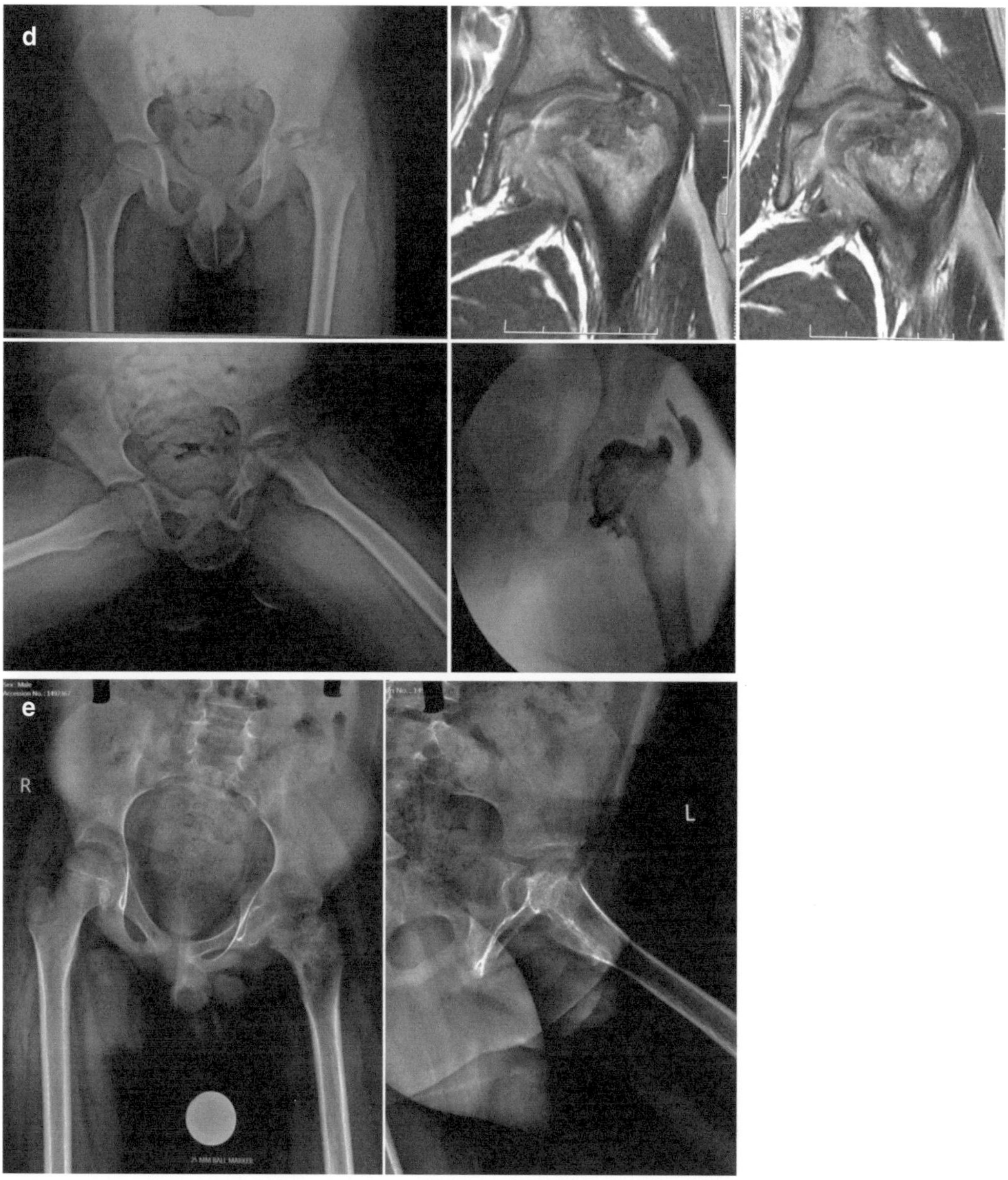


**Fig. 8.2** (continued)

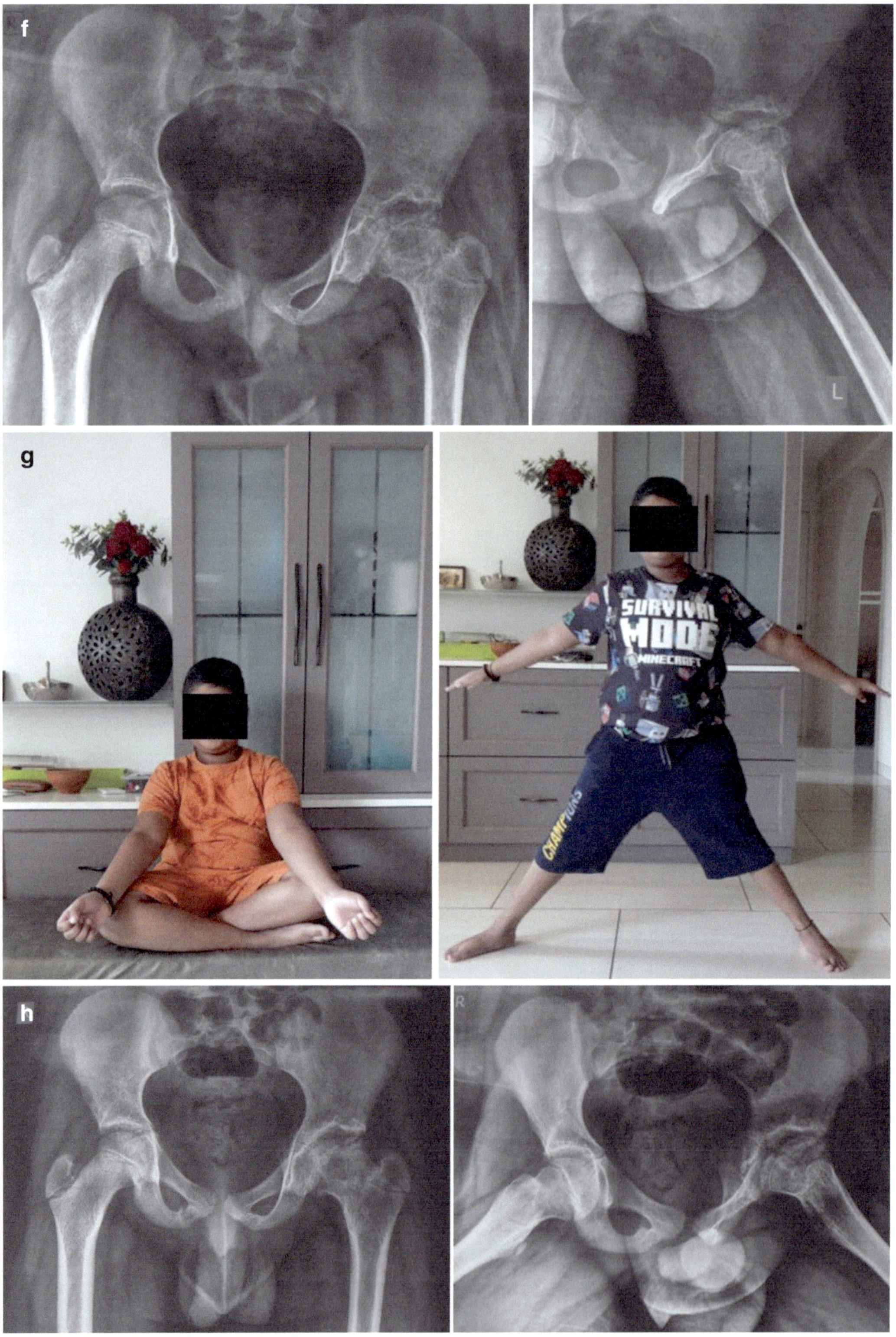


**Fig. 8.2** (continued)

6.4 days). [51] Although a promising approach, hip arthroscopy requires special equipment and training, which may be unavailable routinely.

The minimally invasive procedures may offer several advantages, such as smaller incisions, shorter hospital stays, and better parental acceptance. The minimally invasive approaches have been fraught with the risk of incomplete joint drainage requiring repeat procedures. Studies have shown this risk to be almost five times higher with minimally invasive procedures such as needle aspiration and arthroscopy. In recently published systematic reviews, the risk of redo surgery after open arthrotomy is 3%, arthrocentesis is 15%, and arthroscopy is 14%. [53, 54] This highlights the evolving role of minimally invasive procedures and calls for identifying the correct indications that might minimize the risk of repeat procedures.

## 8.13 Complications

Pediatric musculoskeletal infections can lead to complications. These complications may affect the physeal growth plate, segment of a bone, or the joint and may significantly burden the individual, parental, and healthcare resources. Complications or post-infective sequelae may have long-term effects as they affect growth and can create deformity. There could be physical and psychological consequences leading to disability. In many cases, multiple complex surgeries might be necessary.

The exact prevalence of complications is not clear. The risk factors for the development of complications are infections with MRSA and other highly virulent organisms, complex infections (septic arthritis with osteomyelitis), delay in the treatment, younger children, and positive blood cultures indicating disseminated infection. [39] In addition to a delay in diagnosis, inadequate or inappropriate treatment, and lack of a multidisciplinary care team have been shown to lead to a high prevalence of musculoskeletal infection sequelae. [55–57]. Also, increasing virulence, antibiotic resistance, and changes in epidemiology contribute to adverse outcomes. [58, 59].

A study by McNeil has shown that infection with Accessory Gene Regulator (AGR) III *S. aureus*, duration of fever >4 days after admission, and delayed source control were associated with a significant increase in complications of osteoarticular infections. [60, 61] A-score and C-scores were developed to predict complications. [55] A-score can predict complications within 6 weeks and C-score variables can be used to predict complications at/after 12 weeks. [Tables 8.4 and 8.5] Vij et al. have shown that the A-score, along with clinical judgment, can be useful in determining optimal timing for early care decisions such as the transition to oral antibiotics, the need for further intervention, and discharge. The C-score can be useful while considering the decision specific to the development of chronic osteomyelitis and the need for antibiotics beyond 12 weeks, and to rule out pathological fracture or avascular necrosis. [62].

Complications of pediatric musculoskeletal infection can be acute or chronic, as listed in Table 8.6. [56, 58, 60, 63, 64] [Table 8.6]

**Table 8.4** A-score variables

| | |
|---|---|
| Presence of a bone abscess | 2 |
| Temperature $\geq$ 38 °C for more than 48 h from the start of antibiotics | 2 |
| Suppurative arthritis | 3 |
| Presence of disseminated disease, presence of DVT, septic pulmonary embolism, and endocarditis | 4 |
| Delayed source control (surgical intervention after 3 days) | 4 |
| Maximum score | 15 |

**Table 8.5** C-score variables

| | |
|---|---|
| CRP $\geq$ 100 mg/L at 2–4 days after starting antibiotics | 1 |
| Presence of disseminated disease | 1 |
| Occurrence of bone debridement | 2 |
| Maximum score | 4 |

**Table 8.6** Complications of musculoskeletal infections in children

| Acute complications | Chronic complications |
|---|---|
| Multifocal osteomyelitis | Chronic osteomyelitis |
| Septicemia | Pathological fracture |
| Venous thromboembolism | Osteonecrosis |
| Septic shock | Joint destruction |
| Compartment syndrome | Physeal growth arrest and its sequelae |
| Death | Sequestrum, bone loss |
| | Malignant transformation |

## 8.14 Chronic Osteomyelitis

Chronic osteomyelitis is a long-standing infection characterized by radiographic evidence of dead necrotic bone (sequestrum), reactive new bone formation (involucrum), and signs of long-standing infection. It is associated with repeated episodes of symptoms of infection. In osteomyelitis, 20% form sequestra. [64].

Chronic osteomyelitis poses therapeutic challenges such as the presence of infected bone and/or soft tissue, focal or segmental bone loss, soft tissue loss, physeal damage, joint contracture, and pathological fracture. The commonly used classification systems are the Beit CURE classification and the Cierny–Mader classification. The Beit CURE classification can guide treatment selection. [65, 66] The treatment of this complex problem is multidisciplinary and can vary depending on several host and surgeon factors. The treatment principles include host optimization, antibiotic therapy (systemic antibiotics and/or local antibiotic drug delivery system), and surgical treatment. The surgical treatment involves radical debridement followed by dead space management and the management of focal/segmental bone defects. The local antibiotics delivery systems using various materials have shown encouraging results. [67, 68] Fig. 8.3a–d.

The management principles for treating chronic sequelae of a pediatric musculoskeletal infection are as follows: [37]

- Prevention—early diagnosis and the right treatment—get it right.
- Team approach.
- Comprehensive evaluation—not to miss out on multiple sites of infection, especially in neonates and young children.
- Planning the treatment.
- Creating a problem list.
- Priority list for each problem.
- Taking into consideration family expectations, resources, and surgeon capabilities.
- Discussing reconstructive as well as prosthetic options in detail.
- Biology preservation.
- Follow-up till skeletal maturity and beyond.

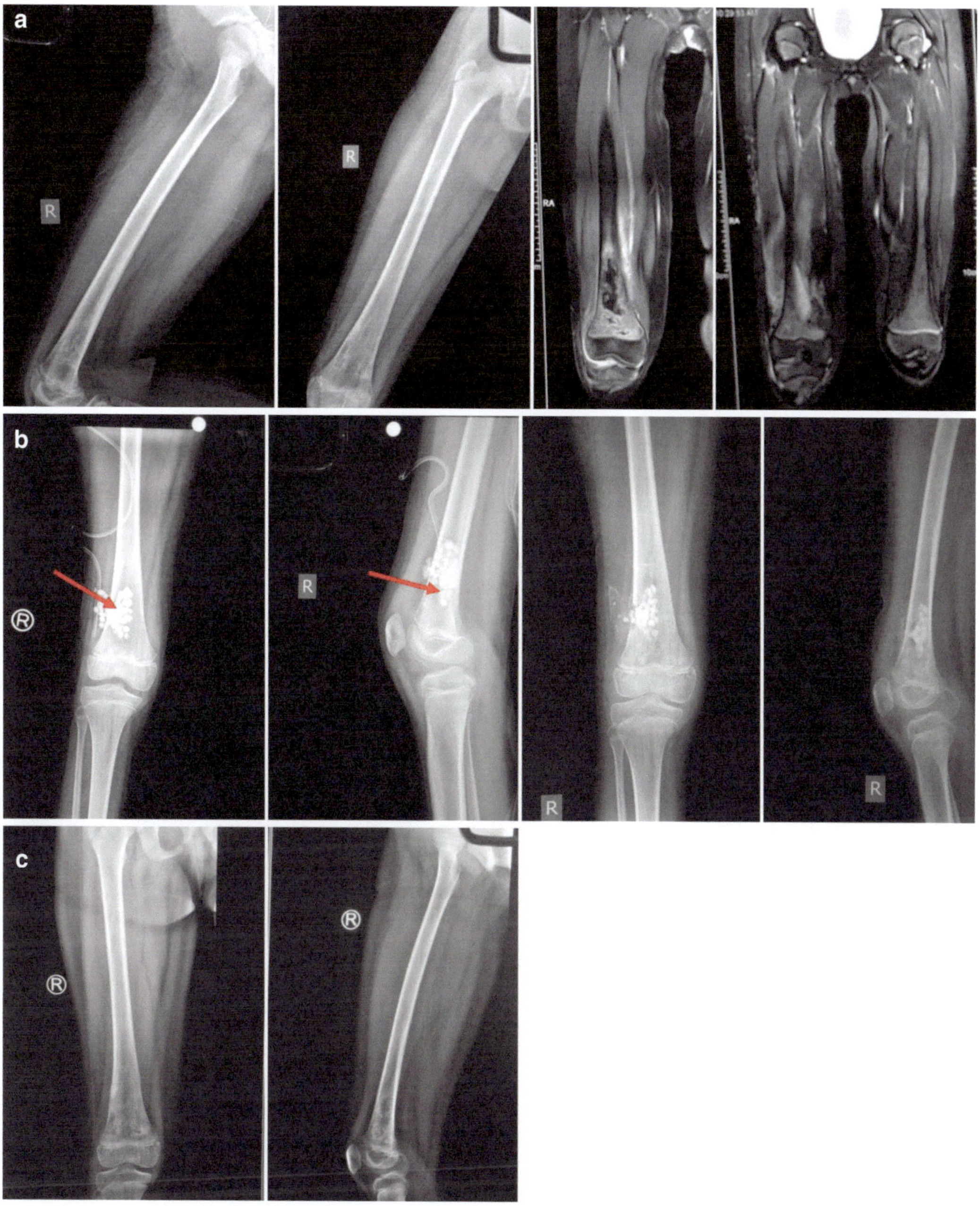

**Fig. 8.3** (**a**). Radiographs and MRI of an 8-year-old girl with chronic osteomyelitis of the right distal femur. She was having recurrent pain, swelling in the right thigh, and fever. (**b**) Immediate postoperative and 1-month post-surgery radiographs. Patient was treated with debridement through a bone window and placement of a local drug delivery system (Vancomycin added to Calcium sulfate). (**c**) Radiographs at 6-month follow-up showing complete absorption of the Calcium sulfate and no signs of recurrence of the infection. (**d**) Radiographs and clinical pictures at 30-month follow-up showing no signs of recurrence and full knee range of motion

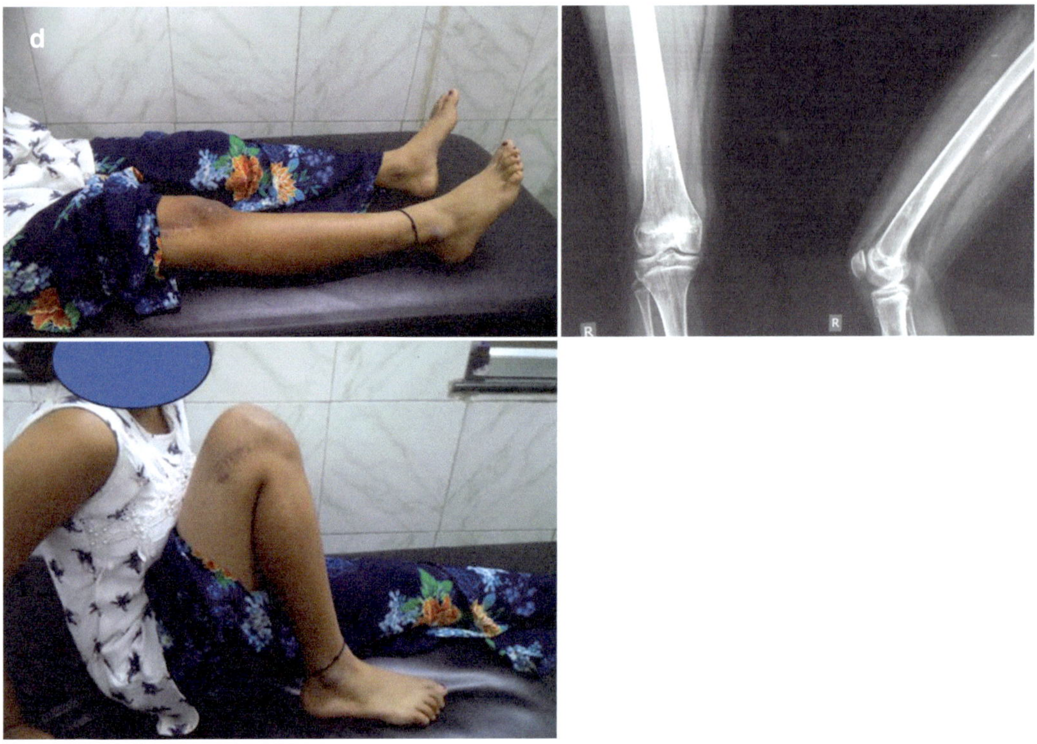


**Fig. 8.3** (continued)

## 8.15 Pathological Fractures

The reported incidence of pathological fractures is 3–5% [69, 70]. The reported risk factors for pathological fractures are infection with a virulent strain (PVL, MRSA, or AGR group III *Staphylococcus aureus*), prolonged fever, more than three debridements, bacteraemia, extent on bone involvement >45% on radiographs at 6 weeks, large subperiosteal abscess, involvement of > two-third length of the bone on the initial MRI and a sharp transitional zone between diseased and normal bone marrow on initial MRI. [30, 38] Inadequate drainage of an intraosseous abscess can be a risk factor. Also, a slot created for bone debridement can act as a stress riser for the development of pathological fractures. It is important to create a slot/window with a small width on the non-tension side of the bone to minimize the risk of pathological fracture. [71–73] The treatment is nonoperative in the majority of cases. Debridement followed by fracture stabilization is necessary for some cases. [70].

## 8.16 Post-infective Segmental Bone Loss

Post-infective segmental bone loss develops due to resorption of bone or destruction of the bone due to infection. Another possibility is during aggressive debridement, after the removal of sequestrum with a weak involucrum done to eradicate infection. [73] The incidence of post-infective bone gap development is 20% [65]. Bone gap management is a daunting task and often needs complex reconstructive surgical treatment. Many times, it may require plastic surgical intervention. The treatment principles include eradication of the infection, optimization of the host condition, soft tissue cover, alignment of the bone segments, dead space management, enhancement of bone healing, achieving bony stability, posttreatment rehabilitation, and protection of the new bone. [74–76]. In general, smaller defects (< 6 cm) can be managed with autologous bone graft and acute shortening. Larger defects need acute or gradual bone transport, induced membrane technique, or fibular graft placement (vascularized or non-vascularized). [74–83].

## 8.17 Post-infective Physeal Growth Arrest

The incidence of post-infective physeal growth arrest is 7–20%. It is more common in the distal and proximal femur. [84] The growth arrest leads to a total or partial closure of the epiphyseal growth plate, leading to limb shortening and/or angular deformity. The severity of the deformity depends on the age of the child and the anatomic location of the physis involved. In general, a peripheral physeal bar involving a smaller area of the physis, and at least 2 years of growth remaining, can be treated with physeal bar resection and fat graft interposition. It is recommended to do simultaneous osteotomy if the deformity is >15 degrees [85, 86]. Physeodesis to be offered if the physeal bar involves >50% of the physeal area and/or the growth remaining is less than 2 years. The associated leg length discrepancy will need to be treated. Figure 8.4a–c The outcomes of post-infective bar resection are unfavorable as compared to posttraumatic bars. [85, 86].

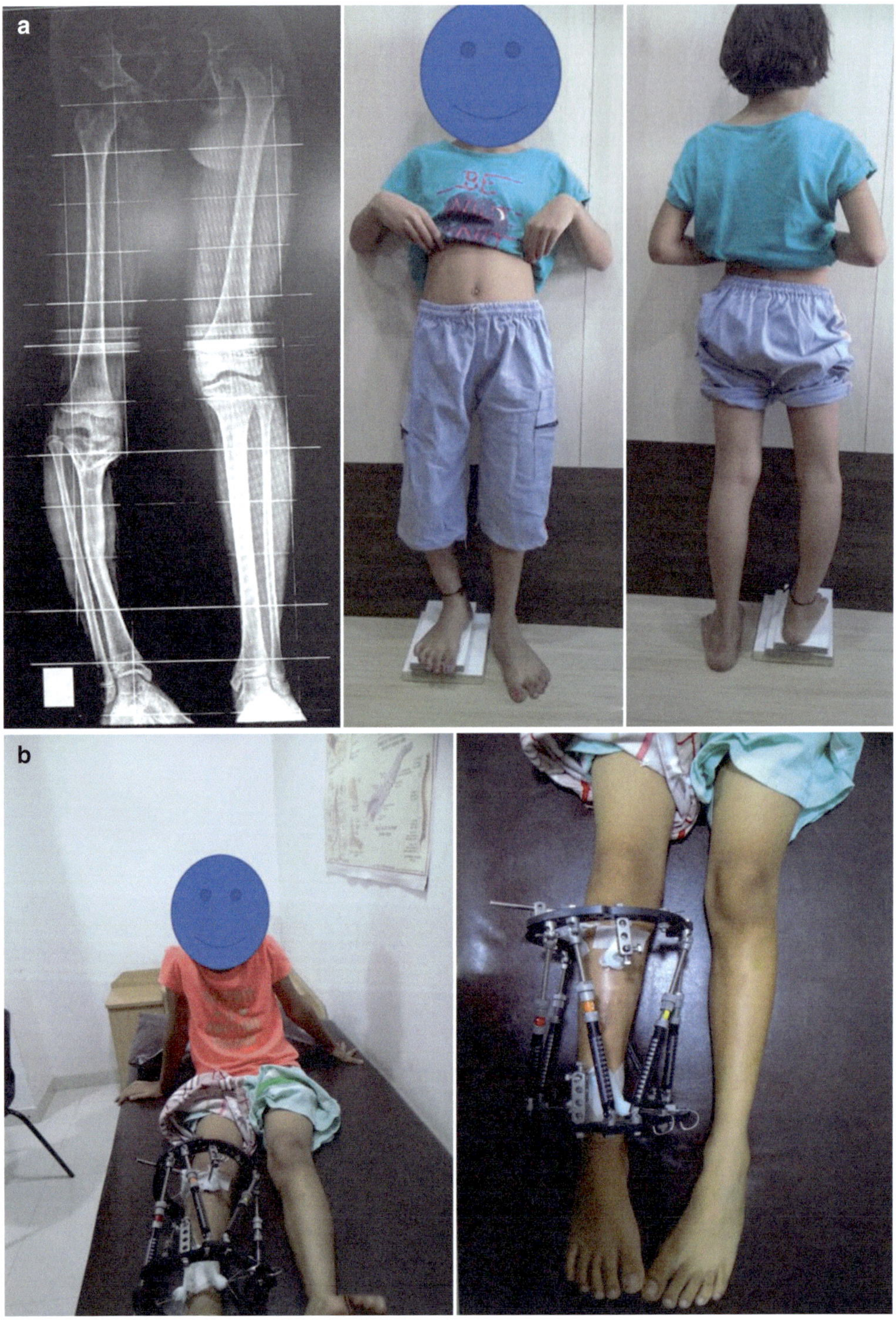

**Fig. 8.4** (**a**) An 8-year-old girl who had right knee septic arthritis and probably right tibial osteomyelitis in early childhood presented with a right tibial varus deformity and 4 cm shortening. (**b**) She underwent completion of the proximal tibial physeodesis, right proximal tibial osteotomy, and tibial lengthening and deformity correction using a six-axis correction system. (**c**) Clinical photographs after the frame removal showing correction of the deformity and leg length equalization. The patient is under regular follow-up, as she will need another leg-length equalization procedure at a later stage

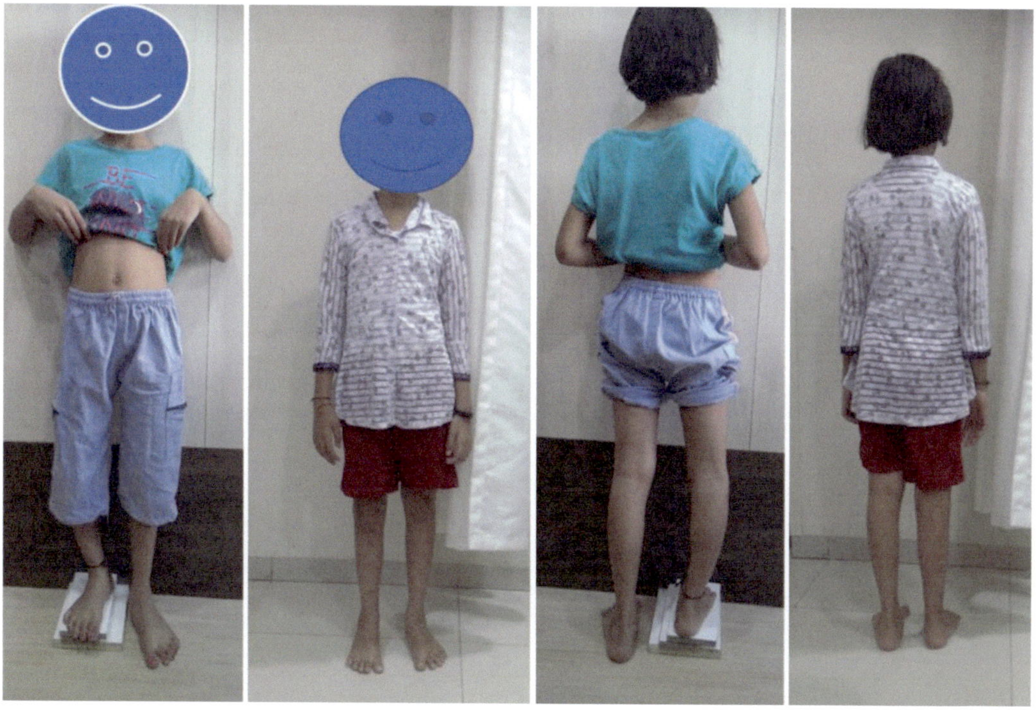


**Fig. 8.4** (continued)

## 8.18 Post-septic Hip Sequelae

The complications of septic arthritis of the hip joint can be varied. They could range from growth disturbance to complete dislocation of the hip and/or destruction of the femoral head and neck. These sequelae are severe if the infection occurs in a neonate and the treatment is delayed or if there is a delay in diagnosis or presentation. Concurrent osteomyelitis and infection with virulent organisms can result in extensive damage to the epiphysis, physis, and metaphysis of the proximal femur, resulting in a spectrum of sequelae. The incidence is approximately 33% [47, 87, 88]. The sequelae are classified by the extent of involvement of the proximal femur. The treatment is complex surgical reconstruction, depending on the involvement of the proximal femur and the status of the hip joint. The treatment offered is dependent on the location and extent of the deformity, the type of deformity, and the vascularity of the femoral head. In addition to symptoms, the range of motion of the hip, age of the child, previous surgical scars, and advanced imaging findings need to be taken into consideration to offer the reconstructive option. [89, 90]. Femoral neck osteomyelitis can give rise to resorption of the neck and creation of a pseudarthrosis with coxa vara. Johari et al. have discussed the management of this condition [91] as a special group (Group 5) in his classification of sequelae of septic hips.

## 8.19 Summary

Pediatric musculoskeletal infections pose a significant challenge for the growing skeleton. It is important to diagnose the infection early and start appropriate, timely treatment to minimize the complications and have optimal outcomes.

This will help to avoid disastrous complications and sequelae. Box 8.1.

**Box 8.1 Key Learning Points**

- A high index of suspicion is necessary for early diagnosis of musculoskeletal infections in children, especially in neonates.
- Consider obtaining an MRI to define the involvement of bone and/or joint and the soft tissues.
- Indications for surgical intervention are the presence of subperiosteal/intramedullary/soft tissue abscess and/or septic arthritis.
- Septic arthritis warrants urgent surgical decompression of the joint.
- A multidisciplinary approach is desirable for the diagnosis and optimal care of a child with a musculoskeletal infection.

## References


1. Kang SN, Sanghera T, Mangwani J, Paterson JM, Ramachandran M. The management of septic arthritis in children: systematic review of the English language literature. J Bone Joint Surg (Br). 2009;91-B:1127–33.
2. Dartnell J, Ramachandran M, Katchburian M. Haematogenous acute and subacute paediatric osteomyelitis: a systematic review of the literature. J Bone Joint Surg (Br). 2012;94-B:584–95.
3. Riise OR, Kirkhus E, Handeland KS, et al. Childhood osteomyelitis-incidence and differentiation from other acute onset musculoskeletal features in a population-based study. BMC Pediatr. 2008;8:45. https://doi.org/10.1186/1471-2431-8-45.
4. Dodwell ER. Osteomyelitis and septic arthritis in children: Current concepts. Curr Opin Pediatr. 2013;25(1):58–63. https://doi.org/10.1097/MOP.0b013e32835c2b42.
5. Yeo A, Ramachandran M. Acute haematogenous osteomyelitis in children. BMJ. 2014;348:1326.
6. Blyth MJ, Kincaid R, Craigen MA, Bennet GC. The changing epidemiology of acute and subacute haematogenous osteomyelitis in children. J Bone Joint Surg (Br). 2001;83-B:99–102.
7. Malcius D, Trumpulyte G, Barauskas V, Kilda A. Two decades of acute hematogenous osteomyelitis in children: are there any changes? Pediatr Surg Int. 2005;21:356–9.
8. Frank G, Mahoney HM, Eppes SC. Musculoskeletal infections in children. Pediatr Clin N Am. 2005;52(4):1083–106.
9. Deshpande SS, Taral N, Modi N, Singrakhia M. Changing epidemiology of neonatal septic arthritis. J Orthop Surg. 2004;12(1):10–3.
10. Carlos JNF, Sartori OC, De Oliveira GE. Epidemiological study of Osteoarticular infections in children. Acta Ortop Bras. 2018;26(3):201–5.
11. Copley LA, Kinsler MA, Gheen T, Shar A, Sun D, Browne R. The impact of evidence-based clinical practice guidelines applied by a multidisciplinary team for the care of children with osteomyelitis. J Bone Joint Surg Am. 2013;95(8):686–93.
12. Ceroni D, Kampouroglou G, Valaikaite R, Anderson della llana R, Salvo D. Osteoarticular infections in young children: what has changed over the last years? Swiss Wkly. 2014;144:w13971.
13. Dohin B, Gillet Y, Kohler R, et al. Paediatric bone and joint infections caused by Panton-valentine leucocidin-positive Staphylococcus aureus. Pediatr Infect Dis J. 2007;26:1042–8.
14. Ritz N, Curtis N. The role of Panton-valentine leukocidin in Staphylococcus aureus musculoskeletal infections in children. Pediatr Infect Dis J. 2012;31(5):514–8. https://doi.org/10.1097/INF.0b013e31824f18cb. PubMed
15. Gijon M, Bellusci M, Petraitiene B, Noguera-Julian A, Zilinskaite V, Sanchez Moreno P, et al. Factors associated with severity in invasive community-acquired Staphylococcus aureus infections in children: a prospective European multicentre study. Clin Microbiol Infect. 2016;22(7):643.e1–6. https://doi.org/10.1016/j.cmi.2016.04.004.PubMed.
16. Dodwell ER. Osteomyelitis and septic arthritis in children: current concepts. Curr Opin Pediatr. 2013;25:58–63.
17. Bruce CE, Rowland DJ, Katchburian M, Dartnell J, Robb JE. British society for children's orthopaedic surgery. The management of acute bone and joint infection in childhood—a guide to good practice http://bscos.org.uk/resources/Downloads/Blue-Book-Infection.pdf
18. Barassi A, Pallotti F, Melzi d'Eril G. Biological variation of procalcitonin in healthy individuals. Clin Chem. 2004;50(10):1878. https://doi.org/10.1373/clinchem.2004.037275.
19. Maharajan K, Patro DK, Menon J, et al. Serum Procalcitonin is a sensitive and specific marker in the diagnosis of septic arthritis and acute osteomyelitis. J Orthop Surg Res. 2013;8:19. https://doi.org/10.1186/1749-799X-8-19.
20. Kocher MS, Zurakowski D, Kasser JR, et al. Differentiating between septic arthritis and transient synovitis of the hip in children: an evidence-based clinical prediction algorithm. J Bone Joint Surg Am. 1999;81-A:1662e70.

21. Caird MS, Flynn JM, Leung L, et al. Factors distinguishing septic arthritis from transient synovitis of the hip in children. A prospective study. J Bone Joint Surg Am. 2006;88-A:1251e7.
22. Copley L, Barton T, Garcia C, et al. A proposed scoring system for assessment of severity of illness in pediatric acute hematogenous osteomyelitis using objective clinical and laboratory findings. Pediatr Infect Dis J. 2014;33:35–41.
23. Mignemi ME, Benvenuti MA, An TJ, Martus JE, Mencio GA, Lovejoy SA, Copley LA, Williams DJ, Thomsen IP, Schoenecker JG. A novel classification system based on dissemination of musculoskeletal infection is predictive of hospital outcomes. J Pediatr Orthop. 2018;38(5):279–86. https://doi.org/10.1097/BPO.0000000000000811.
24. Montgomery NI, Rosenfeld S. Pediatric osteoarticular infection update. J Pediatr Orthop. 2015;35(1):74–81. https://doi.org/10.1097/bpo.0000000000000237.
25. Hollmig ST, Copley LAB, Browne RH, et al. Deep vein thrombosis associated with osteomyelitis in children. J Bone Joint Surg Am. 2007;89:1517e23.
26. Monsalve J, Kan JH, Schallert EK, Bisset GS, Zhang W, Rosenfeld SB. Septic arthritis in children: frequency of coexisting unsuspected osteomyelitis and implications on imaging work-up and management. AJR Am J Roentgenol. 2015;204(6):1289–95. https://doi.org/10.2214/AJR.14.12891.
27. Mignemi ME, Menge TJ, Cole HA, et al. Epidemiology, diagnosis, and treatment of pericapsular pyomyositis of the hip in children. J Pediatr Orthop. 2014;34(3):316–25. https://doi.org/10.1097/BPO.0000000000000106.
28. Courtney PM, Flynn JM, Jaramillo D, Horn BD, Calabro K, Spiegel DA. Clinical indications for repeat MRI in children with acute hematogenous osteomyelitis. J Pediatr Orthop. 2010;30(8):883–7. https://doi.org/10.1097/BPO.0b013e3181fcbae5.
29. Iliadis AD, Ramachandran M. Paediatric bone and joint infection. EFORT Open Rev. 2017;2(1):7–12. https://doi.org/10.1302/2058-5241.2.160027. PMID: 28607765; PMCID: PMC5444236
30. Huang CY, Hsieh RW, Yen HT, Hsu TC, Chen CY, Chen YC, Lee CC. Short- versus long-course antibiotics in osteomyelitis: a systematic review and meta-analysis. Int J Antimicrob Agents. 2019;53(3):246–60. https://doi.org/10.1016/j.ijantimicag.2019.01.007. Epub 2019 Jan 10. PMID: 30639627
31. Hutchinson R, Henman P. Acute musculoskeletal infection in children diagnostic difficulties and when to operate. Orthop Trauma. 2020;34(6):360–8. https://doi.org/10.1016/j.mporth.2020.09.006.
32. Copley B, Lawson A. Pediatric musculoskeletal infection: trends and antibiotic recommendations. J Am Acad Orthop Surg. 2009;17(10):618–26.
33. Elzohairy MM. Primary pyomyositis in children. J Orthop Traumatol: Surg Res. 2018;104:397e403.
34. Mitsionis GI, Manoudis GN, Lykissas MG, et al. Pyomyositis in children: early diagnosis and treatment. J Pediar Surg. 2009;44:2173e8.
35. Rosenfeld SB, Mulpuri K, Copley LA. Evidence-based management of pediatric musculoskeletal infections. In: Belthur MV, Ranade AS, Herman MJ, Fernandes JA, editors. Pediatric musculoskeletal infections: principles & practice. Springer; 2022. p. 151–64.
36. Legister CS, Blumberg TJ, Copley L, Schoenecker J, Sanders J, Miller D. Pediatric musculoskeletal infection roundtable: tips and tricks for streamlining care for common scenarios–Current concept review. JPOSNA. 2022;4(4):570.
37. Belthur MV, Ranade AS, Monsell F, Herman MJ. Controversies in the management of pediatric musculoskeletal infections: an international viewpoint. Instr Course Lect. 2024;73:401–20.
38. Wang B, Cheng W, Liu F, et al. Efficacy and safety of vancomycin-loaded calcium sulfate versus conventional surgical debridement for pediatric acute osteomyelitis: a retrospective study. BMC Musculoskelet Disord. 2022;23(1):1124.
39. Gornitzky AL, Kim AE, O'Donnell JM, Swarup I. Diagnosis and management of osteomyelitis in children: a critical analysis review. JBJS Rev. 2020 Jun;8(6):e1900202.
40. Jain MJ, Bradko V, Zhu H, Inneh I, Shinava VR. Pediatric osteoarticular infection: trend in surgically treated patients and association of methicillin-resistant Staphylococcus aureus with requirement of secondary procedures. J Pediatr Orthop B. 2021 Nov 1;30(6):579–84.
41. Bisht RU, Burns JD, Smith CL, Kang P, Shrader MW, Belthur MV. The modified Kocher criteria for septic hip: does it apply to the knee? J Child Orthop. 2022 Jun;16(3):233–7.
42. Kocher MS, Mandiga R, Zurakowski D, Barnewolt C, Kasser JR. Validation of a clinical prediction rule for the differentiation between septic arthritis and transient synovitis of the hip in children. J Bone Joint Surg Am. 2004 Aug;86(8):1629–35.
43. Brown DW, Sheffer BW. Pediatric septic arthritis: an update. Orthop Clin North Am. 2019 Oct;50(4):461–70.
44. Nunn T, Rollinson P. Haematogenous pyogenic bone, and joint sepsis–Reducing avoidable morbidity. S Afr Med J. 2007;97(6):456–60.
45. Omoke NI, Obasi AA. Childhood pyogenic septic arthritis as seen in a teaching hospital south East Nigeria. Niger J Surg. 2017;23(1):26–32.
46. Chand S, Srivastava S, Afaque SF, Yadav A, Verma V, Qidwai S, Singh A. Late-presenting septic arthritis of the hip in children: variations in presentation and a review of 25 hips after surgical debridement. Cureus. 2023 Oct 26;15(10):e47717.
47. Agarwal A, Kumar KV. Suppurative arthritis of hip in a walking child: effect of patient's age, delay in surgical drainage, and organism virulence. J Orthop Surg (Hong Kong). 2020 Jan-Apr;28(1):2309499020910974.
48. Weigl DM, Becker T, Mercado E, Bar-On E. Percutaneous aspiration, and irrigation technique

for the treatment of pediatric septic hip: effectiveness and predictive parameters. J Pediatr Orthop B. 2016;25(6):514–9.
49. Thompson RM, Gourineni P. Arthroscopic treatment of septic arthritis in very young children. J Pediatr Orthop. 2017;37(1):e53–7.
50. Erkilinc M, Gilmore A, Weber M, Mistovich RJ. Current concepts in pediatric septic arthritis. J Am Acad Orthop Surg. 2021;29(5):196–206.
51. El-Sayed AM. Treatment of early septic arthritis of the hip in children: comparison of results of open arthrotomy versus arthroscopic drainage. J Child Orthop. 2008;2(3):229–37.
52. Saavedra-Lozano J, Falup- Pecurariu O, Faust SN, et al. Bone and joint infections. Pediatr Infect Dis J. 2017;36(8):788–99.
53. Donders CM, Spaans AJ, Bessems JHJM, van Bergen CJA. Arthrocentesis, arthroscopy or arthrotomy for septic knee arthritis in children: a systematic review. J Child Orthop. 2021;15(1):48–54.
54. Donders CM, Spaans AJ, Bessems JHJM, van Bergen CJA. A systematic review of the optimal drainage technique for septic hip arthritis in children. Hip Int. 2022;32(5):685–93.
55. Alhinai Z, Elahi M, Park S, et al. Prediction of adverse outcomes in pediatric acute hematogenous osteomyelitis. Clin Infect Dis. 2020;71(9):e454–e464. 56.
56. Beckles VL, Jones HW, Harrison WJ. Chronic haematogenous osteomyelitis in children: a retrospective review of 167 patients in Malawi. J Bone Joint Surg Br. 2010;92(8):1138–43.
57. Ilharreborde B. Sequelae of pediatric osteoarticular infection. Orthop Traumatol Surg Res. 2015;101(1 suppl):S129–37.
58. Horn A, Wever S, Hoffman EB. Complications following acute severe haematogenous osteomyelitis of the long bones in children. SA Orthop J. 2019;18(3):23–9.
59. Gafur OA, Copley LA, Hollmig ST, Browne RH, Thornton LA, Crawford SE. The impact of the current epidemiology of pediatric musculoskeletal infection on evaluation and treatment guidelines. J Pediatr Orthop. 2008;28(7):777–85.
60. McNeil JC, Vallejo JG, Kok EY, Sommer LM, Hultén KG, Kaplan SL. Clinical and microbiologic variables predictive of orthopedic complications following staphylococcus aureus acute Hematogenous Osteoarticular infections in children. Clin Infect Dis. 2019 Nov 13;69(11):1955–61.
61. El-Sobky T, Mahmoud S. Acute osteoarticular infections in children are frequently forgotten multidiscipline emergencies: beyond the technical skills. EFORT Open Rev. 2021 Jul 8;6(7):584–92.
62. Vij N, Singleton I, Kang P, Esparza M, Burns J, Belthur MV. Clinical scores predict acute and chronic complications in pediatric osteomyelitis: an external validation. J Pediatr Orthop. 2022 Jul 1;42(6):341–6.
63. Belthur MV, Esparza M, Fernandes JA, Choudhary M. Postinfective sequelae of pediatric musculoskeletal infections: overview & management. In: Belthur MV, Ranade AS, Herman MJ, Fernandes JA, editors. Pediatric musculoskeletal infections: principles & practice. Springer; 2022. p. 411–94.
64. Jones HW, Beckles VL, Akinola B, Stevenson AJ, Harrison WJ. Chronic haematogenous osteomyelitis in children: an unsolved problem. J Bone Joint Surg Br. 2011;93(8):1005–10.
65. Stevenson AJ, Jones HW, Chokotho LC, Beckles VL, Harrison WJ. The Beit CURE Classification of Childhood Chronic Haematogenous Osteomyelitis–a guide to treatment. J Orthop Surg Res. 2015 Sep;17(10):144.
66. Cierny G 3rd, Mader JT, Penninck JJ. A clinical staging system for adult osteomyelitis. Clin Orthop Relat Res. 2003 Sep;414:7–24.
67. Arshad Z, Lau EJ, Aslam A, Thahir A, Krkovic M. Management of chronic osteomyelitis of the femur and tibia: a scoping review. EFORT Open Rev. 2021 Sep 14;6(9):704–15.
68. Ellur V, Kumar G, Sampath JS. Treatment of chronic Hematogenous osteomyelitis in children with antibiotic impregnated calcium Sulphate. J Pediatr Orthop. 2021 Feb 1;41(2):127–31.
69. Akinyoola AL, Orimolade EA, Yusuf MB. Pathologic fractures of long bones in Nigerian children. J Child Orthop. 2008;2(6):475–9.
70. Belthur MV, Birchansky SB, Verdugo AA, Mason EO Jr, Hulten KG, Kaplan SL, Smith EO, Phillips WA, Weinberg J. Pathologic fractures in children with acute Staphylococcus aureus osteomyelitis. J Bone Joint Surg Am. 2012 Jan 4;94(1):34–42.
71. Iwai T, Hoshi M, Oebisu N, Orita K, Shimatani A, Takada N, Nakamura H. Exploration of the optimal shape for bone tumour biopsy. Anticancer Res. 2019 Aug;39(8):4191–7.
72. Bickels J, Jelinek JS, Shmookler BM, Neff RS, Malawer MM. Biopsy of musculoskeletal tumors. Current concepts. Clin Orthop Relat Res. 1999 Nov;368:212–9.
73. Daoud A, Saighi-Bouaouina A. Treatment of sequestra, pseudarthroses, and defects in the long bones of children who have chronic hematogenous osteomyelitis. J Bone Joint Surg Am. 1989;71(10):1448–68.
74. Nunn T, Patwardhan S, Hosny GA. Post infective bone gap management of the lower extremity. In: Belthur MV, Ranade AS, Herman MJ, Fernandes JA, editors. Pediatric musculoskeletal infections: principles & practice. Springer; 2022. p. 543–60.
75. Chaudhary MM, Ranade AS, Fernandes JA. Post infective bone gap management of the upper extremity. In: Belthur MV, Ranade AS, Herman MJ, Fernandes JA, editors. Pediatric musculoskeletal infections: principles & practice. Springer; 2022. p. 511–42.
76. Gouron R. Post infective bone gap management: induced membrane technique. In: Belthur MV, Ranade AS, Herman MJ, Fernandes JA, editors. Pediatric musculoskeletal infections: principles & practice. Springer; 2022. p. 561–73.

77. Pierrie SN, Hsu JR. Shortening and angulation strategies to address composite bone and soft tissue defects. J Orthop Trauma. 2017;31:S32–5.
78. Steinlechner CW, Mkandawire NC. Non-vascularised fibular transfer in the management of defects of long bones after sequestrectomy in children. J Bone Joint Surg Br. 2005;87(9):1259–63.
79. Galiwango GW, Loro F. Vascularized fibula flap in the management of segmental bone loss following osteomyelitis in children at a Ugandan hospital. J Bone Jt Infect. 2021;6(6):179–87.
80. Loro A, Loro F, Franceschi F, Brown N. Bone transport in the management of post-osteomyelitis femoral defects in children: a case series with a minimum of 10-year follow-up in Uganda. J Child Orthop. 2022;16(4):313–21.
81. Masquelet AC, Begue T. The concept of induced membrane for reconstruction of long bone defects. Orthop Clin North Am. 2010;41(1):27–37.
82. Cruickshank JA, Graham SM, Harrison WJ. Immediate bone transport: a novel technique for the management of bone defects after chronic osteomyelitis in children. Trop Dr. 2018;48(1):64–6.
83. Khaled A, El-Gebaly O, El-Rosasy M. Masquelet-Ilizarov technique for the management of bone loss post debridement of infected tibial nonunion. Int Orthop. 2022;46(9):1937–44.
84. Tudisco C, Farsetti P, Gatti S, Ippolito E. Influence of chronic osteomyelitis on skeletal growth: analysis at maturity of 26 cases affected during childhood. J Pediatr Orthop. 1991;11(3):358–63.
85. Peterson HA. Partial growth plate arrest and its treatment. J Pediatr Orthop. 1984;4(2):246–58.
86. Ecklund K, Jaramillo D. Patterns of premature physeal arrest: MR imaging of 111 children. AJR Am J Roentgenol. 2002;178(4):967–72.
87. Murphy RF, Plumblee L, Barfield WB, et al. Septic arthritis of the hip-risk factors associated with secondary surgery. J Am Acad Orthop Surg. 2019;27(9):321–6.
88. Forlin E, Milani C. Sequelae of septic arthritis of the hip in children: a new classification and a review of 41 hips. J Pediatr Orthop. 2008;28(5):524–8.
89. Johari AN, Dhawale AA, Johari RA. Management of post septic hip dislocations when the capital femoral epiphysis is present. J Pediatr Orthop B. 2011;20(6):413–21.
90. Choi IH, Yoo WJ, Cho TJ, Chung CY. Operative reconstruction for septic arthritis of the hip. Orthop Clin North Am. 2006;37(2):173–83. vi
91. Johari AN, Hampannavar A, Johari RA, Dhawale AA. Coxa vara in post septic arthritis of the hip in children. J Pediatr Orthop B. 2017;26(4):313–9.

# 9 Osteoarticular Infections in Adults

Ferdinando Da Rin de Lorenzo

Hematogenous joint infections in adults represent a relatively low percentage as the major cause of joint infections is represented by trauma, postsurgical infections, and also local infiltrations, which, in some cases, have been the cause of joint infections. Usually occurs after septicemia or, as with tuberculosis, from a mostly pulmonary focus. I, therefore, thought of treating the tuberculous forms (specific forms), about which little is known, comparing them with the pyogenic (non-specific forms), also giving attention to this pathology which is far from having disappeared and which presents high resistance to normal anti-tubercular drugs. Therefore, the tuberculous joint pathology will be described comparing it with the pyogenic form, highlighting the differences both in diagnosis and in treatment. A typical arthritis in adults is bone tuberculosis which represents approximately 5% of secondary extrapulmonary localizations (Figs. 9.1 and 9.2) [1–4]. In the case of vertebral localization, especially the dorsal one, the infection sometimes occurs due to contiguity from a pulmonary focus. But the "vertebral" topic will not be discussed in this chapter.

Latest tuberculosis estimate: worldwide there were nearly 9 million new cases of tuberculosis and 1.4 million cases of tuberculosis with bone involvement. The World Health Organization (WHO) declared TB a global public health emergency in 1993 (Fig. 9.3) [1, 5, 6].

The arrival of emigrants, especially from Africa, has brought this disease back to Italy, even though most of the subjects come from Eastern Europe (Fig. 9.4).

*Before entering into the diagnosis of the infections, it is important to highlight that there are, in all cases, risk factors that can increase infections.*

*The general risk factors* [9–12] concern the patient's condition rather than the virulence of the germ:

$$\text{Septic risk factors} = \frac{\text{contaminant bacterial load} \times \text{virulence}}{\text{host resistance}}$$

- Poor personal hygiene and an overcrowded environment
- Pathologies with immunodeficiencies (HIV infection: the virus that causes AIDS)
- Corticosteroid therapy (e.g., A.R.)
- Oncological pathologies
- Diabetes mellitus
- Reduced nutritional status
- Older age
- Obesity
- Organ Transplants
- Silicosis
- Skin disorders and/or open wounds
- Smokers (recommended to quit 6 weeks before the eventual intervention)
- Drug intake and alcohol abuse

F. Da Rin de Lorenzo (✉)
Codivilla-Putti Institutes, National Reference Center for the diagnosis and treatment of bone infections, Cortina d'Ampezzo (BL), Italy


P. Ruggieri et al. (eds.), *Bone and Joint Infections*, https://doi.org/10.1007/978-3-031-96383-4_9

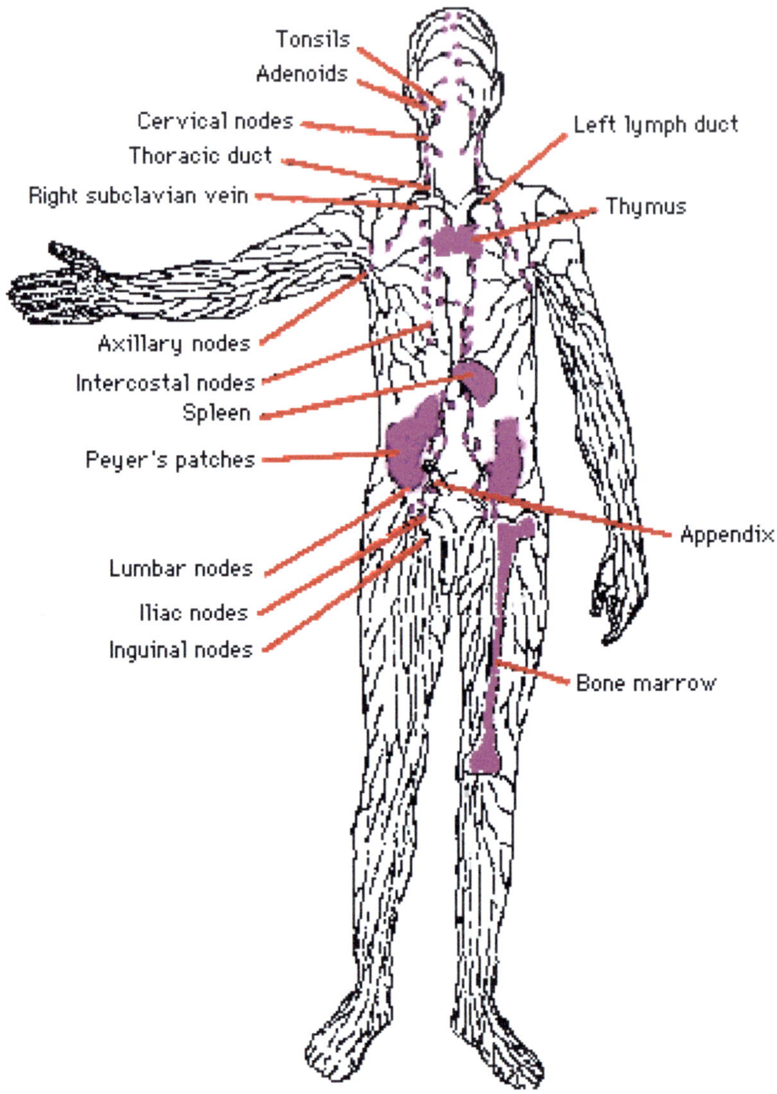


**Fig. 9.1** The relationship between *Mycobacterium tuberculosis* and humans is a complex and delicate balance and is a persistent disease. The lymphatic system and the typical localization

A classification of bone infections identifies the nonspecific forms (Osteomyelitis-Osteoarthritis) with the specific forms (mostly tuberculous) (Fig. 9.5).

Over the years, cases have decreased in our Institute, and nowadays we treat around 40 cases per year in total of all bone localizations (Fig. 9.6).

Out of a total of 4473 cases, these are the percentages of localizations (Fig. 9.7) [8] that remain unchanged to this day, with the prevalence of vertebral localizations followed by the hip and knee.

A different percentage in the pyogenic forms out of a total of 3713 cases (Fig. 9.8) that affect the joints as the long bones are normally affected more.

Types of the most frequently encountered typical and atypical mycobacteria (MB) (Table 9.1) [13]:

- *Typical:*
  - *Mycobacterium tuberculosis hominis* (B.K.)
  - *Mycobacterium bovis e avium*
- *Atypical:*
  - *Mycobacterium kansaii*
  - *Mycobacterium marinum*
  - *Mycobacterium scrofolaceum*
  - *Mycobacterium flavescens*
  - *Mycobacterium avium* complex
  - *Mycobacterium xenopi*
  - *Mycobacterium fortuitum*
  - *Mycobacterium chelone*

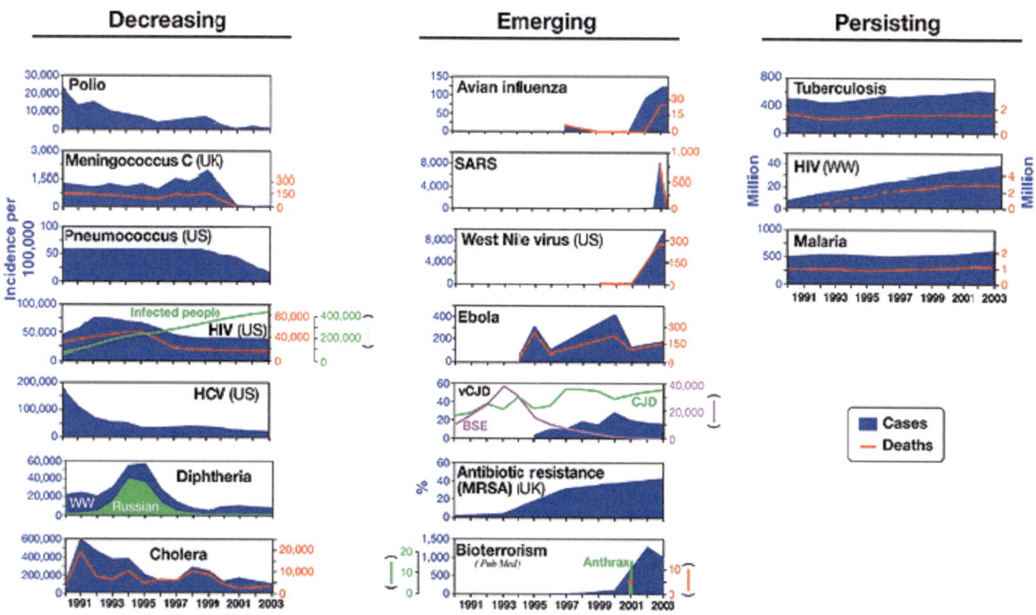


**Fig. 9.2** Area chart displaying trends in disease incidence from 1991 to 2003, categorized into decreasing, emerging, and persisting diseases. The left column shows decreasing diseases like Polio and HIV in the US, with incidence per 100.000. The middle column highlights emerging diseases such as Avian Influenza and SARS, with varying scales. The right column presents persisting diseases like Tuberculosis and Malaria, measured in millions. Blue areas represent cases, and red lines indicate deaths. The chart includes specific labels for diseases and region, with a legend for color coding. Deaths (990,000 among HIV-negative people and 430,000 HIV-associated TB deaths). The latest estimates are that there were almost nine million new cases in 2011 and 1.4 million bone TB. The World Health Organization (WHO) declared TB a global public health emergency in 1993. [5, 6]

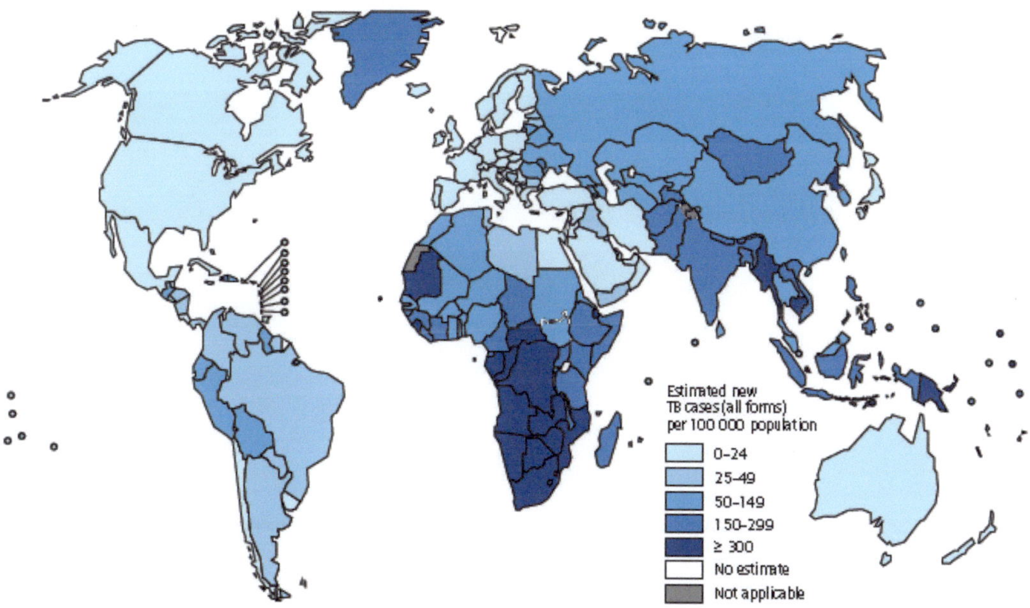


**Fig. 9.3** World map illustrating estimated new TB incidence rates, per 100.000 population by country, 2013 [1, 5, 6]

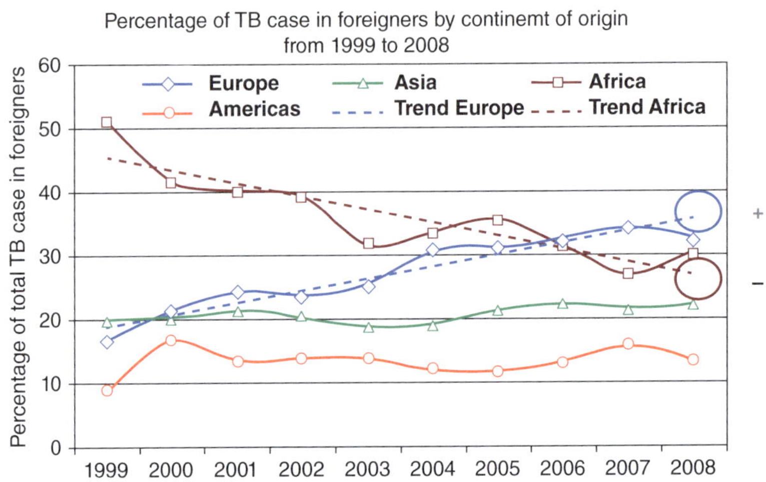


**Fig. 9.4** Line chart showing the percentage of tuberculosis (TB) cases in foreigners by continent of orig froma 1999 to 2008 in Italy. The chart includes data for Europe, Asia, Africa and the Americas, with trend lines for Europe and Africa. The y-axis represents the percentage of total TB cases in foreigners, ranging from 0 to 60%. The x-axis covers the years 1999 to 2008. There has been an improvement regarding the trend from Africa; however, the trend from Europe is negative with an increase of 3–5% Asia and Americas remain relatively stable [5–9]. Before entering into the diagnosis of the infection, it is important to highlight that there are, in all cases, risk factors that can increase infections

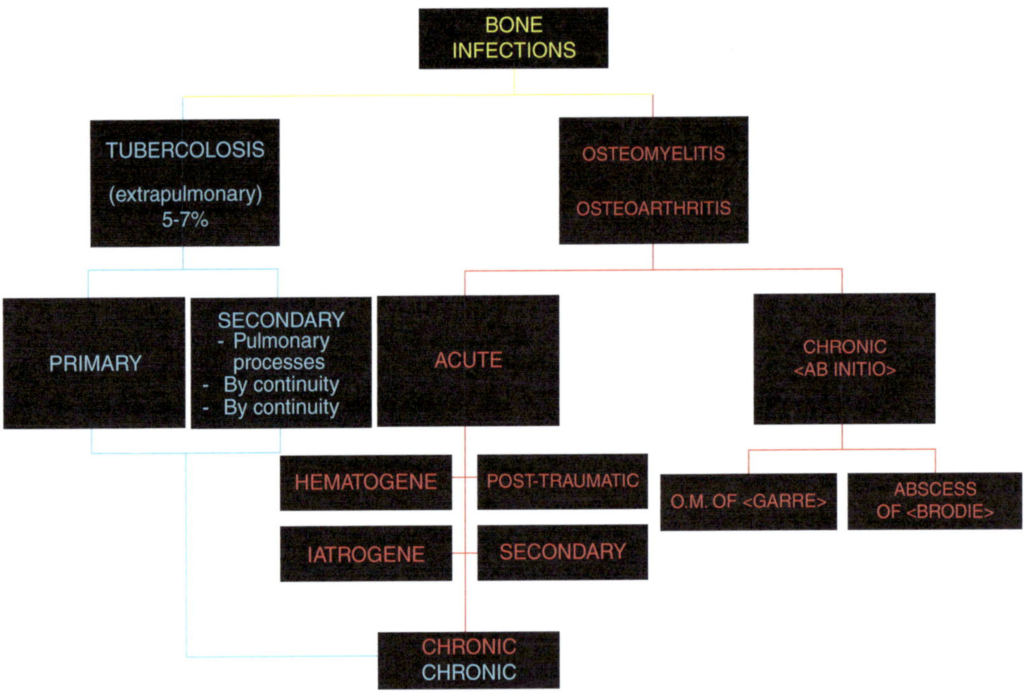


**Fig. 9.5** Classification of bone infections: A flowchart illustrating the classification of bone infections. The diagram begins with "Bone Infections" at the top, then branches out into Tuberculosis (Extrapulmonary-Osseous) 5-7%" and Osteomyelitis-Osteoarthritis. Tuberculosis is then classified into primary, secondary (pulmonary processes by continuity, by contiguity) and finally chronic forms. Osteomyelitis and osteoarthritis are classified as acute or chronic "ab initio" such as Garrè's sclerosing osteomyelitis or Brodie's abscess. Acute forms are divided into hematogenous, post-traumatic, iatrogenic and secondary to a nearby focus. All of these forms can become chronic. The flowchart uses different colors to distinguish the different forms

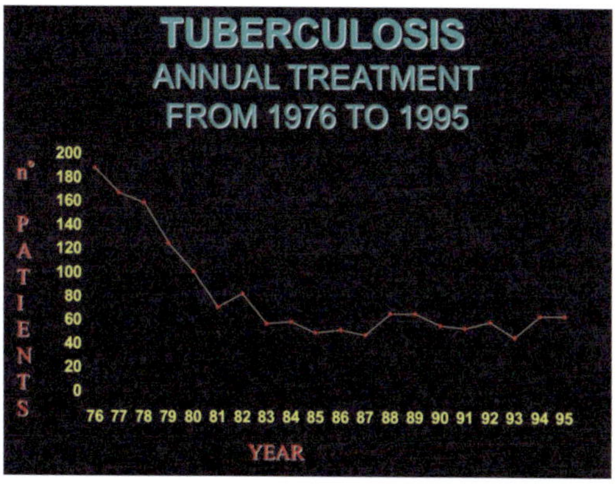


Fig. 9.6 The trend of hospitalizations for bone tuberculosis at the Putti hospital in Cortina in the years. The x-axis represents years from 1976 to 1995, and the y-axis represents the number of patients, ranging from 0 to 200. The chart shows a general decline in the number of patients over the years, with fluctuations

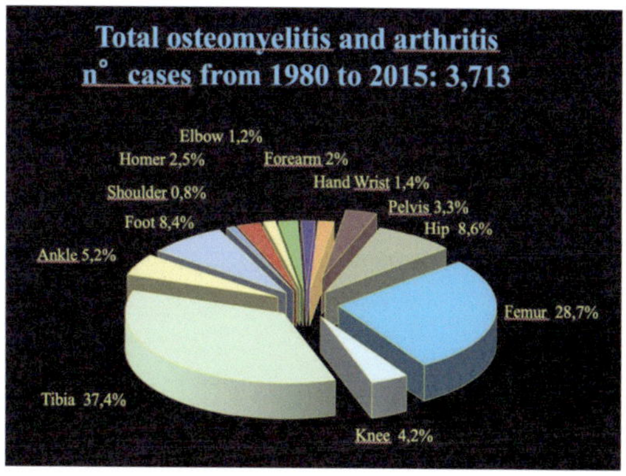


Fig. 9.8 Pie chart illustrating the percentage of localizations of non-tuberculous bone infections (nonspecific) cases from 1980 to 2015, totaling 3.713 cases. The most important localizations involve the long bones and less so the joints, including prosthetics

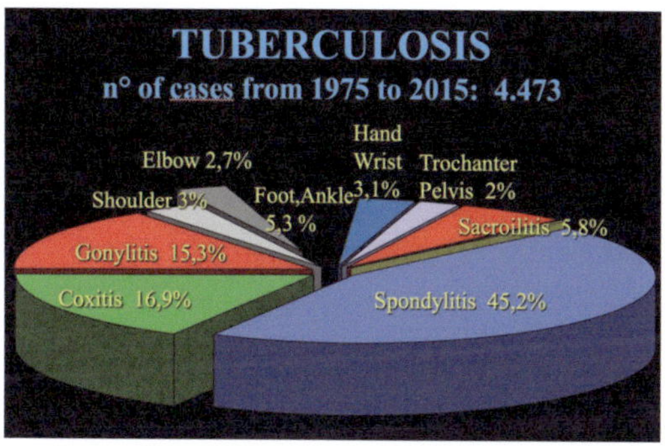


Fig. 9.7 Pie chart illustating the percentage of localizations of tuberculous bone infections (specific) in different part froma 1975 to 2015, totaling 4.473 cases, especially joint. The largest segment is Spondylitis at 45.2%, followed by Coxitis at 16.9% and Gonylitis at 15.3%

**Table 9.1** The different laboratory microbiological highlighting characteristics of MB Atypical

| Ruyon group | organism |
|---|---|
| I (photochromogens) | *M. marinum*<br>*M. kansaii* |
| II (scotochromogens) | *M. szulgai*<br>*M. gordonae* |
| III (nonchromogens) | *M. intracellulare*<br>*M. malmoense*<br>*M. xeopi, M. terrae* |
| IV (rapid growers) | *M. chelonei*<br>*M. fortuitum* |

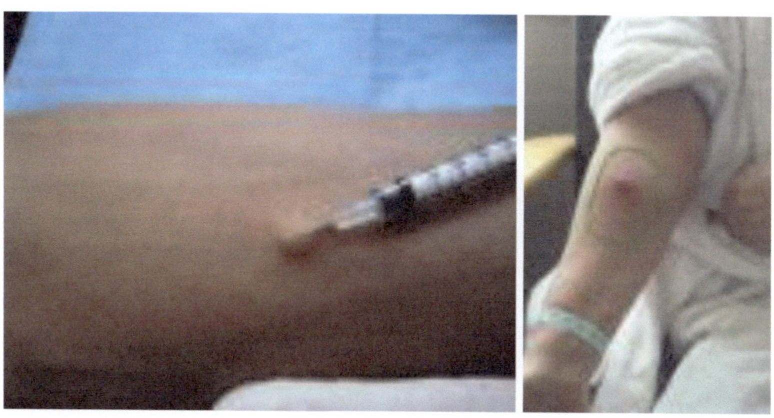

Fig. 9.9 Intradermal Mantoux reaction. Is it a subcutaneous inoculation and on the right positive reaction on the test

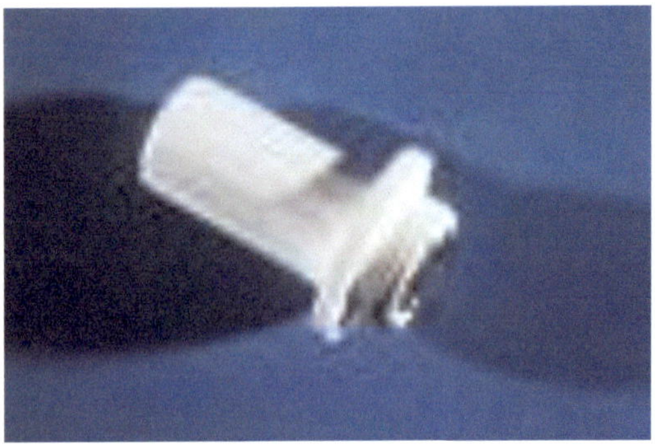

**Fig. 9.10** Tine test. It is a system that olready has the purified protein of the Mycobacterium inside it and is applied directly tothe skin

Pyogenic infections are generally caused and decreasing in percentage by:

- *Staphylococcus aureus*
- *Staphylococcus epidermidis*
- Gram-negative flora
- *Pyocyanus* or *Pseudomonas aeruginosa*
- Anaerobes
- Rarely Mycetes

The history in specific forms is not always helpful unless the patient does not work in contact with meat (e.g., butchers), has not recently had a pulmonary tuberculosis episode, has not come into contact with a tuberculosis patient, or does not come from areas where tuberculosis is endemic. It should be considered that many patients have a calcified primary tuberculosis complex without any symptoms but have a positive Mantoux (Fig. 9.9) or Tine test (Fig. 9.10). The latter is a test consisting of a special disk equipped with four tips previously immersed in a solution of purified bacillary extracts completely free of toxic action; the length of the tips is such as to inoculate a standardized number of units of purified protein derivative, called PPD, into the dermis; after 48 h the inoculation point is examined, where, in the event of a positive reaction, an erythematous infiltrate of proportional extension appears to individual sensitivity.

The tuberculin reaction becomes positive 4–6 weeks after infection.

There is also the "Quantiferon" test [14, 15]. It is a venous blood sample that is placed in test tubes, which detects the quantity of interferon gamma cytokine released following stimulation of T lymphocytes with two specific TB antigens (ESAT-6 and CFP-10) [16–18]. In fact, the laboratory tests are normally different; in the tuberculous form, the erythrocyte sedimentation rate (ESR) and the PCR can be normal unless there is a nonspecific superinfection. Therefore, the tests are the TB test (hematological) and the LCx (in the pus or in the pulmonary secretion). However, ESR, C-reactive protein (CRP), and fibrinogen for nonspecific forms are important. The biopsy as well as the culture examination is very important.

We compared 30 cases of tuberculous arthritis with 19 cases of pyogenic hematogenous arthritis (Table 9.2) and we took into consideration, by comparing them, the different characteristics [16, 19]. The medical history is important in the two pathologies, especially if there was a previous tuberculous episode, if the hygienic conditions are reduced, if the patient has come into contact

**Table 9.2** Comparison between tuberculous bone disease and nontuberculous bone disease

| | Specific (tbc) | Nonspecific (piogenic) |
|---|---|---|
| Anamnesis | 10/30 | 12/19 |
| Clinic | 10/30 | 14/19 |
| Radiographic situation | 10/30 | 6/19 |
| RMN scintigraphy | | |
| With marked leukocytes | 12/19 | |
| Laboratory | 6/30 | 19/19 |
| Mantoux or tine test | 28/30 | ////// |
| Cultural examination | 5/30 | 19/19 |
| Biopsy/histology | 19/30 | ////// |

**Table 9.3** Comparison between tuberculous bone disease and non-tuberculous bone disease

| | Specific | Nonspecific |
|---|---|---|
| Pain | Insidious | Acute |
| Fistolae | Yes (attention overinfection) | Yes |
| Edema | Yes | Yes |
| Thermotouch | No | Yes |
| Reddened skin | No | Yes |
| Functional limitation | Yes | Yes |
| Deformity | Yes | Yes |
| Laboratory | Very altered * | Very altered ** |

* TB test (hematologic)—lcs (pus a/o secreted)
** V.E.S.—PCR—Fibrinogen - Complete blood count with formula

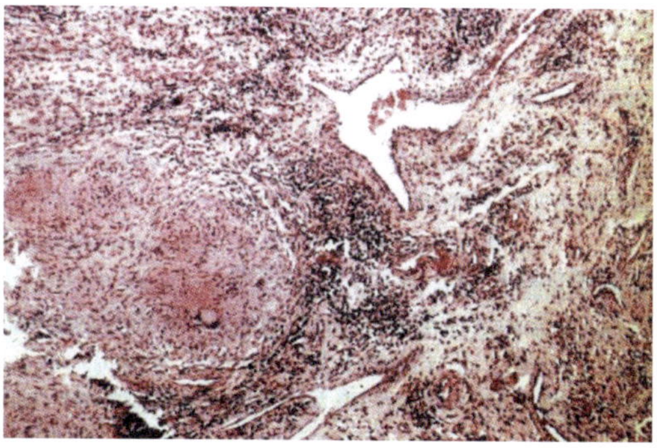

**Fig. 9.11** Typical tuberculoma with central caseous necrosis with the presence of Langerhans cells

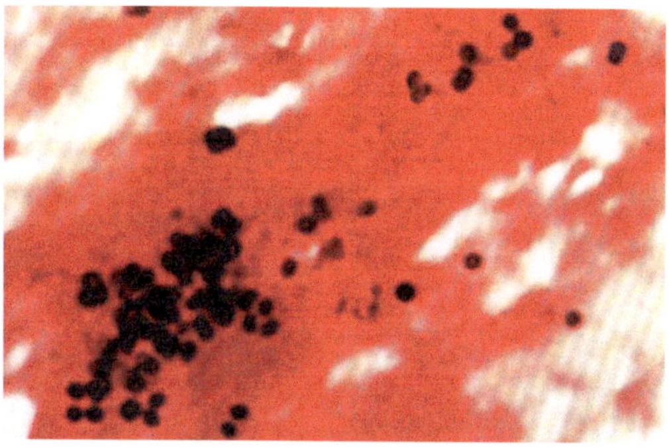

**Fig. 9.12** Culture of pus containing *Staphylococcus aureus*

with a positive person, or if he has risk factors that also concern the pyogenic forms.

The clinic (Table 9.3) highlights how the tuberculous form does not have important septic signs, in fact it does not present the classic signs of inflammation (color, rubor, and dolor et functio lesa) being a "cold" condition, the opposite of the pyogenic pathology. Scintigraphy with marked autologous leukocytes is fundamental for the pyogenic form and less so for the tuberculous form which can, however, give us false positives. The laboratory with the classic signs of infection is derisive for the pyogenic forms, less so for the tuberculous ones. Generally, ESR, PCR, and Fibrinogen were altered in all pyogenic forms only in 1/3 in tuberculous ones. Mantoux and Tine tests were positive in 28 cases. It should be considered that the two cases were anergic subjects and therefore not immunologically active.

The culture examination did not allow us to isolate the mycobacterium in almost all cases but with the biopsy (Fig. 9.11) we managed to obtain all the diagnoses for the tuberculous forms while the culture examination (Fig. 9.12) for the pyogenic forms highlighted 100% of the cases. However, it must be considered that the negativity of the culture test is not an indication of the absence of infection which will be considered after having carried out the entire set of assessments. In fact, the diagnosis is not the outcome of a single piece of data but the overall data collected.

Continuing the clinical comparison between the two pathological forms, first of all, the big difference is the phlogistic aspect, which in the tuberculous form does not present redness and is not hot to the touch, as are the abscesses, which by definition are defined as "cold." Something completely different for nonspecific forms. The TBC forms appear today, so much modified in comparison with classical tables that it is difficult to differentiate the two forms. It is easy to have over-infections in TBC forms or combinations of mixed forms, especially in the super-infections of phytolized tuberculous forms.

Laboratory tests are fundamental for the diagnosis of tuberculosis and are the hematological one, the Tb test (A 60) Serological diagnosis of tbc—IgA, IgM, IgG counts (80% positive) [17] and in the search for mycobacterium antigens in pus or in the pulmonary secretion which is LCx amplification mycobacteria's gene (Ligase reaction at chain) (100% of validity and results are available in 7 days) [18]. The radiographic appearance of a tuberculous arthritic form can be divided into four stages (Figs. 9.13, 9.14, 9.15, and 9.16).

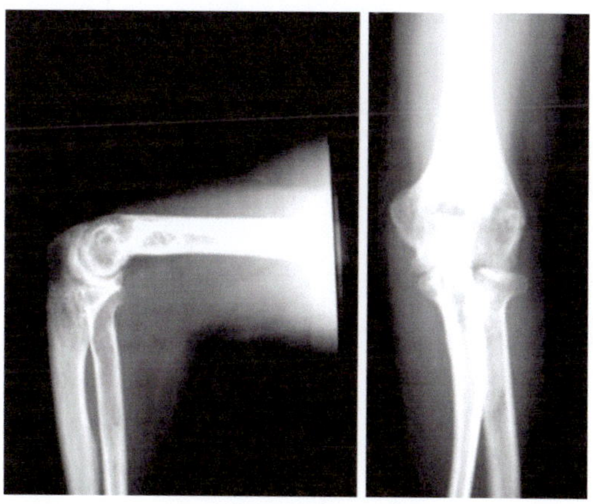

**Fig. 9.13** A radiographic example of stage 1 tubercular arthritis of the elbow with demineralization caused by inflammation of the synovial membrane

## Stage 1

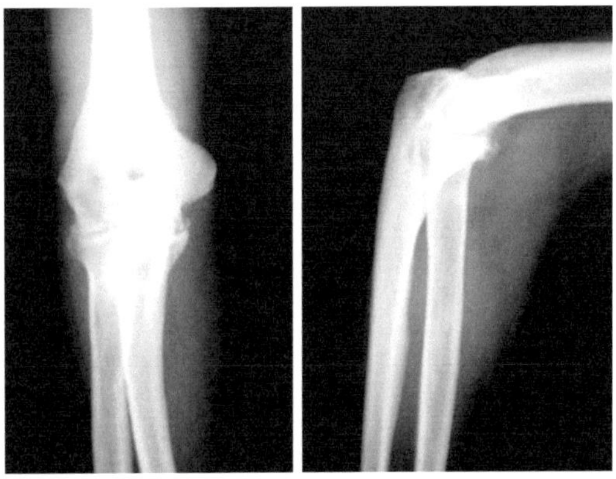

**Fig. 9.14** In the stage 2 is evident narrowing of the articular space due to initial destruction of the cartilage. In this stage, the synovial membrane will hypertrophy and will fill the articular space; bone erosion develops at the sites where the articular capsule is attached

## Stage 2

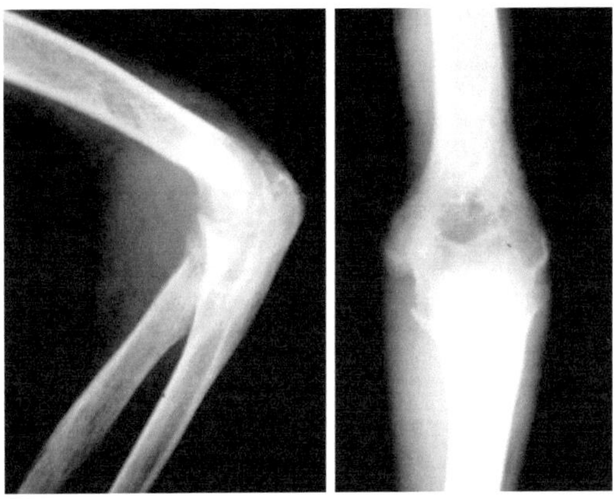

**Fig. 9.15** In the stage 3 the entire joint is affected and presents many bone lesions, and the articular space is narrowing without serious anatomical destruction of the articulation. In this stage, the joint space is filled with hypertrophic synovial membrane and pus. The articular cartilage, the capsule, and the ligaments are destroyed. There could also be abscesses and fistulas

## Stage 3

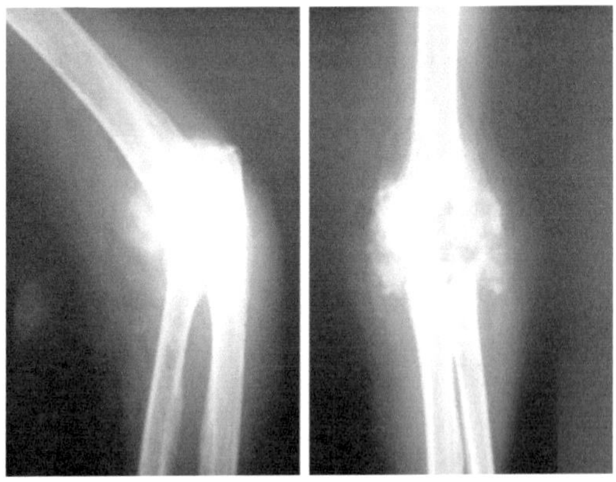

**Fig. 9.16** In the stage 4 the further joint destruction with disruption of the anatomical profile

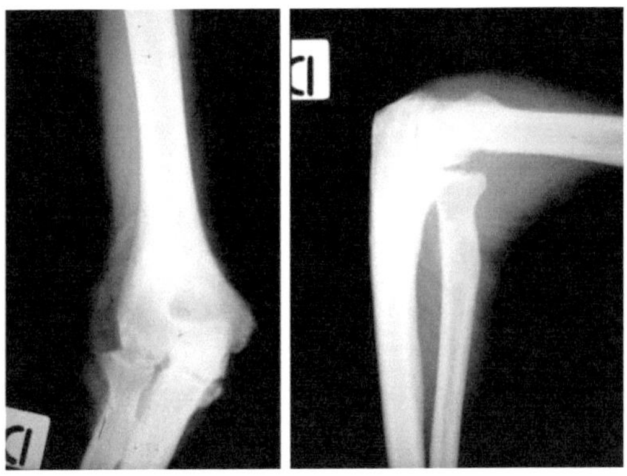

**Fig. 9.17** An apparently normal X-ray....

## Stage 4

A radiological test that can help identify a focus is the CT scan (Figs. 9.17 and 9.18), especially in certain areas such as the pelvis or spine or as in the following case, where the focus was able to be localized in correspondence with the olecranon area.

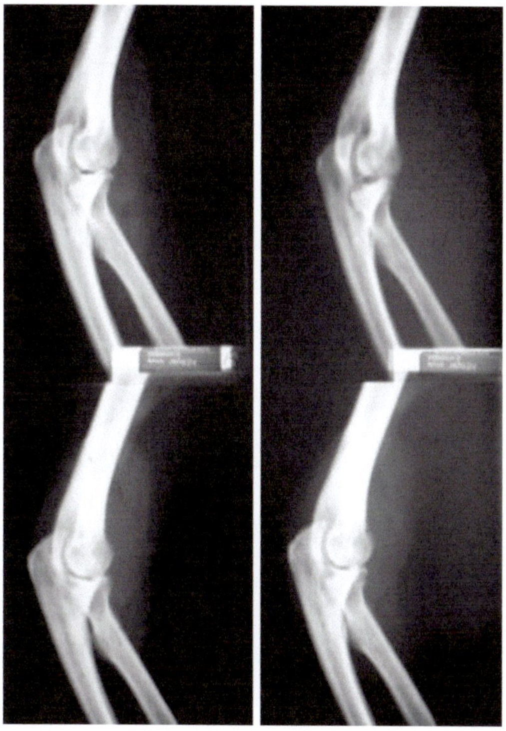

**Fig. 9.18** … but the CT images showing a focus in the olecranon site

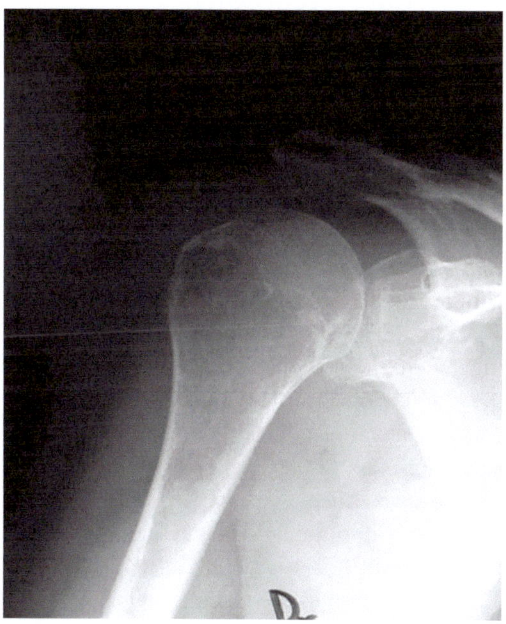

**Fig. 9.19** An apparently normal X-ray of the shoulder …

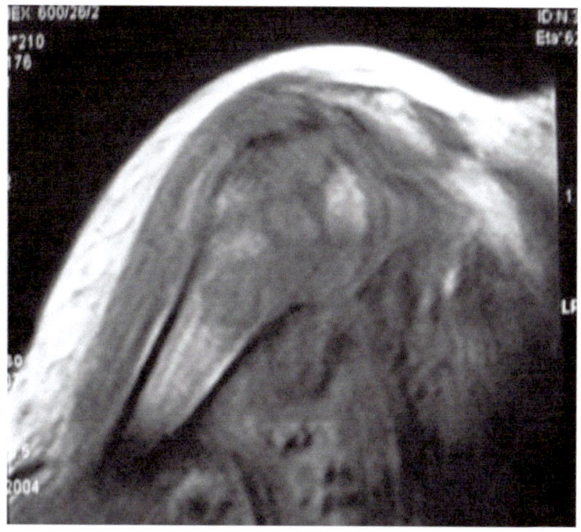

**Fig. 9.20** … but on MRI, there are epiphyseal septic foci

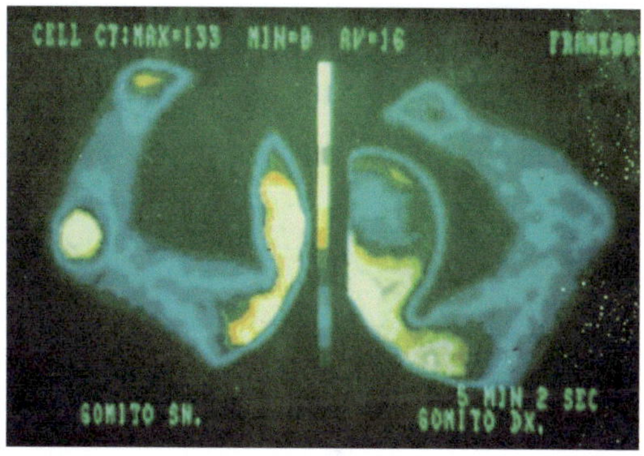


**Fig. 9.21** A scintigraphy with autologous labeled leukocytes showing septic arthritis of the left elbow while the right elbow is normal

Nuclear magnetic resonance (MRI) (Figs. 9.19 and 9.20) [19] is very important because it allows us to identify any septic foci as in the following case, where on the X-ray everything appears normal and instead on the MRI some epiphyseal foci appear.

Furthermore, scintigraphy (Fig. 9.21) with autologous labeled leukocytes.

It should be considered that these radiological tests (conventional radiography, CT scan, MRI, and scintigraphy with technetium) are not specific for the differential diagnosis between the various joint septic forms, but indicate the presence of a septic focus and not the type of infection. The most important test for a differential diagnosis is endoarticular aspiration and biopsy.

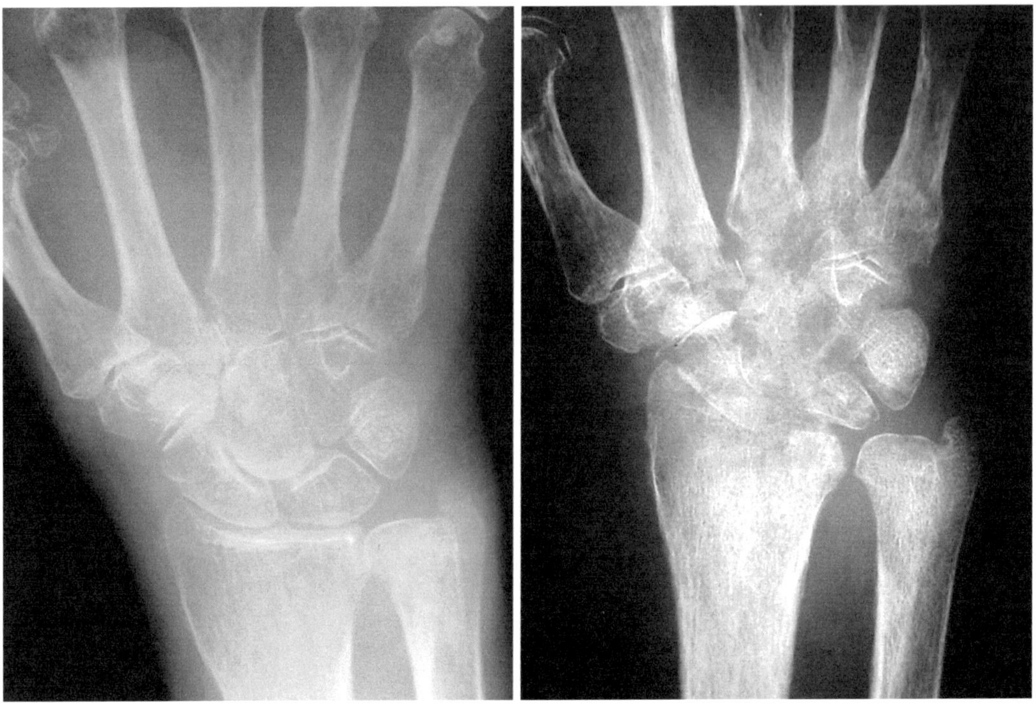

**Fig. 9.22** An example of a tuberculous form of the wrist treated with cortisone for the diagnosis of rheumatoid arthritis that has evolved into carpitis [19. 22]

The biopsy can be performed in joints such as the hip, knee, ankle, shoulder, and wrist, even arthroscopically, which allows the precise collection of any material from the site of the focus, but also capsular parts.

*The differential diagnosis* [20, 21] in tuberculosis pathology is made above all on a percentage basis, from top to bottom, with:

- Non-tuberculous mycobacteria
- Pyogenic arthritis
- Rheumatoid arthritis (Fig. 9.22) [19].
- Osteomyelitis
- Fungal arthritis
- Viral infections
- Sero-negative arthritis
- Gout
- Pseudodogout

We must always suspect a tuberculous form when faced with an X-ray with osteopenia, a reduction in the joint rim, and possibly if there are irregularities on the joint edges, such as nail marks (Phemister's Triad) [4, 18].

## 9.1 Antibiotic Therapy for Osteoarticular Tuberculosis (Table 9.4) [22]

In our experience, we have adopted a local and a general therapy. The first consists of 3-week cycles on alternate days where the antibiotic is introduced into the affected joint by infiltration, which is removed from the general therapy [23–26]. The general therapy is daily, being a therapy with various antibiotics. Therefore, isonicotinic acid, ethambutol, and streptomycin are used to infiltrate while rifampicin (600 mg) is given orally in the morning on an empty stomach with a glass of water to avoid enzymatic induction, which creates drug-induced hepatitis. Recently, it is common to give Rifater ® which contains 50 mg of isoniazid, 120 mg of rifampicin, and 300 mg of pyrazinamide. It is used to administer 3–6 tablets per day, which must be taken all together on an empty stomach and 1–2 h before meals with a little water. This description of antibiotic therapy concerns adults.

**Table 9.4** Recommended doses of first line antituberculosis drugs for adult

| Drug | Recommended dose | | | |
|---|---|---|---|---|
| | Daily | | 3 times per week | |
| | Dose and range (mg/kg body weight) | Maximum (mg) | Dose and range (mg/kg body weight) | Daily maximum (mg) |
| Isoniazid | 5 (4–6) | 300 | 10 (8–12) | 900 |
| Rifampicin | 10 (8–12) | 600 | 10 (8–12) | 600 |
| Pyrazinamide | 25 (20–30) | – | 35 (30–40) | – |
| Ethambutol | 15 (15–20) | – | 30 (25–35) | – |
| Streptomycin[a] | 15 (12–18) | | 15 (12–18) | 1000 |

[a] Patients aged over 60 years may not be able to tolerate more than 500–750 mg daily, so some guidelines recommend reduction of the dose to 10 mg/kg per day in patients in this age group (2). Patients weighing less than 50 kg may not tolearate doses above 500–750 mg daily (*WHO Model Formulary 2008*, www.who.int/selection_medicines/list/en/)

For children, the dosages and antibiotic drugs are obviously not the same. Antibiotic therapy can last from 6 months to 18 months.

Visual and auditory function and liver and kidney function must be checked because these antibiotics can cause damage to the optic nerve [27] and/or acoustic and renal and hepatic dysfunction.

Table 9.4 The antibiogram of mycobacterium is very important because there are some forms that are resistant to common antituberculosis drugs but sensitive to antibiotics used for pyogenic forms [22]. We will now deal with some localizations, always comparing the tuberculous forms with the pyogenic ones.

## 9.2 Locations

### 9.2.1 Tuberculous Arthritis of the Hip (Coxitis) 16.9% TB and 8.6% Pyogenic [28–34]

For diagnosis, in addition to what has been seen previously, it is important to carry out an arthrocentesis which, as we have said, needs to be ultrasound-guided (Figs. 9.23 and 9.24), as the joint is in depth and it is also useful if you want to reach a possible outbreak or spill.

The symptoms of septic arthritis usually appear rapidly and include acute pain in the groin region, swelling and local heat associated with evening fever but chills, tiredness, and generalized weakness, inability to move the limb may also be present, and the inability to walk with weight on the affected limb. The treatment of acute forms generally consists of an arthrotomy, associated with surgical cleaning, especially of the soft parts, and the application of drains for continuous washing for 7–10 days (Fig. 9.25). On the same occasion, samples can be taken for histological examination and analysis of the collected liquid.

Treatment with broad-spectrum antibiotics is started immediately while awaiting the results of the culture tests and the antibiogram associated with anti-inflammatories and antipyretics. Bear in mind that the results of the samples, if it is tuberculosis, can be obtained even after 10–15 days. Rest, the use of braces to avoid direct load which must be maintained for at least a month. In our experience we have used, in cases in which a possible joint collapse was suspected, mobilizations with trans-skeletal traction, in others cases of active and passive mobilizations with the help of the physiotherapist. If the diagnosis results in a tuberculous form, antibiotic therapy (multidrug therapy) [1] must be started immediately and continued for at least a year. Instead, if it is a form, for example, staphylococcal, the therapy, usually with two antibiotics, must be continued for 6–8 weeks, the same treatment if we are faced with a mycobacterium resistant to antitubercular drugs.

Infection of a joint at a young age very often leads, if not treated with the utmost urgency, to the complete destruction of the joint itself. The reinfection rate on prostheses applied in septic arthritis if caused by Gram-negative germs is 20%. In TB of 40%, therefore, we believe that the objective is to perform the prosthesis in two stages [35]. In tuberculous forms, as the biofilm

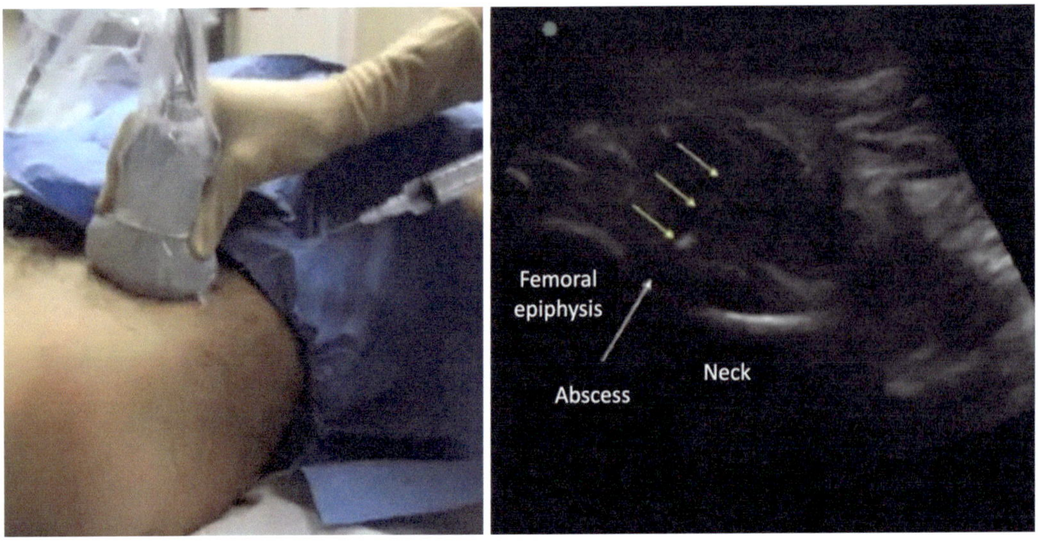


**Fig. 9.23** Ultrasound that highlights an abscess near the femoral epiphysis, that can be aspirated under ultrasound guidance

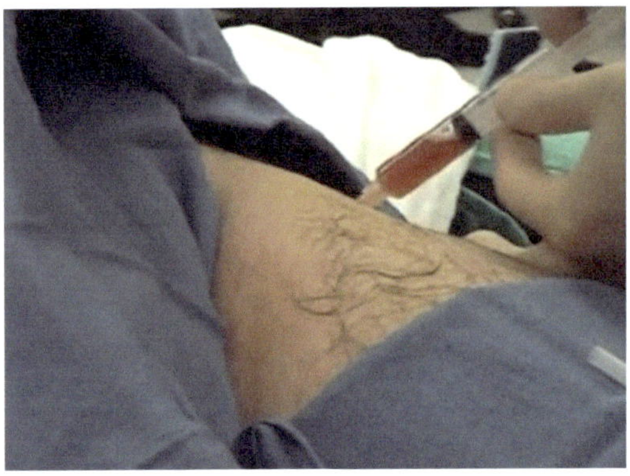

**Fig. 9.24** The aspiration of the material that will be examined

is missing, it is possible to restore the prosthesis in one stage [35–40] but we prefer to do it in two stages, trying to save the bone structures as much as possible [33]. For the prosthesis of pyogenic septic arthritis, once an irreparable lesion has been created in the joint, we intervene by applying a prosthesis and as we have said in our experience, we do it in two stages.

If we carry out an excellent surgical cleaning, we are a little more economical because we want to maintain the vascularization of the neck as much as possible as highlighted in the following case:

A 35-year-old male patient who complained of severe pain and was treated with antibiotics without carrying out emptying and drainage and also favoring weight bearing, and, therefore, as a result, we had osteolysis of the cup and lysis of the epiphyseal area (Fig. 9.26a–b). Upon arthrocentesis, it was found to be *Mycobacterium hominis*. Blood tests showed an ESR of 28 and CRP was normal.

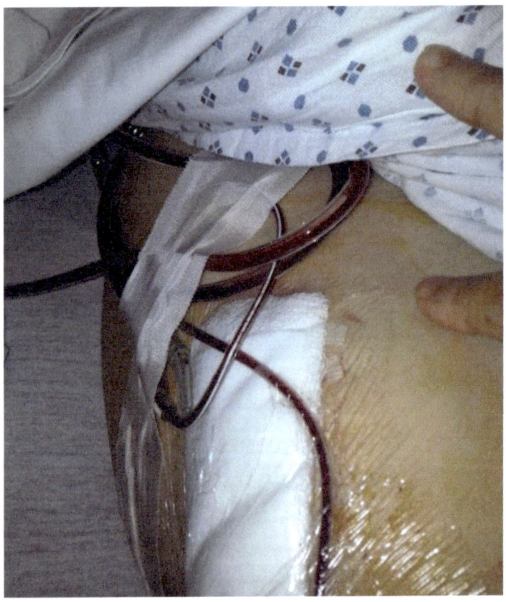

**Fig. 9.25** Arthrotomy and surgical cleaning with application of drains for continuous washing. A DAIR on a the tubercular form

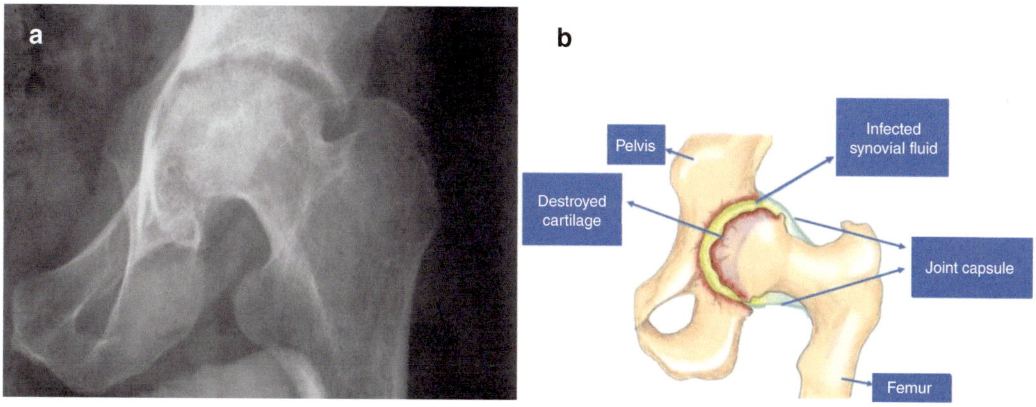


**Fig. 9.26a–b** (Fig. 9.26a) An X-ray showing septic arthritis and the drawing (Fig. 9.26b) reproducing the pathological condition of the hip arthritis

After two cycles of general and local antibiotic therapy, it was decided to carry out the prosthetic surgery in two stages. Therefore, removal of the femoral epiphysis, cleaning and reaming of the cotyle. Cleaning of the remaining part of the neck and multiple samples, both in the central areas and in the remaining neck, for culture examination and antibiogram. A self-made spacer was then applied with the addition of two anti-tuberculosis drugs:

Rifampicin.........10%
Streptomycin......5%

(The percentage is related to 40 g of polymethylmethacrylate powder)

Radiographic data to consider is the osteopenia of the hip and epiphyseal wormholes, as well as reduction of the joint rim (Phemister's Triad) (Fig. 9.27) [32, 33].

After 60 days with negative culture tests, negative laboratory tests, and an almost normal local clinical appearance, the second surgical stage is performed: removal of the spacer (Fig. 9.28) and application prosthesis (Fig. 9.29).

Also, on this occasion, samples are taken for culture and antibiogram examination, and the spacer is sent to the laboratory to carry out the microbiological research test with dithiothreitol, which did not reveal any germs or mycobacteria.

Another case of a 45-year-old male patient presenting with coxalgia that arose after a 10-day feverish period with episodes of 40° resistant to antipyretics and antibiotics given by his doctor. Laboratory tests reveal a significant alteration of ESR, CRP, and fibrinogen as well as an increase in neutrophils.

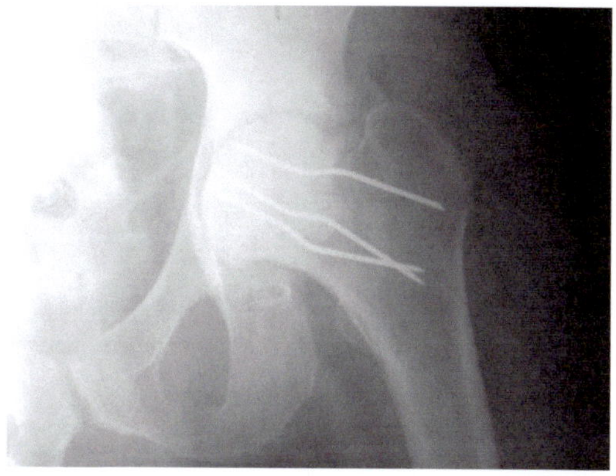

**Fig. 9.27** Radiographic appearance with the antibiotic spacer

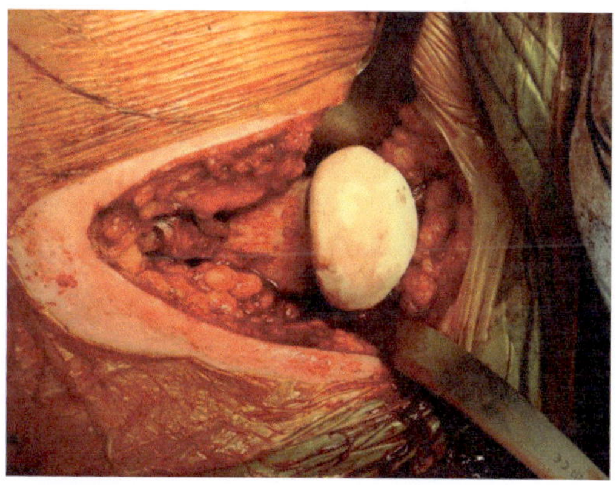

**Fig. 9.28** Surgical removal of the antibiotic spacer

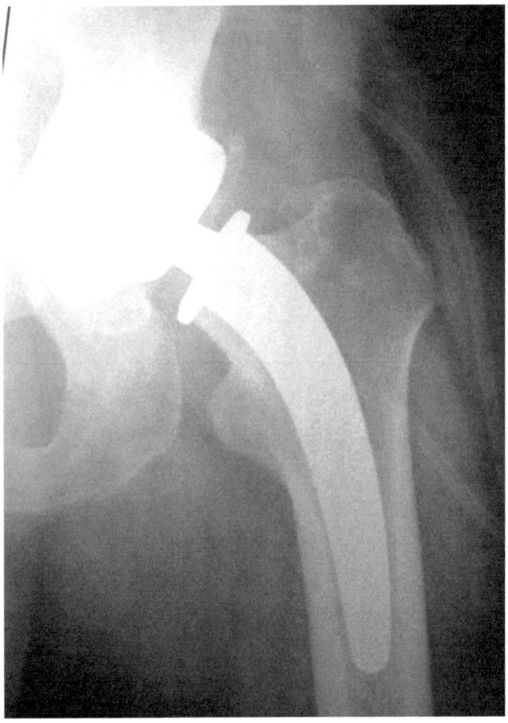

Fig. 9.29 X-ray 10 years later, the result remained unchanged, and the tuberculosis has never reactivated

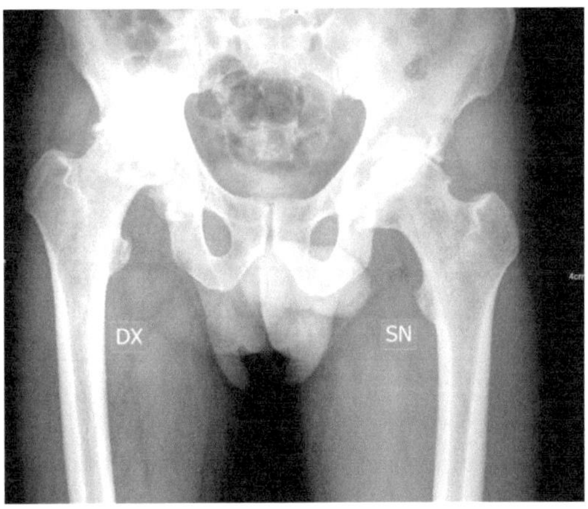


Fig. 9.30 X-ray of suspected septic arthritis of the right hip but only if we find the germ we understand wath type of infection it is and its sensitivity to antibiotics

The differential diagnosis includes tuberculosis, arthrosis, or chondrolysis, but see the comparison with the contralateral hip (Fig. 9.30). The arthrocentesis performed resulted in a pyogenic form due to *Staphylococcus aureus*.

Therefore, after a period of remediation, we decided to intervene in two stages.

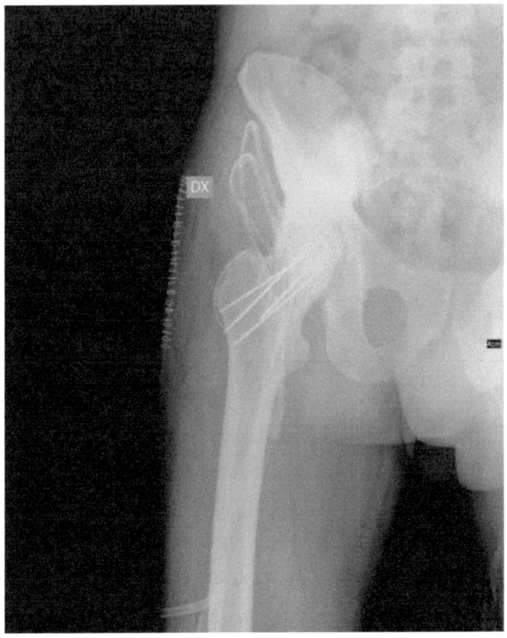


Fig. 9.31 X-ray of surgical cleaning and application of antibiotic spacer

Application of antibiotic spacer (Fig. 9.31) added with antibiotics according to the sensitivity of the antibiogram:

Vancomycin....0.10% Imipenem.........0.5%
Cefotaxime.......0.5%, always in realtion to the cement powerd.

After 4 weeks, still under local and general antibiotic therapy, the spacer was removed and the neck-sparing prosthesis was applied (Figs. 9.32 and 9.33).

Why did we use the neck-sparing prosthesis?

Because its characteristic is to save the neck bone, but also to leave good vascularity, as can be seen from Drawing 9.1.

This would help the arrival of antibiotics and cells predisposed to the immunological action against germs, especially at the site of implantation of the stem on the resected edge, where the previous infection was located.

Some other considerations must be added regarding tuberculosis of the hip, namely that it is a disease that does not produce biofilm, so much so that some authors apply the prosthesis at one time even if the infection is active because they believe that after having done a resection, careful

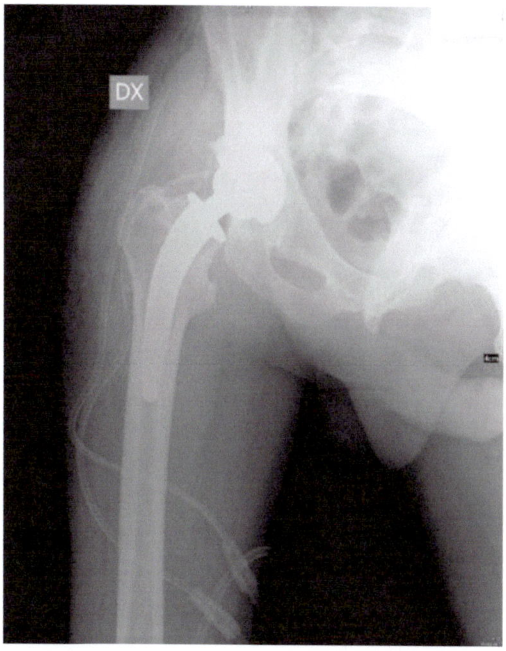


**Fig. 9.32** Radiographic control after surgery

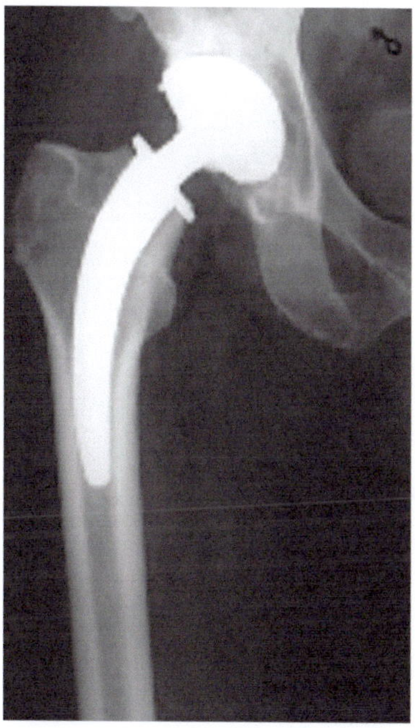

**Fig. 9.33** Radiographic control after 4 years without any sign of septic flare-up

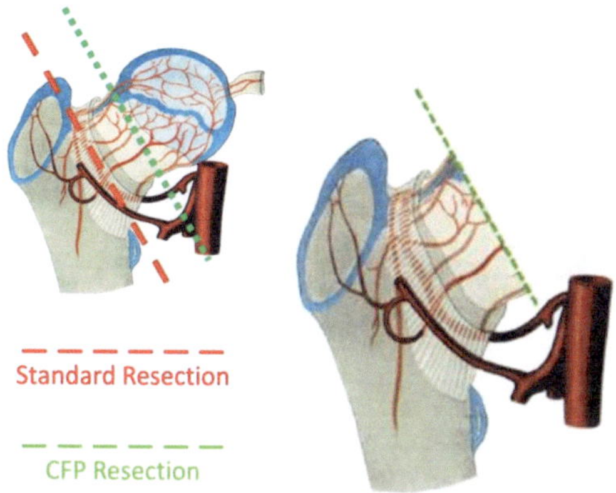


**Drawing 9.1** The resection of the CFP prosthesis maintains the vascularity of the neck

and excellent surgical cleaning, the application of the prosthesis will not result in any reignition of infection [33–39].

From 2008 to 2015, we performed 12 cases of neck-sparing hip prosthesis for septic arthritis.

(6 males and 6 females).

The pathogen was:

- Tuberculosis in four cases,
- *Staphylococcus aureus* in six cases.
- Mixed flora two cases.

*7 patients were drug-dependent.*

The agreement of both basic science and orthopedic surgery has confirmed, through the exposition of the results, the logical foundation, and the main characteristics of the neck-sparing prosthesis, summarized in this «Decalogue» from F. Pipino [40, 41]:

1. The prosthesis must integrate into the natural joint and not replace it
2. Maximum respect for the anatomy
3. Restoration of joint biomechanics
4. Dedicated access routes
5. Dedicated instruments
6. Mini prostheses respecting the bone stock
7. Minimization of blood loss and duration of hospitalization
8. Computer assistance

9. Bone-prosthesis interaction in the field of regenerative medicine
10. Removal of only pathological tissues while respecting healthy tissues: TSS

### 9.2.2 Shoulder Arthritis 3% in TB and 0.8% in Pyogenic (Figs. 9.34, 9.35, 9.36, and 9.37) [42–44]

A case of a 70-year-old patient presenting with an infection of the right shoulder that arose suddenly after a major febrile episode. He complains of pain, low-grade fever and on clinical examination the shoulder appears swollen, internally rotated, and very painful.

A pain spontaneous that at minimal movements. Furthermore, there is a fistula (Figs. 9.34 and 9.35) on the lateral aspect of the shoulder. Blood tests show ESR, CRP, fibrinogen, and white blood cells far above the normal value. Both synovial fluid and bone biopsy samples are taken for culture examination and antibiogram.

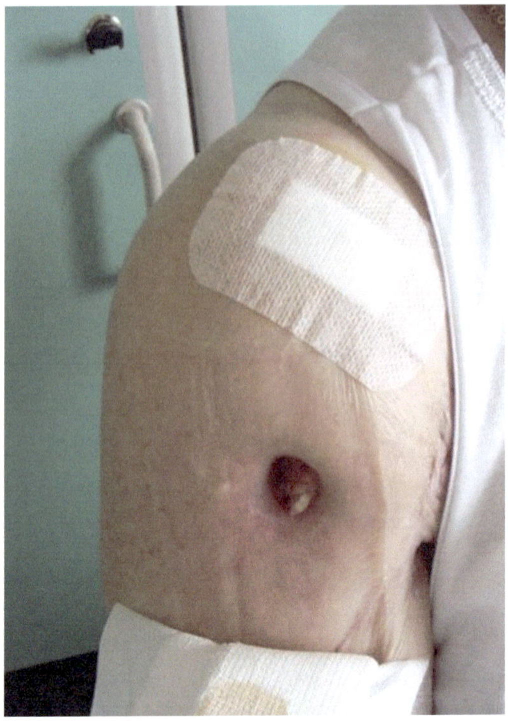

**Fig. 9.34** Treatment is initiated with broad-spectrum antibiotics and daily lavage through the fistula

In the meantime, the culture tests have arrived, and it turns out that it is super-infected tuberculosis. The mycobacterium is sensitive to classic antituberculosis drugs while the discovery of *Staphylococcus aureus* highlights that it is methicillin resistant, and therefore both pathogens will have to be treated. Both local and general treatment is started with teicoplanin, ciprofloxacin, and antituberculosis drugs (rifampicin, streptomycin, isoniazid, and ethambutol), according to the scheme we have adopted for about 40 years. It is decided to carry out the first stage of surgical cleaning, resection of the proximal epiphysis of the humerus, and application of an antibiotic spacer consisting of streptomycin, vancomycin, and clindamycin (Fig. 9.36).

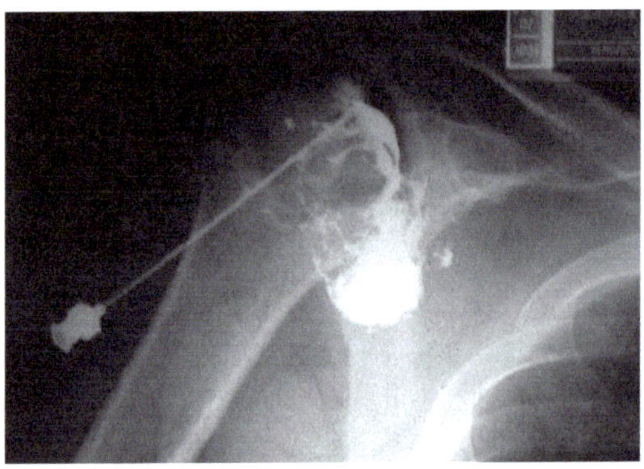

**Fig. 9.35** A fistulography is performed which highlights a collection in the lower part of the glenoid

When the overall picture appears stabilized; the blood tests are normal, no secretions, x-ray does not show any images related to septic re-ignition and the patient is able to make some active movements of the shoulder without pain, with the help of a physiotherapist we move on to the second stage where the spacer is removed and samples are taken for the culture test which will later be negative and a reverse prosthesis is applied (Fig. 9.36). Normally, in these cases, the rotator cuff appears significantly damaged and therefore one is forced to use only this type of prosthesis.

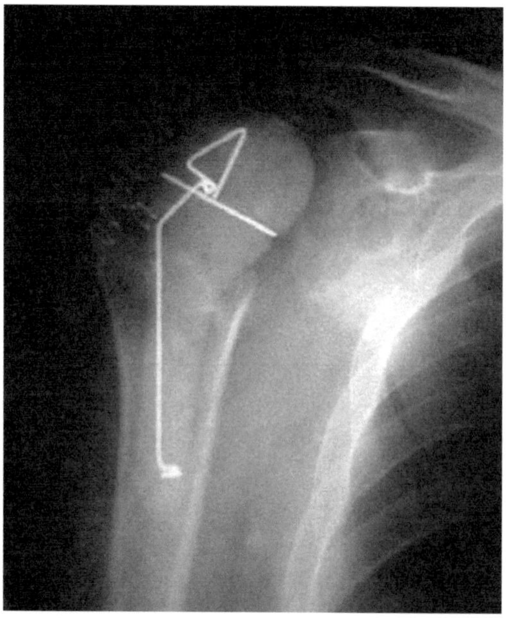

**Fig. 9.36** Radiographic image highlighting the positioning of the antibiotic spacer

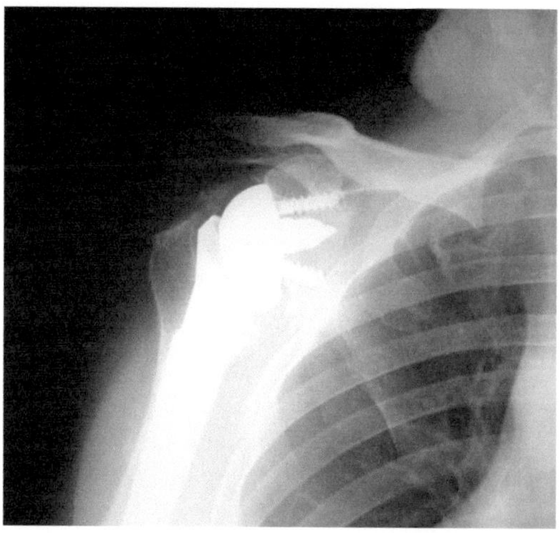

**Fig. 9.37** Radiograph after removal of the antibiotic spacer and application of a reverse prosthesis

### 9.2.3 Arthritis of the Elbow 2 7% in TB and 1 2% in Pyogenic (Figs. 9.38, 9.39, 9.40, 9.41, 9.42, 9.43, 9.44, 9.45, 9.46, 9.47, 9.48, 9.49 and 9.50) [45–49]

The big problem of the elbow is that it tends to stiffen and the bone is superficial to the point that a modest skin lesion can create exposure.

A 42-year-old patient who comes to us with an active infection at the left elbow with the formation of an abscess and plurifistolized. At the beginning, the picture made one suspect a pyogenic form because it presented all the characteristics; the laboratory tests showed an ESR, a CRP, and increased white blood cells. Furthermore, the situation presented, clinically, with signs of classic inflammation. Finally, the X-ray showed a bony detachment of the olecranon which had not been traumatic but due to tearing in supporting oneself (Fig. 9.37). In this case, the anamnesis helps us a lot due to the fact that the patient came from an area endemic for tuberculosis and 20 years earlier he had contracted pulmonary tuberculosis and had no longer been checked. Another fact was the periosteal reaction that had developed in such a short time (start of symptoms 6 months before our observation). Tuberculosis is much more aggressive than the pyogenic form in eutrophic patients.

Given the very active phase, with the presence of an abscess and a lot of purulent secretion, it was decided to immediately perform a surgical cleaning (Figs. 9.39, 9.40, and 9.41). Samples were taken for both culture and tuberculosis.

After 7 days, we had the results of the tests, and we found tuberculosis from an atypical mycobacterium sensitive to rifampicin and trimetroprim-cotrimoxazole.

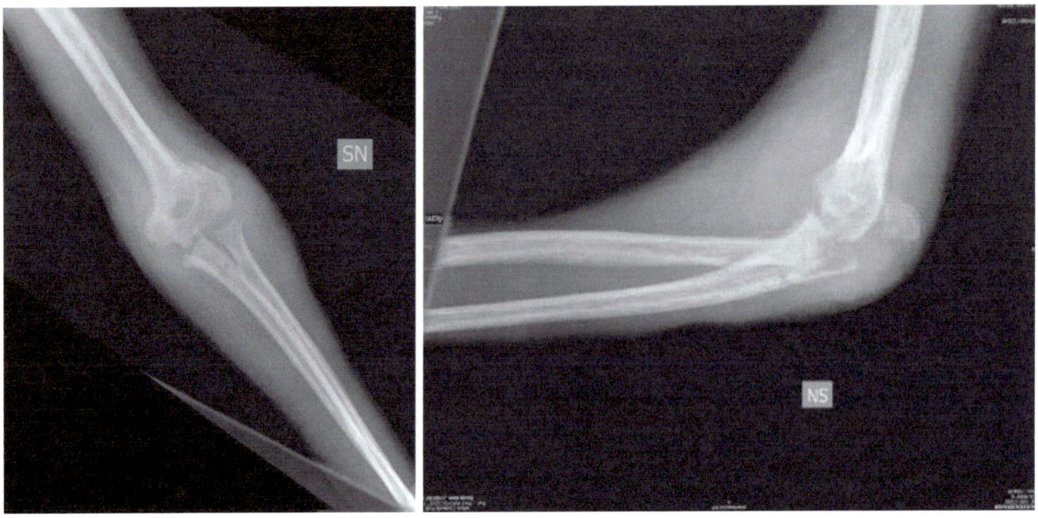


**Fig. 9.38** The X-ray of the elbow show a bony detachment of the olecranon which had not been traumatic but due to tearing in supporting oneself

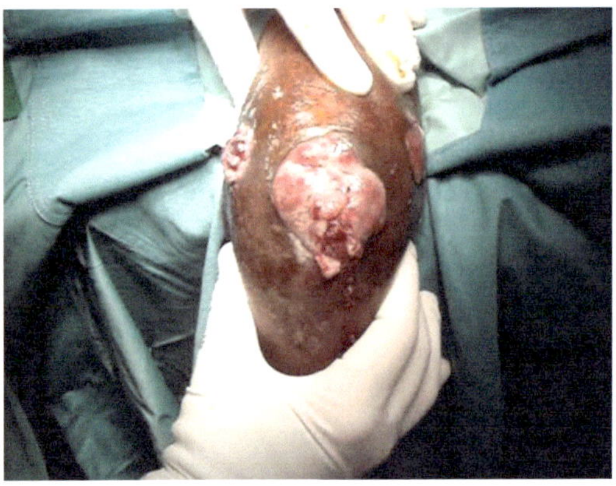

**Fig. 9.39** Abundant discharge of pus when squeezing the elbow

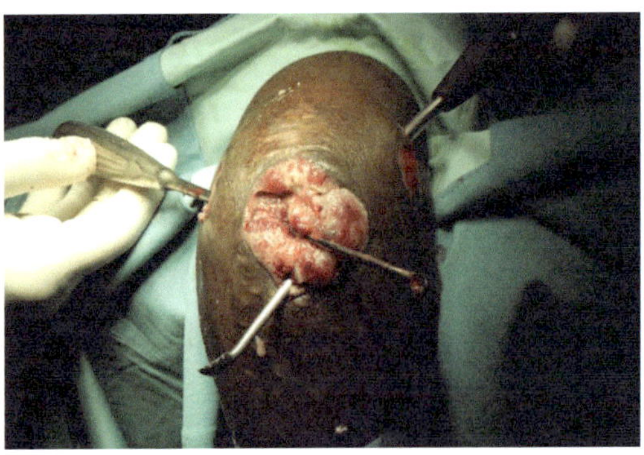

**Fig. 9.40** The ducts of the fistulas

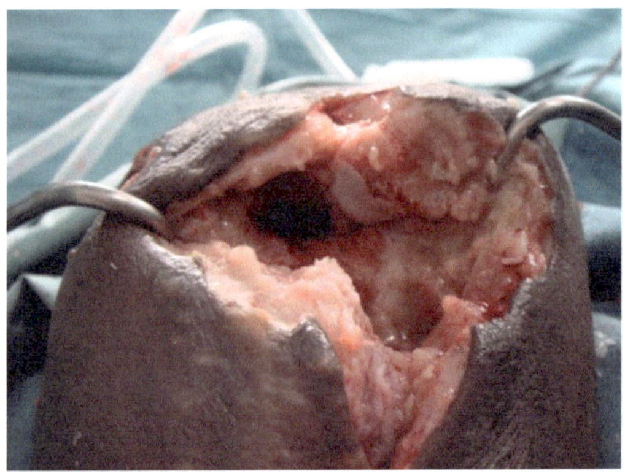

**Fig. 9.41** After the obsessive surgical cleaning, the still vital olecranon fragment can be seen

We carried out the antibiotic treatment with local washings until the situation was stabilized, and the fistulas and the continuous solutions closed as much as possible. Then we managed to perform the synthesis of the olecranon (Fig. 9.42) and the patient regained satisfactory motility.

Typically, the spontaneous outcome of tuberculosis is ankylosis (Figs. 9.42 and 9.43) when the process heals, as can be seen in the following X-ray of a patient who had had tuberculosis of the elbow 10 years earlier and had been treated only with antibiotics and immobilization.

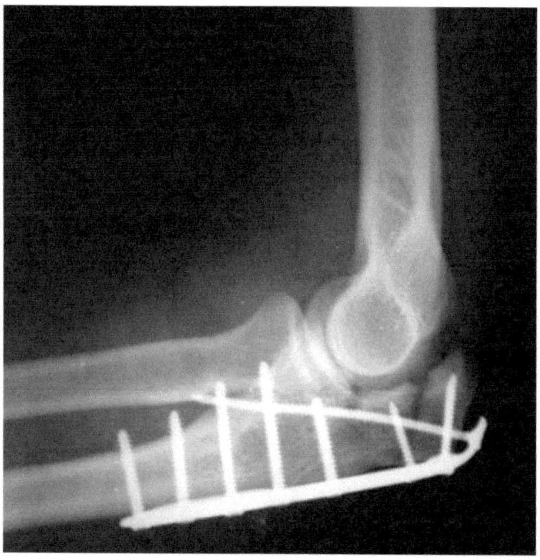

**Fig. 9.42** When the situation was considered stable, from a septic point of view, the detachment of the proximal part of the olecranon was osteynthesized

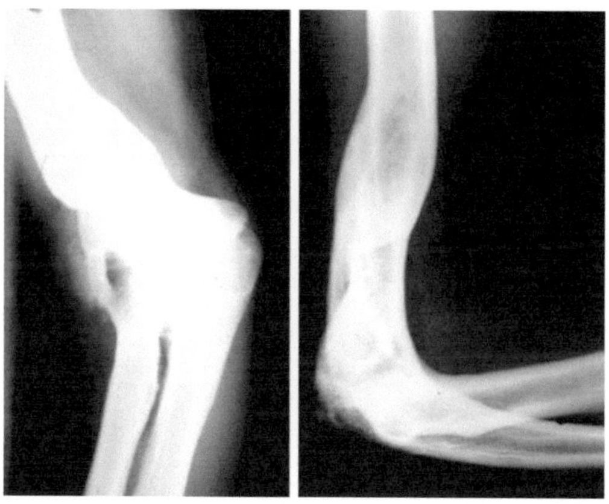

**Fig. 9.43** Radiological aspect of a spontaneous arthrodesis resulting froma a tubercular of the elbow

Since he did not want to undergo surgery again but was trying to have better functionality, since the flexion-extension was absent and the pronation-supination was also absent, we did not try to improve the latter by doing a reverse Sauvè-Kapandji (Figs. 9.45, 9.46, 9.47, and 9.48), that is, not creating a pseudarthrosis on the ulna but making it on the radius, that is, removing the radial head and restoring pronation-supination (Figs. 9.47 and 9.48).

A 78-year-old patient presents with a significant *Staphylococcus aureus* infection of the elbow.

On the X-ray, severe joint disruption (Fig. 9.49).

The blood sample revealed a *Staphylococcus aureus* infection sensitive to many antibiotics.

After a period of local and general antibiotics, we applied an elbow prosthesis (Fig. 9.50) at one time because the infection was not so aggressive, and it was on arthritic terrain. In fact, both the ESR and the CRP were normal, and the patient did not wish to undergo many operations as she was a heart patient and diabetic.

### 9.2.4 Wrist Arthritis 3.1% TB, 1.4% Pyogenic (Figs. 9.51, 9.52, 9.53, 9.54, 9.55, and 9.56) [20, 50–55]

As already mentioned, patients who present with signs of a joint infection are immediately examined for all possible pathogenic agents, and therefore in addition to pyogenic they are also evaluated for tuberculous and fungal infections. A case of a 66-year-old patient suffering from a tuberculosis pathology already diagnosed affecting the right wrist. The X-ray shows a wrist sprain with a large focus on the distal epiphysis of the radius with an alteration of the normal anatomy (Fig. 9.51). There is a volar dislocation of the lunate and clinically the wrist is almost ankylotic.

Begin both general and local antituberculous therapy with infiltration cycles of local antituberculous antibiotics (Fig. 9.52).

A restraint cast shower is applied (Fig. 9.53).

After a period of "cooling" of the infection we intervene by performing a surgical cleaning by removing the entire first chain of the carpus (Fig. 9.54).

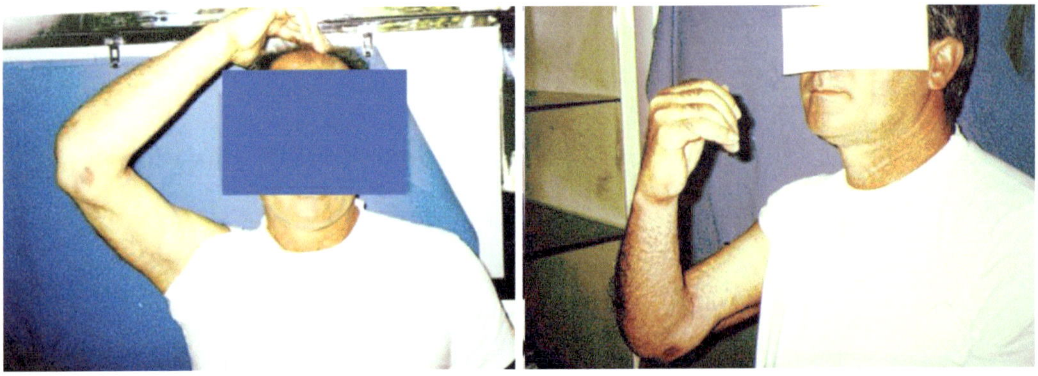

**Fig. 9.44** Clinical aspect of the patient demostraiting arm movements with complete lack of pronation-supination

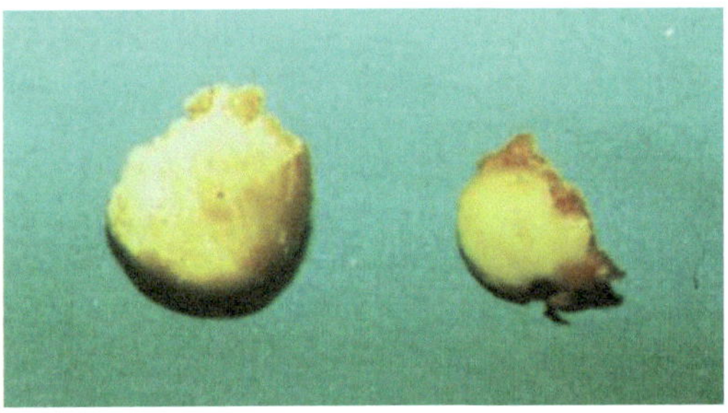

**Fig. 9.45** We removing the radial head to recover at least pronation-supination

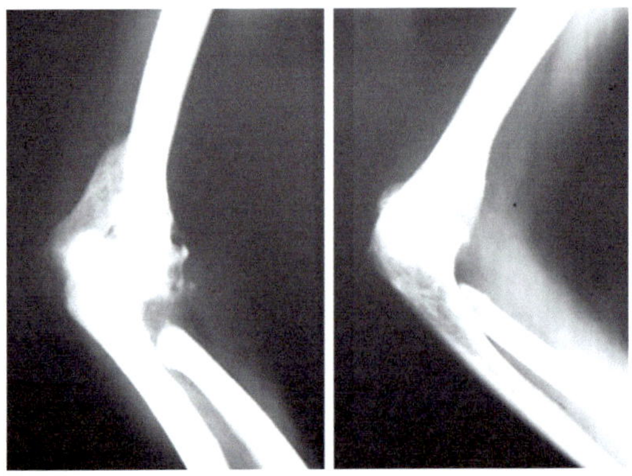

**Fig. 9.46** The x-ray aspect after removal of the radial head

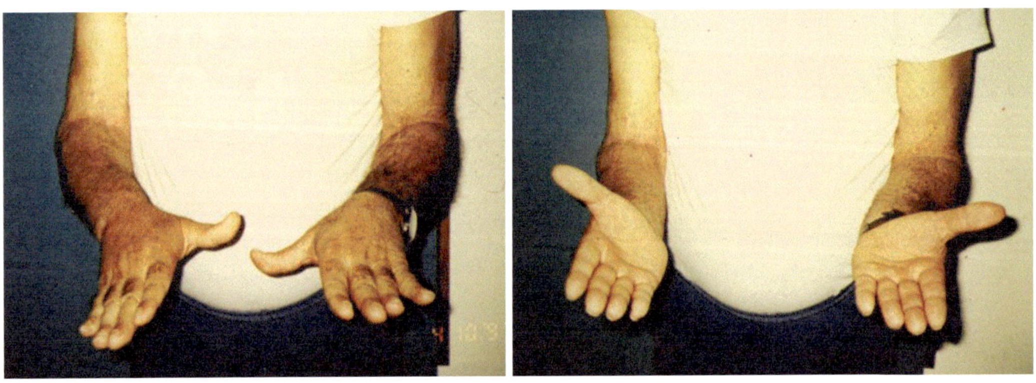

**Figs. 9.47 and 9.48** The clinical aspect with the recovery of pronation-supination

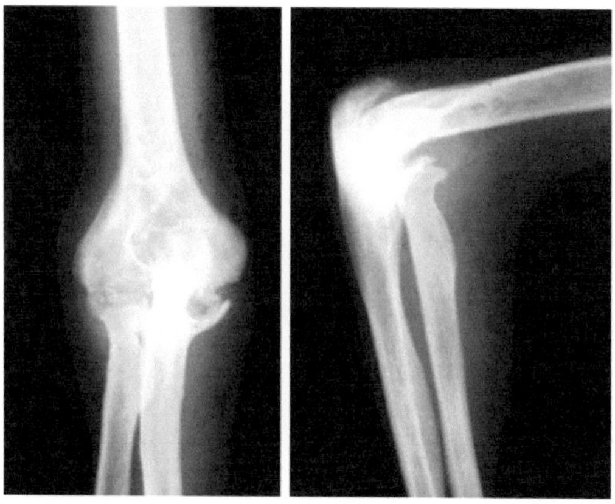

**Fig. 9.49** The X-ray shows a serious joint injury of the elbow

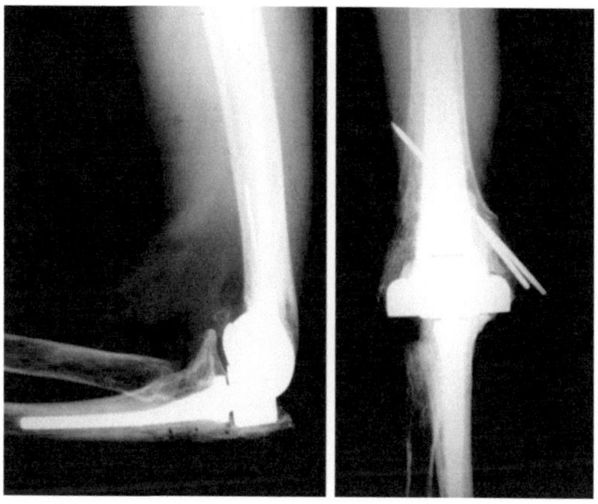

**Fig. 9.50** The X-ray highlights the application of an elbow prosthesis which was done in a single stage

Radiographic check-up at 2 years with no signs of septic flare-up and attempted filling of the epiphyseal focus of the radius (Fig. 9.55). In septic forms, in the residual empty spaces, a fibrous tissue is most often created which acts as a shock absorber, taking away pain and promoting minimal movement.

Finally, the clinical aspect (Fig. 9.54) is that the wrist does not have good motility, but the patient no longer has pain and no longer has signs of infection and is able to use his wrist to carry out normal life functions.

I would like to close this chapter by highlighting some points, especially on tuberculosis, which has not yet disappeared and is always present in our reality as orthopedic specialists and which we forget about:

1. It does not have a preferential age.
2. It is not preceded by sufficiently indicative diagnostic elements.
3. It is often masked at a clinical level by the most varied and, at times, the least predictable symptoms.
4. It is often camouflaged by antibiotic treatments, even those that are not specific in the strict sense.
5. It does not recognize its own morphological characteristics.
6. It must always be treated in poly chemotherapy also locally.
7. The therapy is mainly medical.
8. The therapy must then be continued under medical supervision, at the patient's home, for at least 1 year.
9. Do not hesitate to perform a biopsy and a culture test if you are in doubt about a tuberculous form.
10. It is easily overinfected, especially if fistulized.
11. It is increasingly caused by atypical mycobacteria resistant to common anti-tuberculosis antibiotic therapies.
12. Each joint has its own characteristics, which must be known to provide the most appropriate treatment.
13. Finally, it is a pathology that presents many customizations such as the patient's characteristics (age, sex, comorbidities, immunological and antibiotic reactivity, and the type of life and work that the patient does and his expectations) local characteristics (location, type of bone and soft parts, and characteristics of the lesion).

*Therefore, each patient is a case that must be treated in a personalized way.*

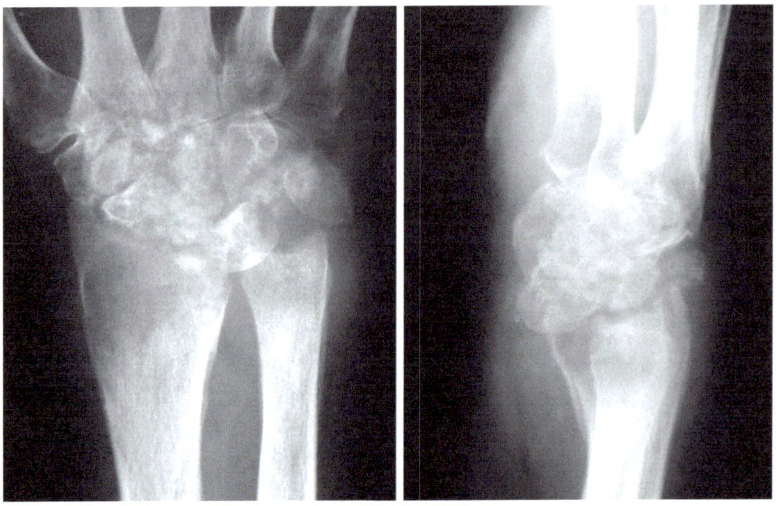

**Fig. 9.51** The X-ray shows a serious lesion of the entire carpus and the radiocarpal with a large focus on the distal epiphysis of the radius

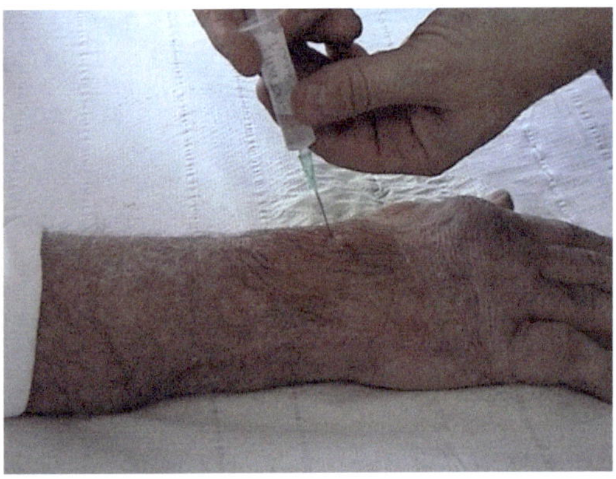

**Fig. 9.52** Local infiltration of targeted antibiotic. Since 1970 we have been using local antibiotic infiltrations for both tubercular and pyogenic articular forms [21, 22, 23]

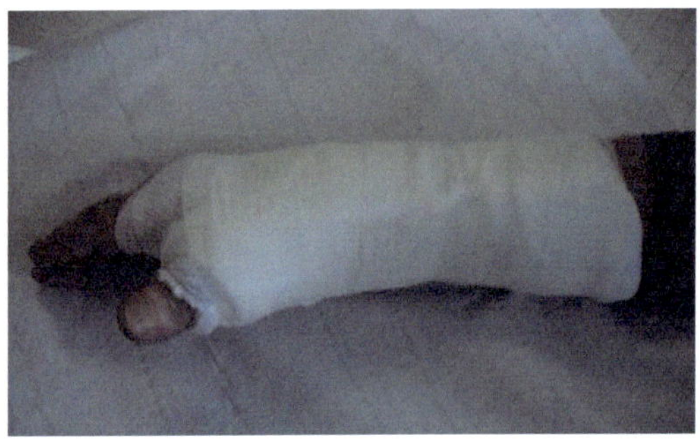

**Fig. 9.53** Application of a position brace removable only to reduce the pain. When the patient is well he can remove the brace and move

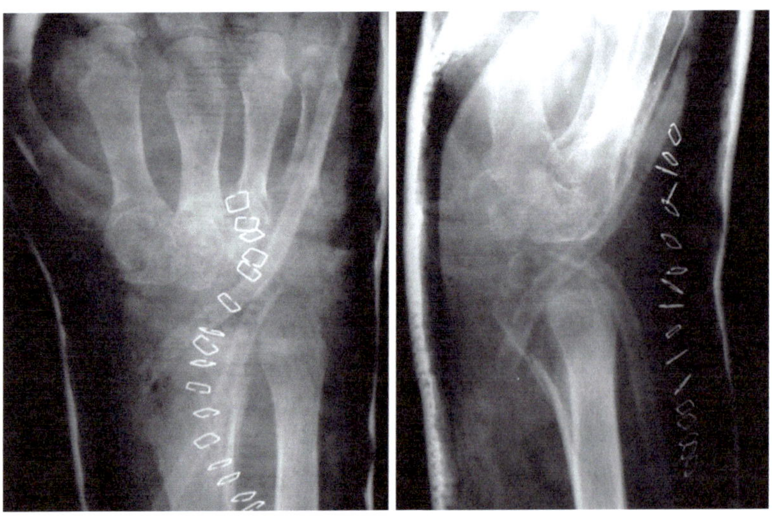

**Fig. 9.54** The X-ray highlights the surgical cleaning with the removal of the first row of the carpus

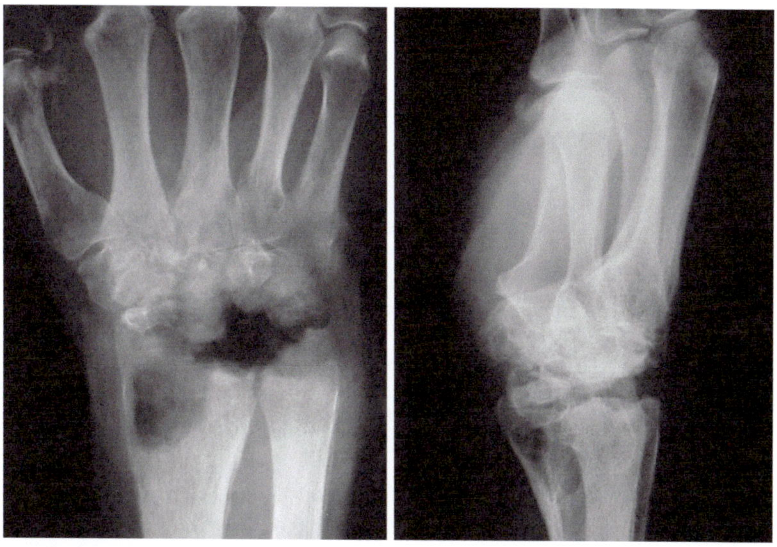

**Fig. 9.55** The X-ray 2 years after surgical cleaning ...

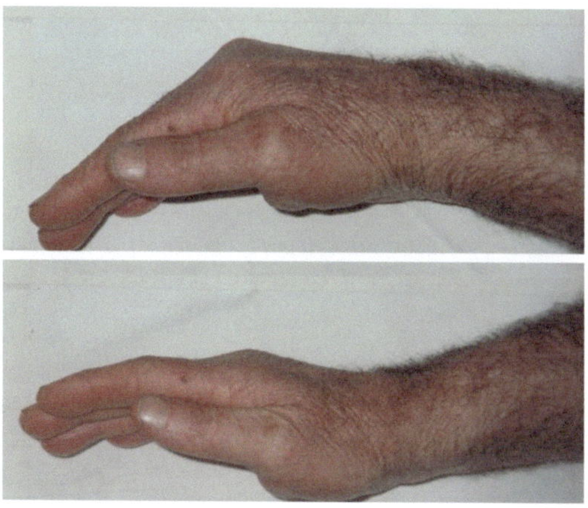

**Fig. 9.56** .... and clinical aspect

## Bibliography


1. Treatment of tuberculosis: guidelines—4th ed. WHO/HTM/TB/2009.420.
2. Marais LC, Nieuwoudt L, Nansook A, Menon A, Benito N. Tuberculous arthritis of native joints – a systematic review and European Bone and Joint Infection Society workgroup report. J Bone Jt Infect. 2023 Aug 28;8(4):189–207. https://doi.org/10.5194/jbji-8-189-2023.
3. Tuli SM. General principles of osteoarticular tuberculosis. Clin Orthop Relat Res. 2002 May;398:11–9. https://doi.org/10.1097/00003086-200205000-00003.
4. Tuli S. Tuberculosis of the skeletal system. New Delhi: JP Medical Ltd.; 2016. p. 57.
5. Yáñez A. The World Health Organization and the control of tuberculosis. Rev Med Chile. 1998;126(7 suppl):61–5. Cited by: 0 articles | PMID: 9838282
6. Didilescu C. The long way of TB eradication versus TB elimination, from utopia to reality. Pneumologia. 2011;60(2):70–3. Cited by: 0 articles | PMID: 21823355
7. Didilescu C, Tănăsescu M. Proportion and site distribution of extrarespiratory tuberculosis in 2007–2010 in Romania. Pneumologia. 2012;61(1):10–4. Cited by: 2 articles | PMID: 22545482
8. Popescu G, Chiotan D, Cioran N, Didilescu C. Prudent optimism and the evolution of the main indicators of endemic tuberculosis in Romania in 2012. Pneumologia. 2013;62(2):72–9. Cited by: 2 articles | PMID: 23894787
9. Risk factors for tuberculosis infection https://www.cdc.gov/
10. Griffith DE, Aksamit T, Brown-Elliott BA, Catanzaro A, Daley C, Gordin F, Holland SM, Horsburgh R, Huitt G, Iademarco MF, Iseman M, Olivier K, Ruoss S, von Reyn CF, Wallace RJ, Winthrop K. ATS mycobacterial diseases subcommittee. American Thoracic Society. Infectious disease Society of America. An official ATS/IDSA statement: diagnosis, treatment, and prevention of nontuberculous mycobacterial diseases. Am J Respir Crit Care Med. 2007 Feb 15;175(4):367–416.
11. Hunter JG, Gross JM, Dahl JD, Amsdell SL, Gorczyca JT. Risk factors for failure of a single surgical debridement in adults with acute septic arthritis. J Bone Joint Surg Inc. 2015;97:558–64.
12. Appelberg R. Pathogenesis of Mycobacterium avium infection: typical responses to an atypical mycobacterium? Immunol Res. 2006;35(3):179–90.
13. Yancey JR, Melchert VE. QuantiFERON-TB gold+ for the diagnosis of mycobacterium tuberculosis infection. Am Fam Physician. 2021;103(3):177–8.
14. Tănăsescu M, Didilescu C, Marica C. The present and future prospects in rapid molecular diagnosis of tuberculosis and MDR-TB (First Part). Pneumologia.

2013;62(3):134–8. Cited by: 1 article | PMID: 24273995
15. Agashe VM, Johari AN, Shah M, et al. Diagnosis of osteoarticular tuberculosis: perceptions, protocols, practices, and priorities in the endemic and non-endemic areas of the world—a waiot view. Microorganisms. 2020;8(9):1312. https://doi.org/10.3390/microorganisms8091312.
16. Alifano M, Del Pezzo M, Lamberti C, Faraone S, Covelli I. ELISA method for evaluation of anti-A60 IgG in patients with pulmonary and extra-pulmonary tuberculosis. Microbiologica. 1994;17:37–44.
17. Tortoli E, Lavinia F, Simonetti MT, Evaluation of a commercial ligase chain reaction kit (Abbott LCx) for direct detecion of Mycobacterium tuberculosis in pulmonary and Extra-pulmonary specimens. JClinMicrobiol. 1997;35:2424–6.
18. Choi J-A, Koh SH, Hong S-H, Koh YH, Choi J-Y, Kang HS. Rheumatoid arthritis and tuberculous arthritis: differentiating MRI features. Am J Roentgenol. 2009;193:1347–53. https://doi.org/10.2214/AJR.08.2164.
19. Mandell G. Mandell, Douglas, and Bennett's principles and practice of infectious diseases. Philadelphia, PA: Churchill Livingstone/Elsevier; 2010.
20. Garcia-Monco JC. Tuberculosis. 2014;121:1485–99. https://doi.org/10.1016/B978-0-7020-4088-7.00100-0. ISSN 0072-9752
21. Newman JH. Review of septic arthritis throughout the antibiotic era. Ann Rheum Dis. 1976;35(3):198–205.
22. Whiteside LA. Prophylactic peri-operative local antibiotic irrigation. Bone Joint J. 2016;98-B(1 Suppl A):23–6. https://doi.org/10.1302/0301-620X.98B1.36357.
23. Whiteside LA, Peppers M, Nayfeh TA, Roy ME. Methicillin-resistant Staphylococcusaureus in TKA treated with revision and direct intra-articular antibiotic infusion. Clin Orthop Relat Res. 2011;469:26–33. https://doi.org/10.1007/s11999-010-1313-9.
24. Fukagawa S, Matsuda S, Miura H, Okazaki K, Tashiro Y, Iwamoto Y. High-dose antibiotic infusion for infected knee prosthesis without implant removal. J Orthop Sci. 2010;15(4):470–6. https://doi.org/10.1007/s00776-010-1487-8.
25. de Lalla F, Novelli A, Pellizzer GP, Milocchi F, Viola R, Rigon A, Stecca C, Dal Pizzol V, Fallani S, Periti P. Regional and systemic prophylaxis with teicoplanin in monolateral and bilateral total knee replacement procedures: study of pharmacokinetics and tissue penetration. Antimicrob Agents Chemother. 1993;37:2693–8.
26. Sogebi OA, Adefuye BO, Adebola SO, Oladeji SM, Adedeji TO. Clinical predictors of aminoglycoside-induced ototoxicity in drug-resistant tuberculosis patients on intensive therapy. Auris Nasus Larynx. 2017;44(4):404–10.
27. Balato G, De Matteo V, Ascione T, De Giovanni E, Marano MRM. Mariconda management of septic arthritis of the hip joint in adults. A systematic review of the literature. BMC Musculoskelet Disord. 2021;22:1006.
28. Mathews CJ, Weston VC, Jones A, Field M, Coakley G. Bacterial septic arthritis in adults. Lancet. 2010;375:846–55.
29. Flores-Robles BJ, Jiménez Palop M, Sanabria Sanchinel AA, Andrus RF, Royuela Vicente A, Sanz Pérez MI, et al. Medical versus surgical approach to initial treatment in septic arthritis: a single Spanish center's 8-year experience. J Clin Rheumatol. 2019;25:4–8.
30. Ascione T, Balato G, Mariconda M, Rotondo R, Baldini A, Pagliano P. Continuous antibiotic therapy can reduce recurrence of prosthetic joint infection in patients undergoing 2-stage exchange. J Arthroplast. 2019;34:704–9.
31. Babhulkar S, Pande S. Tuberculosis of the hip. Clin Orthop Relat Res. 2002 May;398:93–9. https://doi.org/10.1097/00003086-200205000-00013.
32. Kushwaha NS, Kumar D, Gupta RK, Tewari PG, Singh R, Kumar A. Functional outcome of total hip arthroplasty in tubercular hip arthritis: a prospective study. J Clin Orthop Trauma. 2024;48:102337. https://doi.org/10.1016/j.jcot.2024.102337.eCollection. PMID: 38304415
33. Van Le T, Duong TB, Hien KQ, Ton QNQ, Huyn T, Binh TP, Tu DT, Tho PP, Binh LN, Hau HP, Hung TNK. Two-stage revision for treatment of tuberculous prosthetic hip infection: an outcome analysis. Eur J Orthop Surg Traumatol. 2023;33(3):645–51. https://doi.org/10.1007/s00590-022-03317-9. Epub 2022 Jul 2
34. Kim YH, Han DY, Park BM. Total hip arthroplasty for tuberculous coxar-throsis. J Bone Joint Surg Am. 1987;69(5):718–27.
35. Santavirta S, Eskolal A, Konttinen YT, Tallrothl K, Lindholml ST. Total hip replacement in old tuberculosis. A report of 14 cases. Acta Orthop Scand. 1988;59(4):391–5.
36. Yoon TR, Rowe SM, Santosa SB, Jung ST, Seon JK. Immediate cementless total hip arthroplasty for the treatment of active tuberculosis. J Arthroplast. 2005;20(7):923–6.
37. Sidhu S, Singh AP, Singh AP. Total hip replacement in active advanced tuberculous arthritis. J Bone Joint Surg Br. 2009;91(10):1301–4.
38. Neogi DS, Yadav CS, Kumar A, Khan SA, Rastogi S. Total hip arthroplasty in patients with active tuberculosis of the hip with advanced arthritis. Clin Orthop Relat Res. 2010;468:605–12.
39. Zhang Y-c, Zhang H. One-stage total joint arthroplasty for patients with active tuberculosis. Orthopedics. 2013 May;36(5):328–30. https://doi.org/10.3928/01477447-20130426-02.
40. Bi AS, Li D, Ma Y, Wu D, Ma Y. Mycobacterium tuberculosis as a cause of periprosthetic joint infection after total knee arthroplasty: a review of the literature. Cureus. 2019;11(3):e 4325. https://doi.org/10.7759/cureus.4325.

41. Langdon IJ, et al. Cemented hip replacements in patients younger than 50 years: 16-24 years results. Hip Int. 1999;9(3):151–3.
42. Pipino F, Keller A. Tissue sparing surgery (TSS) in hip and knee arthroplasty and tissue-sparing surgery: 25 years experience with femoral neck preserving hip arthroplasty. Orthop Traumatol. 7(1):36–41.
43. Kirchhoff C, Braunstein V, Buhmann KS, Oedekoven T, Mutschler W, Biberthaler P. Stage-dependant management of septic arthritis of the shoulder in adults. Int Orthop. 2009;33(4):1015–24.
44. Lossos IS, Yossepowitch O, Kandel L, Yardeni D, Arber N. Septic arthritis of the glenohumeral joint. Medicine. 1998;77(3):177–87.
45. Leslie BM, Harris JM 3rd, Driscoll D. Septic arthritis of the shoulder in adults. J Bone Joint Surg Am. 1989;71(10):1516–22.
46. Van den Ende KIM, Steinmann SP. Arthroscopic treatment of septic arthritis of the elbow. J Shoulder Elb Surg. 2012;21(8):1001–5.
47. Assunção JH, Noffs GG, Malavolta EA, Gracitelli MEC, Lima ALM, Neto AAF. Septic arthritis of the shoulder and elbow: one decade of epidemiological analysis at a tertiary referral hospital. Rev Bras Ortop. 2018 Nov-Dec;53(6):707–13. https://doi.org/10.1016/j.rbo.2017.08.005.
48. Kennedy N, Chambers ST, Nolan I, Gallagher K, Werno A, Browne M. Native joint septic arthritis: epidemiology, clinical features, and microbiological causes in a New Zealand population. J Rheumatol. 2015;42(12):2392–7.
49. Moon JG, Biraris S, Bilaris S, Jeong WK, Kim JH. Clinical results after arthroscopic treatment for septic arthritis of the elbow joint. Arthroscopy. 2014;30(6):673–8.
50. Domingo A, Nomdedeu M, Tomás X, García S. Elbow tuberculosis: an unusual location and diagnostic problem. Arch Orthop Trauma Surg. 2005;125(1):56–8. https://doi.org/10.1007/s00402-003-0612-y. Epub 2004 Feb 4. PMID: 14760492
51. Mehta P, Schnall SB, Zalavras CG. Septic arthritis of the shoulder, elbow, and wrist. Clin Orthop Relat Res. 2006;451:42–5.
52. Horan TC, Andrus M, Dudeck MA. CDC/NHSN surveillance definition of health care-associated infection and criteria for specific types of infections in the acute care setting. Am J Infect Control. 2008;36(5):309–32.
53. Jennings JD, Zielinski E, Tosti R, Ilyas AM. Septic arthritis of the wrist: incidence, risk factors, and predictors of infection. Orthopedics. 2017 May 1;40(3):e526–31. https://doi.org/10.3928/01477447-20170404-01.
54. Malizos KN, Papadopoulou ZK, Ziogkou AN, Rigopoulos N, Athanaselis ED, Varitimidis SE, Dailiana ZC. Infections of deep hand and wrist compartments. Microorganisms. 2020 Jun 3;8(6):838. https://doi.org/10.3390/microorganisms8060838.
55. Szabo RM, Spiegel JD. Infected fractures of the hand and wrist. Hand Clin. 1988;4:477–89.

# 10 Chronic Osteomyelitis

Yangguan Wu and David Joseph

## 10.1 Introduction

Chronic osteomyelitis, a long-lasting inflammation of the bone and surrounding tissue due to infection by microorganisms, has been around for a long time. Evidence of this disease in animals dates back hundreds of millions of years [3], and discussions about human osteomyelitis can be traced back to the era of Hippocrates (460–370 BC). Over the years, various terms were used to describe bone infection until Nelaton introduced the term "osteomyelitis" in 1844 [3].

Historically, the treatment for osteomyelitis prior to 1976 [4–8] involved a series of steps: sequential debridement, saucing, packing, healing by secondary intention, bypass open bone grafting, followed by prolonged antibiotic therapy [9–12] and long-term external support using orthotics and casts [4, 7, 13, 14]. Bone infection was often tolerated because methods for restoring hard and soft tissue deficits were unreliable. Surgeons were hesitant to remove all infected segments due to the fear of causing fractures, loss of function, and even death. As a result, the criteria for selecting patients for limb salvage were restrictive. Debridement was only intralesional. Deficiencies in wound healing and persistent infections contributed to a low treatment success rate (50–70%) [4, 7, 14].

However, the treatment of chronic osteomyelitis has evolved rapidly over the past three decades. The development of methods to counter biofilm formation, a key mechanism in pathogen colonization of wounds, has been instrumental in shaping modern treatment protocols [15–29].

With the advent of limb salvage protocols, more than 90% of patients with chronic osteomyelitis can now be successfully treated [30–31]. This is particularly impressive given the increasing number of patients with multiple comorbidities that affect wound healing.

Innovations in technology have led to new fixation strategies, such as locking plates and retrograde nails, and improved methods of detecting and isolating biofilm pathogens [32–35]. The development of antimicrobial agents for resistant pathogen strains and innovative approaches to open wound treatment, such as vacuum-assisted closure [36, 37], has broadened the selection criteria for treatment and provided a basis for limb salvage following debridement [38–43].

The successful use of antibiotic depot protocols before final reconstruction has ushered in a new era of treating chronic osteomyelitis with staged treatment protocols [44–48]. This process parallels the staging and treatment of musculoskeletal tumors and requires the same precision and foresight [49–52].

Y. Wu (✉) · D. Joseph
Department of Orthopedic Surgery, Elmhurst Hospital Center, Icahn School of Medicine, NY, New York, USA
e-mail: wuyang@nychhc.org; Josedav@nychhc.org



P. Ruggieri et al. (eds.), *Bone and Joint Infections*, https://doi.org/10.1007/978-3-031-96383-4_10

The prospect of successful reconstruction following infection has helped to overcome early fears of treatment failure among orthopedic surgeons and has provided the confidence to perform thorough debridement [53]. The maintenance or restoration of a competent soft tissue envelope facilitates re-exposure, contains and concentrates locally released antibiotics, revascularizes bone and tendon grafts, and prevents secondary colonization of the wounds.

A currently proposed treatment algorithm for chronic osteomyelitis includes thorough debridement with local antibiotic depots that preserve length, safeguard early wound closure, maintain working dead space, and prepare the wound for reconstruction [54–60]. This is followed by a staged reconstruction strategy tailored to the location, size of soft and bony defects, local soft tissue and vascular supply, and the patient's overall physiological status.

## 10.2 Etiology

The etiology of this condition is multifactorial, involving a complex interplay of host factors, microbial pathogens, and environmental influences. Understanding the underlying causes of chronic osteomyelitis is crucial for effectively managing and preventing this challenging disease [61].

Host factors play a significant role in the development of chronic osteomyelitis. Patients with compromised immune systems, such as those with diabetes, HIV/AIDS, or autoimmune disorders, are at increased risk of developing chronic osteomyelitis. Additionally, individuals with vascular insufficiency or peripheral neuropathy are more susceptible to bone infections due to impaired blood flow and sensation in the affected area. These host factors create an environment conducive to bacterial colonization and proliferation within the bone tissue, leading to chronic inflammation and bone destruction [62].

Microbial pathogens are another key component in the etiology of chronic osteomyelitis. The most common causative agents of chronic osteomyelitis are *Staphylococcus aureus* and *Pseudomonas aeruginosa*, although many other bacteria, fungi, and even mycobacteria can also be implicated. These pathogens can enter the bone tissue through direct trauma, surgical procedures, or hematogenous spread from other sites of infection. Once inside the bone, the pathogens form biofilms, complex communities of bacteria encased in a protective matrix that resist host immune defenses and antibiotic therapy. The presence of biofilms contributes to the chronicity of osteomyelitis by allowing the bacteria to persist and evade eradication [63].

Environmental influences, such as poor wound care, inadequate antibiotic therapy, and foreign body implantation, can also contribute to the development of chronic osteomyelitis. Improper management of acute osteomyelitis or failure to address underlying risk factors can lead to the progression of the infection to a chronic state. Inadequate blood supply to the affected bone, either due to trauma or underlying vascular disease, can impair the delivery of immune cells and antibiotics to the site of infection, further complicating the treatment of chronic osteomyelitis [64].

## 10.3 Epidemiology

The epidemiological landscape of osteomyelitis in the United States is complex and multifaceted [65–70]. While the incidence remains elusive, estimates suggest a rate as high as 1 in 675 hospital admissions per annum, translating to approximately 50,000 cases yearly. Further studies indicate an overall incidence of 21.8 cases per 100,000 person-years [66].

Interestingly, the incidence appears disproportionately higher in males, although the underlying reasons for this disparity remain unclear. Age is another significant factor, with incidence rates escalating primarily due to the increased prevalence of comorbid conditions such as diabetes mellitus and peripheral vascular disease in older populations [66].

The advent of advanced imaging modalities, including magnetic resonance imaging (MRI) and bone scintigraphy, has markedly enhanced our diagnostic capabilities and our understanding of the infection's characteristics [67].

In 2004 alone, the United States witnessed over 110,000 infections stemming from nearly 600,000 artificial joint replacements and two million internal fracture fixations. The financial implications are substantial, with the treatment of implant-related chronic osteomyelitis (COM) projected to cost US hospitals $1.62 billion by 2020 [67].

Moreover, the intersection of osteomyelitis with other conditions presents additional challenges. For instance, chronic diabetic foot ulcers can become infected and lead to diabetic foot osteomyelitis, thereby elevating mortality rates and amputation risks [68].

In summary, osteomyelitis poses a significant public health challenge. It burdens the healthcare system considerably, underscoring the critical need for early detection strategies and effective treatment protocols to manage this condition optimally [69–70].

## 10.4 Pathophysiology

The pathophysiology of chronic osteomyelitis involves a complex interplay of host immune response, bacterial virulence factors, and bone remodeling processes [61].

The initial stage of chronic osteomyelitis begins with introduction of bacteria into the bone tissue through direct trauma, surgery, or hematogenous spread. Once inside the bone, bacteria adhere to the bone matrix and form biofilms [18], which protect host immune defenses and antibiotics [1, 2]. The biofilm structure allows bacteria to evade phagocytosis by immune cells and establish a chronic infection within the bone [1, 2, 62–64].

The host immune response to chronic osteomyelitis is characterized by a persistent inflammatory reaction involving the recruitment of immune cells such as neutrophils, macrophages, and lymphocytes to the site of infection. These immune cells release pro-inflammatory cytokines and chemokines, leading to further tissue damage and bone resorption. Chronic inflammation also disrupts the normal bone remodeling process, impairing bone healing and increasing susceptibility to recurrent infections [62–64].

Bacterial virulence factors play a crucial role in the pathogenesis of chronic osteomyelitis. Some bacteria, such as *Staphylococcus aureus*, produce toxins and enzymes that facilitate tissue invasion and immune evasion. These virulence factors contribute to the formation of biofilms and establish a chronic infection within the bone. In addition, some bacteria can persist within host cells, further complicating the treatment of chronic osteomyelitis [62–64].

Biofilms are structured communities of bacteria embedded in a self-produced extracellular matrix consisting of polysaccharides, proteins, and nucleic acids. Forming biofilms is a critical factor in the pathogenesis of chronic osteomyelitis, as biofilms provide a protective environment for bacteria, allowing them to evade both the host immune response and antibiotic treatment [1, 2].

The biofilm formation process in chronic osteomyelitis typically involves several stages, including the initial attachment of planktonic bacteria to the bone surface, followed by the proliferation and maturation of the biofilm [71]. This maturation phase is crucial, enhancing the biofilm's structural integrity and antibiotic resistance. Studies have shown that biofilms can significantly reduce the efficacy of antibiotic treatments, as the bacteria within biofilms exhibit altered metabolic states and gene expression profiles that confer increased resistance [72, 73]. For instance, *S. aureus* biofilms harbor mutant forms and minor colony variants that complicate treatment efforts [72].

Moreover, the presence of biofilms in osteomyelitis is associated with various clinical challenges, including the need for surgical intervention to remove infected tissue or implants [74]. The chronic nature of these infections often leads to repeated episodes of inflammation and bone destruction, exacerbated by the biofilm's ability to persist in a dormant state, allowing for recurrence even after seemingly successful treatment [1, 2, 75, 76]. This persistence is particularly problematic in patients with compromised immune systems or those with underlying conditions such as diabetes, which can predispose them to chronic infections [73].

The pathophysiology of chronic osteomyelitis also involves alterations in bone metabolism and remodeling. Chronic inflammation and infection disrupt the balance between bone formation and resorption, leading to bone destruction and necrosis. The release of inflammatory mediators and cytokines further exacerbates bone loss and impairs healing. As a result, patients with chronic osteomyelitis often experience persistent pain, deformity, and functional impairment [61].

## 10.5 Clinical Evaluation and Diagnosis

Diagnosing chronic osteomyelitis requires a thorough history and physical examination, as well as imaging studies and laboratory tests to confirm the presence of infection [61].

## 10.6 History and Physical

History taking in patients with suspected chronic osteomyelitis should focus on identifying risk factors for infection, such as recent trauma, surgery, or the presence of underlying medical conditions that may predispose to bone infections. Patients may report persistent pain, swelling, and drainage from the affected area and systemic symptoms such as fever, chills, and malaise. A detailed history of previous treatments, including antibiotics and surgical interventions, is essential for further management [61, 62].

Physical examination of patients with chronic osteomyelitis typically reveals localized tenderness, swelling, and erythema over the affected bone. Sinus tracts, draining wounds, or exposed bone may also be noted. In some cases, the affected limb may be warm to the touch, with limited range of motion and muscle weakness. Careful inspection of the skin and soft tissues surrounding the affected bone is important to assess for signs of cellulitis or abscess formation [61, 62, 77].

Physical examination should also include in the vascular status, deformity, and functional impairment because of the disease. This information helps clinical decision-making.

## 10.7 Laboratory Test

The test pertains to the diagnostic procedures employed in detecting and monitoring osteomyelitis, a bone infection. Here are the key points [78]:

Complete Blood Counts (CBCs): These are crucial in detecting acute infections, where an increase in white blood cells, or leukocytosis, is observed. However, the white blood cell count may remain within normal ranges in chronic osteomyelitis cases.

Inflammatory Markers: Erythrocyte Sedimentation Rate (ESR) and serum C-reactive protein (CRP) escalate during the acute phase of infection and postsurgical intervention. These markers peak on the third and fifth days following manipulation, respectively.

Normalization of CRP and ESR: CRP levels typically revert to baseline within 3 weeks, while ESR normalization is more protracted than CRP. A resurgence in CRP levels 3 days postsurgical intervention or at the commencement of antibiotic therapy could indicate a relapse or unsuccessful treatment. These tests play a pivotal role in diagnosing and monitoring osteomyelitis. However, it is nonspecific because elevated levels of both CRP concentration and ESR can occur due to factors unrelated to osteomyelitis.

Several biomarkers have been studied for their diagnostic value in chronic osteomyelitis, including interleukin-6 (IL-6), defensins, calmodulin, and D-dimer [79–82].

IL-6 is a pro-inflammatory cytokine that plays a key role in the immune response to infection and inflammation. Studies have shown that elevated levels of IL-6 are associated with chronic osteomyelitis, making it a potentially useful biomarker for diagnosing the condition. However, IL-6 is not specific to osteomyelitis and can be elevated in other inflammatory conditions, limiting its diagnostic value [79].

Defensins are antimicrobial peptides that have been implicated in the pathogenesis of chronic osteomyelitis. Studies have shown that defensin levels are elevated in patients with chronic osteomyelitis, suggesting a potential role as a diagnostic biomarker. However, further research is needed to validate the diagnostic value of defensins in this context [80].

Calmodulin is a calcium-binding protein that regulates various cellular processes, including inflammation and immune response. Studies have shown that calmodulin levels are altered in patients with chronic osteomyelitis, indicating a potential role as a diagnostic biomarker. However, more research is needed to establish the diagnostic accuracy of calmodulin in chronic osteomyelitis [81].

D-dimer is a fibrin degradation product that is elevated in conditions associated with hypercoagulability and inflammation, such as chronic osteomyelitis. Studies have shown that elevated D-dimer levels are associated with chronic osteomyelitis, suggesting a potential role as a diagnostic biomarker. However, D-dimer is not specific to osteomyelitis and can be elevated in other conditions, limiting its diagnostic value [82].

In conclusion, IL-6, defensins, calmodulin, and D-dimer are promising biomarkers for diagnosing chronic osteomyelitis. However, further research is needed to validate their diagnostic accuracy and establish their clinical utility in this context.

Laboratory results are also important, offering insights into patient comorbidities that may impact metabolic, immune, or hematopoietic function [61].

## 10.8 Diagnostic Radiology

Radiological Findings: Radiological findings are typically inconclusive during the initial 2 weeks of hematogenous osteomyelitis, considered the disease's acute phase. A fracture, bone callus, or surgical implant can obscure the detection of specific infectious indicators. In contrast, during the late phase of chronic osteomyelitis, there may be unusually well-localized local bone rarefactions or lytic lesions following the destruction of 50–75% of the bone matrix. Other abnormalities that may be observed include visible bone sequestration, bone sclerosis, neoformation, and cortical thickening, periosteal reaction, and sinus tract [77].

Bone Scintigraphy: This diagnostic technique has proven to be valuable for osteomyelitis screening and early diagnosis. It utilizes technetium-99 or indium-labeled white blood cells or gallium-67, markers of bone marrow activity, to highlight areas of inflammatory activity. However, there is ongoing debate regarding which marker would be most sensitive for the early detection of osteomyelitis [83].

Computed Tomography (CT): CT scans can help determine how much bone fragment is involved and extended into soft tissues. CT also provides a more detailed characterization of bone sequestration. They offer comprehensive images of the cortical bone layer, the status of the bone union, bony integrity, and volume. Incorporating deep learning into CT imaging has enhanced its sensitivity and specificity in diagnosing chronic osteomyelitis [84].

Magnetic Resonance Imaging (MRI): MRI provides an in-depth study of the extent of the infection, including its impact on soft tissues. It enables earlier detection of acute changes when simple segmental radiographs are normal. In chronic infections, periosteal reactions can be more accurately verified by visualizing lamellar thickening or "Codman triangle" formation. MRI is a valuable tool for staging [85–87].

Positron Emission Tomography (PET) Scan: PET scan with the 2-[18F]-fluoro-2-deoxy-D-glucose (FDG) marker is another promising imaging modality, with high sensitivity (approximately 95%) and specificity (75–99%). PET Scan provides 3D precision, which helps target disease in surgery for complete eradication. However, this method is limited by its low availability and high cost [88].

## 10.9 Bone Biopsy and Identification of the Pathogen

A bone biopsy is recognized as the definitive method for diagnosing chronic osteomyelitis. The presence of necrotic bone and the replacement of trabecular bone with fibrous tissue infiltrated by inflammatory cells can facilitate the diagnosis of chronic osteomyelitis, even without microorganism isolation. However, isolating a microorganism from a biopsy substantiates the diagnosis and is pivotal in determining the appropriate systemic antimicrobial therapy [89].

Isolation can be achieved through blood cultures, although this method is only validated in acute hematogenous osteomyelitis due to its low yield in a chronic setting. Material obtained from an open sinus tract or other open wounds by swabbing may yield misleading results, as the isolates may include nonpathogenic microorganisms that are colonizing the site [89].

Bone biopsies can be performed percutaneously with the assistance of CT or ultrasonography or via an open biopsy during surgery. Open biopsy is often preferred due to the low yield of percutaneous procedures. When bone biopsies are conducted, it is essential that the samples are processed for both aerobic and anaerobic cultures. If commonly cultured microorganisms are absent and the clinical features are compatible, mycobacterial and fungal culture samples should also be taken and processed [89].

In chronic osteomyelitis culture, many biopsies yield negative results due to long-term antibiotic use and biofilm formation. To maximize diagnostic yield, it was previously recommended that antibiotics be stopped 48 h to 14 days prebiopsy, although there is no consensus on this in the current literature. The specimens should be obtained from up to five sites centered around the disease nidus at the time of debridement [90].

Sonication of dead bone, surrounding tissue, and implanted hardware, extending incubation to at least 14 days, has been reported to increase microbial isolation yields. Mycobacterial cultures take about 6 weeks (approximately one and a half months) to yield results [35, 91, 92].

Recent studies have focused on molecular biology approaches to detect microbial colonization. One advantage of molecular methods for microbial detection is that antibiotic therapy does not affect their results. Techniques such as next-generation sequencing, including 16S rRNA gene profiling, have detected fracture-associated microbiomes in persistent nonunion in 77% of patients not detected by traditional culture [93].

Specimens obtained for histopathology, either by biopsy or during surgery as frozen sections, are also crucial because the presence of neutrophils in significant amounts indicates infection. More than five neutrophils per high-power field indicate infection, with a sensitivity of 43–84% and specificity of 93–97%. Visualization of granulomatous lesions with positive Ziehl-Neelsen staining can lead to the diagnosis of mycobacterial infection earlier than culture results [91].

## 10.10 Classification of the Host and Disease

The primary objective of any treatment is to improve the patient's quality of life. Factors that guide patient selection include the effect of the infection on the patient's physiological well-being and the degree of physical disability caused by the disease. Pain that results in dysfunction and recurrent episodes of sepsis are strong indicators for surgical intervention. The Cierny-Mader classification system, established in 1983, lays down a pioneering framework for understanding the natural history of osteomyelitis, outlining treatment protocols and predicting outcomes [3, 19, 61]. This system categorizes the disease into three host cohorts and four anatomic types of infection, organized sequentially to denote disease complexity and its associated level of treatment strategy [29].

## 10.11 The Host

The physiological health of a patient is a crucial factor in determining their eligibility for treatment. A patient must possess the physiological capacity to resist infection, heal surgical wounds, and withstand the metabolic and psychological stress of sequential procedures, substantial blood loss, and extended hospital stays.

Patients are categorized into three physiological classes based on their health status and the disability caused by their disease (Table 10.1):

1. Class A Hosts: These are healthy individuals with a normal response to stress, trauma, and infection.
2. Class B Hosts: These patients have comorbidities that inherently impair wound healing and their response to treatment.
3. Class C Hosts: These are patients for whom the potential morbidity or functional loss resulting from treatment may exceed the impact of the disease on their quality of life. Observation or palliation alone may be the preferred course of action for such patients [59, 62, 63]. However, if their condition improves or advancements in medical technology present a treatment option that outweighs the risks. These patients may be reevaluated for treatment and reclassified as Class A or B hosts.

**Table 10.1** Physiological class: the host

| Type | Characteristics |
|---|---|
| A | Good immune system and delivery |
| B | Compromised locally (BL) or systemically (BS) |
| C | Requires suppressive or no treatment; Minimal disability; Treatment worse than disease; Not a surgical candidate |

| Factors affecting physiological class | |
|---|---|
| Systemic factors (S) | Local factors (L) |
| Malnutrition Renal or hepatic failure | Chronic lymphedema |
| Diabetes mellitus | Venous stasis |
| Chronic hypoxia | Major vessel compromise |
| Immune disease | Arteritis |
| Extremes of age | Extensive scarring radiation fibrosis |
| Immunosuppression Immune deficiency | Small-vessel disease |
| Tobacco abuse | Neuropathic Ulcer |
| Alcohol abuse | |
| Malignancy | |

## 10.12 The Disease

The Chierny-Mader classification system for osteomyelitis delineates the disease into four distinct types, each escalating in complexity, associated increased level of the treatment modality (Table 10.2):

Type I: This category is characterized by a sequestered nidus confined to the endosteum. It may be associated with an isthmic scar, granulation tissue, sequestered bone (trabeculae and endosteal cortex), or medullary implants. The enveloping soft tissue may also be implicated. Predominantly observed in immunosuppressed adults, this variant of osteomyelitis is more diaphyseal than metaphyseal.

Type II: Termed superficial osteomyelitis, the biofilm nidus in this type is exposed on a bony surface at the base of an atrophic soft tissue defect [61]. The nidus involves only the superficial part of an otherwise healthy osseous segment and does not extend into the medullary canal.

Type III: This type is marked by a full-thickness cortical sequestrum within or adjacent to a stable osseous segment. The canal, like Type I, and the soft tissue envelope may be involved, like Type II, and foreign bodies are common.

Type IV: This permeative form of osteomyelitis exhibits characteristics of Types I, II, and III but additionally features instability. The lesions are either intrinsically unstable or become unstable following debridement.

Each type necessitates a specific treatment modality that aligns with the nature and history of osteomyelitis.

**Table 10.2** Anatomic type of the chronic osteomyelitis (local disease) and treatment strategy

| Type | Description | Graph | Surgery | |
|---|---|---|---|---|
| | | | Debridement | Restoration |
| I | Medullary | 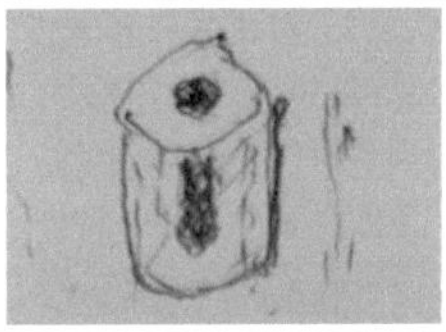 | Unroofing RIA | Dead space management: e.g. Abx beads |
| II | Superficial | 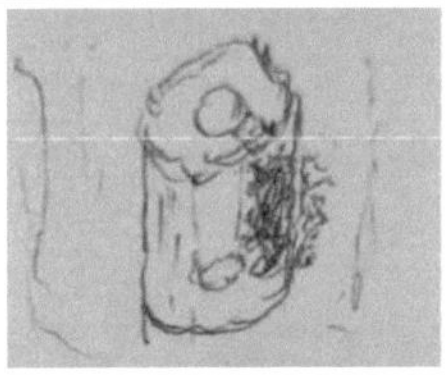 | Unroofing<br>RIA<br>*Decortication* | Soft Tissue Coverage: e.g tissue transfer |
| III | Localized | 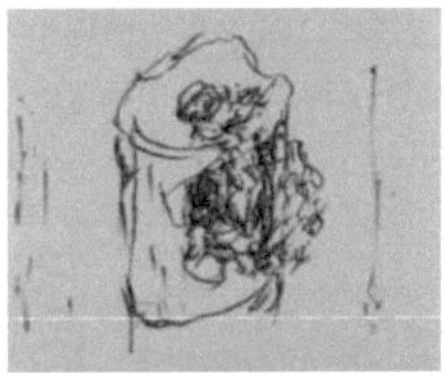 | Unroofing<br>Reaming<br>Decortication<br>*Sequestrectomy* | Dead space management Soft tissue coverage<br>*Bone graft* |
| IV | Diffuse | 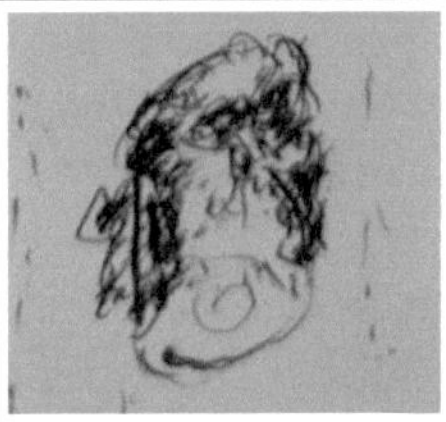 | Unroofing<br>Reaming<br>Decortication<br>Sequestrectomy<br>*Stabilization* | Dead space management<br>Soft tissue coverage<br>*Segmental bone restoration*<br>*Fixation* |

## 10.13 Treatment

Patient selection and decision-making (Fig. 10.1):

Selecting a treatment strategy is a complex process that hinges on various factors. These include the clinical stage of the disease, the anatomical site of infection, wound characteristics, and the proficiency of the healthcare team.

In instances where curative treatment is contraindicated, untimely, or excessively debilitating for the patient, palliative and suppressive therapies are employed to enhance patient well-being. The potential benefits of limb salvage must significantly outweigh those of amputation to warrant the associated morbidity and risk [59, 94, 95].

Limb ablation becomes a consideration when neither limb salvage nor palliative care is deemed safe or feasible. This decision-making process is profoundly influenced by intrinsic patient conditions or comorbidities, heightening the risk of treatment failure. Such risk factors can precipitate metabolic deficiencies, skin and wound breakdown, immune deficiencies, bacteremia, and complications associated with excessive bleeding. Moreover, the presence of multiple comorbidities can exacerbate these risks [3, 58, 94–97]. Therefore, engaging in these discussions with a well-informed healthcare team that can guide these decisions based on the patient's condition and prognosis is crucial.

Upon determining that a patient is at risk due to comorbidities, it is imperative to exhaust all avenues to invoke interventions to optimize the host response, irrespective of the chosen treatment modality [98, 99]. The preoperative rectification of deficiencies in wound healing could enhance the outcome for a Type B host, making it

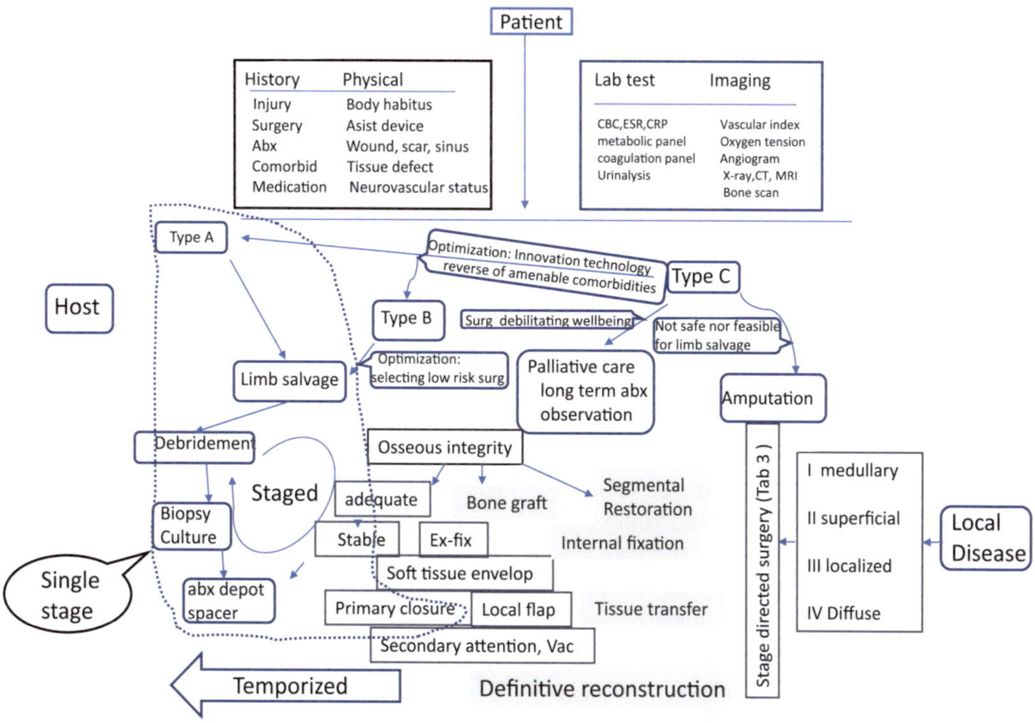


**Fig. 10.1** The diagram depicts the general rule of patient selection and decision-making. A patient was carefully evaluated with history and physical, laboratory test, and diagnostic image. The patient was then divided into three categories: Type A host is a healthy patient with normal repose to stress, trauma, and infection. Type A patient is usually a good candidate for limb salvage. Type B patients have comorbidities that inherently compromise wound healing and response to the treatment. Using less invasive methods should be considered for limb salvage. For type C patients, the treatment causing morbidity and loss of function outweighs the patient's quality of life impacted by disease. Palliative treatment is chosen. However, after reversing some comorbidities and/or new technology can offer a more favorable outcome, C-host can be re-classified to A-host or B-host. Limb salvage is considered. Amputation is recommended if the patient's condition is worsening and/or reversal of the adverse comorbidity is not feasible. Once limb salvage is chosen, A live, clean, manageable wound is established with thorough debridement, which is followed by pathogen-target antibiotics and bone stabilization. A single-stage reconstruction with antibiotic depot can be considered if the patient is healthy, osseous integrity is adequate with simple treatment, the wound is clean without sign of infection, and the soft tissue envelop is healthy and pliable (content in broken line). Otherwise, the I&D, biopsy, and antibiotic depot/spacer with or without temporized fixation can be repeated as many as possible until a viable, clean, manageable wound is achieved. A staged definitive reconstruction was then instituted based on the status of osseous integrity and soft tissue envelope. Cierny-Madar classification provides great help in establishing the treatment strategy (Table 10.2)

akin to that of a Type A host [55]. This underscores the importance of comprehensive patient management, where the focus extends beyond the primary disease to include overall health optimization [3, 96, 97].

As for surgical intervention, methods with low morbidity, such as atraumatic exposure, staged treatment protocols, and reconstruction unlikely to require surgical implants, should be considered first if they provide equivalent results [11–105]. If internal fixation stabilization is an absolute requirement, the final reconstruction may be better staged to follow the interval of local antibiotics therapy [46, 106, 107].

## 10.14 Systemic Antibiotic Therapy

Upon securing an adequate tissue sample for analysis, broad-spectrum antibiotics are initiated, guided by the patient's medical history, frozen section results, and the most probable pathogen. Hematogenous osteomyelitis is typically monomicrobial, while osteomyelitis resulting from contiguous spread or direct inoculation can be either polymicrobial or monomicrobial.

The pathogens most implicated in osteomyelitis vary according to the patient's age. *Staphylococcus aureus* is the predominant cause of both acute and chronic hematogenous osteomyelitis in adults and children. An increasing number of osteomyelitis cases are being attributed to methicillin-resistant *Staphylococcus aureus* (MRSA), which, in some studies, accounted for over a third of all staphylococcal isolates [108].

Other frequently encountered pathogens include coagulase-negative staphylococci, beta-hemolytic streptococci, enterococci, aerobic Gram-negative bacilli (including species of Pseudomonas and Enterobacter, as well as *Escherichia coli*), and anaerobic Gram-negative bacilli (such as Peptostreptococcus, Clostridium species, and Bacteroides).

The less common pathogens in specific epidemiological contexts and in immunocompromised patients are paramount. These include Mycobacterium tuberculosis, which may disseminate to the spine from the lungs; nontuberculous mycobacteria (Mycobacterium avium intracellulare, Bacille Calmette-Guerin, which may complicate intravesical therapy for bladder cancer); Candida species; fungi such as Blastomyces, Coccidioides, Cryptococcus, and Aspergillus. Infections with Actinomyces and Sporothrix typically follow traumatic inoculation. Salmonella and *S. aureus* are implicated in hematogenous osteomyelitis in sickle cell disease, while Brucella and Salmonella occur in spinal infections. *Bartonella henselae* may be associated with HIV-related osteomyelitis, and *Pasteurella multocida* or *Eikenella corrodens* are seen in human or animal bites [108–109].

Nevertheless, if the source of infection is unclear, imperative broad coverage is used, typically vancomycin and Zosyn, until culture and sensitivity results return.

Antibiotic coverage is then tailored to the sensitivities from surgical wound isolates. The optimal antibiotic coverage maintains a 1:1 ratio between a pathogen's mean inhibitory concentration and mean bactericidal concentration, with serum concentrations kept at least six times the mean bactericidal concentration [3].

There appears to be no significant difference in the efficacy of long-term (12 weeks) systemic treatment as compared to short-term treatment (6 weeks) [2, 8]. Similarly, no difference has been observed between parenteral antibiotics and a regimen of 2 weeks of IV antibiotics followed by a switch to oral antibiotics [109].

The efficacy of supplements such as Rifampin, which has previously shown benefit in hardware-related infections, remains inconclusive due to the study's low statistical power [109].

## 10.15 Local Antibiotic Depots

The persistence of planktonic and microscopic fragments of biofilm colony (sessile) cells following debridement, despite extensive lavage, is a significant concern. However, the high local concentrations of antimicrobial agents achieved in the seroma after the implantation of an antibiotic depot can eradicate these residual pathogens.

In the United States, the use of antibiotic depots for infection treatment is primarily limited to handmade antibiotic beads and antibiotic spacers. Only high-dose antibiotic mixtures are utilized in these composites to favor elution kinetics and achieve very high antibiotic concentrations [100, 110–114]. Conversely, commercially available antibiotic-loaded bone cement contains low-dose antibiotic mixtures and is intended solely for prophylactic use in revision total joint arthroplasty.

Polymethylmethacrylate (PMMA) is the most commonly used material in local depot beads and spacers. Palacos bone cement (Zimmer, Warsaw,

IN) is preferred as a PMMA carrier due to its superior release kinetics. Following implantation, these antibiotic implants can either be removed during a separate procedure or left in place indefinitely. However, there is a concern regarding the formation of secondary microbial colonies and biofilms after antibiotic release if the infection persists [106, 113–115].

Tobramycin and vancomycin are the antibiotics most used for PMMA depots. Drugs loaded in PMMA must be water-soluble and heat-tolerant for optimal release kinetics and antibiotic activity. The dose for a PMMA depot can be as high as 8 gm of vancomycin and 4.6 gm of tobramycin per package of bone cement (personal experience).

The utilization of biodegradable materials, specifically calcium sulfate beads (e.g., Osteoset, Wright Medical, Memphis, TN; Stimulant, Biocomposites, Wilmington NC) and calcium phosphate (e.g., Ceramet G or V, Bone Support), has been observed to circumvent concerns associated with the permanent in situ presence of acrylic depots. These biodegradable depots offer improved antibiotic release kinetics and demonstrate comparable clinical efficacy to PMMA depots in infection management. Certain biodegradable materials exhibit osteoconductive and osteo-inductive properties, providing some degree of mechanical support. Using these materials to fill bone defects allows for the potential completion of surgical procedures in a single stage [112].

However, these materials are not without their limitations. They lack the robustness required to function as structural spacers. The quantity and variety of antibiotics they can deliver are restricted due to alterations in their setting time characteristics caused by integration. Wound complications such as fistulas and wound dehiscence may arise due to the substantial byproduct of degradation. These complications are particularly prevalent with calcium-based antibiotic depots but can be mitigated with vacuum-assisted wound closure (incisional vac dressing) [112].

New materials are being explored to reduce wound complications and enhance biofilm treatment's efficacy. Composite materials, a blend of inorganic and biodegradable polymers loaded with antibiotics using nanotechnology, have demonstrated promising results in vitro and in animal studies for eradicating biofilm infection. The medical community eagerly anticipates the outcomes of ongoing clinical trials [116].

## 10.16 Surgical Treatment

Despite recent technological advancements, surgical management of chronic osteomyelitis remains a formidable challenge. The fundamental principle of surgical intervention is the comprehensive eradication of the infectious focus and its associated biofilm, followed by reconstruction of bone defect, restoration and maintenance of the bony stability using either internal or internal fixation, and finally, soft tissue coverage. The procedures can be done in a single stage or multiple stages, depending on the extensiveness and severity of the local disease and the patient's overall health condition [117].

Debridement: Complete eradication of the infection foci and associated biofilm is the key to the successful treatment of Chronic osteomyelitis. Thorough debridement is typically achieved through a meticulous process, which involves the removal of the diseased bone and a small margin of healthy bone to ensure complete removal of the infection. Following debridement, the infected area is meticulously irrigated to eliminate debris, residual pus, and necrotic tissue [117]. A recent study demonstrated that some fluorescent dye may help delineate the margin for complete surgical debridement [118]. Various irrigation methods have been explored, including using different solutions, such as soap and normal saline, with or without antiseptic agents and with varying degrees of force. The current literature supports low-pressure irrigation with a large quantity of normal saline. However, the choice of irrigation method and solution may depend on various factors, including the severity and location of the infection, patient characteristics, and surgeon preference [119].

Reconstruction of the bone defect: Bone defect after debridement is divided into two categories: noncritical size bone defect and critical size bone defect. (Fig. 10.2).

A noncritical size bone defect is defined as a bony defect less than 2.5 cm; this size of the bone defect can be successfully treated with a cancellous bone graft or bone substitute. The various antibiotics have been impregnated into grafts to increase local infection control. This method is currently in clinical trial for its efficacy as a one-stage procedure [120].

Critical size Bone defect [121]: There are several methods to successfully treat a critical size bone defect: Masquelet technique, free vascularized bone graft, bone transport with a universal external fixator or with a lengthening nail, and acute shortening and lengthening.

Masquelet technique: The Masquelet technique, also known as the induced membrane technique, is a two-stage surgical procedure used for the treatment of bone defects. This technique was first described by Masquelet et al. in 1986 and has since gained popularity in the field of orthopedic surgery. The first stage of the Masquelet technique involved the creation of a membrane around the bone defect. This membrane is induced by placing an antibiotic cement spacer in chronic osteomyelitis, which serves as an antibiotic depot and stimulates the formation

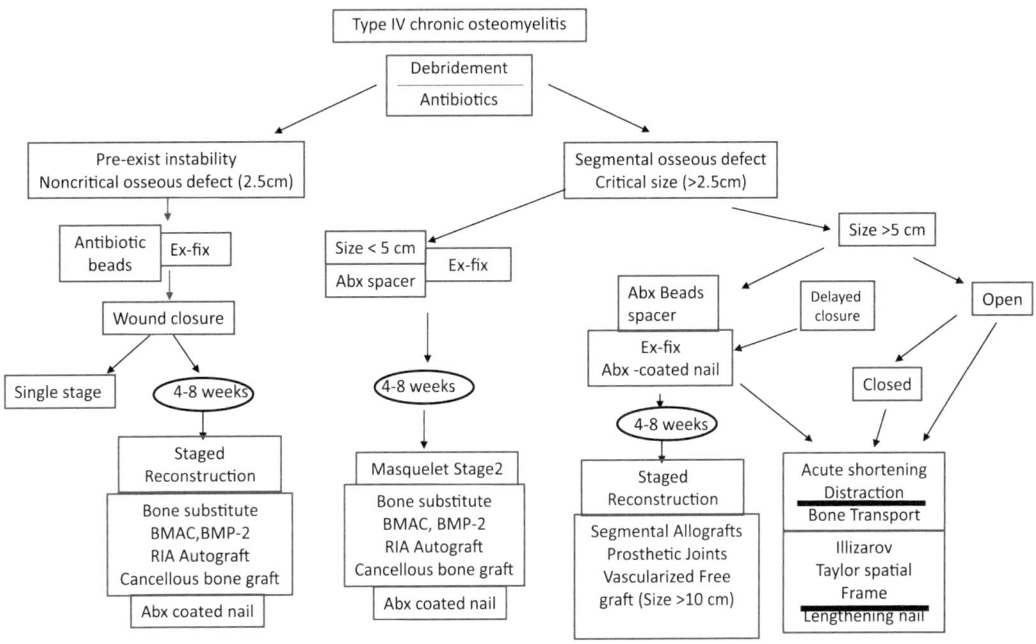


**Fig. 10.2** The diagram illustrates the algorithm for the management of Type IV chronic osteomyelitis. Patients with preexisting osseous instability (e.g., infected nonunion) or noncritical bone defect (size 2.5 cm) due to the debridement. The bone void can be filled with antibiotic-beads, and the medullary canal was reamed with RIA. The osseous stabilized with antibiotic-coated nail or ex-fix, followed by pathogen-target antibiotic. Single-stage management is feasible if the infection is subclinical. Otherwise, the definite treatment waited for 4–8 weeks and staged; the bone defect was filled with antibiotic beads, cancellous bone graft, and other bone substitutes, and osseous stabilization was preferred with antibiotic-coated nails. If the bony defect is a critical size but less than 5 cm, the reconstruction should be staged, and the Masquelet technique should be applied. If the defect is over 10 cm, the staged-free bone graft is the most favorable choice. Size 5–10 cm bone defects have many choices for reconstruction, such as staged segmental allograft, arthroplasty, acute shortening, distraction, and bone transport or Masquelet. Despite their own benefit and risks, they all prove a similar result. Thus, choice one of the reconstructions is solely based on the care provider's experience and the availability of their health care system

of a vascularized membrane. This membrane is a scaffold and stimulator for bone regeneration in the procedure's second stage. The cement spacer is removed in the second stage, and the bone defect is filled with bone graft or substitute material. The membrane is a barrier that prevents soft tissue ingrowth and promotes bone healing. The vascularized membrane also provides a source of growth factors and stem cells, further enhancing bone regeneration. Several studies have reported successful outcomes with this technique in treating significant bone defects due to osteomyelitis, especially for those with less than 5 cm of the critical-size bone defect [121].

Free Vascularized bone grafts involve the microsurgical transfer of healthy bone tissue along with its blood supply to the site of the bone defect. Free fibular transfer is a commonly used procedure, and this is an example of this technique. This technique allows for the delivery of vital nutrients and immune cells to the affected area, prompting bone healing and combating infection. The vascularized nature of the graft also enhanced its ability to integrate with the surrounding bone tissue, leading to improved long-term outcomes. One of the key advantages of vascularized bone grafts is the ability to provide a stable and durable solution for chronic osteomyelitis bone defects. Studies have shown that this technique can achieve high infection eradication rates and bone healing, improving functional outcomes and quality of life. Free vascularized bone is superior to other methods for osteomyelitic bone defects that are more significant than 10 cm. It can reduce the need for multiple surgeries and prolonged antibiotic therapy, thereby minimizing the risk of complications and improving overall treatment efficiency. The drawback of this technique is the requirement for equipment and surgeon proficiency in microsurgery [41, 54, 121].

## 10.17 Stabilization of the Target Bone

External fixation: External fixation in chronic osteomyelitis is particularly beneficial because it facilitates staged treatment protocols. For instance, Chen et al. emphasize that managing chronic osteomyelitis requires a multistage approach to minimize the risk of reinfection, especially following debridement procedures [122]. This is echoed by Lin et al., who describe a staged protocol involving radical debridement followed by applying Ilizarov's apparatus, which allows for distraction osteogenesis and subsequent stabilization with an intramedullary nail once healing is underway [123]. Such techniques highlight the importance of external fixation in providing a temporary yet effective solution that can adapt to the patient's evolving needs. Moreover, external fixation is particularly advantageous in cases with significant soft tissue involvement or when traditional internal fixation methods may exacerbate infection risks.

Additionally, antibiotic-impregnated external fixators have been shown to reduce the incidence of pin tract infections, a common complication associated with external fixation [124]. This antimicrobial strategy can be crucial in managing chronic infections, as it directly addresses one of the significant risks associated with external fixation. The effectiveness of external fixation in limb salvage procedures is further supported by studies that highlight its role in managing diabetic foot ulcers and Charcot osteoarthropathy, both of which are often complicated by osteomyelitis. Paola et al. note that external fixation is considered mandatory in cases of Charcot osteoarthropathy with osteomyelitis, underscoring its critical role in limb preservation [125].

Internal fixation: Internal fixation methods, such as plates and screws and intramedullary nails, are often preferred for their ability to provide stability and facilitate early mobilization. The role of internal fixation in the treatment of chronic osteomyelitis is a complex and evolving topic within orthopedic surgery. One of the primary considerations in using internal fixation for chronic osteomyelitis is the need for adequate debridement to remove necrotic tissue and infected bone. Studies indicate that successful treatment hinges on thorough surgical debridement, which includes the removal of dead bone and scar tissue, followed by stabilization of the remaining bone structure (122; 126). The internal fixation materials can be applied only after confirming that the infection process is under control, emphasizing the importance of a staged approach to treatment [122]. This aligns with findings that highlight the necessity of achieving biomechanical stability to facilitate healing and prevent the recurrence of infection [126]. Recent advancements have introduced the use of antibiotic-loaded bone cement coated with an internal fixation device. This method aims to combat bacterial colonization on implants, which is a significant concern in osteomyelitis cases [127]. Incorporating such materials can help eliminate the residual bacteria embedded in the biofilm and, at the same time, provide osseous stability that encourages early mobility and function recovery.

## 10.18 Soft Tissue Coverage

Primary closure vs. closure with secondary attention: The decision to pursue primary wound closure in patients with chronic osteomyelitis is complex and requires careful consideration of several factors. One of the key considerations is the extent of the infection and the likelihood of successful eradication with surgical intervention; in cases where the infection is localized and can be effectively treated with debridement and antibiotics, primary wound closure may be a viable option.

Another crucial factor to consider is the patient's overall health and immune status. Patients with compromised immune systems or underlying medical conditions may be at risk for complications following primary wound closure, such as wound dehiscence or recurrent infection. In these cases, as delayed wound closure or the use of wound dressings may be more appropriate,

The wound's location must also be considered when considering primary wound closure. Wounds that are large or located in areas with poor blood supply may be at increase for complications and may not be suitable for primary closure. In these cases, alternative management methods, such as negative pressure wound therapy or skin grafting, may be more appropriate.

Primary wound closure in patients with chronic osteomyelitis was associated with a lower rate of wound complications and faster healing compared to delayed wound closure if the correct patient was selected [24].

Primary wound closure with incisional negative pressure therapy broadens the indication of primary wound closure in the treatment of Chronic osteomyelitis.

Tissue transfer (local rotation flap vs. free flap): Tissue transfer is a common surgical technique for treating chronic osteomyelitis. This procedure involves the transfer of healthy tissue from one part of the body to the affected area to promote healing and prevent further infection. In recent years, regional tissue transfer has become an increasingly popular option for patients with chronic osteomyelitis, as it offers several advantages over traditional treatment methods [42, 42].

One of the main benefits of regional tissue transfer is its ability to provide a stable and reliable source of healthy tissue to the affected area. This is particularly important in the case of chronic osteomyelitis, where the infection may have caused significant damage to the surrounding bone and soft tissue. By transferring the healthy tissue from another part of the body, surgeons can ensure that the affected area receives the necessary nutrients and blood supply to promote healing and prevent further infection. In addition to providing a stable source of healthy tissue, regional tissue transfers also offer several other advantages in treating chronic osteomyelitis. For example, this technique can help improve the affected area's overall function and appearance, as the transferred tissue is often more robust and better able to cope with the stress of daily life [42, 43].

Furthermore, tissue transfer can also help reduce the risk of complications such as wound breakdown and infection, which are common in patients with chronic osteomyelitis. Regional tissue transfer is divided into two categories based on the location of its donor: local flaps involve moving tissue from an adjacent area to cover the defect. In contrast, free flaps involve transferring tissue from a distant site with its own blood supply. Local flaps are often preferred for smaller defects that can be covered by tissue from nearby areas. These flaps are further classified based on their blood supply, with options including radom pattern flaps, axial pattern flaps, and pedicle flaps; local flaps are advantageous because they are easier to perform, have a shorter operative time, and typically result in better aesthetic outcomes due to the proximity of the tissue. A typical example of a local flap is a gastronomic flap for the proximal tibia defect [43, 44].

On the other hand, free flaps are used for more extensive defects or when local tissue is not available or inadequate. Free flap involves a microsurgical technique to transfer tissue and blood supply from donor to recipient sites [27]. This requires specialized training and equipment, as well as longer operative times and hospital stays compared to local flaps. However, free flaps are often necessary for complex constructions and can provide better functional and esthetic outcomes in some instances. The free flap provides well-vascularized tissue that can effectively cover the defects, obliterate space, and enhance healing, thereby reducing the risk of recurrence of infection [128, 129].

Negative pressure wound therapy (NPWT) has emerged as a promising adjunct treatment modality in managing chronic osteomyelitis. NPWT, also known as vacuum-assisted closure (VAC) therapy, involves the application of controlled negative pressure to the wound site, promoting wound healing through various mechanisms. The therapy helps to reduce edema, promote granulation tissue formation, and enhance blood flow to the wound bed, ultimately facilitating the removal of infection material and promoting tissue regeneration. Several studies have demonstrated the efficacy of NPWT in treating chronic osteomyelitis. In a study by Xie, NPWT significantly reduced wound size and promoted healing in patients with chronic osteomyelitis. Similarly, a systemic review by Wang et al. reported that NPWT was associated with a higher rate of wound healing and a lower rate of recurrent infection compared to traditional wound care methods [130].

Techniques manage bone defects and soft tissue defects at the same time.

Bone transport with universal external fixator [131]:

The Illizarov method, a sophisticated technique for bone and soft tissue reconstruction, employs a composite bone flap. This process mirrors the action of orthodontic braces aligning teeth in the oral cavity. A healthy portion of the bone is subjected to a subperiosteal transverse osteotomy (cortectomy) to create a transport segment. The dimensions of this segment are dictated by the length of bone necessary to securely engage all bone segments using fixation wires and half pins. The fixator construct is designed to allow controlled relative movement of all segments. It can be adapted to accommodate various scenarios, including compression (shortening), distraction (lengthening), single or multiple bone transports, and simultaneous compression, distraction, and transport. The bone's movement away from its cortectomy site is typically restricted to 0.5 and 1.0 mm per day (distraction rate). The newly formed bone results from distraction osteogenesis, a process where host tissue at the cortectomy site forms new columns of bone when subjected to slow, controlled tension forces, allowing for bone regeneration in the wake of the moving segment. Forces generated by the fixator move the transport segment away from the cortectomy and toward the defect. The transport process is deemed complete when the segment crosses the defect and compresses against the opposing surface, facilitating osteosynthetic healing. While in the fixator, bony continuity is restored, the transported segment eliminates the defect, and intrinsic stability is reestablished when osteosynthesis healing occurs, and regenerated bone consolidates into cortical bone. The pin capture of soft tissue with the transport segment eliminates composite hard and soft tissue defects from within the injured limb segment. This negates the need for complex techniques to harvest living tissue from remote anatomical sites. The disadvantage of the procedure is that long-term wearing the universal ex-fix is cumbersome and uncomfortable, and there is a high chance of pin-side infection. Thus, it is difficult for the patient to comply with the treatment plan.

Bone transportation with lengthening nails: Bone transport with lengthening nails has been increasingly utilized in treating significant bone defects. This method involves gradually distracting the bone segments using an intramedullary nail with an integrated lengthening mechanism instead of the external fixator. Since the hardware is intramedullary, there is no exposed wire and ring outside, and thus relatively easily accepted by the patient. However, the drawback of the procedure is the NWB on distraction state and requires an addition to exchange nails if premature of the regenerate and solid nails after docking [132].

Acute shortening followed by distraction osteogenesis is a novel approach that has been applied in cases where significant bone loss or nonunion is associated with chronic osteomyelitis. This method initially shortens the bone after removing the infected segment, followed by gradual distraction to lengthen the bone over time. This technique has been particularly beneficial in managing complex cases, as it allows for correcting limb length discrepancies and deformity while simultaneously addressing the infection. The distraction process stimulates new bone formation, which is essential for restoring structural integrity and function [133].

The Taylor Spatial Frame (TSF) is an advanced external fixation device that has gained prominence in treating complex orthopedic conditions, including chronic osteomyelitis. Chronic osteomyelitis, characterized by persistent infection and inflammation of the bone, often necessitates intricate surgical interventions for effective management. The TSF's design allows for precise correction of deformities and stabilization of the affected limb, which is crucial in cases where traditional methods may fall short [134]. The TSF operates on the principles of distraction osteogenesis, enabling the gradual correction of bone deformities while maintaining stability. This is particularly beneficial in the context of chronic osteomyelitis, where the structural integrity of the bone is compromised. Studies have shown that the TSF can facilitate limb salvage procedures by allowing for simultaneous correction of angulation, translation, and rotation of the bone thus addressing the multifaceted nature of deformities associated with osteomyelitis [135, 136]. For instance, in a case report involving a large tibial defect due to chronic osteomyelitis, the combination of the TSF with other techniques resulted in successful limb reconstruction and functional recovery [137]. Moreover, the TSF's ability to dynamically adjust during treatment is a significant advantage. This feature allows for real-time modifications based on the patient's healing progress, which is critical in managing the complications often associated with chronic osteomyelitis, such as nonunion and infection recurrence [135, 138]. The frame's design, which includes six adjustable struts, provides the flexibility needed to correct complex deformities without requiring frequent frame adjustments thus minimizing patient discomfort and the risk of complications [138]. Regarding clinical outcomes, the TSF has yielded favorable results regarding limb function and patient satisfaction. A comparative study indicated that the TSF achieved accurate deformity corrections and had fewer complications than traditional external fixators [139, 140]. This is particularly relevant for patients with chronic osteomyelitis, where the stakes are high due to the potential for severe complications if the infection is not adequately managed.

## 10.19 Stage-Directed Treatment Protocols (Table 10.2)

Type I Medullary Osteomyelitis is primarily a surgical condition necessitating debridement. The medullary nidus is accessed via a cortical window, either directly by exposing the cortex to unroof the lesion or indirectly through reaming above and below (Table 10.2). The synthesis reaming aspiration system is an effective tool for debriding the intramedullary disease. This approach is contingent on the disease being confined to an isthmus; otherwise, a combination of reaming and unroofing is required to treat the truncated medullary abscess found at a metaphyseal and diaphyseal junction [3, 19]. This treatment protocol also applies to Type III and IV infections with a medullary component.

Post-debridement, the preferred treatment, involves the implantation of an acrylic or degradable depot within the canal, which typically constitutes the dead space. Primary wound closure can be performed if the infecting organism is identified and the soft tissue remains pliable. In other cases, a delayed closure of 3–5 days is recommended. Following debridement, the surgical site may necessitate protection for 3–6 months to facilitate recovery of the bone and host and prevent an insufficient fracture. The protection can be provided through ambulatory aids, external fixation devices, or internal splints such as rods or plates coated with antibiotic-impregnated composites.

Treating a Type II osteomyelitis lesion characterized by a compromised soft tissue envelope necessitates a meticulous and comprehensive approach. Here is a more professional rendition of the process (Table 10.2):

1. Preoperative Planning: The primary focus is restoring soft tissue. A combination of angiograms, transcutaneous oxygen tension measurements, and vascular indices is employed to evaluate the deficit and pinpoint the location of available portals for reconstruction. The nidus, or the focal point of infection, is optimally mapped using Magnetic Resonance Imaging (MRI) to delineate the zone of injury.
2. Lesion Classification: When a concomitant medullary infection is detected, the lesion is categorized as either Type III or Type IV osteomyelitis.
3. Treatment Initiation: The process commences with the resection of the soft tissue to viable, supple margins. The debridement of the nidus is performed tangentially, aiming for uniform Haversian bleeding—a phenomenon referred to as "the paprika sign" [141].
4. Soft Tissue Management: This phase necessitates significant surgical expertise in tissue transfer, practical application of vascular territories, and interpretation of vascular studies to prognosticate wound healing.
5. Restoration Process: Techniques such as local tissue interposition, free flap transfer, and dead space management with antibiotic depot and bone graft are frequently employed in this phase [30, 31, 142, 143].
6. Contingency Measures: Despite high success rates, there are instances where flaps may fail or are not viable options [144]. In such scenarios, negative pressure wound therapy utilizing vacuum-assisted closure presents a potent alternative if further reconstruction is deemed unnecessary [145–147].

Managing Type III osteomyelitis requires a comprehensive and meticulous approach due to the involvement of both osseous and soft tissue. Here is a more professional rendition of the treatment protocol (Table 10.2):

1. Resection: The initial step involves totally resecting the cortical sequestrum, employing methodologies to treat Type I and Type II osteomyelitis.
2. Debridement: After resection, the wound typically presents as a composite defect, implicating both osseous and soft tissue. In instances where the osseous resection is extensive enough to compromise the integrity of the remaining osseous segment, preventative measures should be instituted to avert an insufficient fracture.
3. Stabilization: Prior to debridement, limb stabilization may be achieved via a bypass bone graft, an external fixator, or a combination of both. Alternatively, in situ stabilization can be executed immediately post-debridement utilizing an antibiotic-coated implant or spacer.
4. Tissue Management: Components characteristic of Type II osteomyelitis found within Type III osteomyelitis are typically managed via tissue transposition or transfer.
5. Reconstruction: In scenarios where osseous reconstruction is indicated, or significant dead space is anticipated post-closure, an antibiotic depot is implanted, and a two or three-stage reconstruction is strategized [148–150].

Conversely, primary closure may be indicated, with or without an antibiotic depot.

The Type IV osteomyelitis lesion's intricate treatment protocol necessitates a multifaceted approach (Table 10.2, Figs. 10.2, 10.3, and 10.4). Initially, debridement is performed, which entails the excision of infected or necrotic tissue, potentially resulting in an unstable wound exhibiting characteristics of Type I, II, and III osteomyelitis (Figs. 10.2 and 10.4). In the other scenarios, osseous instability preexisted due to previous injury (Figs. 10.2 and 10.3).

Restoring the soft tissue envelope can be complicated by an extended zone of injury and concurrent conditions such as a history of compartment syndrome, vascular injury or disease, or radiation injury. Ipsilateral deformities and bone loss may limit fixation options.

A significant proportion (over 50%) of these lesions necessitate a staged approach involving soft tissue or dead space restoration before osseous reconstruction. Post-debridement, the objective is restorative: limb stabilization, reestablishment of a supple soft tissue envelope, and management of any residual dead space with an antibiotic depot (beads or spacer). If the soft tissue is adequate, the first stage can be completed simultaneously with the debridement. Otherwise, completion may be delayed, enabling the coverage team to achieve complex tissue transposition and/or microsurgical transfer [104,

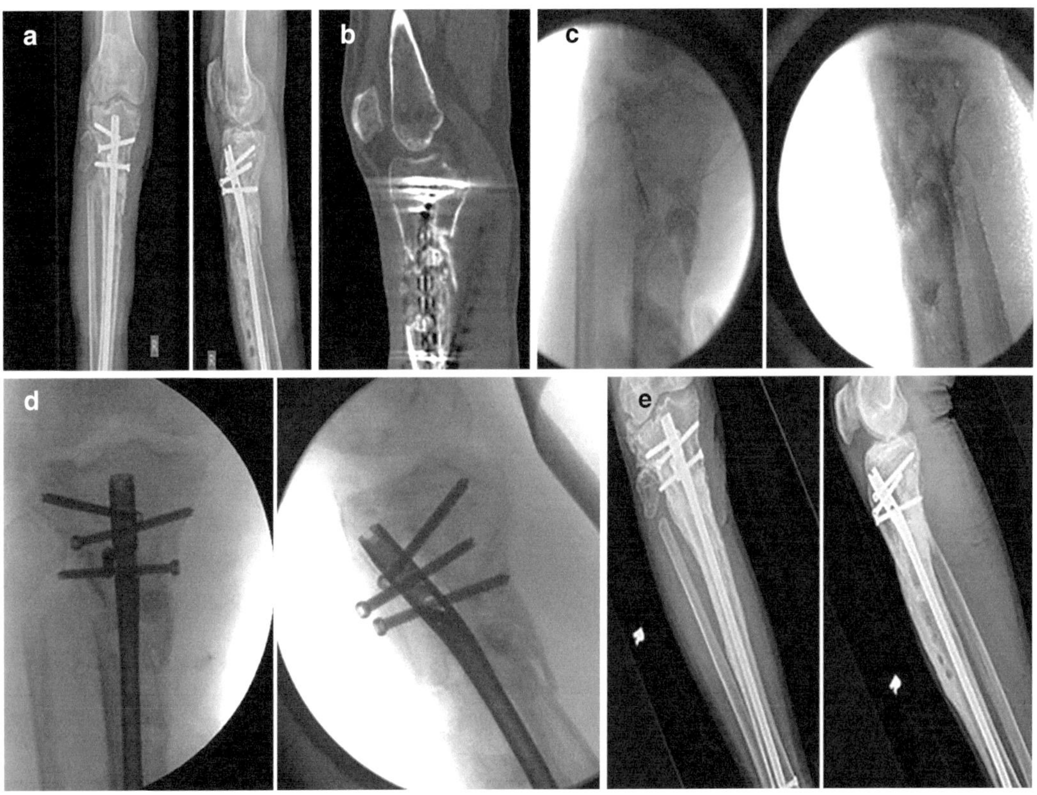


**Fig. 10.3** The case represented managing type IVA chronic osteomyelitis with preexisting osseous instability. (**a**) a pre-op X-ray demonstrating the right bicondylar tibia plateau fracture; the fracture is not healed, and bone destruction and sclerotic change, especially at the metaphyseal and diaphyseal regions. (**b**) Pre-op CT image demonstrated permissive destruction with some extra-bone formation. (**c**) Intra-op image of the first surgery. I noticed that the hardware removed the lytic lesion filled with six beads. (**d**) Intra-op image of a staged second surgery. Please notice that the antibiotic-coated nail was in place; minimal change of antibiotic bead filling

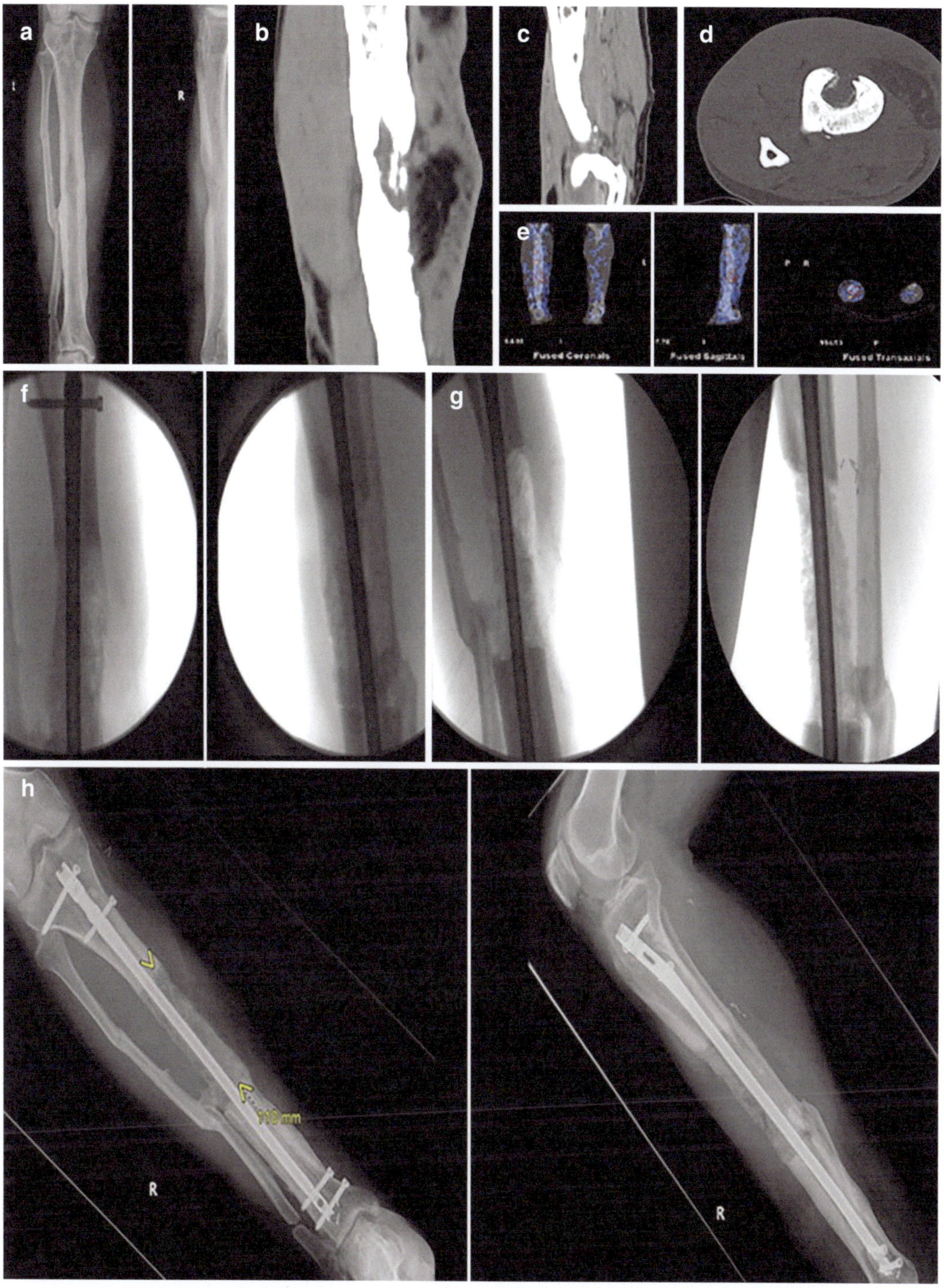


**Fig. 10.4** Case presentation of type IVB chronic osteomyelitis with segmental bone loss after debridement. (**a**) pre-op X-ray depicts a healed tibia shaft fracture with long significant cortical thickening and bone defect on the mid-shaft noticed sequester. (**b**), (**c**), and (**d**): pre-op CT representing coronal, sagittal, and cross-section confirms the significant defect. There is a small sequester. Significant cortical thickening. Fluid collection around disease bone. The medial side under the flap is significant. (**e**) CT Scintigraphy: increased up-take in the diseased segment of the bone. (**f**) Intra-op image of Masquelet stage 1, noticed diseased segment was removed, replaced with cement spacer. Abx-coated nail in place. (**g**) intra-op image of the second stage of the Macquet; Cement was replaced with a graft, and antibiotic-coated nail was in place. (**h**) 9 months after the second stage of the Miquelet. Some healing, no complete consolidation

151]. Once the wound has healed and the patient is able to tolerate further surgery, osseous reconstruction is done as a second stage, using external fixation, bone graft, a prosthetic total joint, or an allograft composite. Hard and soft tissue can be simultaneously restored and reconstructed; following the debridement and stabilization, composite defects can be eliminated by interposing a composite bone flap and bone transport either by Illizarov or lengthening nails [56]; bone transport and acute shortening followed by graduate distraction must use in some complex cases either alone or in combination with other technique in staged fashion (Fig. 10.2). Following cases represents the management of type IV chronic osteomyelitis with/without segmental bone defect in different Host.

**Case 1 (Fig. 10.3)**

A 40-year-old male with a history of major depressive disorder sustained the right type 3b open bicondylar tibia plateau fracture with segmental bone loss and underwent I&D staged ORIF and Masquelet for segmental bone loss and delayed wound coverage with gastronomic flap by plastic. He had the perineal nerve palsy due to accident. The patient had an on-and-off wound issue that was taken care of by plastic surgery. The wound was eventually healed. About 6 weeks ago, the patient had to drain the wound again; lab tests showed CBC 7.2, ESR 41, and CRP 35; the X-ray showed a healing fracture of the proximal plateau but nonunion of at metaphyseal and diaphyseal region with evidence of bone absorption and formation (Fig. 10.3a). This was confirmed with CT, and bone destruction presented multiple small permissive lesions at the metaphyseal diaphyseal junction. Bone formation represents increased density in the same region (Fig. 10.3b). The changes involve all full thickness of the cortex. Small soft tissue collection is also identified (Fig. 10.3b). Based on the patient history and clinical evaluation, the patient is a type A host with chronic osteomyelitis Type IV (infected nonunion) with no segmental bone loss. The treatment strategy included a staged procedure with the first surgery starting with a thorough debridement, removal of all foreign bodies (here is plate and screw), infected tissue, and dead bone and soft tissue till the visualization of a healthy envelope. The type I lesion was cleaned by reaming with RIA and type II lesion was cleared by curettage (decortication). The wound was then irrigated with a large volume of normal saline (12 L), and the bone void was filled with vancomycin and tobramycin-impregnated stimulant beads (Fig. 10.3c). A sample from I&D was sent for culture and pathology. The wound was closed with an incisional vac dressing. The bone was temporarily stabilized with a knee immobilizer. Pathology confirmed chronic osteomyelitis. The culture was positive for *Staphylococcus lugdunensis* and sensitive to vancomycin. The second surgery was restoration, which was scheduled for 3–4 weeks. Again, the wound was debrided. The residue beads were removed. The medullary canal was reamed with RIA, and the wound was much cleaner. No infected tissue was visualized. A bone void filled with vancomycin beads and the Osseous instability was supported by a vancomycin-coated nail (Fig. 10.3d), which delivers high-concentration antibiotics to eliminate the bacterial residue presented in biofilm. The patient continued with IV antibiotics for 6 weeks. Six weeks after the second surgery, the perineal nerve palsy started recovery. He was doing well at the 5-year follow-up and infection-free with hypersensitive CRP of 1.6 and ESR of 12. The fracture was completely healed (Fig. 10.3e). The patient was ambulating without the assistance device. However, he does complain about his knee pain due to traumatic arthritis, which was managed by pain management and physical therapy.

**Case 2 (Fig. 10.4)**

A 35-year-old male with a history of uncontrolled diabetes sustained the right type 3b open tibia shaft fracture, underwent I& D, ex-fix, vac dressing followed by IMN, and delayed wound coverage with free flap by plastic surgery. The patient developed post-op infection and underwent I&D with an antibiotic nail and/or antibiotic beads about eight times in the past 5 years. Each time, the patient's wound was closed after I&D. However, the wound started draining again about 10–12 months. The last surgery was about 12 months ago; at the time, the medullar canal was reaming with RIA to a size of 13. The flap was open to expose the diseased segment. The segment was deroofing and decorticated till they saw the bleeding bone. The medullary canal and bone defect were filled with antibiotic stimulant beads, the sinus tract was excised, and the wound was closed with the incisional vac. The patient's symptom was resolved. About 6 weeks ago, the patient experienced pain, swelling, and a draining wound again. A physical exam demonstrated the right leg swelling erythema and two open wounds on the medial side of the leg. One had the sinus tract appearance at the junction of the flap and normal skin above the ankle. The other one appeared to be a recent breakthrough on the superior edge of the flap, with noticeable purulent discharge. On blood exams, CBC 5.34, CRP 65, ESR 26, A1C 13. The blood sugar fluctuated between 230 and 450 mg/dl. X-ray demonstrated significant thickening of the cortex of the right tibia shaft with a noticeable sequestrum and sizable bony defect in the mid-section (Fig. 10.4a). CT confirmed a bony defect with significant sequestrum. Abnormal bone involves segmental bone around it with extension to soft tissue represented as a collection around the bone (Fig. 10.4b, c, and d). CT Scintigraphy also suggested radio nuclear uptake around the diseased segment of the bone (Fig. 10.4e). Based on clinic evaluation, this is B Host with type IV chronic osteomyelitis with segmental bone loss after a thorough debridement. A staged protocol was chosen to avoid recurrent infection. Masquelet reconstruction was chosen over free tissue transfer, which proves similar efficacy but is more invasive. Because the patient is B type host, low-invasive surgery is preferred. Other reconstruction modalities, such as acute shortening followed by distraction and bone transport, could be a good choice. However, we have limited experience with this technique. Furthermore, the patient prefers not wearing the ex-fix for a long period of time due to his experience at the time of injury. The patient is optimized by diabetes control consulting the endocrinology. The first surgery started with extensive debridement, including the removal of a segment of the diseased bone. The surrounding, infected soft tissue and sinus tract were excised, and adjacent bone was decorticated with high-speed bur till healthy bleeding bone was visualized. The entire medullary canal was reamed with RIA, and the wound was irrigated with 12 liters of normal saline. The antibiotic-coated nail was inserted to stabilize the bone fragment. The segment with done defect was then filled with antibiotic-impregnated cement spacer. A tissue sample was sent for biopsy and culture. The wound was closed with an assisted incisional vac dressing (Fig. 10.4f). Empirical IV antibiotic was given after surgery and switched to a culture-sensitive brand. Seven weeks after surgery, the second surgery was scheduled. The antibiotic spacer was removed, no significant infection was observed, and a formed membrane was noticed around the cement spacer. A small fragment of the bone at the distal segment was removed, and an old nail was also removed. The medullary canal was reamed with RIA; the wound was then irrigated with 3 liters of normal saline. The segmental defect was filled with graft collected from the femur, BMAC, cancellous bone chip DBM, BMP-2, and antibiotic-impregnated beads (kitchen sink technique). The graft material was protected with a membrane formed around the spacer. The antibiotic-coated nail was then inserted to provide stability while releasing the antibiotic locally in high concentration to eliminate residue. The microbe was resigned in the biofilm (Fig. 10.4g). Culture-sensitive antibiotics were given for 6 weeks post-op. Paitent was doing well in the 6 months post-op, then had another episode of the infection, which was controlled by the exchange of the antibiotic-coated nail. The final X-ray shows the patient's last visit 9 months after the Masquelet (Fig. 10.4h). He is infection-free with CRP 0.6 and ESR 1.6. He will be monitored closely for recurrent infection.

## 10.20 Results

Overall, the success rate, defined as survival with an infection-free segment that met all functional expectations, was 84% following the first treatment attempt, as Cherny reported [151]. This included 96% of A-hosts and 73% of B-hosts. No significant differences were found between the outcomes of patients treated using internal or external fixation strategies, patients with a monomicrobial or polymicrobial infection, or patients with a sensitive or resistant pathogen. The infection-free survival rates were similar after all biological treatment methods, including bone transport and lengthening, bypass bone grafting, microvascular transfer of segmental bone grafts, and massive cancellous bone graft. However, the success rate decreased by an average of 6% if internal hardware was used for both the methods of fixation and the form of reconstruction. The initial treatment failed in 315 (16%) of the 1966 patients, including 22% of the C-hosts, 19.5% of the patients undergoing ablation, and 17% of the patients who underwent a limb salvage attempt. The reasons for treatment failure included septic nonunion (43%), recurrent sepsis (12%), unexpected functional impairment (15%), wound breakdown (28%), and unrelated death. Retreatment to achieve cure was attempted in 275 of the 308 surviving patients, and a retreatment success rate of 87% boosted the overall 2-year success rate to 95%. In contrast to Cherny's report, a recent study demonstrated that the size of the bony defect is an important determinant for choosing certain reconstruction strategies to obtain better outcomes. Size 2.5 cm bone defect can be successfully treated with a cancellous bone graft, 2.5–5 cm may be successfully treated with Masquelet technique, 5–10 cm is suitable for both bone transport on free bone graft, and more than 10 cm defect get better result with free bone graft. A recent study reported improved outcomes using the combined Masquelet and bone transport [152].

## 10.21 Summary

Chronic osteomyelitis is a condition that can be difficult to treat without surgical intervention. This is due to the presence of a resilient nidus that harbors sessile, matrix-protected pathogens bound to the substrate surface. The clinical stage of the disease plays a crucial role in determining surgical planning, identifying suitable candidates for treatment, and establishing a means of comparing outcomes.

Curative treatment requires the complete removal of the entire biofilm colony. Therefore, the limb is stabilized, and residual pathogens are eliminated using both local and systemic antibiotics. Every effort is made to optimize the host response.

The reconstruction process is guided by wound parameters affecting outcomes such as bone integrity, fixation requirements, and soft tissue adequacy. These factors are critical in supporting both wound closure and its subsequent reconstruction.

## References

1. Gristina AG. Biomaterial–centered infection: microbial adhesion versus tissue integration. Science. 1987;237:1588–95.
2. Costerton JW, Stewart PS, Greeberg EP. Bacterial biofilms: a common cause of persistent infection. Science. 1999;284:1318–22.
3. Schmitt SK. Osteomyelitis. Infect Dis Clin North Am. 2017;31(2):325–38.
4. Cllawson DK, Dunn AW. Management of common bacterial infection of bones and joints. J Bone Joint Surg Am. 1967;49:164–82.
5. Taylor AR, Maudsley H. Installation –suction technique in chronic osteomyelitis. J Bone Joint Surg Br. 1970;52:88092.
6. Burri C, Passler HH, Henkemeyer H. Treatment of post-traumatic osteomyelitis with bone, soft tissue, and skin defects. J Trauma. 1973;13:7799–810.
7. Shannon JG, Woolhouse FM, Eisinger PJ. The treatment of chronic osteomyelitis by saucerization and immediate skin grafting. Clinic Orthop Relat Res. 1973;96:98–107.
8. Kelly PJ, Wilkowske FM, Washington JAII. Chronic osteomyelitis in adult. Curr Pract Orthop Surg. 1975;6:120–7.
9. Harmon PJ. A simplified surgical approach to the posterior tibia for bone grafting and fibular transfer. J Bone Joint Surg Am. 1945;27:496–7.
10. Campanacci M, Zaaoli S. Double tibiofibular synostosis (fibula pro tibia) for nonunion and delayed union of tibia: result review of one hundred seventy-one cases. J Bone Joint Surg Am. 1966;48:48–56.
11. Papineau LJ. Osteocutaneous resection reconstruction in diaphyseal osteomyelitis. Clin Orthop Relat Res. 1974;101:306.

12. Waldvogel FA, Papageogiou PS. Osteomyelitis: last decades. N Engl J Med. 1980;303:360–70.
13. Kelly PJ, Martin WJ, Conventry MB. Chronic osteomyelitis II: treatment with closed irrigation and suction. JAMA. 1970;213:1843–7.
14. Clawson DK, Davis FJ, Hansen ST Jr. Treatment of chronic osteomyelitis with emphasis on closed suction-irrigation technique. Clin Orthop Relat Res. 1973;96:88–97.
15. Whiteside LA, Lesker PA. The effect of extraperitoneal and subperiosteal dissection: I. On blood flow in muscle. J Bone Joint Surg Am. 1978;60:23–30.
16. Mathes SJ, Alpert BS, Chang N. Use of the muscle flap in chronic osteomyelitis: experimental and clinical correlation. Plast Reconst Surg. 1983;69:815–29.
17. Mathes SJ, Feng LJ, Hunt TK. Coverage of the infected wound. Ann Surg. 1983;198:420–9.
18. Chritina AG, Casterton JW. Bacterial adherence, the glycocalyx, and the rolling musculoskeletal infection. Orthop Clin Noth Am. 1984;15:517–35.
19. Cierny G, Mader JT, Pennick JJ. A clinical staging for adult osteomyelitis. Clin Orthop Relat Res. 2003;414:7–24.
20. Perry CR, Pearson RL, Miller GA. Accuracy of cultures of material from swabbing of the superficial aspect of the wound and needle biopsy in preoperative assessment of osteomyelitis. J Bone Joint Surg Am. 1991;73:745–9.
21. Chang CC, Meritt K. Infection at the site of the implant material with and without pre-adherent bacteria. J Ortho Res. 1994;12:526–31.
22. Patzakis MJ, Wilkins J, Kunar J, et al. Comparison of the results of bacterial cultures from multiple sites in chronic osteomyelitis of long bone: a prospective study. J joint and Bone Surg. 1994;76:664–6.
23. Happenstall RB, Goodwin CW, Brighton CT. Fracture healing in the presence of chronic hypoxia. J Bone Joint Surg Am. 1976;58:11531156.
24. Damholt VV. Treatment of chronic osteomyelitis: a prospective study of 55 cases treated with radical surgery and primary wound closure. Acta Ortho Scand. 1982;53:715–526.
25. Lortat Jacob A, Guilio B, Ramadier JO. Septic leg fracture: the value of cancellous bone graft without skin closure, alignment on the fibula. Rev Chir Orthop Reparative Appar Mot. 1985;71:515–26.
26. Esatehia JL, Jr Sennett B, Gelb H, et al. Treatment of chronic osteomyelitis complicating nonunion and segmental defects of tibia with open cancellous bone graft, posterolateral bone graft, and soft tissue transfer. J Trauma. 1990;30:49–54.
27. Gayle LB, Lineaweaver WC, Oliva A, et al. Treatment of chronic osteomyelitis of the lower extremities with debridement and microvascular muscle transfer. Clin Plast Surg. 1992;19:895–903.
28. Swiontkowswski MF, Hanel DP, Vedder NB, Scwappack JR. A comparison of short and long term intravenous antibiotic therapy I the postoperative management of adult osteomyelitis. J Bone Joint Surg Br. 1999;81:1046–50.
29. Simpson AH, Deakin M, Latham JM. Chronic osteomyelitis: the effect of the extent of surgical resection on infection-free survival. J Bone Joint Surg Br. 2001;83:403–7.
30. Illizarov GA. The tension stress effect of the genesis and growth of tissue: part I the influence of fixation stability and soft tissue preservation. Clin Orthop Relat Res. 1989;238:249–81.
31. Illizarov GA. The tension stress effect on the genesis and growth of tissues. Part II: the influence of the rate and frequency of distraction. Clin Orthop Relat Res. 1989;239:263–85.
32. Selan L, Passarlelo L, Rizzo L, et al. Diagnosis of vascular graft infection with antibodies against staphylococcal slime antigens. Lancet. 2002;359:2166–8.
33. Balban N, Stookey P, Fux CA, et al. Prevention of staphylococcal biofilm-associated infection by the quorum sensing inhibition RIP. Clin Orthop Rela Res. 2005;437:48–54.
34. McDowell A, Patrick S. Evaluation of nonculture methods for the detection of prosthetic hip biofilm. Clin Orthop Relat Res. 437:74–82.
35. Kobayashi M, Baer TW, Tuohy MJ, Fuji Shiro T, Procopio GW. Brief ultrasonication improves the detection of biofilm formative bacteria around metal implants. Clin Orhtop Relat Res. 2007;457:210–3.
36. Greer S, Kasabian A, Thorne C, Borud L, Sime CDS, Hsu M. The use of a sub-atmospheric pressure dressing to salvage a Castillo grade IIB open tibia fracture with concomitant osteomyelitis to avert a free flap. Ann Plastic Surg. 1998;41:687.
37. Webb LX. New techniques in wound management: vacuum assistant wound closures. J Am Acad Orthop Surg. 2002;10:303–11.
38. McCraw JB, Dubbel DG, Garraway JH. Clinical definition of independent myocutaneous vascular territories. Plast Reconstr Surg. 1977;60:341–52.
39. O'Brien BM, Henderson PN, Nennert RC, Crock GW. Microvascular surgical techniques. Med J Aust. 1970;1:722–5.
40. Mclean DH, Bucke HJ. Auto-transplantation of Omentum to a large scalp defect, with microsurgical revascularization. Plast Reconstr Surg. 1972;49:268–74.
41. Taylor GI, Miller GD, Ham FJ. The free vascularized bone graft: a clinical extension of microvascular technique. Plast Reconstruct Surg. 1975;55:533–44.
42. Vaconez LO, Bostwick J II, McCraw J. Coverage of exposed bone by muscle transposition and skin grafting. Plast Reocst Surg. 1974;53:526–31.
43. Ger R. Muscle transposition for treatment and prevention of chronic post-traumatic osteomyelitis of the tibia. J Bone Joint Surg Am. 1977;59:784–79.
44. Klemm K. Die Behandlung Chronischer Knowechen infekioenen Mit Gentamicin PMMA ketten und Kulgem. In: Contzen HE, editor. Gentamycin PMMA ketten: symposium. Munich: Verlag fur Lehrmitel,Wissenschaft und Forschung; 1976. p. 202–22.

45. Wahlig H, Dingeldein E, Bergmann R, Reuss K. The release of gentamycin from polymethylmethacrylate beads: an experimental and pharmacokinetic study. J Bone Joint Sur Br. 1978;60:270–5.
46. Walenkamp GH. Gentamycin PMMA beads a clinical pharmacokinetic and toxicologic study. Amsterdam: Drukkerij Clietur; 1983. p. 19–22.
47. Cierny G III. Infection tibia non-unions (1981–1995) the evolution of change. Clin Orthop Relat Res. 1999;360:97–105.
48. Bernard F, Gandon J. Postoperative wound infection: the influence of ultraviolet irradiation of the operating room and of various other factors. Ann Surg. 1964;160(suppl):21–192.
49. Cierny G III. Managing the debridement defect. In: Combs R, editor. Infection in the orthopedic patient. London: England Butterworth Publishers; 1989.
50. Hovellius L, Josefsson G. An alternative method for exchange operation of infected arthroplasty. Acta Orthop Scans. 1979;50:93–6.
51. Salvati EA, Cherkasky KM, Brause BD, Wilson PD Jr. Reimplantation in infection: a 12 years' experience. Clin Orthop Relat Res. 1982;170:62–75.
52. Enneking WF, Spanier SS, Goodman MA. A system for the surgical staging of the musculoskeletal sarcoma. Clin Orthop Relat Res. 1980;153:106–20.
53. Klemm K, Winter Klemm B. Unconscious guilt in the treatment of infection patients. In: Coombs R, Fitzgerald R, editors. Infection in the orthopedic patient. London: Butterworth Publisher; 1989.
54. Yajima H, Tami S, Dipas M, Inada Y. Vascularized fibular graft in the treatment of osteomyelitis and infected nonunion. Clin Orthop Relat Res. 1993;293:256–64.
55. Cierny G III, DiPassqual D. Treatment of chronic infection. J AAOS. 2006;14:105S–S110.
56. Cierny G III, Zorn K. Segmental tinea defects: comparing conventional and Illizarov methodologies. Clin Orthop Relat Res. 1994;301:118–23.
57. Sen C, Kocaglu M, Eralp L, Gulsen M, Cinar M. Bifocal compression distraction in the acute treatment of grade IIB open tibia fracture with bone and soft tissue loss. A report of 24 cases. JOT. 2004;18:150–7.
58. Younger AS, Duncan P, Mari BA. Treatment of infection associated with the segmented bone loss in the proximal part of the femur in two stages with the use of an antibiotic-loaded internal prosthesis. J Bone Joint Surg Am. 1998;80:60–9.
59. Cierny G III, Di Pasquale D. Periprosthetic total joint infection: staging, treatment, and outcomes. Clin Orthop Relat Res. 2002;403:23–4.
60. Cobos JA, Lindsey RW, Gugas Z. The cylindrical mesh cage for treatment of long bone segmental defect and usual aspects. N Engl J Med. 1970;282:198–316.
61. Lew DP, Waldvogel FA. Osteomyelitis. Lancet. 2004;364(9431):369–79.
62. Cierny G III, Mader JT. Adult chronic osteomyelitis. Orthopedics. 1984;7(11):1557–64.
63. Kalinka HM, Geraci J, et al. Staphylococcus aureus isolates from chronic osteomyelitis are characterized by high host cell invasion and intracellular adaptation but still induced inflammation. Int J of Med Microbial. 2017;304:1038–49.
64. Hatzenbuehler J, Pulling TJ. Diagnosis and management of osteomyelitis. Am Acad Fam Physician. 2011;84(9):1027–33.
65. Lew DP, Waldvogel FA. Osteomyelitis. N Engl J Med. 1997;336:9.
66. Walter N, Baert S, Alt V, Rupp M. What is the burden of osteomyelitis in Germany? BMC Infect Dis. 2021;21:55.
67. Kremers HM, Nwojo ME, Ransom JE, Wood-Wentz CM, Melton LJ 3rd, Huddleston PM 3rd. Trends in the epidemiology of osteomyelitis: a population-based study, 1969 to 2009. J Bone Joint Surg Am. 2015;97:837–45.
68. Lindbloom BJ, James ER, McGarvey WC. Osteomyelitis of the foot and ankle: diagnosis, epidemiology, and treatment. Foot Ankle Clin. 2014;19:569–88.
69. Cunha BA. Osteomyelitis in elderly patients. Clin Infect Dis. 2002;35:287–93.
70. McNeil JC, Vallejo JG, Kok EY, Sommer LM, Hultén KG, Kaplan SL. Clinical and microbiologic variables predictive of orthopedic complications following staphylococcus aureus acute hematogenous osteoarticular infections in children. Clin Infect Dis. 2019;69:1955–61.
71. Nishitani K, Sutipornpalangkul W, Bentley KLDM, et al. Quantifying the natural history of biofilm formation in vivo during the establishment of chronic implant-associated staphylococcus aureus osteomyelitis in mice to identify the critical pathogen and host factors. J Orthop Res. 2015;33(9):1311–9.
72. Johansen LK, Koch J, Frees D, et al. Pathology and biofilm formation in a porcine model of staphylococcal osteomyelitis. J Comp Pathol. 2012;147:343–53.
73. Zhao Z, Zhang Y, Cheng Y, Li J, et al. Thermosensitive nanotherapeutics for localized photothermal ablation of MRSA-infected osteomyelitis combined with chemotherapy. ACS Appl Mater Interfaces. 2023;15(10):12842–54.
74. Stoodley P, Ehrlich D, Sedghizadeh P, et al. Orthopedic biofilm infections. Curr Orthop Pract. 2011;22(6):558–63.
75. Racenis K, Rezevska D, Madelāne M, et al. Use of phage cocktail bfc 1.10 in combination with ceftazidime-avibactam in the treatment of multidrug-resistant pseudomonas aeruginosa femur osteomyelitis—a case report. Front Med. 2022;9:9.
76. Zhang Y, Cheng Y, Zhao Z, Jiang S, et al. Enhanced chemoradiotherapy for MRSA-infected osteomyelitis using immunomodulatory polymer-reinforced nanotherapeutics. Adv Mater. 2024;36(19):e2304991.
77. Berbari EF, Steckelberg JM, Osmon DR. Osteomyelitis. In: Mandell GL, Bennett JE, Dolin R, editors. Mandell, douglas, and Bennett's

principles and practice of infectious diseases. 8th ed. Philadelphia: Elsevier Saunders; 2015. p. 1282–97.
78. Ma X, Han S, et al. Epidemiology, microbiology and therapeutic consequences of chronic osteomyelitis in northern China: a retrospective analysis of 255 patients. Nature. 2018;8:148–95.
79. Smith A, Jones B. The role of interleukin-6 in chronic osteomyelitis. J Bone Infect. 2018;3(2):69–75.
80. Brown C, White D. Defensins as biomarkers for chronic osteomyelitis. J Infect Dis. 2019;205(4):589–96.
81. Johnson E, Smith G. Calmodulin levels in chronic osteomyelitis: a potential diagnostic biomarker. Bone Res. 2020;7(3):201–8.
82. Williams H, Davis R. D-dimer as a diagnostic biomarker for chronic osteomyelitis. J Clin Microbiol. 2021;45(6):123–30.
83. Palestro CJ. Radionuclide image of musculoskeletal infection: a review. JNM. 2016;57(9):1406–12.
84. Wu Y, Lu X, et al. Detection of the extremity chronic traumatic osteomyelitis by machine learning based on computed-tomography image: a retrospective study. Medicine. 2020;99:1–9.
85. Erdman WA, Tamburro F, Jayson HT, et al. Osteomyelitis: Characteristics and pitfalls of diagnosis with MRI imaging. Radiology. 1991;180:533–9.
86. Gross T, Kaim AH, Regazzoni P, Widmer AF. Current concepts in post-traumatic osteomyelitis: a diagnostic challenge new imaging options. J Trauma. 2002;52(12):1210.
87. Aydingoz U. Imaging osteomyelitis: an update. Fortschr Röntgenstr. 2023;195:297–308.
88. Lee SH, Kim MB. Localization of osteomyelitis lesion for operative eradication of chronic osteomyelitis of the lower extremity. Int Orthop. 2023;47(1):5–15.
89. Perry CR, Pearson RL, Miller GA. Accuracy of cultures of material from swabbing of the superficial aspect of the wound and needle biopsy in the preoperative assessment of the osteomyelitis. J Bone Joint Surg Am. 1991;73:745–9.
90. Patzakis MJ, Wilkins J, Kumar J, Holtom P, Greenbaum B, Ressler R. Comparison of the results of bacterial cultures from multiple sites in chronic osteomyelitis of long bones: a prospective study. J Bone Joint Surg Am. 1994;76:664–6.
91. Tunney MM, Patrick S, Gorman SP, et al. Improved detection of infection in hip replacement: a current under-estimated problem. J Bone Joint Surg Br. 1998;80:56.
92. Wagner RK, Mees P, et al. Characteristics and outcome of occult infections in presumed aseptic nonunion: a retrospective cohort study. JOT. 2024;38:452–8.
93. Bouchiat C, Ginevra C, et al. Improving the diagnosis of bacterial infections: evaluation of 16S rRNA nanopore metagenomics in culture negative samples. Front Microbiol. 2022;13:341.
94. McPherson EJ, Tontz WT, Patzakis M, et al. Outcome of the infected total knees utilizing a seating system for prosthetic joint infection. Am J Orthop. 1999;28:161–85.
95. Lain K, Bohn ER, Burnel C, Helden DR. Presence of medical comorbidities in patients with infected primary hip or knee arthroplasties. J Arthroplast. 2007;22:651–6.
96. Patzakis MJ, Zalavras CG. Chronic post-traumatic osteomyelitis and infected nonunion of the tibia: current management concepts. J AAOS. 2005;13:417–27.
97. Cierny G III. Infection following open fracture. In: Levin LS, editor. Complications in orthopedics: open fractures. Rosemont: The American Academy of Orthopaedic Surgeons. In press.
98. Kunisda T, Morgan SY, Powell G, Choong PF. Wound complication following pre-op radiotherapy for soft tissue sarcoma. Eur J Surg Oncol. 2002;28:75–9.
99. Cireny G III. Chronic osteomyelitis: results of treatment. Intr Course Lect. 1990;39:495–508.
100. Cierny GIII, Matava M, Zorn KE. Cancellous bone grafting in the presence of bacterial contamination: indications, methods, long term results. Ortho Trans. 1990;13:633.
101. Matava M, Cierny G, Zorn KE. Papineau Grafting: Still a treatment option. Orthop Trans. 1991;15:616–7.
102. Cieny G III, Nahai F. Dialogue: lower extremity reconstruction. Part 2, vol. 2. Perspect Plast Surg; 1988. p. 109–21.
103. Cierny G III. The classification and treatment of the adult osteomyelitis. In: Evarts CM, editor. Surgery of the musculoskeletal system. 2nd ed. New York: Churchill Livingstone; 1990. p. 4337–79.
104. Cierny GIII, Aelod B, Mader JT. Ipsilateral fibular transfers in the treatment of tibia osteomyelitis defects. Orthop Trans. 1987;13:535.
105. Cierny G III, Byrd SH, Jonc RE. Primary versus delayed soft tissue coverage for severe open tibia fractures. A comparison of results. Clin Orthop Relet Res. 1983;178:54–63.
106. Osetrmann PA, Seligson DM, Henry SL. Local antibiotic therapy for severe open fracture: a review of 1085 consecutive cases. J Bone Joint Surg By. 1995;77:93–7.
107. Enggesaaeter LB, Lie SA, Espehauug B, et al. Antibiotic prophylaxis in total hip arthroplasty: effect of antibiotic prophylaxis systemically and in bone cement on the revision rate of 22,179 primary hip placements followed 0-14 years in Norwegian arthroplasty register. Acta Orthop Scand. 2003;74:644–51.
108. Emori TG, Gaynes RP. An overview of nosocomial infection, including the role of the microbiology laboratory. Clin Microbial Rev. 1993;6:428–4.
109. Besal R, Adamic P, et al. Systemic antimicrobial treatment of chronic osteomyelitis in adults: a narrative review. Antibiotics. 2023;12:944.
110. Adams K, Couch L, CieG II, et al. Invitro and in vivo evaluation of antibiotic diffusion from

antibiotic-impregnated poly-methyl methacrylate beads. Clin Ortho Relat Res. 1992;278:244–52.
111. Younger AS, Duncan CP, Masri BA. Treatment of infection associated with segmental bone loss in the proximal part of the femur in two stages with the use of two stages of an antibiotic-loaded interval prosthesis. J Bone Joint Surg Am. 1998;80:60–9.
112. Mckee MD, Wild LM, Schemitsch EH, Wadell JP. The use of an antibiotic-impregnated, osteoconductive, bioabsorbable bone substitute in the treatment of long bone defects: early results of a prospective trial. JOT. 2002;16:22–627.
113. Paly D, Herzenberg JE. Intramedullary infection treated with antibiotic cement rods: preliminary results in nine cases. J Orthop Trauma. 2002;16:723–9.
114. Hanssen AD. Local antibiotic delivery vehicles in the treatment of musculoskeletal infection. Clin Orthop Relat Res. 2005;437:91–6.
115. Henry SI, Seligson D. Management of open fractures and osteomyelitis with the antibiotic beads pouch technique. South Med J. 1990;83:98–104.
116. Ly X, Zhou DM, Sun XH, Zhao Z. Nanosized hydroxyapatites-polycystic acid-vancomycin in the alleviation of chronic osteomyelitis. Drug Des Devel Ther. 2022;16:1983–93.
117. Hashmi M, Norman P, Saleh M. The management of chronic osteomyelitis using the Lautenbach method. J Bone Joint Surg. 2004;86(2):269–75.
118. Huang H, Zhao N, Li Q, et al. The therapeutic effectiveness using fluorescence-guided surgery for MRONJ. BioMed Res Int. 2022:1–9.
119. Yasheng T, Mijiti A, Yushan M, Liu Z, et al. Ozonated water lavage and physiological saline irrigation combined with vacuum-sealed drainage in the treatment of 18 cases of chronic osteomyelitis. J Int Med Res. 2021;49(3):300060521999530.
120. Schemitsch EH. Size matters: defining critical in bone defect size. JOT. 2017;31:S20–2.
121. Klifio KM, PharmD DO, et al. Treatment of post-traumatic tibia Diaphyseal bone defects: a systemic review and meta-analysis. JOT. 2022;36:55–62.
122. Chen L, Hou H, Zhang L, Pan Q. Refractory chronic osteomyelitis of femur: a case report. Med Case Rep and Rev. 2021;3:3.
123. Lin CC, Chen C, Chiu F, Su Y, Liu CL, Chen TH. Staged protocol for the treatment of chronic tibial shaft osteomyelitis with Illizarov's technique followed by the application of intramedullary locked nail. Orthopedics. 2012;3:5–12.
124. Ismat A, Walter N, Baert S, et al. Antibiotic cement coating in orthopedic surgery: a systematic review of reported clinical techniques. JOT. 2021;22(1):56.
125. Dalla Paola L, Carone A, Boscarino G, Scavone G, Vasilache L. Combination of open subtotal calcanectomy and stabilization with external fixation as limb salvage procedure in hindfoot-infected diabetic foot ulcers. Int J Low Extrem Wounds. 2016;15(4):332–7. https://doi.org/10.1177/1534734616667865.
126. Sharma P, Baghel A. Outcome of intramedullary nail coated with antibiotic-impregnated cement in chronic osteomyelitis. Ann Afr Med. 2023;22(4):434–9.
127. Shi J, Yang X, Song M, Zhang X, Xu Y. Clinical effects of early debridement, internal fixation, and Masquelet technique for childhood chronic hematogenous osteomyelitis of long bones. J Orthop Surg Res. 2023;18:12.
128. Huffman SS, Berger LE, Li K, et al. Muscle versus fascia free tissue transfer for treatment of chronic osteomyelitis in the comorbid population. J Reconstr Microsurg. 2023;40:253–26.
129. Imai H, Yoshida S, Mese T, et al. Osteocutaneous superficial circumflex iliac perforator flap for the lower extremity bone and soft tissue reconstruction with perforator-to-perforator anastomosis after radical debridement of tibia osteomyelitis: a case report. Microsurgery. 2023;43:713–8.
130. Li J, Zhang H, Qi B, Pan Z. Outcomes of vacuum sealing drainage treatment combined with skin flap transplantation and antibiotic bone cement on chronic tibia osteomyelitis: a case series study. Med Sci Monit. 2019;25:5343–9.
131. Bari M, Islam S. Trifocal bone transport by Illizarov technique for large post-traumatic tibial bone defects: a single center Bari-Illizarov experience of 46 cases. MOJ Orthop Rheumatol. 2020;12:12–4.
132. Brinker MR, Amirian A, O'Connor DP, Laughlin MS. Efficacy of precise nail in the treatment of adult patients with posttraumatic femoral leg length discrepancy. J Orthop Trauma. 2021;35:304–8.
133. Salih S, Mills EJ, McGregor-Riley J, Dennison M, Royston S. Transverse debridement and acute shortening followed by distraction histogenesis in the treatment of open tibial fractures with bone and soft tissue loss. Strateg Trauma Limb Reconstr. 2018;13:129–35.
134. Naude J, Manjra MA, Birkholtz F, et al. Outcomes following treatment of complex tibial fractures with circular external fixation: a comparison between the Taylor spatial frame and truelock-hex. Strateg Trauma Limb Reconstr. 2020;14(3):142–7.
135. Abuomira IEA, Sala F, Elbatrawy Y, Lovisetti G, Alati S, Capitani D. Distraction osteogenesis for tibial nonunion with bone loss using combined Illizarov and Taylor spatial frames versus a conventional circular frame. Strateg Trauma Limb Reconstr. 2016;11:153–9.
136. Krkovic M, Geetala R, Zhang J, Maghsoudi D, Madigasekara A. The use of the Taylor spatial frame in treating tibial osteomyelitis following traumatic tibial fracture. Strateg Trauma Limb Reconstr. 2024;19:32–5.
137. Pan H, Ding Y, Xu R, Rai S, Liu R, Li J. A combination of Illizarov frame, externalized locking plate and tibia bridging for an adult with large tibial defect and severe varus deformity due to chronic osteomyelitis in childhood: a case report. Medicina. 2023;59(2):262.

138. Khunda A, Al-Maiyah M, Eardley W, Montgomery RJ. The management of tibial fracture non-union using the Taylor spatial frame. J Orthop. 2016;13:360–3.
139. Dammerer D, Kirschbichler K, Donnan L, Kaufmann G, Krismer M, Biedermann R. Clinical value of the Taylor spatial frame: a comparison with the Illizarov and orthodox fixators. J Child Orthop. 2011;5(5):343–9.
140. Rozbruch SR, Segal KL, Illizarov S, Fragomen AT, Illizarov G. Does the Taylor spatial frame accurately correct tibial deformities? Clin Orthop Relat Res. 2010;468:1352–61.
141. Sachs BL, Shaffer JW. Abstract: osteomyelitis of the tibia and femur: a critical evaluation of the effectiveness of the Papineau technique in a prospective study. In: 50th annual meeting Proceedings Park. Ridge: American Academy of Orthopedic Surgeons; 1993.
142. Lutz DA, Hallock GG. Microsurgical transfer of vascularized tissue to close problem wounds. AORN J. 1995;62:234–48.
143. Koker AR, Kasabian AK, Karp NS, Gottlieb JJ. Fate of the free flap micro anastomosis distal to the zone of injury in lower extremity trauma. Plast Reconstr Surg. 1997;99:1068–73.
144. Archdeacon MT, Herscovici D Jr, Sanders RW. Wound care: debridement, coverage, and antibiotic utilization. Tech Orthop. 2001;16:398–408.
145. Argenta LC, Morykwas MJ. Vacuum-assisted closure: a new method for wound control and treatment: clinical experience. Ann Plast Surg. 1997;38:563–77.
146. Datiashvili RO, Knox KR. Negative pressure dressing: an alternative to free tissue transfers? Wounds. 2005;17:206–12.
147. Lam WL, Garrido A, Staley PRW. Use of topical negative pressure in the treatment of chronic osteomyelitis: a case report. J Bone Joint Surg Am. 2005;87:622–4.
148. Harmon PJ. A simplified surgical approach to the posterior tibia for bone grafting and fibular transference. J Bone Joint Surg Am. 1945;27:496–8.
149. Campanacci M, Zaanola S. Double tibiofibular synostosis (fibula pro-tibia) for nonunion and delayed union of the tibia: end result review of one hundred seventy-one cases. J Bone Joint Surg Am. 1966;48:440–56.
150. Fodor L, Ullmann Y, Choudry M, Calif E, Lerner A. Prophylactic external fixation and extensive debridement for chronic osteomyelitis. Acta Orthop Belg. 2006;72:448–53.
151. Cherny G III, Fitzgerald RH. Adult osteomyelitis and septic arthritis. In: Fitzgerlad RH, Kaufer H, Malkani AL, editors. Orthopedic. St Louis: Mosby; 2002. p. 718–27.
152. Khaled A, El-Gabay O, EL-Rosasy M, et al. Masquelet- Illizarov technique for the treatment of bone loss post debridement of infected tibia non-union. Int Orthop. 2022;46:1937–44.

# 11 Fungal Infections in Orthopedics

Yazan Kadkoy, Claire Park, Joseph A. Ippolito, and Joseph Benevenia

## 11.1 Diagnosis

### 11.1.1 History and Physical

Diagnosis of FOAI can be difficult given the variety of different presentations. Most common symptoms include pain, swelling, erythema, and may progress to sinus tract. Fever can be present, but is found to only to occur in 31% of patients with candida osteomyelitis [1]. Such infections typically present like bacterial infections, as well as occur in conjunction with bacterial infections, although FOAI is often more subacute and progresses more indolently [3]. A careful history should be acquired noting any recent procedures, surgical manipulation, or traumas. Patient history of antibiotic use, chemotherapy, and immune-modulating medications should point to the possibility that an infection could be fungal in origin [4].

### 11.1.2 Labs

Labs for FOAI typically involve inflammatory markers such as erythrocyte sedimentation rate (ESR), C-reactive protein (CRP), along with standard complete blood count and differential. In a large systematic review of candida osteomyelitis, these markers were shown to be variable and only mildly elevated with an average WBC of 900–3600 cells/mm^3 with 73% neutrophils. Median ESR and CRP were found to be 65 mm/h and 8.8 mg/dl, respectively. For fungal periprosthetic joint infections (FPJI), laboratory cutoffs for diagnosis of infection follow the Musculoskeletal Infection Society (MSIS) criteria [2]. Tests like CRP, while helpful in the setting of more virulent bacteria, can show lower values for yeast with false positive rates as high as 50%, stressing the importance of clinical judgment when treating patients suspected of having a fungal infection [5]. Although they are present more sporadically, certain endemic mycoses can be tested for in the serum. Coccidioides can be tested with a serum antibody test and Cryptococcus can be tested with serum cryptococcal antigen. Additionally, both Histoplasma and Sporothrix can be tested utilizing enzyme-linked immunosorbent assay (ELISA) and polymerase chain reaction (PCR) [6].

### 11.1.3 Synovial Fluid

If a fungal infection is suspected in a joint space, the joint should undergo aspiration. For FPJI again, MSIS criteria denote WBC > 3000 cells/

Y. Kadkoy (✉) · C. Park · J. A. Ippolito · J. Benevenia
Department of Orthopaedic Surgery, Rutgers New Jersey Medical School, Newark, NJ, USA
e-mail: Yk399@gsbs.rutgers.edu; cp906@njms.rutgers.edu; ippolija@njms.rutgers.edu; benevejo@njms.rutgers.edu


P. Ruggieri et al. (eds.), *Bone and Joint Infections*, https://doi.org/10.1007/978-3-031-96383-4_11

mL and PMN % > 80 as suggestive of chronic PJI [7]. While these numbers are widely accepted in the total joints' literature for the diagnosis of PJI, there is little evidence to validate these cutoffs in the setting of FPJI. Additionally, data on the efficacy of alpha-defensin for detecting fungal infection is limited. With a sample size of six isolated yeast infections, no differences in alpha defensin levels were detected when compared to more virulent bacteria [8]. A case series by Zhang et al. utilized metagenomic next-generation sequencing (mNGS) to help aid in the diagnosis of FPJI when cultures were negative for growth. Twelve cases in the series were tested with mNGS and results correlated with cultures for six patients and revealed fungal infections in five patients who were culture negative. Additionally, mNGS was able to aid in ruling out bacterial contaminants in one patient [9].

### 11.1.4 Culture

Culturing of fungi can be challenging with up to 46% of fungal PJI being culture negative [10]. In the case of osteomyelitis, direct culturing is the mainstay for diagnosis. The difficulty with fungal cultures pertains to both isolation of the organism as well as lead time for growth. Although cultures can show growth at around 1–2 weeks, Assessment for growth should be allowed to culture for 4–6 weeks [11]. This growth can be improved by collecting cultures in blood culture bottles, which decreased the inhibitory effects of antibiotics or inflammatory mediators [12].

### 11.1.5 Histopathology

Frozen sections have been proven effective for the diagnosis of bacterial PJI but are less effective for fungi. Affected patient populations are typically immunocompromised and have a weaker response. In the chronic phase of infection, granuloma formation is the only histologic hallmark with polymorphonuclear leukocyte numbers remaining stagnant [13]. In a case series by Miller et al., histopathology was only able to detect organisms in 1 of 23 cases [3].

### 11.1.6 Imaging

Imaging can be useful in assessing FOAI, with the most common finding being bone destruction. MRI can show decreased signal on T1-weighted imaging and increased signal on T2-weighted images. MRI can also be useful for assessing soft tissue extension of infection. Other radiographic findings of infection like periosteal reaction and technician nuclear scan uptake are less prevalent with FOAI occurring in around 7% and 23%, respectively [1].

## 11.2 Risk Factors

A precise list of risk factors for FOAI and FPJI is not currently agreed on. Most listed risk factors in the literature include immunosuppression from medication or disease, use of broad-spectrum antibiotics, prior surgeries, and parenteral hyperalimentation, among others [14, 15]. FPJI has also been associated with prolonged antibiotic use and prior revision for bacterial PJI [16–18].

## 11.3 Common Species

Candida species is by far the most common pathogen implicated in FOAI and is best described in the literature. This species is a natural part of the skin flora and has been well documented to cause infection in both IV drug users as well as patients receiving total parenteral nutrition. Infection is spread hematogenously in 70% of cases and clinical presentation typically is more indolent, taking weeks to become apparent [19]. Antifungal regimen for this pathogen is regularly selected based on sensitivities, with fluconazole most commonly reported [20]. This species, like many fungi produces a robust biofilm that can make medical treatment alone difficult, essentially around implants [21]. Echinocandins have shown promise in combating biofilm through their noncompetitive inhibition of 1,3-β-glucan synthesis with one study, and showed micafungin was able to reduce biofilm by 80% at a concentration of 4 μg/ml [22]. The literature on FPJI lists *C. Albicans* and *C. Parapsilosis* as the most common causative organism appearing in upto 49% and 27% of FPJI, respectively [17]. A case series of 29 patients by Karczewski et al. showed worse implant survival for candida PJI when compared to non-candida PJI with 26.7% infection-free survival vs. 72.41%, respectively [23].

Aspergillus species, namely *A. Fumigatus* and *A. Flavus*, represent a minority of fungal infections, but are often more virulent causing focal infections in immunocompromised patients. These infections can start in the pulmonary system and spread to nearby locations, especially in the pediatric population. Medical treatment of this organism most often involves the use of voriconazole and itraconazole, which have particularly high penetration in bone, with levels of the drug reaching around five times higher concentration in bone from plasma [24].

Cryptococcus species have been implicated in osteomyelitis and PJI, although rarely. This fungus often affects immunosuppressed patients, as seen in transplant recipients and those with HIV/AIDS [25]. Infection in bone can be the result of disseminated infection or primary infection in bone. Musculoskeletal involvement is most commonly seen in the skull and lower extremities. Patients can present with constitutional symptoms and elevated inflammatory markers. Imaging most commonly demonstrates multiple areas of sclerosis and periosteal reaction [26]. Treatment recommendations involve fluconazole for 6–12 months for patients with mild or asymptomatic disease and amphotericin B + 5-flucytosine for disseminated disease [27].

Endemic Dimorphic fungi represent a small subset of FOAI, usually tied to a geographic niche. These fungi usually do not cause systemic symptoms, but when they do can affect the musculoskeletal system. The farthest-reaching of these fungi is Sporothrix. This fungus is primarily limited to the skin, with bone being the second most common location. Lesions can be multiple if spread hematogenously or isolated in contiguous spread. Imaging can show nodular granulomas or large cavitary lesions like a bacterial infection [28]. Disseminated coccidiomycosis has been documented to involve bone, occurring in almost 60% of patients. Lesions are typically multifocal and involve axial skeleton [29]. Blastomyces infection in bone most commonly affects the lower extremity and axial skeleton. These lesions can occur with or without pulmonary symptoms and are often confused with a potential neoplasm [30]. For many of these dimorphic fungi, treatment involves treatment with an azole (fluconazole or itraconazole) for 12 months, with the addition of amphotericin B for 2–6 weeks for severe infections, along with surgical debridement.

## 11.4 Types of Infection

### 11.4.1 Soft Tissue

Although many fungal infections spread hematogenously, the spread from bone to soft tissue and vice versa is evident in the literature. Gamalestou et al. found a 23% incidence of soft tissue extension in patients with candida osteomyelitis [1]. Likewise, in the hand literature, deep fungal infections present a challenging problem to solve that is associated with significant morbidity and mortality for immunocompromised patients. Aspergillosis infection of the hand has been described in immunocompromised patients. Infections start off as small vesicles or necrotic lesions but can quickly spread into the surrounding tissue and the flexor compartment. Treatment here involves early diagnosis by biopsy and repeated debridement. Newer generation azoles, like voriconazole, can be helpful in treating these infections [31].

### 11.4.2 Bone

In the case of candida osteomyelitis, Gamaletsou et al. analyzed over 207 cases of candida osteomyelitis in both adults and children. They concluded that much like bacterial osteomyelitis, the axial skeleton is frequently involved in adults, and patients often have infection in multiple sites. The most infected location in adults was the lumbar vertebrae in adults. For the pediatric population, the femur and humerus were most commonly involved. Additionally, pediatric fungal osteomyelitis typically affects the metaphysis of bone, compared to adults, where the epiphysis is commonly implicated.

In the same review by Gamaletsou et al., treatment response for fungal osteomyelitis varied. Most patients were treated with antifungal and surgical intervention (48%), with antifungal agents only following as a close second (44%). Here, there were no differences found between what antifungal agents were used; however, in practice, this decision should be tailored to the causative pathogen. Treatment duration averaged around 90 days and was successfully treated in around 32%, with a partial response in 59% and failure in 7% of patients [1].

### 11.4.3 Joint

Like many of the other fungal infections, fungal septic arthritis is most commonly associated with Candida species. These infections can be seen in healthy patients but are most often associated with immunosuppression. The majority of patients will present with acute constitutional symptoms and effusion similar to bacterial septic arthritis, but over 30% of patients will have a more indolent course, which can be mistaken for progression of arthritis [32]. Treatment involves early detection, systemic antifungal, and repeated drainage.

### 11.4.4 Periprosthetic

FPJI represents 1% of all PJI diagnoses. This rare infection can have devastating consequences with significant morbidity and mortality for patients. Risk factors include revision total joint surgery and antibiotic use. Treatment can be difficult due to the robust biofilm fungi produced around implants. FPJI can involve a coinfection with bacterial pathogens. These coinfections are often difficult to treat and require multiple staged procedures to treat. From the literature, most surgical interventions start with resection of all implants and irrigation and debridement (Fig. 11.1).

Debridement, antibiotics, and implant retention (DAIR) has been used to treat acute bacterial PJI with moderate success for infections diag-

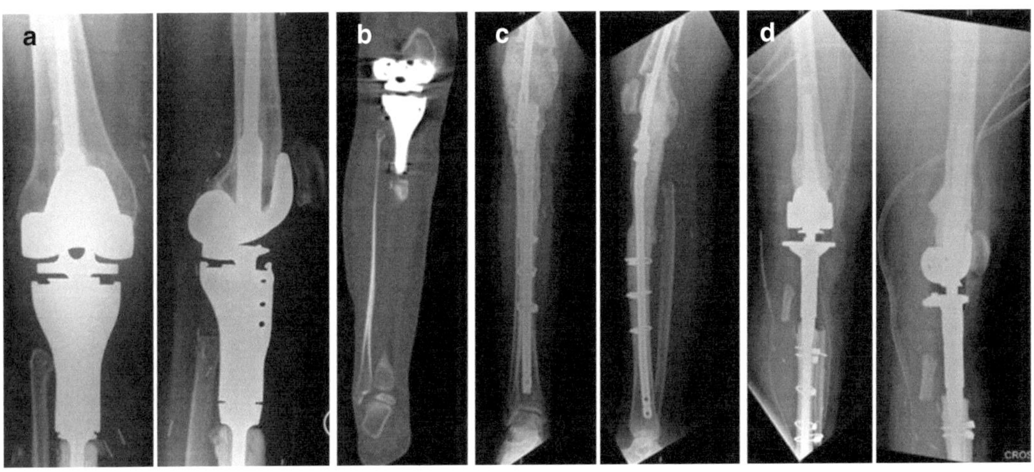

**Fig. 11.1** (**a**) Radiographs of a patient with the history of proximal tibia sarcoma treated with hinged proximal tibia replacement. (**b**) Patient was found to have a fluid collection around the device, which was cultured and grew *C. Parapsilosis*. (**c**) Patient underwent explant and antibiotic and antifungal spacer. (**d**) Patient underwent reconstruction with a hinged mega prosthesis and a vascularized fibular graft

nosed less than 4 weeks postoperatively [33]. Several case series have shown little efficacy with this treatment for FPJI. Rates are even lower for patients treated with DAIR in the setting of coinfections [34]. Success rates for infection eradication with FPJI ranged from 0 to 28% [18, 34–38]. This could be because of the biofilm produced by bacteria, as well as the time frame of infection. Because fungal infections typically move slower than bacterial infections and they are so rare, FPJI is usually diagnosed late. Large series have shown low success rates with this type of surgical intervention, and most patients go on to have staged procedures.

One-stage revision has become increasingly popular. Some studies have used this approach for FPJI with success, although these samples are small in the literature. Ji et al. retrospectively analyzed a cohort of 11 patients, all treated with one-stage revision for FPJI. Of the 11 patients, five had a history of bacterial PJI and 7 had an overall satisfactory result with no need for further operation. The study covered both bacterial and fungal pathogens, both at the site of infection as well as systemically. The investigators also treated patients with intra-articular injections of fluconazole every 12 h for 15 days [39]. Klatte et al. retrospectively analyzed 14 patients treated with one-stage revision for FPJI. Four patients in the study were excluded. Successful eradication of infection was achieved in 9 patients, with 1 patient becoming reinfected. The benefit of this approach is the lack of a second procedure, which allows patients to avoid the risk associated with additional surgery and begin an earlier range of motion. The key step for success with this approach involves extensive debridement of all necrotic tissue, bone, and residual cement. When supported by reliable cultures and sensitivity, this method shows promise, but larger studies do not exist in the literature.

Two-stage revisions are still the gold standard for the treatment of PJI. The staged procedure uses a cement spacer that can be loaded with both antibacterial and antifungal agents. The elution of these antifungal agents is debated, and their efficacy has not been fully tested. One study found less than 0.03% elution of Amphotericin B from polymethylmethacrylate(PMMA) cement after 1 week [40]. Similar results are present between studies regardless of whether antifungal-loaded cement was used. In fact, because many FPJIs have a bacterial component, many studies incorporated both antifungal and antibacterial agents into their PMMA cement [4, 38, 39, 41]. Success rates defined as successful eradication of infection vary greatly between studies, ranging from 38 to 100%, depending on patient demographics and the incidence of bacterial coinfection [9, 36, 42–44].

Although studies have described patients receiving multiple staged procedures either for persistent or recurrent infection, the largest study reporting outcomes for a three-stage revision arthroplasty was by Baeker et al. In this case series of only 18 patients, 39% of patients had a bacterial coinfection. The first stage of the procedure involved the removal of all implants and the placement of an antifungal and antibacterial-loaded cement spacer. This spacer was then exchanged for another cement spacer before the patient's new device was reimplanted. Patients were treated systemically with medication tailored to the latest cultures taken at each stage. Time between explant and reimplantation was 6 weeks, the same as the recommended 2-week interval for two-stage revisions. The study found an 88.8% infection eradication rate with three patients receiving arthrodesis and two receiving a girdle stone [41].

Fungal infections in orthopedics continue to be a difficult problem to diagnose and treat. It is important to recognize risk factors for these types of infections early and test accordingly. It is also important to realize that by the time these infections present, they may have been present for some time. Early recognition and a multidisciplinary approach are helpful for ensuring the best outcomes for patients.

## References


1. Gamaletsou MN, Kontoyiannis DP, Sipsas NV, Moriyama B, Alexander E, Roilides E, et al. Candida osteomyelitis: analysis of 207 pediatric and adult cases (1970–2011). Clin Infect Dis. 2012;55(10):1338–51.
2. Nace J, Siddiqi A, Talmo CT, Chen AF. Diagnosis and management of fungal periprosthetic joint infections. J Am Acad Orthop Surg. 2019;27(18):e804–e18.
3. Miller AO, Gamaletsou MN, Henry MW, Al-Hafez L, Hussain K, Sipsas NV, et al. Successful treatment of Candida osteoarticular infections with limited duration of antifungal therapy and orthopedic surgical intervention. Infect Dis (Lond). 2015;47(3):144–9.
4. Kuiper JW, van den Bekerom MP, van der Stappen J, Nolte PA, Colen S. 2-stage revision recommended for treatment of fungal hip and knee prosthetic joint infections. Acta Orthop. 2013;84(6):517–23.
5. Deirmengian CA, Citrano PA, Gulati S, Kazarian ER, Stave JW, Kardos KW. The C-reactive protein may not detect infections caused by less-virulent organisms. J Arthroplast. 2016;31(9, Supplement):152–5.
6. Kohli R, Hadley S. Fungal arthritis and osteomyelitis. Infect Dis Clin N Am. 2005;19(4):831–51.
7. Higuera CA, Zmistowski B, Malcom T, Barsoum WK, Sporer SM, Mommsen P, et al. Synovial fluid cell count for diagnosis of chronic periprosthetic hip infection. J Bone Joint Surg Am. 2017;99(9):753–9.
8. Deirmengian C, Kardos K, Kilmartin P, Gulati S, Citrano P, Booth RE. The alpha-defensin test for periprosthetic joint infection responds to a wide spectrum of organisms. Clin Orthop Relat Res. 2015;473(7):2229–35.
9. Zhang C, Lin Y, Huang C, Huang Z, Fang X, Bai G, et al. Metagenomic next-generation sequencing assists the diagnosis treatment of fungal osteoarticular infections. Front Cell Infect Microbiol. 2022;12:1072539.
10. Yoon HK, Cho SH, Lee DY, Kang BH, Lee SH, Moon DG, et al. A review of the literature on culture-negative periprosthetic joint infection: epidemiology, diagnosis and treatment. Knee Surg Relat Res. 2017;29(3):155–64.
11. Perfect JR, Dismukes WE, Dromer F, Goldman DL, Graybill JR, Hamill RJ, et al. Clinical practice guidelines for the management of cryptococcal disease: 2010 update by the infectious diseases society of America. Clin Infect Dis. 2010;50(3):291–322.
12. She RC, Romney MG, Jang W, Walker T, Karichu JK, Richter SS. Performance of the BacT/Alert Virtuo Microbial Detection System for the culture of sterile body fluids: prospective multicentre study. Clin Microbiol Infect. 2018;24(9):992–6.
13. Geng L, Xu M, Yu L, Li J, Zhou Y, Wang Y, Chen J. Risk factors and the clinical and surgical features of fungal prosthetic joint infections: a retrospective analysis of eight cases. Exp Ther Med. 2016;12(2):991–9.
14. Pappas PG, Kauffman CA, Andes DR, Clancy CJ, Marr KA, Ostrosky-Zeichner L, et al. Clinical practice guideline for the management of candidiasis: 2016 update by the infectious diseases society of America. Clin Infect Dis. 2016;62(4):e1–50.
15. Jakobs O, Schoof B, Klatte TO, Schmidl S, Fensky F, Guenther D, et al. Fungal periprosthetic joint infection in total knee arthroplasty: a systematic review. Orthop Rev (Pavia). 2015;7(1):5623.
16. Phelan DM, Osmon DR, Keating MR, Hanssen AD. Delayed reimplantation arthroplasty for candidal prosthetic joint infection: a report of 4 cases and review of the literature. Clin Infect Dis. 2002;34(7):930–8.
17. Sambri A, Zunarelli R, Fiore M, Bortoli M, Paolucci A, Filippini M, et al. Epidemiology of fungal periprosthetic joint infection: a systematic review of the literature. Microorganisms. 2022;11(1):84.
18. Azzam K, Parvizi J, Jungkind D, Hanssen A, Fehring T, Springer B, et al. Microbiological, clinical, and surgical features of fungal prosthetic joint infections: a multi-institutional experience. J Bone Joint Surg Am. 2009;91(Suppl 6):142–9.
19. Wu M-H, Hsu K-Y. Candidal arthritis in revision knee arthroplasty successfully treated with sequential parenteral-oral fluconazole and amphotericin B-loaded cement spacer. Knee Surg Sports Traumatol Arthrosc. 2011;19(2):273–6.
20. Henry MW, Miller AO. Management of fungal osteoarticular infections. Curr Fungal Infect Rep. 2023;17(1):25–35.
21. Pereira R, dos Santos Fontenelle RO, de Brito EHS, de Morais SM. Biofilm of Candida albicans: formation, regulation and resistance. J Appl Microbiol. 2021;131(1):11–22.
22. Guembe M, Guinea J, Marcos-Zambrano LJ, Fernández-Cruz A, Peláez T, Muñoz P, Bouza E. Micafungin at physiological serum concentrations shows antifungal activity against Candida albicans and Candida parapsilosis biofilms. Antimicrob Agents Chemother. 2014;58(9):5581–4.
23. Karczewski D, Ren Y, Andronic O, Akgun D, Perka C, Muller M, Kienzle A. Candida periprosthetic joint infections – risk factors and outcome between albicans and non-albicans strains. Int Orthop. 2022;46(3):449–56.
24. Felton T, Troke PF, Hope WW. Tissue penetration of antifungal agents. Clin Microbiol Rev. 2014;27(1):68–88.
25. Shah NB, Shoham S, Nayak S. Cryptococcus neoformans prosthetic joint infection: case report and review of the literature. Mycopathologia. 2015;179(3):275–8.
26. Zhou HX, Lu L, Chu T, Wang T, Cao D, Li F, et al. Skeletal cryptococcosis from 1977 to 2013. Front Microbiol. 2014;5:740.
27. Baddley JW, Forrest GN, Practice tAIDCo. Cryptococcosis in solid organ transplantation—guidelines from the American Society of Transplantation

Infectious Diseases Community of Practice. Clin Transpl. 2019;33(9):e13543.
28. Barros MB, de Almeida PR, Schubach AO. Sporothrix schenckii and Sporotrichosis. Clin Microbiol Rev. 2011;24(4):633–54.
29. Taljanovic MS, Adam RD. Musculoskeletal coccidioidomycosis. Semin Musculoskelet Radiol. 2011;15(05):511–26.
30. Jain R, Singh K, Lamzabi I, Harbhajanka A, Gattuso P, Reddy VB. Blastomycosis of bone: a clinicopathologic study. Am J Clin Pathol. 2014;142(5):609–16.
31. Amirtharajah M, Lattanza L. Fungal infections of the hand. Curr Orthop Pract. 2010;21(6):564–7.
32. Cuellar ML, Silveira LH, Espinoza LR. Fungal arthritis. Ann Rheum Dis. 1992;51(5):690.
33. Qasim SN, Swann A, Ashford R. The DAIR (debridement, antibiotics and implant retention) procedure for infected total knee replacement – a literature review. SICOT J. 2017;3:2.
34. Sidhu MS, Cooper G, Jenkins N, Jeys L, Parry M, Stevenson JD. Prosthetic fungal infections: poor prognosis with bacterial co-infection. Bone Joint J. 2019;101-B(5):582–8.
35. Escolà-Vergé L, Rodríguez-Pardo D, Lora-Tamayo J, Morata L, Murillo O, Vilchez H, et al. Candida periprosthetic joint infection: a rare and difficult-to-treat infection. J Infect. 2018;77(2):151–7.
36. Hwang BH, Yoon JY, Nam CH, Jung KA, Lee SC, Han CD, Moon SH. Fungal peri-prosthetic joint infection after primary total knee replacement. J Bone Joint Surg Br. 2012;94(5):656–9.
37. Kuo FC, Goswami K, Shohat N, Blevins K, Rondon AJ, Parvizi J. Two-stage exchange arthroplasty is a favorable treatment option upon diagnosis of a fungal periprosthetic joint infection. J Arthroplast. 2018;33(11):3555–60.
38. Yang HY, Shin HH, Kim JW, Seon JK. The fate of fungal periprosthetic joint infection after total knee arthroplasty. Int Orthop. 2023;47(11):2727–35.
39. Ji B, Zhang X, Xu B, Guo W, Mu W, Cao L. Single-stage revision for chronic fungal periprosthetic joint infection: an average of 5 years of follow-up. J Arthroplast. 2017;32(8):2523–30.
40. Goss B, Lutton C, Weinrauch P, Jabur M, Gillett G, Crawford R. Elution and mechanical properties of antifungal bone cement. J Arthroplast. 2007;22(6):902–8.
41. Baecker H, Frieler S, Gessmann J, Pauly S, Schildhauer TA, Hanusrichter Y. Three-stage revision arthroplasty for the treatment of fungal periprosthetic joint infection: outcome analysis of a novel treatment algorithm : a prospective study. Bone Jt Open. 2021;2(8):671–8.
42. Theil C, Schmidt-Braekling T, Gosheger G, Idelevich EA, Moellenbeck B, Dieckmann R. Fungal prosthetic joint infection in total hip or knee arthroplasty: a retrospective single-centre study of 26 cases. Bone Joint J. 2019;101-B(5):589–95.
43. Saconi ES, de Carvalho VC, de Oliveira PRD, Lima A. Prosthetic joint infection due to Candida species: case series and review of literature. Medicine (Baltimore). 2020;99(15):e19735.
44. Anagnostakos K, Kelm J, Schmitt E, Jung J. Fungal periprosthetic hip and knee joint infections clinical experience with a 2-stage treatment protocol. J Arthroplast. 2012;27(2):293–8.

## Further Readings

Bariteau JT, Waryasz GR, McDonnell M, Fischer SA, Hayda RA, Born CT. Fungal osteomyelitis and septic arthritis. J Am Acad Orthop Surg. 2014;22(6):390–401.

Henry MW, Miller AO, Walsh TJ, Brause BD. Fungal musculoskeletal infections. Infect Dis Clin N Am. 2017;31(2):353–68.

Slenker AK, Keith SW, Horn DL. Two hundred and eleven cases of Candida osteomyelitis: 17 case reports and a review of the literature. Diagn Microbiol Infect Dis. 2012;73(1):89–93.

# Bone and Joint Infection in Immunocompromised Patients

# 12

Luísa Paganini Martins

## 12.1 What Is Immunodeficiency?

Immunodeficiency is the loss of one or several defense mechanisms and can happen due to a number of different factors. It is commonly divided between primary and secondary deficiencies. In this chapter, we will explore the most common causes for both primary and secondary deficiencies and go through the most common musculoskeletal infections they present with, based on the published literature.

## 12.2 What Are Primary Immunodeficiencies?

The primary immunodeficiencies are those genetically determined and may affect up to 1% of the population, in all its combined forms [1]. Some examples are the Autoimmune Lymphoproliferative Syndrome (ALPS), APS-1 (APECED), BENTA Disease, Caspase 8 Deficiency State (CEDS), Caspase Recruitment Domain-Containing Protein 9 (CARD9) deficiency and other syndromes of susceptibility to Candidiasis, Chronic Granulomatous Disease (CGD), Common Variable Immunodeficiency (CVID), Congenital Neutropenia Syndromes, Leukocyte Adhesion Deficiency (LAD), and Severe Combined Immunodeficiency (SCID). There are more than 450 primary immunodeficiencies, and they range from mild to severe, being detected in various stages of life.

One of the most severe forms, the SCID, is included in newborn screening in the United States [2].

## 12.3 What Are Secondary Immunodeficiencies?

Secondary immunodeficiencies occurs when the immune system is weakened by environmental factors [3]. They are the most prevalent cause of immune weakness, affecting millions of people annually. The most common exemples include Human Immunodeficiency Virus (HIV), various types of cancer, medications (notably chemotherapy schemes, radiation therapy, stem cell or organ transplants, and corticosteroid therapy), malnutrition [4], diabetes [5], and obesity [6].

Each of these deficiencies contributes to a higher incidence of infection overall, and a bigger number of publications can be found on more prevalent infections (i.e., pulmonary, skin, and urinary) than on skeletal disorders, given their more rare form.

L. P. Martins (✉)
Einstein Israelite Hospital, Sao Paulo, SP, Brazil



P. Ruggieri et al. (eds.), *Bone and Joint Infections*, https://doi.org/10.1007/978-3-031-96383-4_12

## 12.4 Musculoskeletal Infections and Primary Immunodeficiencies

Given the rarity of primary immunodeficiencies and their many forms, not many studies have been made linking them to musculoskeletal infections. However, it has been shown that joint complications are a well-recognized finding in these patients, many of those being infectious in etiology. Noninfectious abnormalities, similar to rheumatoid arthritis, have also been shown and demonstrated to be an underlying infectious trigger [10].

Bacterial organisms are the most common cause of infectious arthritis in humoral immunodeficiencies (such as common variable immunodeficiency and X-linked agammaglobulinemia), but mycoplasmas and ureaplasmas are also of particular importance. In non-humoral immunodeficiencies, noninfectious inflammatory arthritis is more prevalent [7]. In many cases, septic arthritis is the first sign of a primary immunodeficiency, and the growth of unusual organisms (such as *s. pneumoniae*) may be what triggers the care team to investigate further.

A 2016 review [8] shows that, in patients with primary immunodeficiencies, septic arthritis due to pyogenic bacteria or mycoplasmal arthritis is the most common osteoarticular manifestation. However, there are other uncommon manifestations, such as osteomyelitis, due to tuberculosis [9] (Fig. 12.1).

These patients have elevated rates of bone and joint infections, with and incidence of 33% of patients with TWEAK (TNF-like weak inducer of apoptosis) deficiency [12], 27% of patients with isolated IgG subclass deficiency [16], 10% of patients with Warts, Hypogammaglobulinemia, Infections, and Myelokathexis Syndrome (WHIM) and 1% in CD40 ligand deficiency [13] presenting with osteomyelitis in their lifetime. Eleven percent of the latter had aseptic arthritis, while 7% of patients with Activation-Induced Cytidine Deaminase (AICDA) deficiency had it as well [14, 15].

Keep in mind that the overall age and sex-adjusted annual incidence of osteomyelitis was 21.8 cases per 100,000 person-years, which adds up to 0.022% [17], and the incidence of septic arthritis incidence varies between 2 and 10 per 100,000 patient years in the United States and Western Europe [18], which corresponds to 0.002–0.01% of the population. The rates for immunodeficient patients are much higher, even if we consider the milder forms, with 1% rate of osteomyelitis.

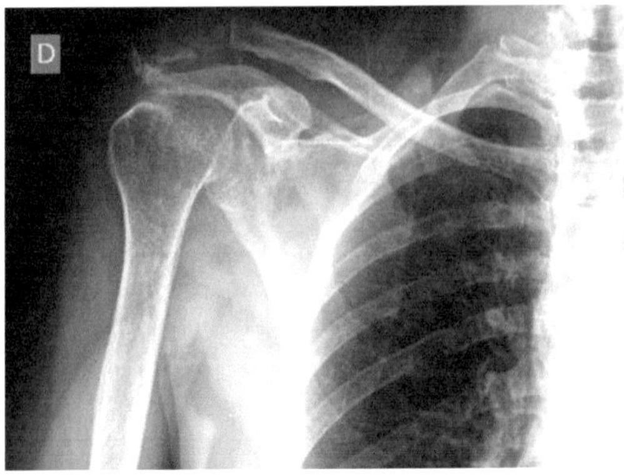


**Fig. 12.1** A 52-year-old female, HIV positive, presenting with lytic acromial lesion due to a tuberculosis infection. (Personal archive)

## 12.5 Musculoskeletal Infections and Secondary Immunodeficiencies

When talking about secondary immunodeficiencies, the most recent publications tend to focus on specific diseases/causes of immunodeficiency and their developments, rather than musculoskeletal diseases and their underlying causes. Such is the case with a number of papers on HIV and infections [19–22], on oncological patients [23], and hematologic malignancies [24]. There has also been a lot more focus on the relation between obesity and increased infection rates, especially after joint replacements [25–30], as well as the role of diabetes as a key factor [31–34].

Recent papers show, for instance, that 24% of patients admitted due to musculoskeletal infections have diabetes, which amounts to twice as many as the general adult hospitalized patients [31].

Obesity, in turn, is associated with a twofold increased risk of surgical site infections in orthopedics, as shown in a 2013 meta-analysis [25]. In a study with almost 20,000 patients, BMI > 40 was directly associated with increased infection risk on both total knee and total hip arthroplasties [28].

Studies trying to determine whether or not there is a BMI-threshold are inconclusive until now, but *Parvizi* et al. have demonstrated that, for each 2 unit decrease in BMI, chance of infection within 90 days of surgery dropped by 10% [29].

Type 2 diabetes is considered a global problem, affecting an estimated 8.5% of the world's population in 2014. From 1980 to 2014, there was a fourfold increase in its numbers (108–422 million), according to the World Health Organization.

Overweight and obesity, in turn, have tripled since 1975. There were an estimated 1.9 billion overweight people in 2022, accounting for 43% of the population being overweight, and 16% clinically obese [35]. With an increased growth of type 2 diabetes and obesity in the general population, orthopedic infections tend to rise in the upcoming years as well, presenting yet another challenge for orthopedic surgeons worldwide. With the expected increase in incidence, it is urgent that more studies are done on the subject, so we can obtain clearer results in terms of risk factors, as well as better protocols for avoiding them.

Another big cause of immunodeficiency is HIV, which is commonly overlooked as a disease of the past, but remains highly prevalent in African countries, and has had recent increases in infection rates globally. It is estimated to affect 39.9 million patients at the end of 2023, and infects another 1.3 million people every year [36]. Six hundred and thirty thousand people have died from HIV-related diseases in 2023.

A small study performed in 1995 studied HIV patients with both closed and open fractures, showing an astonishing rate of 72% infection after open fractures, and 28% rate of mal union. In spite of the high numbers, the infections presented with usual organisms (non MRSA), and were treated conventionally, without further complications [19].

A more recent paper on the subject, published in 2011 [21], cites rates of up to 30% musculoskeletal infection in HIV patients in Thailand, but varying greatly, with a 0% rate reported in the United States, 0.34% in Italy, and 6.6% in Spain. This incidence has declined in recent years, with anti-retroviral drug therapy becoming increasingly more used.

Septic arthritis remains a leading cause of musculoskeletal manifestation of HIV in some centers. Bacterial and septic arthritis are more commonly caused by *S. Aureus* all over the world, with infections by *S epidermidis*, *H. influenzae*, *N. gonorrhea*, *N. meningitidis*, *Salmonella* spp., *S. pneumoniae*, *S. pyogenes*, *S sanguis*, *Bacteroides melaninogenicus*, *Burkholderia pseudomallei*, *and Pseudomonas* spp. also being reported, depending greatly on endemic bacteria for each region. For unknown reasons, the sacroiliac, sternocostal, and sternoclavicular joints are commonly more affected than usual, but hips and knees remain the main places of commitment. The presence of HIV does not seem to affect clinical presentation or treatment of these infections [21].

These numbers urge us to investigate further when apparently healthy individuals present with a spontaneous joint infection, with appropriate testing for uncommon organisms, as well as proper infectious triage for HIV.

## 12.6 Conclusion

Bacterial organisms are the most common cause of infectious arthritis in humoral immunodeficiencies

A 2016 review [8] shows that, in patients with primary immunodeficiencies, septic arthritis due to pyogenic bacteria or mycoplasmal arthritis is the most common osteoarticular manifestation.

In spite of the high numbers, the infections presented with usual organisms (non MRSA), and were treated conventionally, without further complications [19].

For unknown reasons, the sacroiliac, sternocostal, and sternoclavicular joints are commonly more affected than usual, but hips and knees remain the main places of commitment. The presence of HIV does not seem to affect clinical presentation or treatment of these infections [21].

From the data collected, we can also infer that the organisms causing these infections also tend to be common organisms, with a higher incidence of *S. aureus* than any other bacteria, and without an elevated incidence of drug-resistant bacteria so far. Thus, the regular antibiotic regimens tend to heal these infections when properly applied.

Special attention needs to be paid to postoperative patients presenting with any type of immunodeficiency, as oftentimes the clinical response to infection can be diminished, postponing the diagnosis and treatment of these complications. Active research for complications, such as frequent post-op visits and close monitoring of Reactive C-protein and ESR rates, seems to be the safer approach in high-risk patients.

Furthermore, additional measures can be taken to reduce post-op infections in more susceptible patients. Adequate pre-op skin preparation and antibiotic prophylaxis before the incision and up to 48 hours post-op should be scrutinously observed (as per international consensus on musculoskeletal infections). More recently, the role of negative-pressure wounds and their decrease in postoperatory infection has also been studied, with promising results [37–40]. Although this is a high-cost prevention strategy (at an estimated US$ 495 per use), the estimated cost reduction from infectious complications tends to be higher than the price paid for the utilization of such dressings, making this a cost-effective tactic [41].

Lastly, patients presenting with uncommon manifestations of musculoskeletal infections, such as opportunistic bacteria, fungi, or mycobacteria in cultures (either local or blood samples), uncommon age or site of infection or spontaneous septic arthritis should be thoroughly investigated for underlying causes of immunodeficiency, and properly treated for both the present infection and the factor leading up to it. The concomitant action of other medical specialties such as infection specialists, rheumatologists, and immunologists is of foremost importance in some cases, and should be seeked whenever possible.

## 12.7 Biography

**Protocols and Guidelines**

- Infectious Diseases Society of America (IDSA) Guidelines for the Diagnosis and Treatment of Bone and Joint Infections: https://www.idsociety.org/practice-guideline/bone-and-joint-infections/
- IDSA Guidelines for the Management of Asymptomatic Bacteriuria: https://www.idsociety.org/practice-guideline/asymptomatic-bacteriuria/
- American Academy of Orthopaedic Surgeons (AAOS) Clinical Practice Guideline on the Diagnosis of Periprosthetic Joint Infections of the Hip and Knee: https://www.aaos.org/globalassets/quality-and-practice-resources/pji-guideline-9-6-18.pdf
- IDSA Guidelines for the Prevention of Opportunistic Infections in HIV-Infected Adults and Adolescents: https://www.idsociety.org/practice-guideline/opportunistic-infections-prevention/

## References


1. Quinn J, Modell V, Orange JS, et al. Growth in diagnosis and treatment of primary immunodeficiency within the global Jeffrey Modell Centers Network. Allergy Asthma Clin Immunol. 2022;18:19. https://doi.org/10.1186/s13223-022-00662-6.
2. cdc.org.
3. https://www.aaaai.org/.
4. França T, Ishikawa L, Zorzella-Pezavento S, Chiuso-Minicucci F, da Cunha M, Sartori A. Impact of malnutrition on immunity and infection. J Venom Anim Toxins Incl Trop Dis. 2009;15(3):374–90. https://doi.org/10.1590/S1678-91992009000300003.
5. Berbudi A, Rahmadika N, Tjahjadi AI, Ruslami R. Type 2 diabetes and its impact on the immune system. Curr Diabetes Rev. 2020;16(5):442–9. https://doi.org/10.2174/1573399815666191024085838. PMID: 31657690; PMCID: PMC7475801
6. de Heredia FP, Gómez-Martínez S, Marcos A. Obesity, inflammation and the immune system. Proc Nutr Soc. 2012;71(2):332–8. https://doi.org/10.1017/S0029665112000092. Epub 2012 Mar 20. PMID: 22429824
7. Bloom KA, Chung D, Cunningham-Rundles C. Osteoarticular infectious complications in patients with primary immunodeficiencies. Curr

Opin Rheumatol. 2008;20(4):480–5. https://doi.org/10.1097/bor.0b013e3282fd6e70.
8. Gharib A, Gupta S. Skeletal and joint manifestations of primary immunodeficiency diseases. SOJ Immunol. 2016;4(1):1–13. https://doi.org/10.15226/2372-0948/4/1/00145.
9. Hugosson C, Harfi H. Disseminated BCG-osteomyelitis in congenital immunodeficiency. Pediatr Radiol. 1991;21(5):384–5.
10. Sordet C, Cantagrel A, Schaeverbeke T, Sibilia J. Bone and joint disease associated with primary immune deficiencies. Joint Bone Spine. 2005;72(6):503–14.
11. Akman IO, Ostrov BE, Neudorf S. Autoimmune manifestations of the Wiskott-Aldrich syndrome. Semin Arthritis Rheum. 1998;27(4):218–25.
12. Wang HY, Ma CA, Zhao Y, Fan X, Zhou Q, Edmonds P, et al. Antibody deficiency associated with an inherited autosomal dominant mutation in TWEAK. Proc Natl Acad Sci USA. 2013;110(13):5127–32. https://doi.org/10.1073/pnas.1221211110.
13. Winkelstein JA, Marino MC, Ochs H, Fuleihan R, Scholl PR, Geha R, et al. The X-linked hyper-IgM syndrome: clinical and immunologic features of 79 patients. Medicine (Baltimore). 2003;82(6):373–84.
14. Quartier P, Bustamante J, Sanal O, Plebani A, Debré M, Deville A, et al. Clinical, immunologic and genetic analysis of 29 patients with autosomal recessive hyper-IgM syndrome due to Activation-Induced Cytidine Deaminase deficiency. Clin Immunol. 2004;110(1):22–9.
15. Jimenez MJ, Steele RW. Recurrent severe arthralgia. Clin Pediatr. 2013;52(9):882–5.
16. Castrignano SB, Carlsson B, Carneiro Sampaio MS, Söderström T, Hanson LA. IgA and IgG subclass deficiency in a poor population in a developing country. Scand J Immunol. 1993;37(4):509–14.
17. Kremers HM, Nwojo ME, Ransom JE, Wood-Wentz CM, Melton LJ 3rd, Huddleston PM 3rd. Trends in the epidemiology of osteomyelitis: a population-based study, 1969 to 2009. J Bone Joint Surg Am. 2015;97(10):837–45. https://doi.org/10.2106/JBJS.N.01350. PMID: 25995495; PMCID: PMC4642868
18. Vassallo C, Borg AA, Farrugia D, Mercieca C. The epidemiology and outcomes of septic arthritis in the Maltese Islands: a hospital-based retrospective cohort study. Mediterr J Rheumatol. 2020;31(2):195–205. https://doi.org/10.31138/mjr.31.2.195. PMID: 32676557; PMCID: PMC7362118
19. Jellis JE. Viral infections: musculoskeletal infection in the human immunodeficiency virus (HIV) infected patient. Baillieres Clin Rheumatol. 1995; https://doi.org/10.1016/S0950-3579(05)80149-9.
20. Authier FJ, Gherardi RK. Complications musculaires de l'infection par le virus de l'immunodéficience humaine (VIH) à l'ère des trithérapies. Rev Neurol. 2005; https://doi.org/10.1016/S0035-3787(06)74984-0.
21. Pattamapaspong N, Louthrenoo W. Musculoskeletal infection in acquired immunodeficiency syndrome. Semin Musculoskelet Radiol. 2011; https://doi.org/10.1055/s-0031-1293499.
22. Steinbach LS, Tehranzadeh J, Fleckenstein JL, Vanarthos WJ, Pais MJ. Human immunodeficiency virus infection: musculoskeletal manifestations. Radiology. 1993; https://doi.org/10.1148/RADIOLOGY.186.3.8430195.
23. Emmanouilides C, Glaspy JA. Opportunistic infections in oncologic patients. Hematol Oncol Clin North Am. 1996; https://doi.org/10.1016/S0889-8588(05)70372-5. S-0031-1293499
24. Papanicolaou GA, Mehta J. Infections in patients with hematologic malignancies. 2010; https://doi.org/10.1007/978-1-60761-644-3_3.
25. Yuan K, Chen H-L. Obesity and surgical site infections risk in orthopedics: a meta-analysis. Int J Surg. 2013; https://doi.org/10.1016/J.IJSU.2013.02.018.
26. Zhongxi M, Fengjin G, Jun Q, Wei X, Jinming Z. Meta-analysis shows that obesity may be a significant risk factor for prosthetic joint infections. Int Orthop. 2016; https://doi.org/10.1007/S00264-015-2914-4.
27. O'Toole P, Maltenfort M, Chen AF, Parvizi J. Projected increase in periprosthetic joint infections secondary to rise in diabetes and obesity. J Arthroplasty. 2015; https://doi.org/10.1016/J.ARTH.2015.07.034.
28. Jung P, Morris AJ, Zhu M, Roberts SA, Frampton C, Young SW. BMI is a key risk factor for early periprosthetic joint infection following total hip and knee arthroplasty. N Z Med J. 2017;130(1461):24–34.
29. Shohat N, Fleischman AN, Tarabichi M, Tan TL, Parvizi J. Weighing in on body mass index and infection after total joint arthroplasty: is there evidence for a body mass index threshold? Clin Orthop Relat Res. 2018; https://doi.org/10.1007/S11999.0000000000000141.
30. Nocon AA, Henry MW, Russell C, Westrich GH, Brause BD, Miller A. The influence of obesity on the infection risk of prosthetic joint infection in the geriatric orthopedic population. Open Forum Infect Dis. 2017; https://doi.org/10.1093/OFID/OFX163.076.
31. Al-Mayahi MA-B, Cian A, Kressmann B, De Kalbermatten BA, Rohner P, Egloff M, Jafaar J, Malacarne S, Howard H, Uçkay MI. Associations of diabetes mellitus with orthopaedic infections. Infect Dis. 2015; https://doi.org/10.3109/23744235.2015.1082620.
32. La Fontaine J, Crisologo PA. Diabetes mellitus—infections and fracture healing. 2019. https://doi.org/10.1016/B978-0-12-820605-8.00006-1.
33. Judit K, Róbert M, Géza B. Treatment of musculoskeletal infections of the foot in patients with diabetes. Therapy. 2005; https://doi.org/10.1586/14750708.2.2.287.
34. Zhou K, Cecilia Lansang M. Diabetes mellitus and infections. In: Endotext. South Dartmouth: MDText.com, Inc; 2021.
35. WHO 2025: https://www.who.int/news-room/fact-sheets/detail/obesity-and-overweight.

36. WHO 2024: https://www.who.int/news-room/fact-sheets/detail/hiv-aids.
37. Higuera-Rueda C, Emara AK, Nieves-Malloure Y, et al. The Effectiveness of closed incision negative pressure therapy versus silver-impregnated dressings in mitigating surgical site complications in high-risk patients after revision knee arthroplasty: The PROMISES randomized controlled trial. J Arthroplast. 2021;36(7S):S295–S302.e14.
38. Newman JM, Siqueira MBP, Klika AK, et al. Use of closed incisional negative pressure wound therapy after revision total hip and knee arthroplasty in patients at high risk for infection: a prospective, randomized clinical trial. J Arthroplasty. 2019;34(3):554–9.
39. Manoharan V, Grant A, Harris A, et al. Closed incision negative pressure wound therapy vs conventional dry dressings after primary knee arthroplasty: a randomized controlled study. J Arthroplast. 2016;31(11):2487–94.
40. Pachowsky M, Gusinde J, Klein A, et al. Negative pressure wound therapy to prevent seromas and treat surgical incisions after total hip arthroplasty. Int Orthop. 2012;36(4):719–22.
41. Frisbie JJ, Bordoli SJ, Simmons JM, Zuiderveen SK. Utilizing closed incisional negative pressure therapy reduces peripheral bypass infection rates without increasing costs. Cureus. 2020;12(7):e9217. https://doi.org/10.7759/cureus.9217. PMID: 32821568; PMCID: PMC7430538

# Vertebral Osteomyelitis and Tuberculosis

13

Luisa Paganini Martin, Andrea Angelini, and Pietro Ruggieri

## 13.1 Vertebral Osteomyelitis

### 13.1.1 History

Osteomyelitis, mainly after a fracture, is a disease that has been described since Hippocrates (460–370 BC). Acute hematogenous osteomyelitis, in its term, was only much later described in 1773, by Bromfield, as bone that "may become carious, first in its internal parts and that from external injury, as well as from a vitiated state of the animal fluids." He called this an *abscessus in medulla*, and advised to drain the infected bone as soon as possible [1].

The first published paper on the theme dates back to 1948, already showing a massive difference in prognosis after the advent of penicillin, with deadly incidence reducing from 33% to 10% after 1940, although the treatment—both surgical and clinical—was still very erratic at the time [2]. Over 2000 years have passed since Hippocrates, some 250 since Bromfield and another 80 since penicillin started being used. The treatment basis for this disease remains mainly unaffected, with proper antibiotic therapy and mechanical debridement being the most important parts of it, to this day.

Vertebral osteomyelitis, in its turn, is rarer than its long bone counterpart, accounting for 1% of skeletal infections, a number which seems to be growing as IV drug users and age expectancy numbers rise [3]. It has been progressively better studied as both radiological and laboratory tests have gotten better, making it easier to diagnose and treat this condition.

### 13.1.2 Epidemiology

Most common studies show that vertebral osteomyelitis affects approximately 0,059/100.000 people, with 60% of those being male, with a mean age of 66 years [4]. Although it tends to present in older patients, there is a trend toward younger patients, which corresponds to IV drug users, with a mean age of 35 years [3]. In general, patients presenting with vertebral osteomyelitis have underlying diseases, reportedly more than one per patient. These were mainly diabetes mellitus (24%), intravenous drug abuse (11%), immunosuppression (7%), malignancy (6%), alcoholism (5%), and rheumatic disease (5%), with lower percentages in patients with liver cirrhosis, renal failure, and previous deficit of the vertebrae, such as radiation or osteopenic fracture. Other underlying medical illnesses, such as

L. P. Martin
Orthopedics and Rheumatology, Hospital Israelita Albert Einstein, Sao Paulo, Brazil

A. Angelini · P. Ruggieri (✉)
Department of Orthopedics and Orthopedic Oncology, University of Padova, Padova, Italy
e-mail: andrea.angelini@unipd.it; pietro.ruggieri@unipd.it


P. Ruggieri et al. (eds.), *Bone and Joint Infections*, https://doi.org/10.1007/978-3-031-96383-4_13

pulmonary fibrosis, heart conditions, malnutrition, myelodysplasia, sarcoidosis, septic phlebitis, or partial gastrectomy, occurred in 10% of the patients [3].

### 13.1.3 Pathophysiology

Vertebral osteomyelitis occurs mainly due to two mechanisms: direct inoculation or hematogenous seeding [5]. In half of the cases, arterial or venous conduits at the intervertebral disks or endplates allow bacteria to access the vertebral column. These areas have slower blood flow, which allows the bacteria to extend from the disk to the adjacent endplate, and vice versa.

Direct inoculation is another common method of bacterial colonization, and can occur after routine procedures such as lumbar puncture, discography, laminectomy, discectomy, or any other spinal intervention. Less commonly, bacterial inoculation occurs through local extension from adjacent areas of infection (3% of cases), including retropharyngeal abscesses or infected aortic grafts [6].

Staphylococcal infections (*S. aureus* and *S. epidermidis*) are the most common organisms found, with an incidence of 32–67%. Loibl et al. [7] noted worse outcomes in patients who had to be admitted to the ICU (58% vs. 34.7%). As for Gram-negative infections, Graham et al. [8] noted a 12.7% incidence of *Escherichia coli*, *Pseudomonas aeruginosa*, *Haemophilus influenzae,* and *Klebsiella pneumoniae*. Approximately 9% of cases will display a polymicrobial etiology [3]. Although positive cultures are helpful for targeted antibiotic therapy, Yoon and colleagues [9] noted similar outcomes, duration of treatment, and normalization of labs between culture-positive and culture-negative patients, as well as Lora-Tamayo et al. [10]. The latter noted a higher rate of sepsis, fevers, and elevated labs on culture-positive patients, indicating that positivity (as well as clinical symptoms) seems to be linked to a higher number of circulating bacteria.

### 13.1.4 Most Common Manifestations

Most patients present with back pain (85%), which can be acute (approximately 10 days) or chronic (up to 2 months), as well as fever in 60% of cases. In a large systematic review, with over a 1000 patients, 34% also had neurological symptoms, ranging from radiculopathy to urine retention, and even paralysis [3]. Neurological compromise tends to increase when diagnosis is delayed [10]. Concomitant infections (urinary tract infection, abscesses, skin infections, pneumonia, etc.) are relatively common, and are found in 47% of culture-positive and 4% of culture-negative Pyogenic Vertebral Osteomyelitis (PVO) [4]. That being said, it presents as back pain in older patients, predominantly male, with underlying diseases. Younger patients are most commonly IV drug users (Fig. 13.1). Diagnosis seems to be made earlier on patients presenting with either fever or neurological symptoms, as back pain alone can have a myriad of other diagnostic possibilities.

### 13.1.5 Diagnosis

Lumbar vertebrae seem to be more commonly involved (58%), followed by thoracic and cervical areas (30% and 11%, respectively). Three to fifteen percent of patients present with multiple level involvement [3]. In a study with IV drug users, those numbers change dramatically, with up to 68% of patients presenting with multiple levels of infection [11]. Routine laboratory analysis of complete blood count, erythrocyte sedimentation rate (ESR), and CRP is helpful in the infectious workup. Blood cultures can reveal the microbiological etiology in 58% of patients and should be obtained during febrile episodes if possible [3].

Bone biopsies, both CT-guided and open, result in a positive diagnosis in a mean of 77% (47–100%) of cases, while blood cultures yield a positive result in 58% of cases on average (ranging from 30% to 78%). We would recommend doing both, whenever possible. *S. aureus*

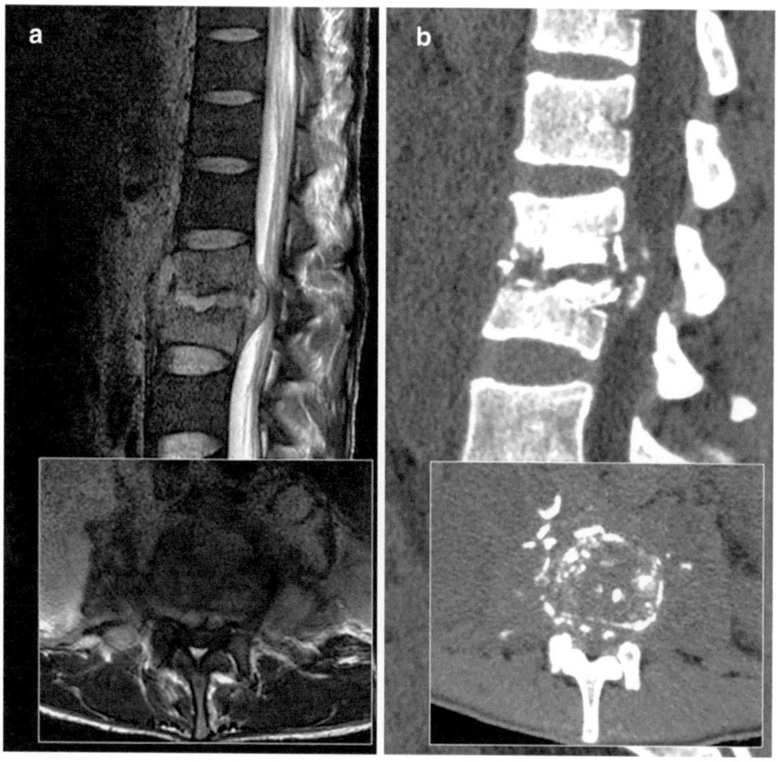


**Fig. 13.1** L2–L3 Spondylodiscitis in a young 46-year-old drug user. (**a**) MRI and (**b**) CT scan show extensive destructione of the disk and adjacent vertebral bodies

remains the most common organism, as with other forms of osteomyelitis, with an incidence of 32–67% in a major literature review. Streptococcus shows in second place in most studies, with an incidence of up to 23% [3]. Some studies seem to show a trend toward infection by Pseudomonas aeruginosa in IV drug users, accounting for up to 38% of cases in this particular population [11]. In 85% of the cases, a single organism was identified, with multiple organisms appearing in 9% [3].

### 13.1.6 Imaging Studies

Usually, the first exam to be performed are traditional x-rays (up to 95% of cases), and, although they take longer to show abnormalities, there were alterations on 89% of them [3]. Early findings (2–3 weeks) are commonly unremarkable and may only reveal endplate blurring, erosion of the endplate corners, disk height loss, and paraspinal soft-tissue swelling. Vertebral body destructive changes on x-ray are only seen after more than a third of the bone structure has been destroyed. Late vertebral osteomyelitis can demonstrate signs of bone formation including sclerosis, osteophytosis, and osteolytic lesions [12]. The high incidence of altered x-rays can be explained due to the fact that most diagnostics seem to be on a later stage, given that it usually presents only with back pain in older males with more than one comorbidity—a common symptom for this population. Bone scanning was performed in over half of the cases (58%), with a 94% positivity. CT scans and MRIs were not always performed (ranging from 0% to 100% in different studies), but showed positive findings in 94% of the cases [3], including specificities as to levels involved, epidural or vertebral abscesses, vertebral and disc destruction (Fig. 13.2). CT-guided biopsy can be a useful adjunct in the diagnosis. Recent studies demonstrate a CT-guided biopsy-positive culture rate of 19–60% in patients with suspected osteomyelitis [13–15]. Antibiotics before CT biopsy can significantly affect culture yields. De Lucas et al. [15] identified a causative organism in 60% of

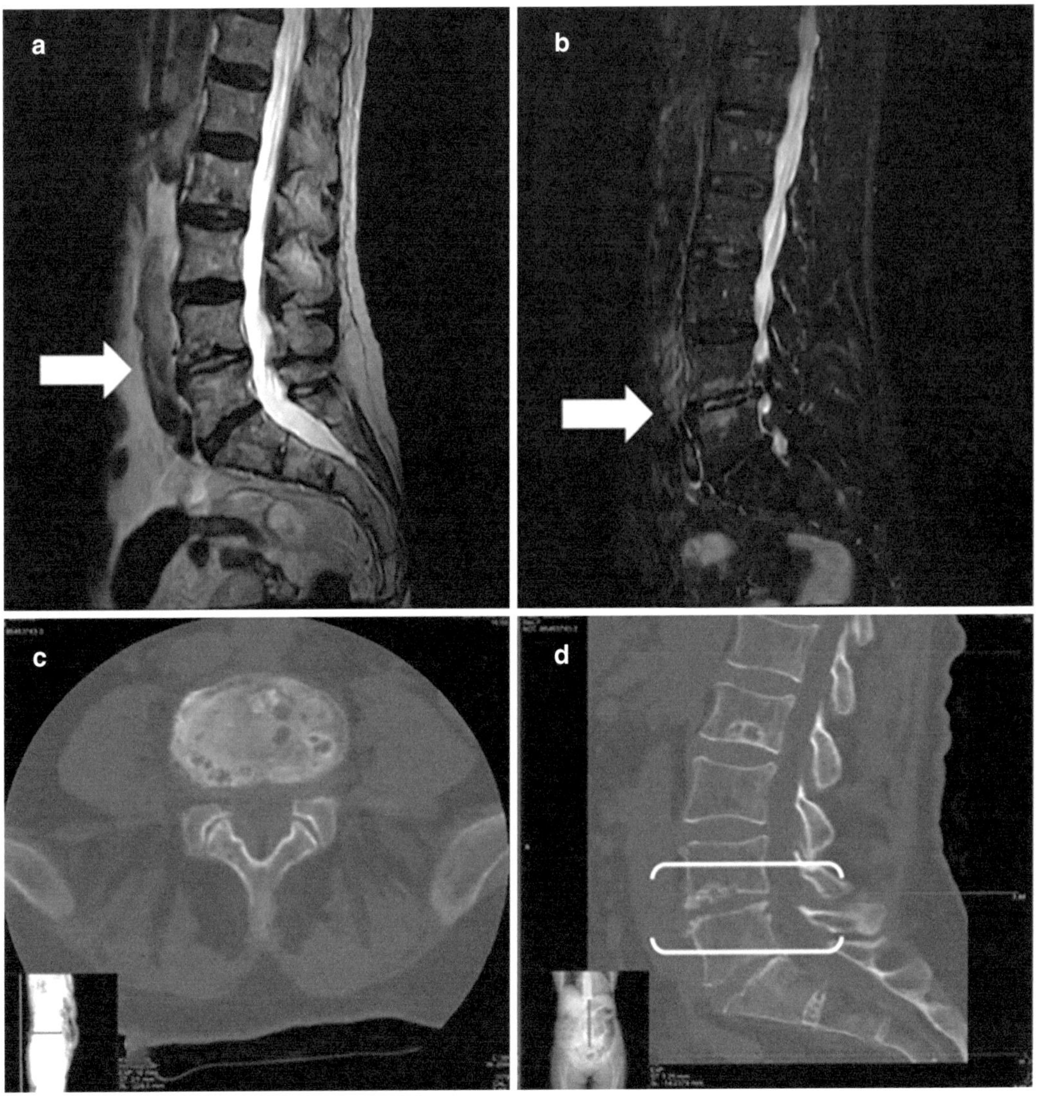


**Fig. 13.2** L4–L5 Spondylodiscitis in a 82-year-old male caused by *S. aureus* (white arrow) (**a**) MRI changes display low T1 signal intensity in affected disk and (**b**) high T2 in disk and adjacent vertebrae. (**c**) Axial CT shows disk degeneration; (**d**) Sagittal CT scan show lytic and sclerotic changes of the adjacent vertebral bodies

patients not previously treated with antibiotics, compared with 23% of patients who had received antibiotics. Early MRI changes display high T2 and low T1 signal intensity in affected disks and adjacent vertebrae. High T2 signal in the paraspinal soft tissues, with inflammation and edema visualized more clearly with fat saturation or short tau inversion recovery sequences, is also associated with early MRI changes. Contrast is often used to display the diffuse enhancement of the subchondral bone and disk. The early MRI findings of high T2 disk signal with disk height loss and contrast uptake within the disk are highly sensitive (70–100%) for diagnosis [3].

### 13.1.7 Treatment

Consultation with infectious disease specialists is useful for recommendations on duration of treatment, dosing, route, and antibiotic selection. Duration of treatment is controversial and ultimately is guided by individual clinical evaluation. Antibiotic therapy is done in all cases, worldwide, ever since the advent of penicillin. Today, as opposed to the 1950s, the drugs used are, when possible, guided by the positivity of organisms found and their respective antibiograms, with dose and drug delivery means being adjusted according to clinical response. Risk factors for failure of treatment were ESR > 55 mm/h and CRP > 2.75 after 4 weeks of antibiotic treatment [9]. There seem to be no significant changes in prognosis between 6 and 12 weeks of treatment, nor between less than or greater than 7 days of IV treatment [12]. Surgical treatment, on the other hand, has evolved a lot during the last years, mainly with minimally invasive approaches, better fixation methods, surgical planning and guided procedures, as well as substances for on-site use that can be bacteriostatic and/or have local antibiotic, enhancing direct drug delivery.

In patients treated nonoperatively, bracing for comfort and prevention of deformity is a reasonable treatment option, although there is no clinical evidence to support whether or not bracing affects outcome. Surgical management should be considered in patients who are refractory to antibiotic treatment or display neurological deficits, spinal instability, or progressive deformity with vertebral body destruction [16].

Approximately half of patients on a large systematic review [3] were subjected to surgical treatment (48%) as initial treatments for biopsies and cultures as well as for spinal stabilization and abscess drainage (23% and 21%), compression relief (13%), debridement, excision of sinuses, removal of infected hardware, resection of infected aneurysms, or grafts (2%). Correction of postinfection deformity is less common (2%), but is also cited [3]. In a study with over 800 cases, previous vertebral osteomyelitis resulted in hospital stays, blood loss, and fusion levels higher, but did not seem to affect any other aspect after 1 year post operation [17]. Although no definitive threshold for surgical management of PVO based on spinal instability or kyphotic deformity exists, Dietze et al. recommend using the following parameters to suggest spinal instability: vertebral body collapse >50%, >20 degrees of angulation, and >5 degrees of vertebral translation [6].

As to different approaches to the spine, an anterior approach affords a more complete debridement, but posterior approaches tend to be less morbid. Apart from debridement itself, which is consensus in the literature, much controversy exists as to the use of instrumentation, one vs two-step procedures, and allograft vs autograft use. Despite controversy, many studies suggest it is safe to use instrumentation in the surgical treatment of vertebral osteomyelitis. Bydon et al. [18] reported on 118 patients, noting similar rates of recurrent infection (8.3% for debridement and 9.8% for debridement with instrumentation) and reoperation (19.4% for debridement and 17.1% for debridement with instrumentation). The use of cages with bone graft placed into vertebral defects after debridement is a helpful adjunct in reconstruction. Robinson et al., Kuklo et al., and Sundara et al. [19–21] reported successful outcomes in small series of patients submitted to cage placement, with good outcomes after 36–44 months of follow-up. Bone grafting is commonly used in these cases to increase the rate and probability of fusion. Common autograft sources are tricortical iliac crest, rib, and fibular strut, as well as humeral and femoral struts after extensive debridement and/or corpectomy. Although allograft avoids the morbidity of donor site harvesting, autograft is theorized to have superior rates of incorporation. However, there is concern about introducing an allograft into the infected surgical field. Some small case series suggest a similar recurrence rate of infection and clinical outcomes when compared to autograft [12].

The mortality rate is low (6%), and most occur due to *S. aureus* septicemia, but the relapse percentage is about 32% [3]. Twenty-seven percent had life-quality affecting complications, in the same meta-analysis. Factors associated with an increased mortality include elevated C-reactive protein (CRP) at admission, advanced age, and a Charlson Comorbidity index of >2 [7]. The most common complications were persistent pain

(28%), motor weakness or paresis (16%), and bowel or bladder dysfunction (7%). Of 128 patients (from two different studies), the majority (80%) had a favorable outcome, while 20% had unaltered or deteriorated functional status [22, 23]. We have found only one study comparing functional outcome between nonsurgically and surgically treated patients, reporting that nonsurgical patients had a 64% chance of disabling pain or relapse, versus 26% of surgically treated patients [24].

## 13.2 Vertebral Tuberculosis

### 13.2.1 History

Tuberculous bacilli have lived among mankind for—arguably—as long as human beings have walked the earth. Proof of this is that there is Paleopathological evidence of tuberculosis of bones, joints, and spine in prehistoric humans [25]. The ancient texts of Rig Veda and the Atharva Veda (3500–1800 BC), in India, mention it by the name of "Yakshama" [26]. Spinal tuberculosis was first scientifically described in the Western world by Percivall Pott, in 1799, as "That kind of palsy of lower limbs which is frequently found to accompany a curvature of the spine" [27–29]. From then on, the actual bacilli were identified in 1870, and the use of the Bacilli Calmette Guerin (BCG) vaccine was introduced in 1945. The first antitubercular drugs appeared in 1948. In most developing countries, intradermal BCG vaccination is used for all newborns, and the protection afforded by it is about 80%. For healthcare students (such as myself a long time ago), immunity is checked, and we re-vaccinate the nonimmune in the first year of studies. The World Health Organization (WHO) has stated, in the 1990s, that tuberculosis should remain present in human populations as long as there are conditions that reduce innate immunology and cell-mediated immunity, such as malnutrition, poor sanitation, crowded living conditions, exanthematous fevers, repeated pregnancies, alcohol and substance abuse, diabetes, and advanced age [29–31].

### 13.2.2 Epidemiology

We have seen a recent increase in cases, particularly among the immunosuppressed population, secondary to a global migration phenomenon. WHO has reported a global increase in international migrants from 173 to 244 million between 2000 and 2015. There has also been an increased occurrence of multidrug-resistant bacterial strains of tuberculosis in developing countries [32]. The latest WHO report on tuberculosis (WHO, November 2023) estimates 40 million people treated for TB between 2018 and 2022, being the second cause of death from infectious disease in 2022 (behind COVID); 7.5 million were diagnosed in 2022 alone.

Spinal tuberculosis constitutes 50% of skeletal tubercular infections, and the incidence of extrapulmonary TB is about 3% [33]. That would amount to approximately 112,500 new cases of spinal TB diagnosed in 2022, worldwide.

### 13.2.3 Pathophysiology

Spinal TB is usually secondary to hematogenous spread from a primary site of infection, usually the lungs. The most common site is paradiscal, because the paradiscal vessels tend to supply the subchondral bone, on either side of the disc space. That also amounts to a common clinical characteristic, which is the tubercular infection "skipping" the discs and involving the vertebrae. As for the specific regions of the bone, it tends to include the vertebral body, the posterior structures, and form paravertebral abscesses. The progressive destruction of the bony structure leads to instability and deformity, most commonly in kyphosis [33].

### 13.2.4 Most Common Manifestations

As in pyogenic vertebral osteomyelitis, the patients typically present with back pain. The latter presentation involves deformity, instability, and neural deficit. The back pain is directly correlated to the disease's activity, its bone destruction, and consequent instability. The pain is present even while the patient is resting. Constitutional symptoms, including weight or appetite loss, fever, and fatigue, are less commonly present than in patients with pulmonary disease [34, 35]. The abscesses formed in the disease are called "cold," because they typically lack all the inflammatory signs that are more obvious in abscesses. They can present in the retropharyngeal space, anterior or posterior triangles of the neck or axilla when affecting the cervical spine (Fig. 13.3), as pre- or paravertebral abscesses in the thoracic spine, and may track down along the psoas muscle, Petit's triangle, Scarpa's triangle, or the gluteal region in lumbar cases [36].

As the greater part of cases involve the anterior portion of the spine, the most common deformity found is kyphosis, especially in the thoracic and thoracolumbar spine. Jain et al. observed that kyphotic deformity greater than 60 degrees leads to significant disability and can potentially inflict neurological déficits [37]. The neurological deficits can occur at the active stage of the disease, from direct compression from abscesses, instability, or sequestrum, or afterwards, secondary to mechanical traction or later [38].

The initial compression in tuberculosis involvement tends to be secondary to anterior vertebral body collapse [39], leading to anterior spinal tract involvement, which involves hyperreflexia of deep tendons, positive Babinski sign, (exaggerated deep tendon reflexes and Babinski sign), and progression to upper motor neuron syndrome. As the disease progresses, the lateral spinal tracts are progressively involved, with loss of crude touch, pain, and temperature, followed by posterior column deficit, with sphincter disturbances and complete sensory loss.

There are five classical stages of Pott paraplegia, as defined by the modified Tuli classification, as follows [40, 41]:

- *Stage 1:* Deficit only appears upon clinical examination: ankle clonus, exaggerated deep tendon reflexes, and Babinski or plantar extensor
- *Stage 2:* Patient has upper motor neuron-type of motor deficit, with spasticity; however, he/she remains ambulatory. The anticipated motor score in tetraparesis is 60–100, and in paraparesis the score is between 80 and 100; sensory deficit involves the lateral column

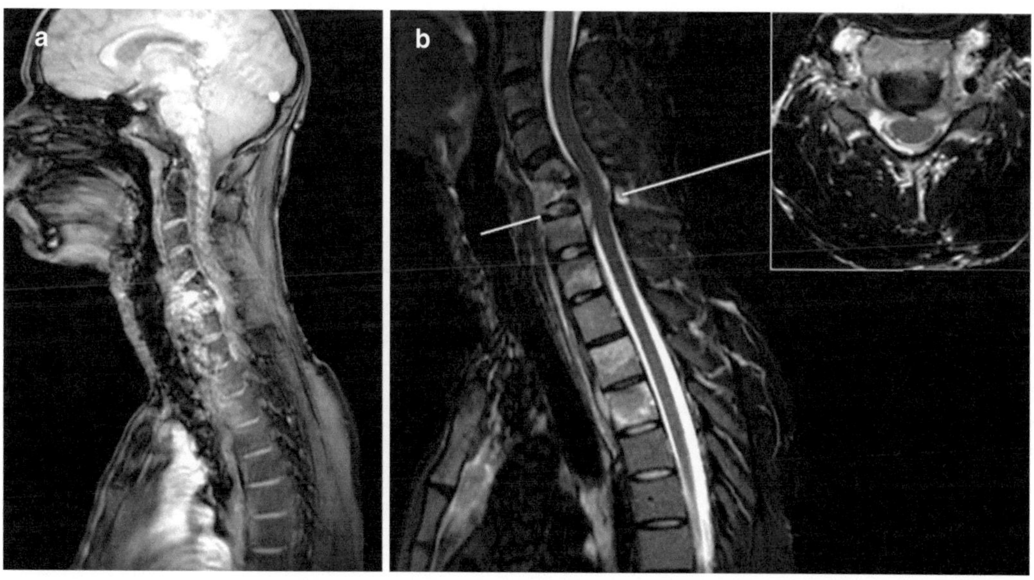


**Fig. 13.3** Tubercular spondylodiscitis in a 32-year-old male affecting the cervical spine. (**a**, **b**) extensive destruction of the anterior vertebral body with spinal cord compression

- *Stage 3:* Bedridden and spastic patient. Anticipated motor score in tetraparesis is 0–30, and in paraparesis is between 50 and 80; sensory deficit involves the lateral column
- *Stage 4:* Bedridden, severe sensory loss/pressure scores. Anticipated motor score in tetraplegia is 0 and in paraplegia is between 0 and 50; sensory deficit involves posterior and lateral columns
- *Stage 5:* Similar to stage 4 +/− bladder/bowel involvement +/− flexor spasms/flaccid tetraplegia/paraplegia

Most of the neural deficits should fit into this classification, but neural deficits in intraspinal granulomas, cauda equina, or other atypical manifestations may not correctly correspond to these stages.

### 13.2.5 Pediatric Spinal Tuberculosis

It is useful to note that, due to the immaturity and increased flexibility of the spine in children, they are more prone to developing a severe progression of the deformity. This worsening can also occur after the disease has healed, so these patients should be followed until they reach skeletal maturity. Rajasekaran et al. described four signs of "spine at risk" in children, which include retropulsion of the posterior aspect of the involved vertebra, facet subluxation, lateral translation of vertebrae, and the toppling of one vertebra over the other. He proposed that children with two or more of these signs had posterior facet disruption and required surgical intervention.

He also proposed a classification system for the progression of the deformity in children:

- *Type 1:* curvature increases until skeletal maturity, and surgical intervention was required
- *Type 2*: deformity decreased with growth progression
- *Type 3*: minimal change in the deformity either during active or healed phases of the disease [42, 43]

### 13.2.6 Diagnosis

The gold standard in the diagnosis is having a positive culture for Mycobacterium. However, the mycobacteria are fastidious, and the cultures typically show poor sensitivity. Other standards for diagnosis are caseating granulomas found on histopathological analysis, serological inflammatory markers, molecular diagnosis, and smear staining for acid-fast bacilli.

***Imaging Modalities*** As in pyogenic osteomyelitis, plain radiographs tend to show signs of vertebral involvement in later stages, and computer tomography and magnetic resonance have been progressively more helpful over the Years (Fig. 13.4). Particularly in TB involvement, it is important to inspect the chest cavity, either by plain X-rays or CT scans, as up to a third of these patients will also present with pulmonary disease [44].

***Laboratory Tests*** Although there are more common (and nonspecific) serum tests, such as erythrocyte sedimentation rate (ESR) and hemo sedimentation velocity (HSV), it is important to note that there are specific tests for latent tuberculosis, such as the Mantoux test, the Interferon-gamma release assay, and ELISA.

The Mantoux test has 40–55% sensitivity and 75% specificity, and it has a low cost. However, it is not accurate in endemic countries or immunodeficient patients.

The Interferon-gamma release assay has 50–65% sensitivity and 85% specificity, and it measures the interferons produced in response to the tubercular antigens. For this reason, it is also not very useful in endemic regions.

Interferon-gamma release assay (50–65% sensitivity and 85% specificity): Measuring interferons produced in response to tubercular antigens; not useful in endemic regions [45, 46].

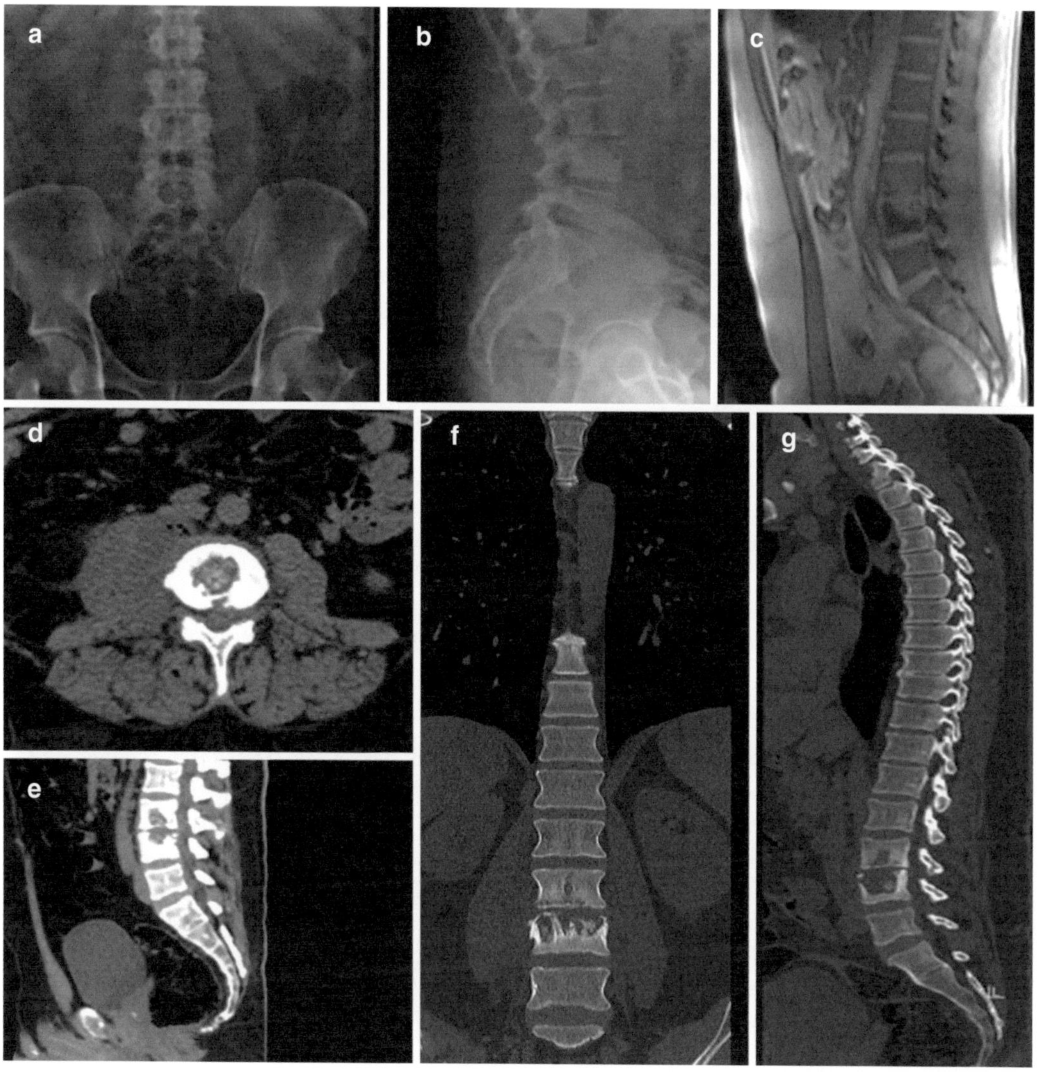


**Fig. 13.4** L3-L4 Spondylodiscitis in a 41-year-old male caused by *Mycobacterium tubercolosis*. (**a**, **b**) radiograph in AP and lateral view; (**c**) sagittal MRI confirm that the infection is limited to the vertebral bodies without involvement of the spinal canal; (**d**, **e**) Axial and sagittal CT scan show lytic erosion in L3 and L4 vertebra… (**f**, **g**) that improved after 1 month of follow-up

### 13.2.7 Treatment

The basis of tuberculosis treatment is always chemotherapy, with multidrug treatment. WHO's most recent guidelines [47] recommend a six to nine-month treatment with four drugs, 9–12 months on regimens that do not include rifampin and/or for patients with extensive or advanced disease, particularly if it is difficult to assess the response to therapy (Fig. 13.5) [48]. Local guidelines should be followed, especially in regions with a high incidence of the disease, especially because of local drug-resistant strains. More importantly for orthopedic surgeons, spinal tuberculosis—as their pyogenic counterpart—should be classified as to spinal stability and the need for surgical intervention. About surgery, the traditional approach to treatment, described since the 1950s, was to perform radical debridement through an anterior approach [49]. However, with

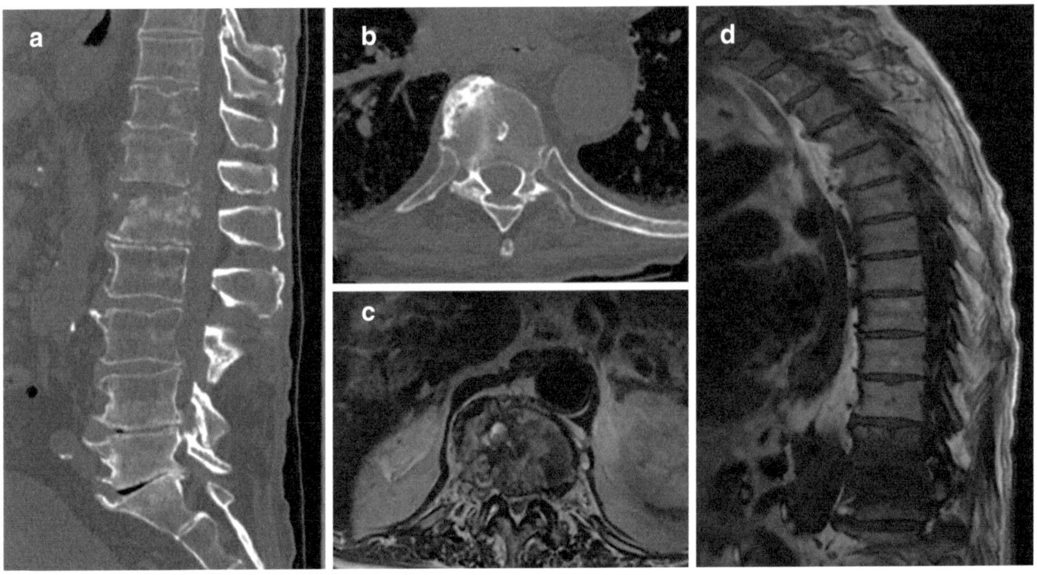


**Fig. 13.5** T12-L1 Spondylodiscitis in an 87 years-old male caused by *Mycobacterium tubercolosis*. (**a**, **b**) CT scan and (**c**, **d**) MR images show the infective process in a degenerative spinal column that increase the difficulty in assessment of response to therapy

the advance of following multidrug chemotherapy and the good clinical results it obtains, Tuli et al. introduced the idea of operating only in patients with specific conditions [50]. These include spinal instability, severe pain, deformity, recurrent disease or disease that is nonresponsive to chemotherapy, severe neurological weakness, and either static or progressive neural deficits. Surgical intervention should drain existing abscesses, debride infected tissues, and provide stability to the spine, as well as correct deformities. As tuberculous bacilli do not form biofilm, it is considered safe to stabilize them with surgical implants. These can be done through anterior, posterior, or combined approaches, depending on vertebral involvement, location of abscesses, and deformities [33].

**Declarations Author Contributions:** Conceptualization, project administration: AA, LPM; data curation and formal analysis: AA, LPM; supervision: PR; writing original draft: LPM; writing review and editing: AA, LPM; figures: AA; All authors have read and agreed to the published version of the manuscript.

**Funding:** There was no external funding source in support of this study.

**Institutional Review Board Statement:** Not applicable.

**Informed Consent Statement:** Written informed consent was obtained from patients at the time of admission to our Institute. However, all pictures have been reported anonymized.

**Consent for Publication (Include Appropriate Statements)**

We confirm that this chapter, including related data, figures, and tables, has not been published previously, it is not under consideration for publication elsewhere, and, if accepted, it will not be published elsewhere in the same form, in English or in any other language, without the written consent of the publisher.

**Conflicts of Interest/Competing Interests (Include Appropriate Disclosures)**

Ruggieri P is a consultant for Stryker and Exactech (not relevant to the present manuscript). The other Authors declare that there are no relationships/conditions/circumstances that present a potential conflict of interest with the present manuscript

**Availability of Data and Material (Data Transparency)**

Manuscript data are embedded in the text and fully available on specific request

## References


1. Bromfield W. Chirurgical observations and cases, vol. II. London: T. Cadall; 1773. p. 19–24.
2. Klenerman L. A history of osteomyelitis from the Journal of Bone and Joint Surgery: 1948 TO 2006. J Bone Joint Surg Br. 2007;89(5):667–70. https://doi.org/10.1302/0301-620X.89B5.19170.
3. Mylona E, Samarkos M, Kakalou E, Fanourgiakis P, Skoutelis A. Pyogenic vertebral osteomyelitis: a systematic review of clinical characteristics. Semin Arthritis Rheum. 2009;39(1):10–7. https://doi.org/10.1016/j.semarthrit.2008.03.002.
4. Lora-Tamayo J, Euba G, Narváez JA, Murillo O, Verdaguer R, Sobrino B, Narváez J, Nolla JM, Ariza J. Changing trends in the epidemiology of pyogenic vertebral osteomyelitis: the impact of cases with no microbiologic diagnosis. Semin Arthritis Rheum. 2011;41(2):247–55. https://doi.org/10.1016/j.semarthrit.2011.04.002.
5. Tsantes AG, Papadopoulos DV, Vrioni G, Sioutis S, Sapkas G, Benzakour A, Benzakour T, Angelini A, Ruggieri P, Mavrogenis AF. World Association Against Infection in Orthopedics and Trauma W A I O T Study Group on bone and joint infection definitions. Spinal infections: an update. Microorganisms. 2020;8(4):476. https://doi.org/10.3390/microorganisms8040476.
6. Dietze DD Jr, Fessler RG, Jacob RP. Primary reconstruction for spinal infections. J Neurosurg. 1997;86:981–9.
7. Loibl M, Stoyanov L, Doenitz C, Brawanski A, Wiggermann P, Krutsch W, Nerlich M, Oszwald M, Neumann C, Salzberger B, Hanses F. Outcome-related co-factors in 105 cases of vertebral osteomyelitis in a tertiary care hospital. Infection. 2014;42(3):503–10. https://doi.org/10.1007/s15010-013-0582-0.
8. Graham SM, Fishlock A, Millner P, Sandoe J. The management gram-negative bacterial haematogenous vertebral osteomyelitis: a case series of diagnosis, treatment and therapeutic outcomes. Eur Spine J. 2013;22(8):1845–53. https://doi.org/10.1007/s00586-013-2750-4.
9. Yoon SH, Chung SK, Kim KJ, Kim HJ, Jin YJ, Kim HB. Pyogenic vertebral osteomyelitis: identification of microorganism and laboratory markers used to predict clinical outcome. Eur Spine J. 2010;19(4):575–82. https://doi.org/10.1007/s00586-009-1216-1.
10. Khan IA, Vaccaro AR, Zlotolow DA. Management of vertebral diskitis and osteomyelitis. Orthopedics. 1999;22(8):758–65.
11. Patzakis MJ, Rao S, Wilkins J, Moore TM, Harvey PJ. Analysis of 61 cases of vertebral osteomyelitis. Clin Orthop Rel Res. 1991;264:178–83.
12. Boody BS, Jenkins TJ, Maslak J, Hsu WK, Patel AA. Vertebral osteomyelitis and spinal epidural abscess: an evidence-based review. J Spinal Disord Tech. 2015;28(6):E316–27. https://doi.org/10.1097/BSD.0000000000000294.
13. Garg V, Kosmas C, Young PC, Togaru UK, Robbin MR. Computed tomography-guided percutaneous biopsy for vertebral osteomyelitis: a department's experience. Neurosurg Focus. 2014;37(2):E10. https://doi.org/10.3171/2014.6.FOCUS14134.
14. Sehn JK, Gilula LA. Percutaneous needle biopsy in diagnosis and identification of causative organisms in cases of suspected vertebral osteomyelitis. Eur J Radiol. 2012;81:940–6.
15. de Lucas EM, González Mandly A, Gutiérrez A, Pellón R, Martín-Cuesta L, Izquierdo J, Sánchez E, Ruiz E, Quintana F. CT-guided fine-needle aspiration in vertebral osteomyelitis: true usefulness of a common practice. Clin Rheumatol. 2009;28(3):315–20. https://doi.org/10.1007/s10067-008-1051-5.
16. Swanson AN, Pappou IP, Cammisa FP, et al. Chronic infections of the spine: surgical indications and treatments. Clin Orthop Relat Res. 2006;444:100–6.
17. Tretiakov PS, Joujon-Roche R, Williamson T, Imbo B, Bennett-Caso C, Dave P, McFarland K, Mir J, Dinizo M, Schoenfeld AJ, Passias PG. Assessing the effects of prior history of vertebral osteomyelitis on peri-operative factors and post-operative recovery in adult spinal deformity patients. J Clin Med. 2022;11(21):6488. https://doi.org/10.3390/jcm11216488.
18. DE LA Garza-Ramos R, Bydon M, Macki M, Abt NB, Rhee J, Gokaslan ZL, Bydon A. Instrumented fusion in the setting of primary spinal infection. J Neurosurg Sci. 2017;61(1):64–76. https://doi.org/10.23736/S0390-5616.16.03302-6.
19. Robinson Y, Tschoeke SK, Kayser R, Boehm H, Heyde CE. Reconstruction of large defects in vertebral osteomyelitis with expandable titanium cages. Int Orthop. 2009;33(3):745–9. https://doi.org/10.1007/s00264-008-0567-2.
20. Kuklo TR, Potter BK, Bell RS, Moquin RR, Rosner MK. Single-stage treatment of pyogenic spinal infection with titanium mesh cages. J Spinal Disord Tech. 2006;19(5):376–82. https://doi.org/10.1097/01.bsd.0000203945.03922.f6.
21. Sundararaj GD, Babu N, Amritanand R, Venkatesh K, Nithyananth M, Cherian VM, Lee VN. Treatment of haematogenous pyogenic vertebral osteomyelitis by single-stage anterior debridement, grafting of the defect and posterior instrumentation. J Bone Joint Surg Br. 2007;89(9):1201–5. https://doi.org/10.1302/0301-620X.89B9.18776.
22. McHenry MC, Easly KA, Locker GA. Vertebral osteomyelitis: long-term outcome for 253 patients from 7 Cleveland-area hospitals. CID. 2002;34:1342–50.

23. Osenbach RK, Hitchon PW, Menezes AH. Diagnosis and management of pyogenic vertebral osteomyelitis in adults. Surg Neurol. 1990;33:266–75.
24. Hadjipavlou AG, Mader JT, Necessary JT, Muffoletto AJ. Hematogenous pyogenic spinal infections and their surgical management. Spine. 2000;25:1668–79.
25. Lichtor J, Lichtor A. Paleopathological evidence suggesting pre-Columbian tuberculosis of spine. J Bone Joint Surg Am. 1957;39-A(6):1938–9.
26. Duraiswami PK, Orth M, Tuli SM. 5000 years of orthopaedics in India. Clin Orthop Relat Res. 1971;75:269–80. https://doi.org/10.1097/00003086-197103000-00032.
27. Bick KM. Classics of orthopaedics. Philadelphia: JB Lippincott Co.; 1976.
28. Tuli SM. Tuberculosis of the skeletal system. 4. New Delhi: Jaypee Brothers Medical Publishers; 2010.
29. Barnes PF, Barrows SA. Tuberculosis in the 1990s. Ann Intern Med. 1993;119(5):400–10. https://doi.org/10.7326/0003-4819-119-5-199309010-00009.
30. Patel S, Collins DA, Bourke BE. Don't forget tuberculosis. Ann Rheum Dis. 1995;54(3):174–5. https://doi.org/10.1136/ard.54.3.174.
31. Scott JE, Taor WS. The changing pattern of bone and joint tuberculosis. J Bone Joint Surg Br. 1982;64:250.
32. Viswanathan VK, Subramanian S. Pott disease. [Updated 2023 Aug 8]. In: StatPearls [Internet]. Treasure Island: StatPearls Publishing; 2024.
33. Rajasekaran S, Soundararajan DCR, Shetty AP, Kanna RM. Spinal tuberculosis: current concepts. Global Spine J. 2018;8(4 Suppl):96S–108S.
34. Su SH, Tsai WC, Lin CY, Lin WR, Chen TC, Lu PL, Huang PM, Tsai JR, Wang YL, Feng MC, Wang TP, Chen YH. Clinical features and outcomes of spinal tuberculosis in southern Taiwan. J Microbiol Immunol Infect. 2010;43(4):291–300.
35. Hayes AJ, Choksey M, Barnes N, Sparrow OC. Spinal tuberculosis in developed countries: difficulties in diagnosis. J R Coll Surg Edinb. 1996;41(3):192–6.
36. Faure E, Souilamas R, Riquet M, Chehab A, Le Pimpec-Barthes F, Manac'h D, Debesse B. Cold abscess of the chest wall: a surgical entity? Ann Thorac Surg. 1998;66(4):1174–8.
37. Jain AK, Aggarwal PK, Arora A, Singh S. Behaviour of the kyphotic angle in spinal tuberculosis. Int Orthop. 2004;28(2):110–4.
38. Subramani S, Shetty AP, Kanna RM, Shanmuganathan R. Ossified ligamentum flavum causing neurological deficit above the level of post-tuberculous kyphotic deformity. J Clin Orthop Trauma. 2017;8(2):174–7.
39. Angelini A, Mosele N, Gnassi A, Baracco R, Rodà MG, Cerchiaro M, Ruggieri P. Vertebra Plana: a narrative clinical and imaging overview among possible differential diagnoses. Diagnostics (Basel). 2023;13(8):1438. https://doi.org/10.3390/diagnostics13081438.
40. Jain AK, Sinha S. Evaluation of systems of grading of neurological deficit in tuberculosis of spine. Spinal Cord. 2005;43(6):375–80.
41. Jain AK, Kumar J. Tuberculosis of spine: neurological deficit. Eur Spine J. 2013;22(Suppl 4):624–33.
42. Rajasekaran S. The natural history of post-tubercular kyphosis in children. Radiological signs which predict late increase in deformity. J Bone Joint Surg Br. 2001;83(7):954–62.
43. Rajasekaran S. Buckling collapse of the spine in childhood spinal tuberculosis. Clin Orthop Relat Res. 2007;460:86–92.
44. Dharmalingam M. Tuberculosis of the spine-the Sabah experience. Epidemiology, treatment and results. Tuberculosis (Edinb). 2004;84(1–2):24–8.
45. Kumar R, Das RK, Mahapatra AK. Role of interferon gamma release assay in the diagnosis of Pott disease. J Neurosurg Spine. 2010;12(5):462–6.
46. Brodie D, Lederer DJ, Gallardo JS, Trivedi SH, Burzynski JN, Schluger NW. Use of an interferon-gamma release assay to diagnose latent tuberculosis infection in foreign-born patients. Chest. 2008;133(4):869–74.
47. World Health Organization. WHO operational handbook on tuberculosis. Module 4: treatment – drug-resistant tuberculosis treatment. Geneva: World Health Organization; 2020. Licence: CC BY-NC-SA 3.0 IGO.
48. Blumberg HM, Leonard MK Jr, Jasmer RM. Update on the treatment of tuberculosis and latent tuberculosis infection. JAMA. 2005;293(22):2776–84. https://doi.org/10.1001/jama.293.22.2776. Erratum in: JAMA. 2005 Jul 13; 294(2): 182. Dosage error in article text. PMID: 15941808
49. Hodgson AR, Stock FE. Anterior spinal fusion a preliminary communication on the radical treatment of Pott's disease and Pott's paraplegia. Br J Surg. 1956;44(185):266–75.
50. Tuli SM. Severe kyphotic deformity in tuberculosis of the spine. Int Orthop. 1995;19(5):327–31.

# Algorithm on Treatment in Fracture-Related Infections

14

Rohan Parwani

## 14.1 Introduction

Infection is the most dreaded complication in orthopedics. As implants have become an important part of orthopedic practice, wound infections, and osteomyelitis have become a common occurrence [1]. This is especially true after a fracture fixation surgery, where the tissue is already traumatized with injury, and it becomes susceptible to infection. The presence of a dead space and hematoma provides an active breeding ground for infection. Also, there might be a direct contamination from the external environment if there has been a compound fracture.

The presence of an infection with a fracture is a double injury to the patient. It prolongs the rehabilitation time after injury and adds to the potential costs of treatment to the patient [2]. It becomes the treating physician's duty to get the patient back to his activities as soon as possible. The physician is faced with conflicting dilemmas and has to navigate through them to get the patient back to a pre-injury routine as soon as possible. There are different options available considering different scenarios. The treatment needs to be strategized depending on the clinical scenario, available resources, and financial freedom of the treating physician. An early infection in a closed injury is different from a delayed infection after the fracture is united. In this chapter, we will discuss various factors that influence the treatment and then how to decide on the best possible treatment strategy.

R. Parwani (✉)
Pediatric Orthopedic Surgeon, Shaishav Children Orthopedic Hospital, Rajkot, India

Department of Orthopedics, PDU Medical College, Rajkot, India

## 14.2 Factors Influencing the Treatment of FRI

Once a fracture gets infected, we need to identify and understand at the earliest, the nature and quantum of the problem to effectively manage it. The following factors help us understand this.

### 14.2.1 Establishing an Early Diagnosis

We perform multiple trauma surgeries in orthopedics. Not all of them develop infection, but the ones that do get infected result in a significant increase in morbidity and duration of rehabilitation. As such, early and reliable diagnosis of infection becomes critical because the patient pays the price in terms of time and finance if the fracture surgery becomes infected. The diagnosis needs to be accurate to optimize the use of antibiotics and the need for revision surgery. A consensus article was published by Metsemakers WJ,



P. Ruggieri et al. (eds.), *Bone and Joint Infections*, https://doi.org/10.1007/978-3-031-96383-4_14

Morgenstern M, et al. in the Injury Journal and Journal of Orthopedic Trauma. The article gives two sets of criteria to establish the diagnosis of fracture-related infection [3]. These diagnostic pointers are divided into two sets of criteria. The sets consist of suggestive and confirmatory criteria and give indicators of when to start treatment in anticipation of infection after orthopedic surgery. Suggestive criteria should alert the caregiver team to the possibility of infection and to start appropriate remedial measures. Confirmatory criteria indicate established infection and should trigger aggressive management strategies.

| Confirmatory criteria | Suggestive criteria |
|---|---|
| Clinical signs | Clinical signs |
| Fistula | Local/systemic (e.g., local redness, swelling, fever) |
| Sinus | New-onset joint effusion |
| Wound breakdown | Persistent, increasing, or new-onset wound drainage |
| Purulent drainage or the presence of pus | |
| Microbiology | Laboratory signs |
| Phenotypically indistinguishable pathogens identified by culture from at least two separate deep tissue/implant specimens | Increased serum inflammatory markers (ESR, WBC, CRP) |
| Histopathology | Radiological and/or nuclear imaging signs, microbiology, pathogenic microorganisms identified from a single deep tissue/implant specimen |
| Presence of microorganisms in deep tissue specimens, confirmed by using specific staining techniques for bacteria and fungi presence of >5 PMNs/HPF in chronic/late-onset cases (e.g., fracture nonunion) | |

*ESR* erythrocyte sedimentation rate, *WBC* white blood cell count, *CRP* C-reactive protein, *PMNs* polymorphonuclear neutrophils, *HPF* high-power field

### 14.2.2 Primary Injury

An open or compound injury is more likely to be infected after fixation [4]. The initial injury determines the extent of soft tissue devascularization, exposure of bone to the external environment, the type of contamination, and the presence of foreign bodies inside the wound. We can also predict the nature of the infecting organism. The nature of primary injury influences not only the primary management of injury but also the management of subsequent complications. Different types of compound injuries have different problems. For example, a blast injury involves the presence of multiple shrapnel and microscopic contaminants. Therefore, the wound has a high chance of developing a persistent infection that is resistant to debridement [5]. The presence of infection after a blast injury is likely to require Gram-negative coverage and a more extensive debridement [6]. On the other end, even a compound injury with bone penetrating the skin envelope (compound grade 1 tibia fracture) might be minimally contaminated. If an infection develops after surgery, it can be treated as an infection after a closed injury. Infection after surgery in a closed fracture would likely be caused by a Gram-positive *staphylococcal coccus* or by a pathogen present as a result of comorbid conditions [7]. It is less likely to need a soft tissue coverage procedure like flap surgery. A crush injury or a degloving injury, on the other hand, could have an intact-looking soft tissue envelope, but the underlying bone would have been devascularized and likely to turn into sequestrum.

Therefore, knowing the primary injury can help us predict the nature of the complication and its further management.

**Case 1** This case shows the benefit of considering the nature of primary injury when analyzing the reason for delayed union.

Figure 14.1 shows the trauma scan of 14-year-old child. She sustained a fall from a height of sixth floor. She had a compound grade 3b shaft of femur fracture with ipsilateral neck of femur fracture.

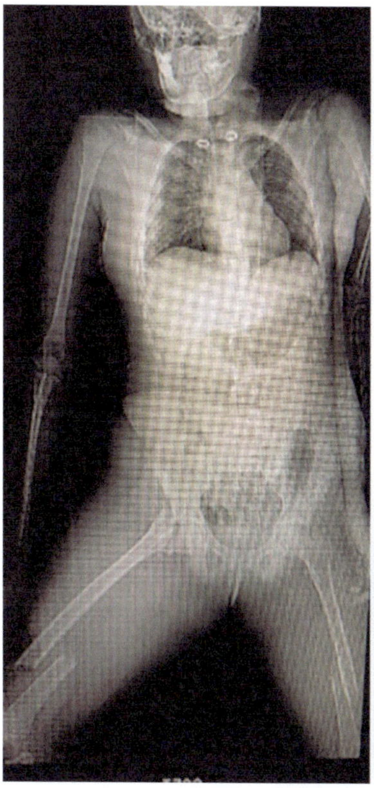

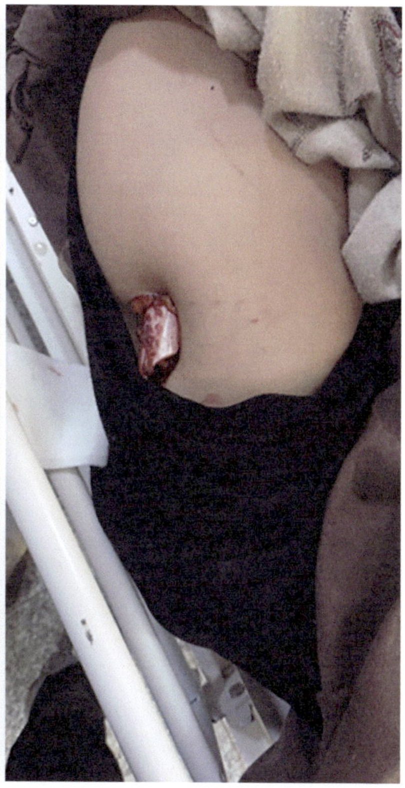

**Fig. 14.1** The trauma scan of 14-year-old child. She sustained a fall from a height of sixth floor. She had a compound grade 3b shaft of femur fracture with ipsilateral neck of femur fracture

Figure 14.2 shows postoperative X-Ray. We had fixed femur diaphysis fracture with titanium elastic nailing and the neck femur fracture with a pediatric dynamic hip screw. She had a routine post-operative course, the neck of femur fracture united at 4 months, and shaft of femur fracture showed partial union at 6 months. She was allowed full weight bearing at 6 months.

Figure 14.3 shows X-Ray at 6 months.

After waiting for 1 year, her knee could not flex more than 90 degrees and the shaft femur fracture showed deficient posterior cortex union. Figure 14.4 shows X-Ray after 1 year of primary surgery. Considering her primary compound fracture, despite no postoperative symptoms and signs of fracture-related infection, we suspected a fracture-related infection. We opened the fracture site and sure enough, the bone that had been exposed to the environment had turned to sequestrum and there was a low-grade infection. We did debridement, removed the loose sequestrum, and put in vancomycin and gentamicin-loaded calcium sulfate beads. No external fixator was required since the anterior

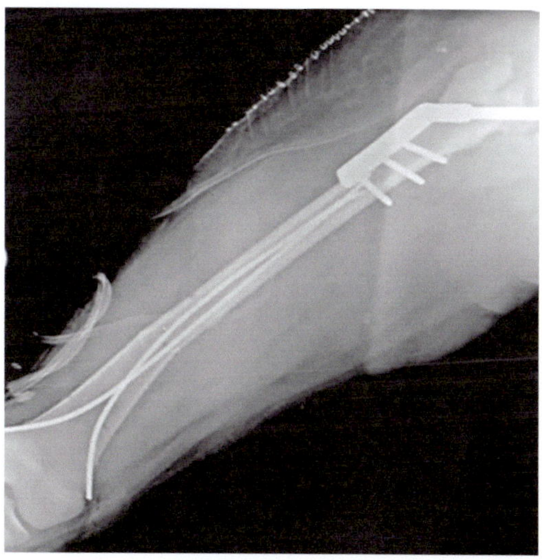

**Fig. 14.2** Postoperative X-Ray. We had fixed femur diaphysis fracture with titanium elastic nailing and the neck femur fracture with a pediatric dynamic hip screw. She had a routine post-operative course, the neck of femur fracture united at 4 months, and shaft of femur fracture showed partial union at 6 months. She was allowed full weight bearing at 6 months

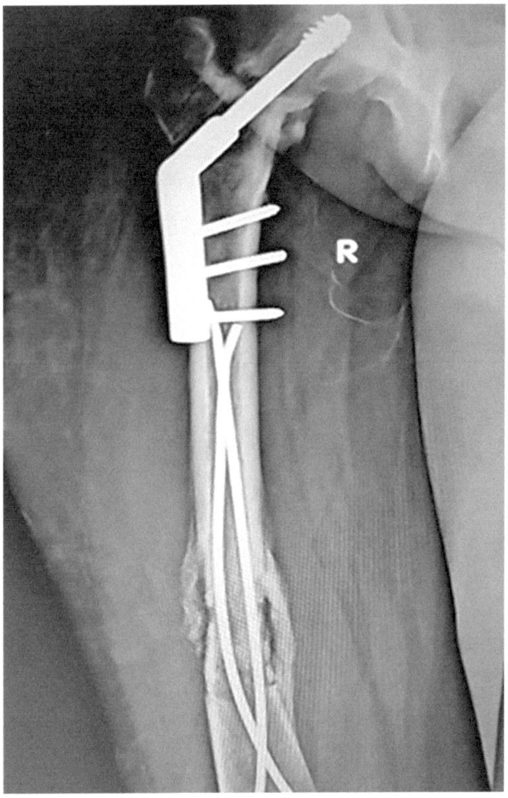

**Fig. 14.3** X-Ray at 6 months

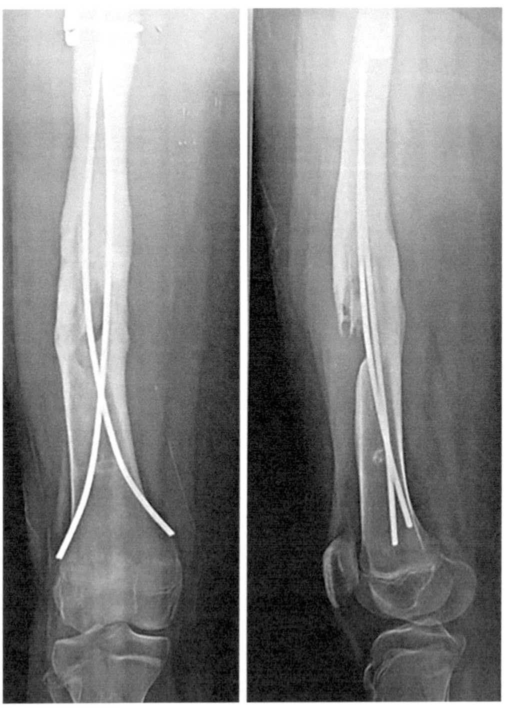

**Fig. 14.4** X-Ray after 1 year of primary surgery. There is persistent posterior gap

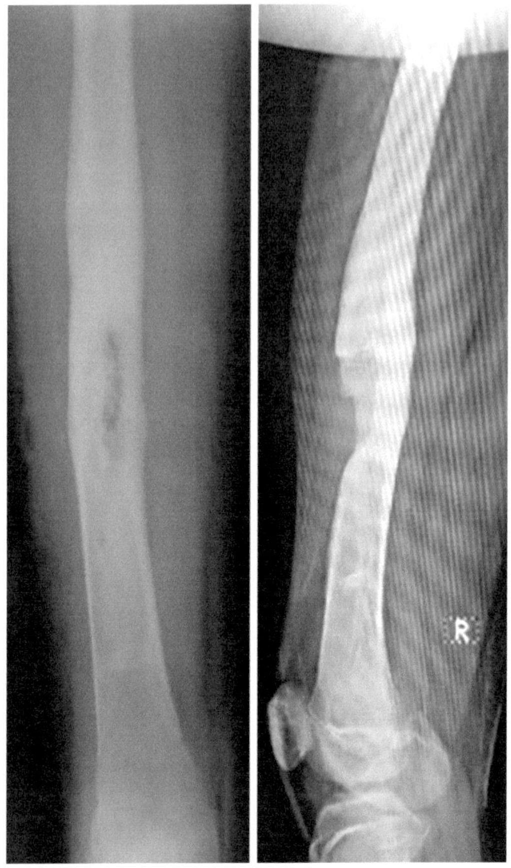

**Fig. 14.5** Last follow up x-ray after debridement and sequestrectomy

half of the fracture had a solid callus. The patient recovered well and regained full function.

Figure 14.5 shows the last follow up X-Ray.

### 14.2.3 Early Versus Late Infection

The duration for which infection is present near the implant site plays a critical role in determining the outcome of treatment of fracture-related infection. This is because of the development of a microscopic structure called biofilm [4]. Biofilm is a thin layer of an extracellular matrix made of polymeric substances excreted by the bacteria themselves [8]. Adherent to this layer are adherent inactive or dormant forms of bacteria. These bacteria are resistant to antibiotics simply because they are dormant and surrounded by an extracellular matrix. Various microbiological studies have demonstrated that biofilms form early after the onset of infection in surgical wound. Therefore, infections should be treated as early as possible [9, 10].

Acute infections that happen within a short period of implantation of fracture fixation devices are likely to have planktonic, metabolically active form of bacteria. They are more likely to be managed successfully with systemic antibiotics and dead space management. If the implants are firm, they may be retained for the time being, till the bone has united [11]. Late infections are likely to be insidious and associated with biofilm formation. Very few antibiotics are known to effectively penetrate the biofilm, some examples being rifampicin for Gram-positive bacteria and fluoroquinolones for Gram-negative bacteria [12]. Once a biofilm is expected to be formed, there are very limited options other than implant removal. If the fracture is not united by this time, the fracture will have to be stabilized with external fixation.

Figure 14.6 shows stages of formation of biofilm. Planktonic form is the form when bacteria are free in tissues and are most likely to be susceptible to antibiotics. Once a mature biofilm forms, usually within 4–6 weeks, the bacteria have built up defense barriers to evade the host immune system and antibiotics.

The presence of biofilm acts as a source of chronic infection and inhibits the process of fracture union. Therefore, once we suspect early infection after fracture surgery, there is a race against time to achieve bone union before the biofilm matures. Various studies have examined the outcome of treatment of early infection with debridement, antibiotics, and implant retention (DAIR). Morgensten et al. published a meta-analysis of six studies [13]. They found 86–100% success rates if this strategy was used within 3 weeks of primary surgery. As time progresses success rates drop off with less than 67% good outcomes in infections that are more than 10-weeks old. However, it should be noted that, once an infection has set in, the strategy of DAIR is only suppressive and not curative, that is, it only works and buys time till the fracture unites. The implant almost always has to be removed after bone union when the function of the limb is not likely to be hampered [13].

### 14.2.4 Identifying the Pathogen

Various bacteria are known to cause persistent infection after orthopedic surgery. The source of bacteria may be from a coexisting chronic illness, it may be a hospital-acquired infection, or from environmental contamination at the time of trauma. The identity of the pathogen is required

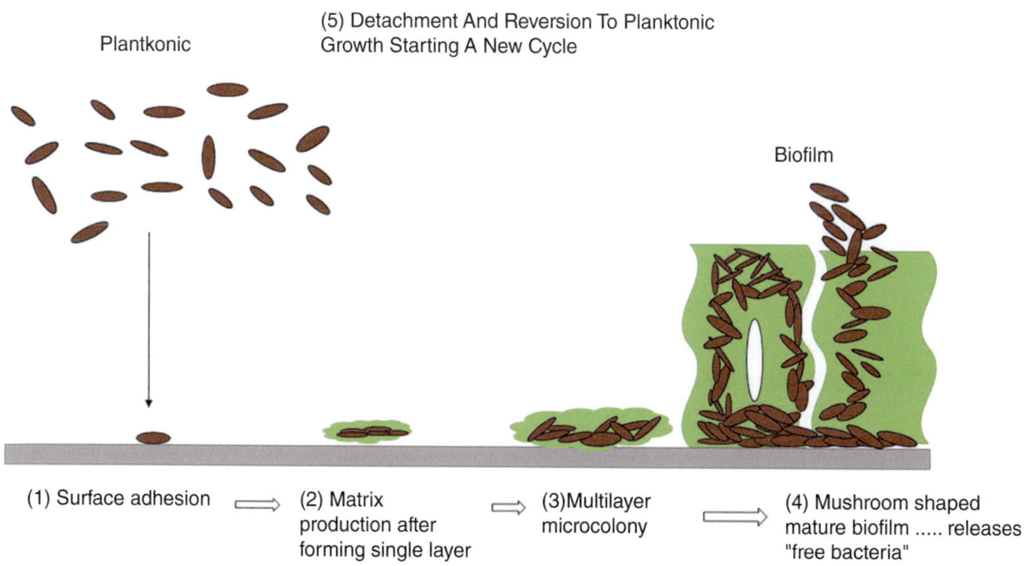


**Fig. 14.6** Biofilm formation

to determine the choice of antibiotics. Timely and accurate identification of the pathogen and the corresponding drug-resistance characteristics is challenging in chronic infections. Various microbiological studies have reported a 70–80% success rate in positively confirming the pathogen [14].

Staphylococcus remains the predominant causative organism in monomicrobial surgical site infections after orthopedic surgery [7]. this bacteria is of particular concern because of its ability to rapidly develop antibiotic resistance to evade both the antibiotics and the host immune response. It is also known to form biofilms and act as a source of persistent infection. It is isolated in up to 60% of orthopedic infections, in both early and late-onset infections. It is more likely to cause a purulent discharge, and sinus/fistulas after an orthopedic infection. If staphylococcus is identified, 60–80% of them are likely to be resistant to penicillin, erythromycin, and fluoroquinolone group of antibiotics [7]. Vancomycin was found to be effective in majority of cases.

Other Gram-positive bacteria, commonly isolated in monomicrobial and polymicrobial infections are staph epidermidis and coagulase-negative staphylococcus epidermidis [7]. Their antibiotic susceptibility usually matches the *s. aureus* species, with vancomycin being regarded as the most effective antibiotic.

Polymicrobial infections are more likely in chronic orthopedic infections. Gram-negative bacilli are more common in this setting and are likely to be susceptible to the piperacillin-tazobactam combination. Gram-negative bacilli are also more likely to be isolated after open fractures, indicating some role of environmental contamination in the development of fracture-related infection.

## 14.2.5 Status of Fracture Union

When faced with an infection after trauma surgery, the stage of fracture union plays the most important role in deciding the future course of action. Removal of implants may solve all problems in a late infection. But if the bone has not united, and the infection has been there for a significant duration of time, the implants need to be replaced with another implant, as a mobile fracture is not conducive to healing infection in soft tissues. The presence of infection either in the implant or soft tissues causes macrophage apoptosis, inhibits osteoblast differentiation, and generally inhibits the biology of fracture healing [15]. Therefore, the presence of a nonunion complicates the treatment of infection and all options should be carefully reviewed before planning for treatment. The bone union can sometimes be difficult to judge on X-ray, especially in cases where we expect a primary bone union [16]. Advanced methods like CT scans or appropriate bone scans can be used to give a better idea of the status of union [17].CT scans have a low specificity in confirming fracture union, mainly because of "beam hardening" artifact from external or internal fixation devices [17]. Bone scan is another important tool, that can identify the site of infection in the bone-implant interface and help identify if the infection is present at the nonunion site [18].

### 14.2.5.1 Sequestrum

Sequestrum is defined as a dead bone present in live bone. It often acts as a source of persistent infection. Its presence also delays bone union. Therefore, when considering a revision for infected nonunion, the sequestrum if present must be removed. The size of the sequestrum must be evaluated before surgery and if after removal, the fracture is further destabilized, appropriate measures like antibiotic spacer with or without external fixation should be considered.

## 14.2.6 Patient Comorbid Factors

Any patient undergoing trauma surgery should have their bio-physiological profile checked. This is required not only for a safe anesthesia but also for postoperative care and rehabilitation. The immunocompetence of the host at the systemic as well as local soft tissue level plays an important role in the ability of the host to resist infection.

The patient is assessed for comorbid factors like poor nutritional status, obesity, smoking, diabetes, and peripheral vascular disease [19]. Peripheral pulse and sensation should be assessed in all patients where surgery is planned especially after infection. We should assess the patient's preoperative glycemic control, as during the physiological stress of surgery, hyperglycemia is known to be independently associated with poor clinical outcomes like wound infections [20]. Hyperglycemia induces increased expression of proinflammatory cytokines like TNF, which inhibit osteoblast activity. Perioperative glycemic control should be assessed with Hba1c and if found elevated, appropriate corrective measures should be started. They should undergo a dietary as well as endocrine consultation and perioperative insulin should be started if required. Similarly, obesity, defined as BMI of more than 30 is known to be associated with adverse postoperative outcomes like thromboembolism and infection. It is not possible or advisable to suggest a drastic weight loss regimen before surgery, but we should consider it as a contributing factor.

Multiple investigators have proven the risk associated with smoking and its relation to fracture union and wound infection rates [21]. A meta-analysis published by Smolle et al. shows the significant risk of orthopedic infections in fractures of the tibia, hip, calcaneum, elbow, distal femur, and spinal surgery [22]. It might be best to initiate cessation of smoking in patients undergoing treatment for fracture-related infection.

Thus, when considering the treatment of a patient with a fracture-related infection, the entire host should be optimized. Depending on the presence of comorbid conditions, the patient's physiology is classified into three categories, according the University of Texas Medical Branch protocol [23].

| | | |
|---|---|---|
| *Anatomic type* | | |
| Type I | — | Medullary osteomyelitis |
| Type II | — | Superficial osteomyelitis |
| Type III | — | Localized osteomyelitis |
| Type IV | — | Diffuse osteomyelitis |
| *Physiologic class* | | |
| A-host | — | Good immune system and delivery |
| B-host | — | Compromised locally ($B^L$) or systemically ($B^S$) |
| C-host | — | Requires suppressive or no treatment minimal disability; treatment worse than disease; not a surgical candidate |
| *Clinical stage* | | |
| Type + class = clinical stage | | |
| Example: Stage IV$B^S$ osteomyelitis = a diffuse lesion in a systemically compromised host | | |

## 14.3 Treatment Options

After identifying the various host factors influencing the treatment of infection, we can then start analyzing the various treatment options that can be offered to the patient. Therefore, we need to acquaint ourselves with the various treatment modalities available. Depending on our understanding of indications for different treatment options we can formulate a cohesive strategy.

### 14.3.1 Choice of Antibiotics

Antibiotics will be the mainstay of our treatment of infection. The choice of antibiotics and duration of antibiotics is determined by the clinical picture with which the patient presents. In case of early infection, where only the suggestive criteria are met, a deep tissue culture should be obtained, with or without formal debridement of the surgical wound. It has been an international consensus, not to start empirical intravenous antibiotics without taking deep tissue samples unless the patient is in systemic sepsis [24]. The choice of empirical antibiotics depends on the epidemiology of local pathogens most likely to be involved and their antibiotic susceptibility properties. The individual risk factors of the patient like existing comorbidities, known allergies, other previously isolated organisms, and their resistance profiles should all be considered. The empirical antibiotic chosen should cover both Gram-positive cocci and Gram-negative bacilli.

There is no clear consensus on the duration of antibiotics and depends on the overall strategy decided by the multidisciplinary team. If the antibiotics are being used as a part of suppressive therapy with implant retention, they should be continued till the fracture consolidates. Intravenous antibiotics are recommended till there are clinical signs of resolution of systemic septicemia, and healing of acute inflammatory changes in the soft tissue. Oral antibiotics can then be started [24]. By this time, clear susceptibility and resistance profiles of the isolated organism are usually identified. The strategy of using antibiotics only is unlikely to eradicate infection and is likely to be suppressive only [25].

### 14.3.2 Debridement with or Without Revision of Fixation

Debridement, as used in this discussion, means the surgical exposure of the whole pathological zone and the removal of all necrotic, contaminated, damaged, and/or infected tissue, whether bone or soft tissue [26]. A good debridement is usually required once an infection sets in after fracture surgery. This is because of the presence of a latent infection in bone and soft tissue. Debridement should be thorough and start from skin to bone. It should be planned properly, keeping in mind the need for future reconstruction and salvage. A multidisciplinary team adapted to the available resources, consisting of an orthopedic surgeon, plastic surgeon, microbiologist, and infectious disease specialist, should be constituted early [26]. The patient should also be counseled about the likely need for further intervention or debridement if necessary.

Tissue samples for culture and histopathology should be sent. At least two specimens from different sites should be sent for culture and sensitivity [27]. If the infected implant is removed, it can be directly sent to a microbiological lab to obtain samples for culture and sensitivity. There have been multiple innovations to improve the culture yield from removed implants. Techniques like sonification use high-frequency sound waves to dislodge bacteria from the biofilm present on the retrieved implants [28]. Multiple studies have shown that this technique significantly improves the culture yield. The debridement procedure may be combined with sequesterectomy. High-flow irrigation is used for the removal of microscopic infected tissue [29]. The choice of irrigation fluid is subjective, and various studies comparing normal saline, distilled water, and iodine solutions show similar outcomes [29]. There is no definitive advantage of high-pressure lavage over low-pressure lavage, as shown by FLOW trials.

If the fracture gets destabilized by the procedure, some form of external fixation may be required [30, 31]. The use of antibiotic spacers may be considered if there is considerable dead space after performing debridement. This method of slow, sustained delivery of high concentrations of antibiotics is effective in controlling local infections [32]. Antibiotic spacers can also be subsequently converted to a membrane-induced osteogenesis technique.

In the case of infected intramedullary nails, the use of a reamer irrigator aspirator system after implant removal has been shown to produce significantly better outcomes [33]. The removed implant can be replaced with either an antibiotic-loaded nail, a new nail, or an external fixation device, depending on the severity of the infection.

### 14.3.3 Soft Tissue Coverage

The nutrition of bones lies in soft tissue. Antibiotics given by the systemic route need good vascularity to reach bones. Soft tissues primarily get damaged after trauma or infection, and once debrided for infection, the bone becomes denuded and lacks vascularity. When analyzing a fracture-related infection and planning its treatment, we need to provide adequate soft tissue coverage to improve the chances of healing of infection and facilitate fracture union. There are multiple options, like flap surgery and negative pressure wound therapy, which help improve the soft tissue cover of the infected wound. When planning a revision of fracture-related infection, a plastic surgeon should be included in the team to plan an appropriate local, pedicled, or free flap surgery. Negative pressure wound therapy has shown promising results in gradually draining the wound and enhancing granulation tissue formation, and improving soft tissue coverage. However, its use as a definitive treatment for coverage of soft tissue defects is not clear [34]. Both methods have their benefits and drawbacks. Flap surgery provides primary closure and rapid return of vascularity of tissues. Negative pressure wound therapy system is a simple method that can be applied at all anatomical sites and can be used even if the flap surgery fails [35]. It has a low cost compared to a free flap and is easily available. Flap coverage surgery requires a specialist consultation with a high skill level to successfully perform a flap surgery, something which might not be available in a low-resource setting hospital. Negative pressure wound therapy requires regular dressing changes, and the patient needs to remain bedridden for a prolonged time, thereby increasing anxiety levels and depression [36]. Whatever the method, a vital soft tissue cover, after a thorough and judicious debridement of infection, remains the cornerstone of managing fracture-related infections.

### 14.3.4 External Fixation

External fixation is a powerful tool in the treatment of orthopedic infections. It provides a so-called implant holiday to the local soft tissues to allow them to heal. Pathogens form a biofilm on internal fixation devices and resist the action of antibiotics. This biofilm inhibits the biology of fracture union and can gradually turn the bone into a sequestrum. The only reliable way to treat the biofilm is to remove the associated internal fixation device with it. The internal implant has to be replaced with an external fixation device. External fixation devices have minimal contact with infected tissues and hence are unlikely to provide a surface for the formation of biofilm [4, 37]. Despite being cumbersome and heavy, external fixation devices can serve as a temporary or definitive method of treatment.

Various types of external fixation devices are available. It may be a monolateral fixator or an Illizarov ring fixator. Ring fixators are considered to be more stable and can be used for definitive fixation [37]. They can also be used for alternate strategies like bone transport as and when required. There is multiple high-level evidence to support the use of external fixation as a gold standard in reconstructing residual bone defects after treating bone infections.

The use of external fixation devices for fracture stabilization has multiple drawbacks. Apart from being bulky and cumbersome, they restrict the joint range of movement and prolong the time for limb rehabilitation. They require regular dressings and sometimes the patient may have to be bedridden for a prolonged period of time. However, given the mandatory requirement of maintaining bone alignment and stability, external fixation plays a unique role in managing fracture-related infections.

**Case 2** Example of Ring fixator being used as definitive treatment of middle third tibia posttraumatic osteomyelitis.

A 55-year-old male patient with sustained compound grade 3b tibia fracture. He was managed initially with ex fixator and soft tissue coverage, and presented to us with middle third tibia osteomyelitis and draining sinus through the flap (Fig. 14.7).

Figure 14.8 is X-Ray after doing debrifdement, sequestrectomy, fixing with illizarov ring fixator, and doing corticotomy.

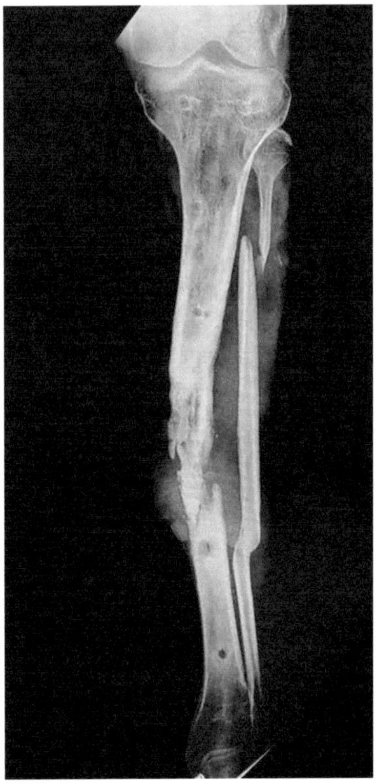

**Fig. 14.7** A 55-year old male patient with sustained compound grade 3b tibia fracture. He was managed initially with ex fixator and soft tissue coverage. Hepresented to us with middle third tibia osteomyelitis and draining sinus through the flap

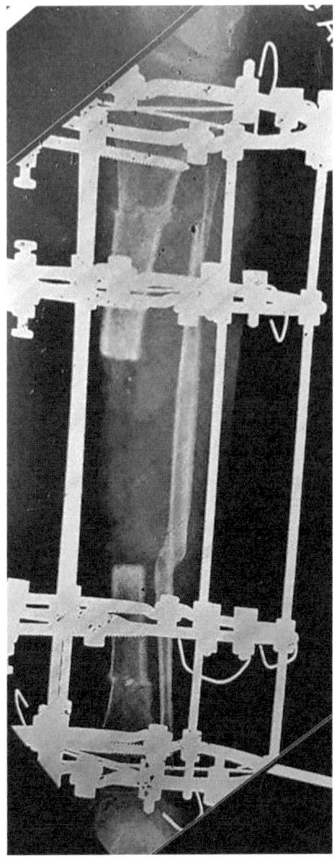

**Fig. 14.8** X-Ray after doing debrifdement, sequestrectomy, fixing with illizarov ring fixator, and doing corticotomy

Figure 14.9 is X-Ray at end of bone transport with both segments meeting at center.

Figure 14.10 is X-Ray after consolidation of regenerate, taken before frame removal.

Figure 14.11 is X-Ray of complete union.

### 14.3.5 Antibiotic Loaded Cement/Bioceramics

Orthopedic infections involve bone and implants and are known to respond slowly to antibiotics. The effective management of orthopedic infections requires the sustained presence of antibiotics in the soft tissue, in a high enough concentration near the bone–implant interface [32]. This high level of serum concentration is difficult to sustain by administering antibiotics through the oral or intravenous routes and may lead to systemic complications. Such high concentrations are best achieved with some form of local antibiotic delivery system. Antibiotic cement, polymethyl methacrylate (PMMA), was the first such biocompatible material discovered that could serve as a vehicle to provide sustained elution of antibiotics to maintain a soft tissue concentration of antibiotics well above the minimum inhibitory concentration (MIC) of bacteria. Thus, PMMA was the first local antibiotic delivery system to be developed commercially. Vancomycin and gentamicin are the most popular antibiotics that are combined with PMMA. It is available in an antibiotic mixed pre-constituted form or antibiotics can be mixed during surgery as well. The antibiotic-loaded PMMA is known to provide the highest in situ diffusion of antibiotics and is considered to be the gold standard. Antibiotic-loaded cement coated onto intramedullary implants can provide fracture stability in the absence of formal implants [39, 40]. This can act as a temporary measure, while high concentrations of antibiotics eluted into soft tissue allow the tis-

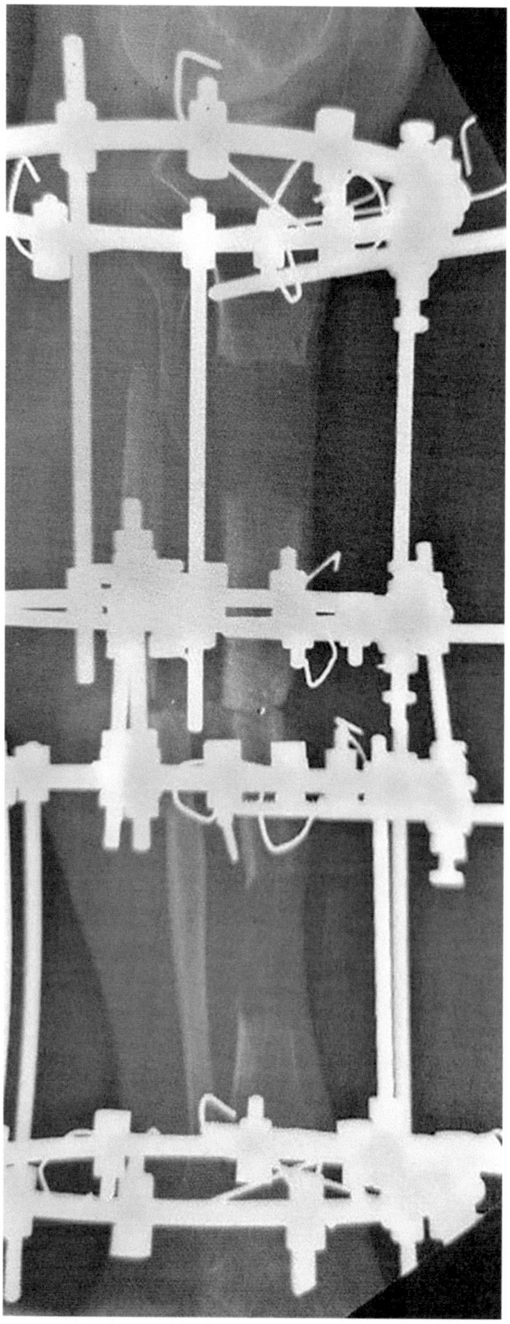

**Fig. 14.9** X-Ray at end of bone transport with both segments meeting at center

sues to regenerate. They have been proven very effective in (1) early suppression of infection, (2) showing a several-fold reduction in the recurrent infection incidence, (3) minimizing the risk of pathological fracture due to internal reinforcement, (4) providing early recovery of extremity's function, and (5) creation of favorable conditions for bone structures restoration [40].

However, there have been some concerns about the heat of polymerization of PMMA, which may inactivate the active antibiotic [41]. It also requires a second surgery for cement removal, since it is a nonbiodegradable product. Vancomycin and gentamicin are the most popular antibiotics that are combined with PMMA. Insertion of properly shaped PMMA models can help provide accurate stability to the infection site by acting as temporizing spacers.

Various other materials, which can act as vehicles for local antibiotic delivery, called bio ceramics, have been discovered. Some examples like calcium sulfate, calcium phosphate, and hydroxyapatite are effective. They were found to have similar properties without the drawbacks of PMMA. The newer systems combine osteoinductive and osteoconductive properties, which enhance bone union by facilitating osteoblast proliferation and osteoclast differentiation. Bioceramics are combined with antibiotics and constituted as scaffolds to provide a controlled, sustained release of antibiotics to the local soft tissue [42]. The biocomposite material is arranged in a porous matrix and, being biocompatible, provides a structure for the neighboring cells to infiltrate and differentiate into osteoblasts and provide osteoinductive properties. As the scaffold dissolves, the material gets absorbed without any local reaction thus obviating the need for a second surgery to remove the product. The various commercially available products and their regulatory approval are listed below.

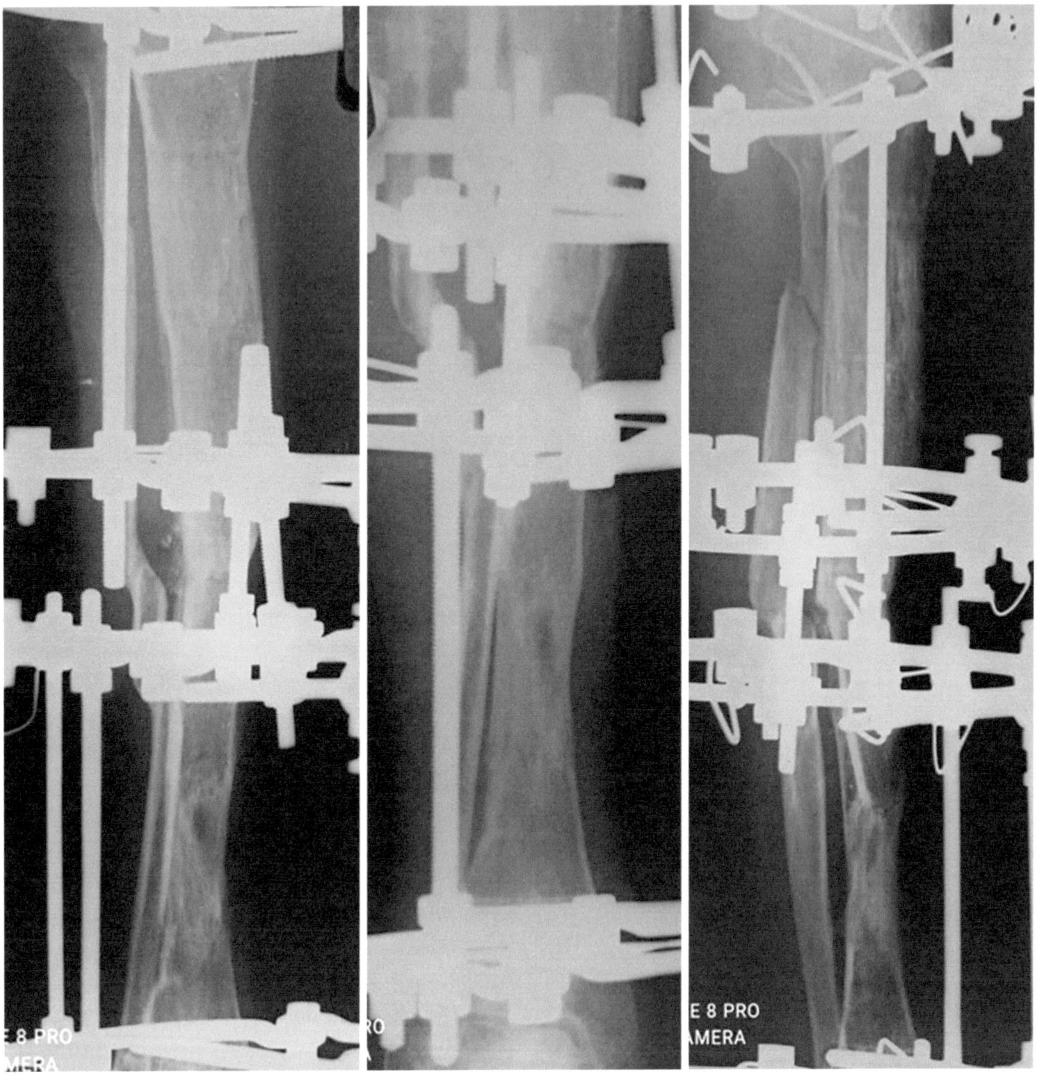

**Fig. 14.10** X-Ray after consolidation of regenerate, taken before frame removal

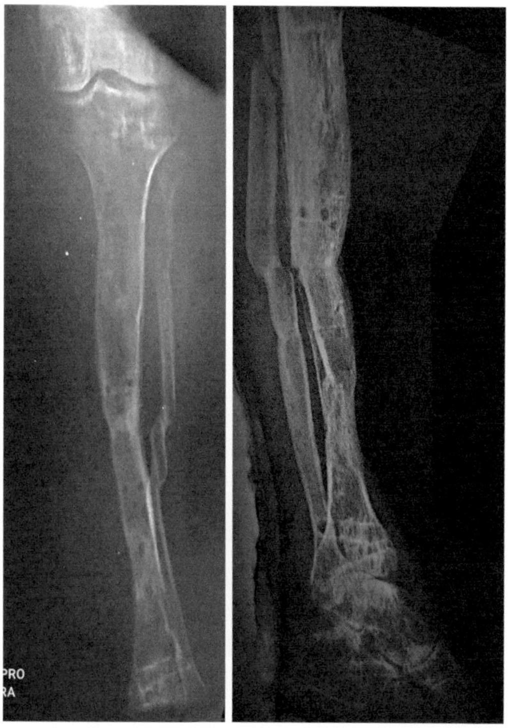


**Fig. 14.11** X-Ray of complete union

| S.n. | Carrier | Antimicrobial agent | From | Commercial products | Official approval |
|---|---|---|---|---|---|
| 1. | PMMA | Gentamicin | Beads impregnated with the antibiotic | Palacios G® | FDA, 2003 |
| | | Tobramycin | Bone cement incorporating the antibiotic | Simplex P® | FDA, 2007 |
| | | Gentamicin and Clindamycin | Bone cement incorporating the antibiotic | Copal® G + C | FDA, 2019 |
| | | Gentamicin and vancomycin | Bone cement incorporating the antibiotic | Copal® G + V | FDA, 2019 |
| | | Gentamicin | Beads impregnated with the antibiotic | Septopal® | The Therapeutic Goods Administration, Australia, 2020 |
| 2. | Hydroxyapatite | – | Xenograft granules that can be preloaded with suitable antibiotic | Endobon® | FDA, 2011 |
| 3. | Hydroxyapatite/calcium sulfate | Gentamicin | Synthetic bone substitute incorporated with the antibiotic | Cerament® G | Health Canada, 2018 |

| S.n. | Carrier | Antimicrobial agent | From | Commercial products | Official approval |
|---|---|---|---|---|---|
| 4. | Calcium sulfate | Tobramycin | Bone graft substitute incorporating the antibiotic | Osteoset® | FDA, 2004 |
| | | – | Synthetic bone substitute that can be preloaded with suitable antibiotic | Stimulan® | FDA, 2015 |
| 5. | Calcium phosphate | – | Synthetic bone substitute that can be preloaded with suitable antibiotic | Cerasorb® M | FDA, 2012 |
| | | – | Synthetic bone cement that can be preloaded with suitable antibiotic | Biopex-R® | The Pharmaceutical and Medical Devices Agency, Japan, 2000 |
| 6. | Calcium phosphate/collagen | | Synthetic bone substitute that can be preloaded with suitable antibiotic | Cerasorb® Ortho Foam | FDA, 2020 |
| 7. | Collagen | Gentamicin | Matrix impregnated with the antibiotic | Callatamp® | Health Canada, 2008 |

### 14.3.6 Membrane-Induced Osteogenesis (Masquelet Technique)

Management of posttraumatic or infected bone defects is a challenging job because of the presence of latent infection, poor soft tissue healing, and regenerative capabilities. If these defects are present in the bones of the lower limb, they can cause significant shortening which will result in some form of permanent disability to the patient. One of the techniques that is a good alternative to bone transport is the membrane-induced osteogenesis technique. The method was popularized by Alain Masquelet in the late 1970s for aseptic nonunion in bones of lower limbs, especially tibia [43]. Over time, the technique has been adapted for treating long bone defects in all long bones and a variety of etiologies.

The technique is essentially a two-step procedure and does not need specialized implants. The first step consists of a good debridement, sequestrectomy, soft tissue coverage, and placement of antibiotic-loaded cement to act as a spacer and internal splint. After a variable period of time of one to one and a half months, when the defect site is surgically opened, a distinct soft tissue membrane is found surrounding the cement spacer [43]. This membrane is incised longitudinally, and the cement spacer is removed. The residual space is filled up with autologous or heterologous bone grafts, and appropriate internal fixation is used to provide stability. After the second step, the fracture consolidates and unites well.

Various animal studies have shown the presence of increased vascularity and mesenchymal stem cells that secrete growth factors in the induced membranes [43]. This method is useful in the osteogenesis of all long bones, including the femur, humerus, and tibia. Animal model studies have shown good vascularity and thicker membranes when the technique is used in bones having better muscular envelope.

Membrane-induced osteogenesis best works in situations of short-segment defects and/or noncircumferential defects [44]. The defects of more than 10 cm require excessive autologous bone grafts and should be considered for bone transport or vascularized bone grafts. Draining wounds, poor soft tissue coverage, and smoking are relative contraindications [44].

It is critical to know when to use the membrane-induced osteogenesis technique. We believe the bone defects should be at least 50% of the diameter of the long bone, and a gap of at least 1–2 cm should be present. Santolina et al. identified 10 risk factors of nonunion. The presence of four or more risk factors should be an indication for considering the Masquelet technique [45]. Some researchers are working on a method of combining two methods—membrane-induced osteogenesis and bone transport—to achieve better union rates and improve the quality of regeneration. Thakeb et al. have shown a better outcome for managing larger bone defects with a combination of induced membrane and bone transport, with better union rates [46].

## 14.4 Algorithm of Approach to Infection

The primary aims of the treatment of fracture-related infection are

1. Fracture consolidation.
2. Eradication of infection as the outcome (in certain cases, initial suppression of infection until fracture consolidation is achieved).
3. Healing of the soft tissue envelope.
4. Restoration of function.
5. Prevention of chronic infection/osteomyelitis. [37]

There have been multiple attempts by various study groups across the world to develop algorithms to treat orthopedic infections. But a consensus remains elusive. This is because of a lack of standardization of diagnostic criteria, classification, and treatment regimens. Some good publications include the review article published by Sylvian et al. [47] We have developed our algorithm, which looks to manage fractures, implants, soft tissue defects, bone gaps, and comorbid factors. We emphasize the role of shared decision-making in a team comprising the orthopedic surgeon, plastic surgeon, and infectious disease specialist (Figs. 14.12 and 14.13).

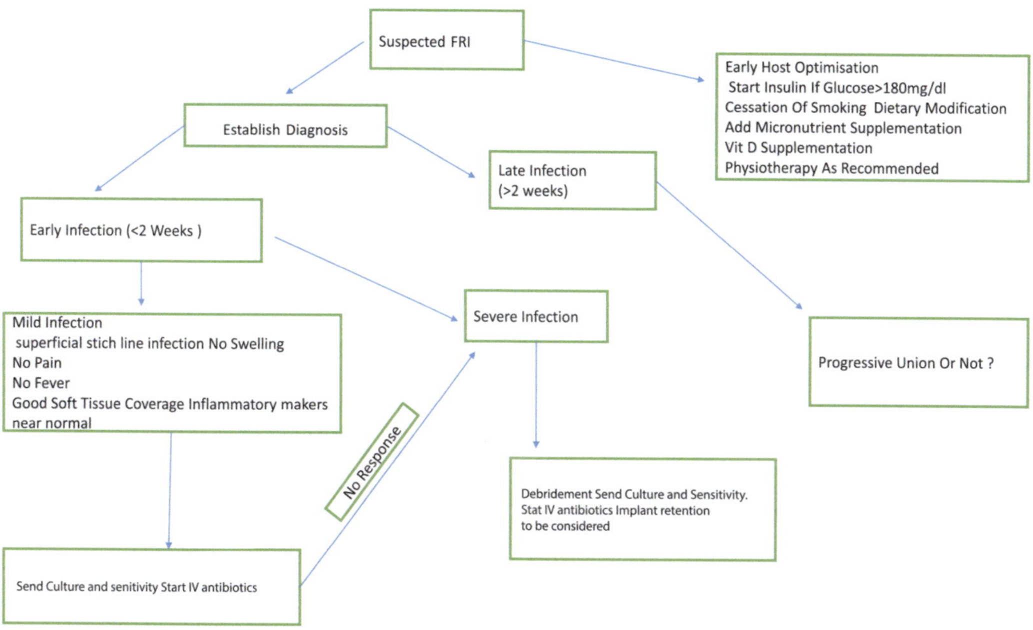


**Fig. 14.12** Flow chart depicting the diagnosis and management of suspected FRI (Fracture-Related Infection)

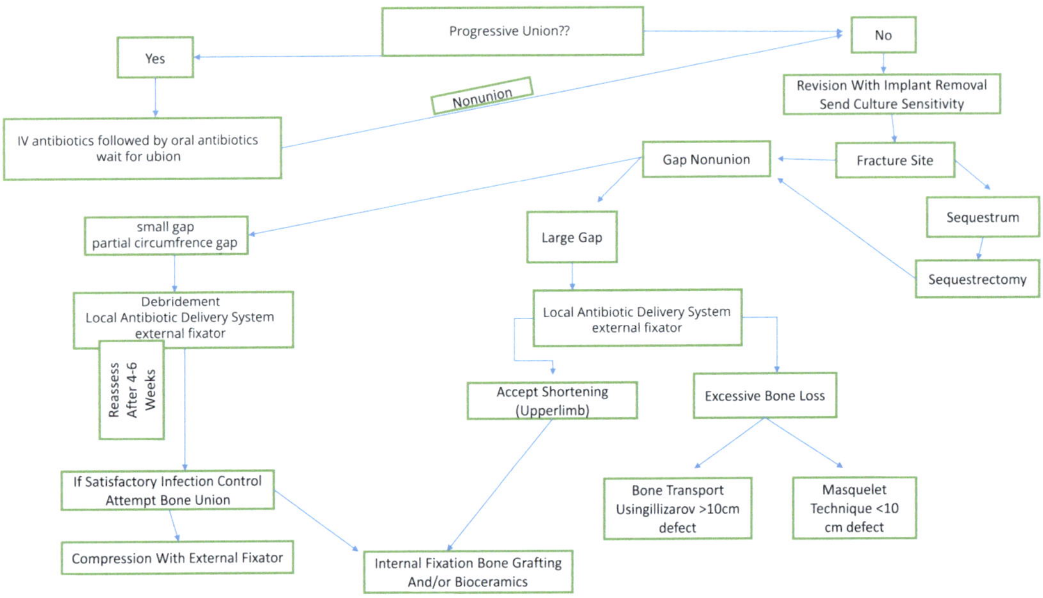


**Fig. 14.13** Flow chart depicting a decision-making process for treatment of infected nonunion

## References


1. Pilskog K, Høvding P, Inderhaug E, Fevang JM, Dale H. Fracture-related infection: prevalence and application of the new consensus definition in a cohort of 1004 surgically treated ankle fractures. Injury. 2023;54(3):841–7. https://doi.org/10.1016/j.injury.2022.12.030. Epub 2023 Jan 6. PMID 36610943
2. O'Connor O, Thahir A, Krkovic M. How much does an infected fracture cost? Arch Bone Jt Surg. 2022;10(2):135–40. https://doi.org/10.22038/abjs.2021.53590.2665. PMID 35655742, PMCID PMC9117895.
3. Metsemakers WJ, Morgenstern M, McNally MA, Moriarty TF, McFadyen I, Scarborough M, et al. Fracture-related infection: a consensus on definition from an international expert group. Injury. 2018;49(3):505–10, ISSN 0020-1383. https://doi.org/10.1016/j.injury.2017.08.040.
4. Depypere M, Morgenstern M, Kuehl R, Senneville E, Moriarty TF, Obremskey WT, et al. Pathogenesis and management of fracture-related infection. Clin Microbiol Infect. 2020;26(5):572–8. https://doi.org/10.1016/j.cmi.2019.08.006. ISSN 1198-743X. PMID 31446152
5. Gordon W, Kuhn K, Staeheli G, Dromsky D. Challenges in definitive fracture management of blast injuries. Curr Rev Musculoskelet Med. 2015;8(3):290–7. https://doi.org/10.1007/s12178-015-9286-7. PMID 26104316, PMCID PMC4596208
6. Wetterslev M, Rose-Larsen K, Hansen-Schwartz J, Steen-Andersen J, Møller K, Møller-Sørensen H. Mechanism of injury and microbiological flora of the geographical location are essential for the prognosis in soldiers with serious warfare injuries. Dan Med J. 2013;60(9):A4704. PMID 24001466
7. Depypere M, Sliepen J, Onsea J, Debaveye Y, Govaert GAM, IJpma FFA, et al. The microbiological etiology of fracture-related infection. Front Cell Infect Microbiol. 2022;12:934485. https://doi.org/10.3389/fcimb.2022.934485. PMID 35873162, PMCID PMC9300981
8. Li J, Cheung WH, Chow SK, Ip M, Leung SYS, Wong RMY. Current therapeutic interventions combating biofilm-related infections in orthopaedics: a systematic review of in vivo animal studies. Bone Joint Res. 2022;11(10):700–14. https://doi.org/10.1302/2046-3758.1110.BJR-2021-0495.R3. PMID 36214177, PMCID PMC9582863
9. Percival SL, McCarty SM, Lipsky B. Biofilms and wounds: an overview of the evidence. Adv Wound Care (New Rochelle). 2015;4(7):373–81. https://doi.org/10.1089/wound.2014.0557. PMID 26155379, PMCID PMC4486148
10. Merritt JH, Kadouri DE, O'Toole GA. Growing and analyzing static biofilms. Curr Protoc Microbiol. 2005;Chapter(1)(1):Unit 1B.1. https://doi.org/10.1002/9780471729259.mc01b01s00. PMID 18770545, PMCID PMC4568995
11. Sutter ST, Frei R, Dangel M, Balmelli C, Schaefer D, Weisser M, et al. Validation of a treatment algorithm for orthopaedic implant-related infections with device-retention-results from a prospective

observational cohort study. Clin Microbiol Infect. 2016;22(5):457.e1–9. https://doi.org/10.1016/j.cmi.2016.01.004. PMID 26806134
12. Coiffier G, Albert J-D, Arvieux C, Guggenbuhl P. Optimizing combination rifampin therapy for staphylococcal osteoarticular infections. Joint Bone Spine. 2013;80(1):11–7. https://doi.org/10.1016/j.jbspin.2012.09.008. PMID 23332140
13. Morgenstern M, Kuehl R, Zalavras CG, McNally M, Zimmerli W, Burch MA, et al. The influence of duration of infection on outcome of debridement and implant retention in fracture-related infection. Bone Joint J. 2021;103-B(2):213–21. https://doi.org/10.1302/0301-620X.103B2.BJJ-2020-1010.R1. PMID 33517743.
14. Dudareva M, Barrett LK, Morgenstern M, Atkins BL, Brent AJ, McNally MA. Providing an evidence base for tissue sampling and culture interpretation in suspected fracture-related infection. J Bone Joint Surg. 2021;103(11):977–83. https://doi.org/10.2106/JBJS.20.00409.
15. Ward CL, Sanchez CJ Jr, Pollot BE, Romano DR, Hardy SK, Becerra SC, et al. Soluble factors from biofilms of wound pathogens modulate human bone marrow-derived stromal cell differentiation, migration, angiogenesis, and cytokine secretion. BMC Microbiol. 2015;15:75. https://doi.org/10.1186/s12866-015-0412-x. PMID 25886581
16. Wade R, Richardson J. Outcome in fracture healing: a review. Injury. 2001;32(2):109–14. https://doi.org/10.1016/s0020-1383(00)00126-1. PMID 11223041
17. Bhattacharyya T, Bouchard KA, Phadke A, Meigs JB, Kassarjian A, Salamipour H. The accuracy of computed tomography for the diagnosis of tibial nonunion. J Bone Joint Surg Am. 2006;88(4):692–7. https://doi.org/10.2106/JBJS.E.00232. PMID 16595457
18. Wenter V, Müller JP, Albert NL, Lehner S, Fendler WP, Bartenstein P, et al. The diagnostic value of [18 F] FDG PET for the detection of chronic osteomyelitis and implant-associated infection. Eur J Nucl Med Mol Imaging. 2016;43(4):749–61. https://doi.org/10.1007/s00259-015-3221-4. PMID 26547722
19. Buckwalter JA, Einhorn TA, Marsh JL, Gulotta L, Ranawat A, Lane J. Bone and joint healing. In: Rockwood and green's fractures in adults. Philadelphia: Lippincott Williams & Wilkins; 2001. p. 245–71.
20. Jiao H, Xiao E, Graves DT. Diabetes and its effect on bone and fracture healing. Curr Osteoporos Rep. 2015;13(5):327–35. https://doi.org/10.1007/s11914-015-0286-8. PMID 26254939, PMCID PMC4692363
21. Castillo RC, Bosse MJ, MacKenzie EJ, Patterson BM, LEAP Study Group. Impact of smoking on fracture healing and risk of complications in limb-threatening open tibia fractures. J Orthop Trauma. 2005;19(3):151–7. https://doi.org/10.1097/00005131-200503000-00001. PMID 15758667
22. Smolle MA, Leitner L, Böhler N, Seibert FJ, Glehr M, Leithner A. Fracture, nonunion and postoperative infection risk in the smoking orthopaedic patient: a systematic review and meta-analysis. EFORT Open Rev. 2021;6(11):1006–19. https://doi.org/10.1302/2058-5241.6.210058. PMID 34909221, PMCID PMC8631245
23. Cierny G III, Mader JT, Penninck JJ. A clinical staging system for adult osteomyelitis. Clin Orthop Relat Res. 2003;414:7–24. https://doi.org/10.1097/01.blo.0000088564.81746.62. PMID 12966271.
24. Depypere M, Kuehl R, Metsemakers WJ, Senneville E, McNally MA, Obremskey WT, et al. Recommendations for systemic antimicrobial therapy in fracture-related infection: a consensus from an international expert group. J Orthop Trauma. 2020;34(1):30–41. https://doi.org/10.1097/BOT.0000000000001626. PMID 31567902, PMCID PMC6903362
25. Zimmerli W, Sendi P. Orthopaedic biofilm infections. APMIS. 2017;125(4):353–64. https://doi.org/10.1111/apm.12687. PMID 28407423
26. Infection. Available from: aofoundation.org.
27. Moojen DJF. The “Magic Number” for microbiological testing for fracture-related infection: commentary on an article by M. Dudareva, BMBCh, MRCP, et al.: “Providing an evidence base for tissue sampling and culture interpretation in suspected fracture-related infection”. J Bone Joint Surg Am. 2021;103(11):e46. https://doi.org/10.2106/JBJS.21.00251. PMID: 34038398
28. Esteban J, Sandoval E, Cordero-Ampuero J, Molina-Manso D, Ortiz-Pérez A, Fernández-Roblas R, et al. Sonication of intramedullary nails: clinically related infection and contamination. Open Orthop J. 2012;6:255–60. https://doi.org/10.2174/1874325001206010255. Epub 2012 Jun 29. PMID 22848337, PMCID PMC3406279
29. The FLOW Investigators. A trial of wound irrigation in the initial management of open fracture wounds. N Engl J Med. 2015;373:2629–41.
30. Schmidt AH, Swiontkowski MF. Pathophysiology of infections after internal fixation of fractures. J Am Acad Orthop Surg. 2000;8(5):285–91. https://doi.org/10.5435/00124635-200009000-00002.
31. Sabaté-Brescó M, Berset CM, Zeiter S, Stanic B, Thompson K, Ziegler M, Richards RG, O'Mahony L, Moriarty TF. Fracture biomechanics influence local and systemic immune responses in a murine fracture-related infection model. Biol Open. 2021;10(9):bio057315. https://doi.org/10.1242/bio.057315. Epub 2021 Oct 1. PMID: 34240122; PMCID: PMC8496694
32. Sliepen J, Corrigan RA, Dudareva M, Wouthuyzen-Bakker M, Rentenaar RJ, Atkins BL, Govaert GAM, McNally MA, IJpma FFA. Does the use of local antibiotics affect clinical outcome of patients with fracture-related infection? Antibiotics (Basel). 2022;11(10):1330. https://doi.org/10.3390/antibiotics11101330. PMID: 36289989; PMCID: PMC9598690

33. Cox G, Jones E, McGonagle D, Giannoudis PV. Reamer-irrigator-aspirator indications and clinical results: a systematic review. Int Orthop. 2011;35(7):951–6. https://doi.org/10.1007/s00264-010-1189-z. Epub 2011 Jan 18. PMID: 21243358; PMCID: PMC3167404
34. Haidari S, IJpma FFA, Metsemakers WJ, Maarse W, Vogely HC, Ramsden AJ, McNally MA, Govaert GAM. The role of negative-pressure wound therapy in patients with fracture-related infection: a systematic review and critical appraisal. Biomed Res Int. 2021;2021:7742227. https://doi.org/10.1155/2021/7742227. PMID: 34722772; PMCID: PMC8548908
35. Quintero JI, Cárdenas LL, Achury AC, Vega-Hoyos D, Bermúdez J. Negative pressure wound therapy as a salvage procedure in venous congestion of microsurgical procedures. Plastic Reconstr Surg Global Open. 2021;9(8):e3725. https://doi.org/10.1097/GOX.0000000000003725.
36. Upton D, Stephens D, Andrews A. Patients' experiences of negative pressure wound therapy for the treatment of wounds: a review. J Wound Care. 2013;22(1):34–9. https://doi.org/10.12968/jowc.2013.22.1.34. Erratum in: J Wound Care 2013 Feb;22(2):73. PMID: 23299356
37. Metsemakers WJ, Morgenstern M, Senneville E, Borens O, Govaert GAM, Onsea J, Depypere M, Richards RG, Trampuz A, Verhofstad MHJ, Kates SL, Raschke M, McNally MA, Obremskey WT, Fracture-Related Infection (FRI) Group. General treatment principles for fracture-related infection: recommendations from an international expert group. Arch Orthop Trauma Surg. 2020;140(8):1013–27. https://doi.org/10.1007/s00402-019-03287-4. Epub 2019 Oct 29. PMID: 31659475; PMCID: PMC7351827
38. Saridis A, Panagiotopoulos E, Tyllianakis M, Matzaroglou C, Vandoros N, Lambiris E. The use of the Ilizarov method as a salvage procedure in infected nonunion of the distal femur with bone loss. J Bone Joint Surg Br. 2006;88-B(2):232–7. https://doi.org/10.1302/0301-620X.88B2.16976.
39. Webb JCJ, Spencer RF. The role of polymethylmethacrylate bone cement in modern orthopaedic surgery. J Bone Joint Surg Br. 2007;89-B(7):851–7. https://doi.org/10.1302/0301-620X.89B7.19148.
40. Dzyuba G, Reznik L, Erofeev S, Odarchenko D. Efficiency of local cement reinforcing antibacterial implants in surgical treatment of long bones chronic osteomyelitis. Khirurgiia. 2016;5:31–6.
41. van Vugt TAG, Arts JJ, Geurts JAP. Antibiotic-loaded polymethylmethacrylate beads and spacers in treatment of orthopedic infections and the role of biofilm formation. Front Microbiol. 2019;10:1626. https://doi.org/10.3389/fmicb.2019.01626. PMID: 31402901; PMCID: PMC6671866
42. Ferguson J, Diefenbeck M, McNally M. Ceramic biocomposites as biodegradable antibiotic carriers in the treatment of bone infections. J Bone Jt Infect. 2017;2(1):38–51. https://doi.org/10.7150/jbji.17234. PMID: 28529863; PMCID: PMC5423569
43. Masquelet AC, Begue T. The concept of induced membrane for reconstruction of long bone defects. Orthop Clin North Am. 2010;41(1):27–37. https://doi.org/10.1016/j.ocl.2009.07.011; table of contents. PMID: 19931050.
44. Mühlhäusser J, Winkler J, Babst R, Beeres FJP. Infected tibia defect fractures treated with the Masquelet technique. Medicine (Baltimore). 2017;96(20):e6948. https://doi.org/10.1097/MD.0000000000006948. PMID: 28514314; PMCID: PMC5440151
45. Hoit G, Kain MS, Sparkman JW, Norris BL, Conway JD, Watson JT, Tornetta P 3rd, Nauth A. The induced membrane technique for bone defects: basic science, clinical evidence, and technical tips. OTA Int. 2021;4(2 Suppl):e106(1-5). https://doi.org/10.1097/OI9.0000000000000106. PMID: 37608856; PMCID: PMC10441675
46. Thakeb MF, Kozman MA, ElGebeily MA, Baraka MM, Al Kersh MA. Bone transport through induced membrane versus conventional bone transport in management of infected long-bone defects of lower limbs: a randomized controlled trial. J Orthop Trauma. 2023;37(9):462–8. https://doi.org/10.1097/BOT.0000000000002613. PMID: 37074808
47. Steinmetz S, Wernly D, Moerenhout K, Trampuz A, Borens O. Infection after fracture fixation. EFORT Open Rev. 2019;4:468–75. https://doi.org/10.1302/2058-5241.4.180093.

# 15 Orthoplasty in the Management of Lower Limb BJI

Cesare Tiengo, Francesca Mazzarella, Daniele Brunelli, Pasquale Zona, Franco Bassetto, Mariachiara Cerchiaro, Andrea Angelini, and Pietro Ruggieri

## 15.1 Introduction

Osteomyelitis, a severe and debilitating bone infection, poses a significant challenge to both patients and healthcare professionals, necessitating innovative approaches for effective treatment and reconstruction. In the realm of plastic surgery, the management of osteomyelitis has witnessed a transformative change with the evolution of both microsurgical and non-microsurgical approaches. Through an in-depth analysis of the current literature, case studies, and expert insights, this chapter seeks to bridge the gap between theoretical knowledge and practical application, facilitating a nuanced understanding of the intricacies involved in the plastic surgical treatment of osteomyelitis, providing perspectives on the multifaceted strategies employed to address incapacitating bone infections.

The integration of microsurgery into the plastic surgeon's armamentarium has revolutionized the treatment of osteomyelitis by providing precision and flexibility in reconstructive options. Vascularized bone grafts, free flaps, and composite tissue transfers have become instrumental in not only eradicating infection but also restoring form and function. This chapter will delve into the intricate details of microsurgical and non-microsurgical interventions, exploring the selection criteria, surgical techniques, and outcomes associated with these cutting-edge procedures.

Furthermore, a holistic understanding of osteomyelitis demands an exploration of the underlying etiology, diagnostic modalities, and antimicrobial therapies that form the foundation of any successful treatment plan.

Concurrently, non-microsurgical approaches to osteomyelitis have also demonstrated significant advancements, offering viable alternatives in certain clinical scenarios. Local and regional flaps, antibiotic impregnated bone cement and bioengineered scaffolds are among the non-microsurgical techniques that have gained success [1].

While dehiscence of the soft tissue overlying the incision may occur, most patients undergoing arthroplasty or osteosynthesis have a

C. Tiengo (✉)
Reconstructive and Aesthetic Surgery at the University of Padua, Padua, Italy
e-mail: cesare.tiengo@unipd.it

F. Mazzarella
Loughborough University, London, UK
e-mail: francesca.mazzarella@aopd.veneto.it

D. Brunelli
University of Modena, Modena, Italy
e-mail: daniele.brunelli@aopd.veneto.it

P. Zona · F. Bassetto
University of Padua, Padua, Italy
e-mail: franco.bassetto@unipd.it

M. Cerchiaro · A. Angelini · P. Ruggieri
Department of Orthopedics and Traumatology and Oncological Orthopedics, University of Padua, Padua, Italy
e-mail: andrea.angelini@unipd.it; pietro.ruggieri@unipd.it




P. Ruggieri et al. (eds.), *Bone and Joint Infections*, https://doi.org/10.1007/978-3-031-96383-4_15

straightforward postoperative wound healing course. A soft tissue, bone, or implant infection may exacerbate the ensuing abnormalities in 1–12% of patients. Severe soft tissue loss or superficial skin loss may coexist with such infections. Therefore, the presence of exposed metal or bone frequently adds to the complexity of the issue. There is no universal agreement on how to treat wound exposure, despite the fact that it puts the implant and the bone at danger. The numerous factors affecting the management alternatives are mostly to blame for this.

### 15.1.1 Conservative Approach

We have witnessed an increased number of infections resulting from surgical procedures related to these traumatic lesions, which frequently take the form of posttraumatic osteomyelitis and serious soft tissue infections. This is due to high-energy trauma with extensive damage to soft tissues, necessitating more aggressive treatments for open and closed fractures. In the given situation, osteomyelitis, especially posttraumatic osteomyelitis, is a serious public health concern due to the steady rise in traumatic injuries and the consequences they cause [2].

Treatment for osteomyelitis, especially those involving implants, is largely dependent on both appropriate antibiotic therapy and significant surgical debridement. The hazards of bacteremia resulting from surgical manipulation of infection without sufficient antibiotic coverage are mitigated by initiating empirical antibiotics during anesthetic induction. However, it has no effect on the positive cultures obtained during the process. When non-septic patients' culture samples are collected, empirical antibiotics can also be administered. Given the significance of *Staphylococcus aureus* in epidemiology, empirical coverage of this agent is advised. Even in cases that were community-acquired, the local prevalence of methicillin resistance varies and needs to be monitored. Initial treatment for acute infections may need thorough surgical cleansing followed by 4–6 weeks of antibiotic administration.

Treatment for chronic infections should involve extensive surgical debridement, implant removal, and a 3–6 month course of antibiotics.

For more than 30 years, the reconstructive ladder has operated in its contemporary, conventional form. Its gradually more complex procedures to treat wounds and other soft tissue defects are still valid, as long as closure stays within these three categories: (1) direct closure (primary or secondary); (2) nonoperative, topical wound healing (advanced secondary intention methods, including NPWT); and (3) tissue transfer, which includes both vascularized and nonvascularized transfers (e.g., split- or full-thickness skin grafts, fat transfer, cartilage or bone grafts, etc.) [3].

A guide for varying degrees of open wound interventions is the reconstructive ladder. The use of the ladder is altered by NPWT and, more recently, NPWTi-d, as it is now simpler to move between the ladder's "rungs" by altering the initial defect during initial wound care. The parameters of the defect will frequently change during the strategy selection process for wound treatment, making a less invasive method possible. As a result, the reconstructive plan becomes more flexible and is modified at each NPWTi-d review. Additionally, NPWTi-d can improve closure and minimize the use of certain reconstruction techniques.

### 15.1.2 Reconstructive Approach

While some authors have recommended free tissue transfers or pedicled fasciocutaneous flaps, such as an anterolateral thigh flap for the treatment of periprosthetic infections of the knee, local muscle flaps are considered the most useful for reconstruction in cases of an exposed prosthesis. Primary soft tissue coverage with a medial or lateral gastrocnemius transposition flap has become the primary reconstructive method of choice. The proximally based gracilis and semimembranosus muscles have been used for supplemental coverage after detachment of their tendon distally [4].

The gracilis muscle has been used both as a free flap and as a proximally based pedicled flap, secondary to the adequacy of its proximal vascular pedicle and minimal associated morbidity. A distally based gracilis muscle flap nourished by distal vascular pedicles has been proposed to cover areas of proximal tendon exposure in the knee. In cases where a lateral or medial gastrocnemius flap is not available, or to treat large defects of the soft tissues in combination with the use of a gastrocnemius flap, we proposed the use of an extended reversed gracilis flap based on secondary pedicles (the GReSP flap) for the reconstruction of large defects of the knee.

## 15.2 Pedicled Flaps

### 15.2.1 Rectus Abdominis Musculocutaneous Flap

The rectus abdominis musculocutaneous flap is type III according to the Mathes and Nahai classification. It can be used as a muscular or as a musculocutaneous flap, allowing several types of reconstructions. Depending on the orientation of its skin paddle, it is divided into transverse rectus abdominis musculocutaneous (TRAM) flap and vertical rectus abdominis musculocutaneous (VRAM) flap. It is based on two main pedicles: the deep inferior epigastric artery (DIEA) and the superior epigastric artery. The rectus abdominis muscle measures about 30 x 10 cm and can be used as pedicled or microsurgical flap. The principal vessel, the DIEA, measures 14–18 cm in length and has a caliber of about 3–4 mm [5]. It arises from the external femoral artery and travels superomedially in the extraperitoneal tissue piercing the transversalis fascia. After leaving several branches, it enters the rectus sheath anterior to the arcuate line. Normally, it divides into two or three major vessels that run cranially into the muscle belly, originating several muscular or musculocutaneous perforators. These vessels, which are usually bigger when originating from the medial raw, supply the skin paddle. The main venous drainage is granted by the deep inferior epigastric vein, which is connected to the external iliac vein. Preoperatively, an angio-TC is advisable to investigate the abdominal wall vessels. The VRAM is one of the principal solutions for periacetabular reconstructions (Fig. 15.1).

#### 15.2.1.1 Surgical Technique

*Patient Positioning*: The patient is placed in the supine position.

*Incision:* The orientation of the skin paddle is tailored to the extension and on the orientation of the defect.

*Harvest*: The flap is raised medially to laterally, in the subfascial plan, isolating the chosen perforator.

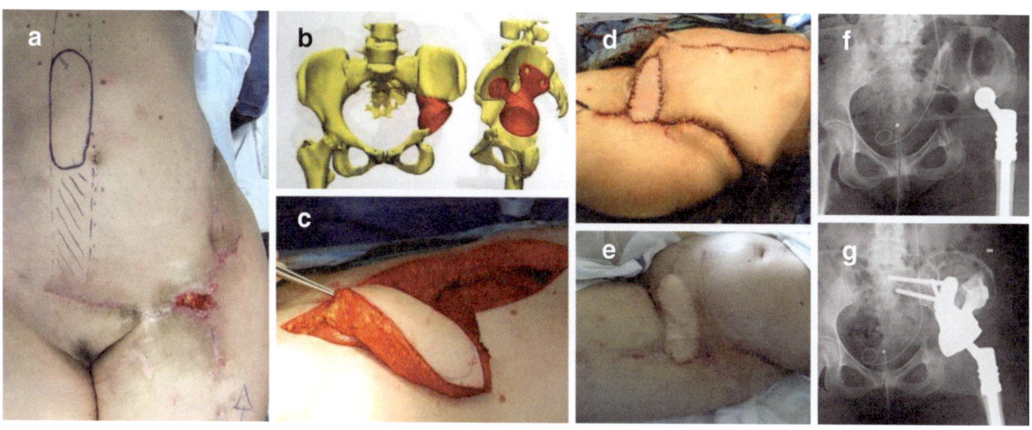


**Fig. 15.1** Management of an acetabular chronic infection using a VRAM pedicled flap (**a**), together with an acetabular custom prosthesis (**b**). The flap is harvested and inset (**c**, **d**), with postoperative outcomes demonstrating total coverage of the initial defect (**e**). Radiographic pre- and postoperative images are shown in images (**f**) and (**g**)

*Vascular Pedicle Dissection*: Usually, the rectus sheath is approached medially, far from the skin paddle, in order to preserve the skin perforators. The muscle can be easily separated from the posterior fascia, but care must be taken when handling the pedicle, which usually lies on the posterior surface of the muscle belly.

*Flap Transfer*: The flap is then inset to the recipient site. For acetabular defects, the flap is tubulized onto the inguinal area and inset at the desired site; the insetting of the flap must be tension-free to avoid necrosis, flap loss, or dehiscences. In case a free flap is necessary, the pedicle is ligated proximally and transferred to cover the damage.

*Closure*: In the case of large defects, a synthetic mesh or an acellular dermal matrix can be used to restore the integrity of the donor site. Even though both alternatives have been described, most authors prefer the synthetic options, especially to avoid long-term hernias or bulging, which are costly and may be challenging to manage. It is very important that the mesh does not decubitate on the pedicle and its course is regular and without twistings or kinkings.

*Postoperative Care*: To minimize dehiscences, the patient is placed in a semi-orthostatic position with the bed inclined at 45 degrees for the first 3 days after the operation. Additional abdominal girdle must be worn for approximately 40–60 days.

### 15.2.2 Reversed Gracilis Pedicle Flap for Coverage of a Total Knee Prosthesis

Total knee arthroplasty (TKA) is a common procedure for end-stage knee arthritis. However, complications such as wound dehiscence, infection, and exposure of the prosthesis can occur, necessitating soft tissue coverage. The reversed gracilis pedicle flap, introduced by Masquelet et al. in 2018, has gained popularity for its simplicity and reliability in providing soft tissue coverage around the knee. The flap is based on the descending branch of the medial circumflex femoral artery (MCFA), which supplies the gracilis muscle. The pedicle is dissected in a retrograde manner, preserving the main trunk of the MCFA. The flap is then rotated 180 degrees and tunnelled subcutaneously to cover the exposed prosthesis. The gracilis muscle provides a robust and well-vascularized soft tissue cover, reducing the risk of infection and promoting wound healing. The reversed gracilis pedicle flap has been shown to have a low complication rate and excellent functional outcomes in patients undergoing TKA.

The gracilis muscle belly is depicted during its mobilization as a reversed flap based on its secondary pedicles. The muscular dissection is carried to the entry of the proximal secondary pedicle. The proximal tendon of the gracilis muscle is then transected to provide the maximal length for the muscle flap. After adequate blood flow is confirmed, the main vascular and nervous pedicles are ligated. The muscle flap is reversed 180 degrees and tunnelled under the residual skin of the anterior aspect of the distal part of the thigh, in order to reach the exposed prosthesis.

**Clinical Case** Total knee prosthesis exposition in a 72-year-old woman with preliminary CT angiographic study and its repair through reversed gracilis pedicle flap.

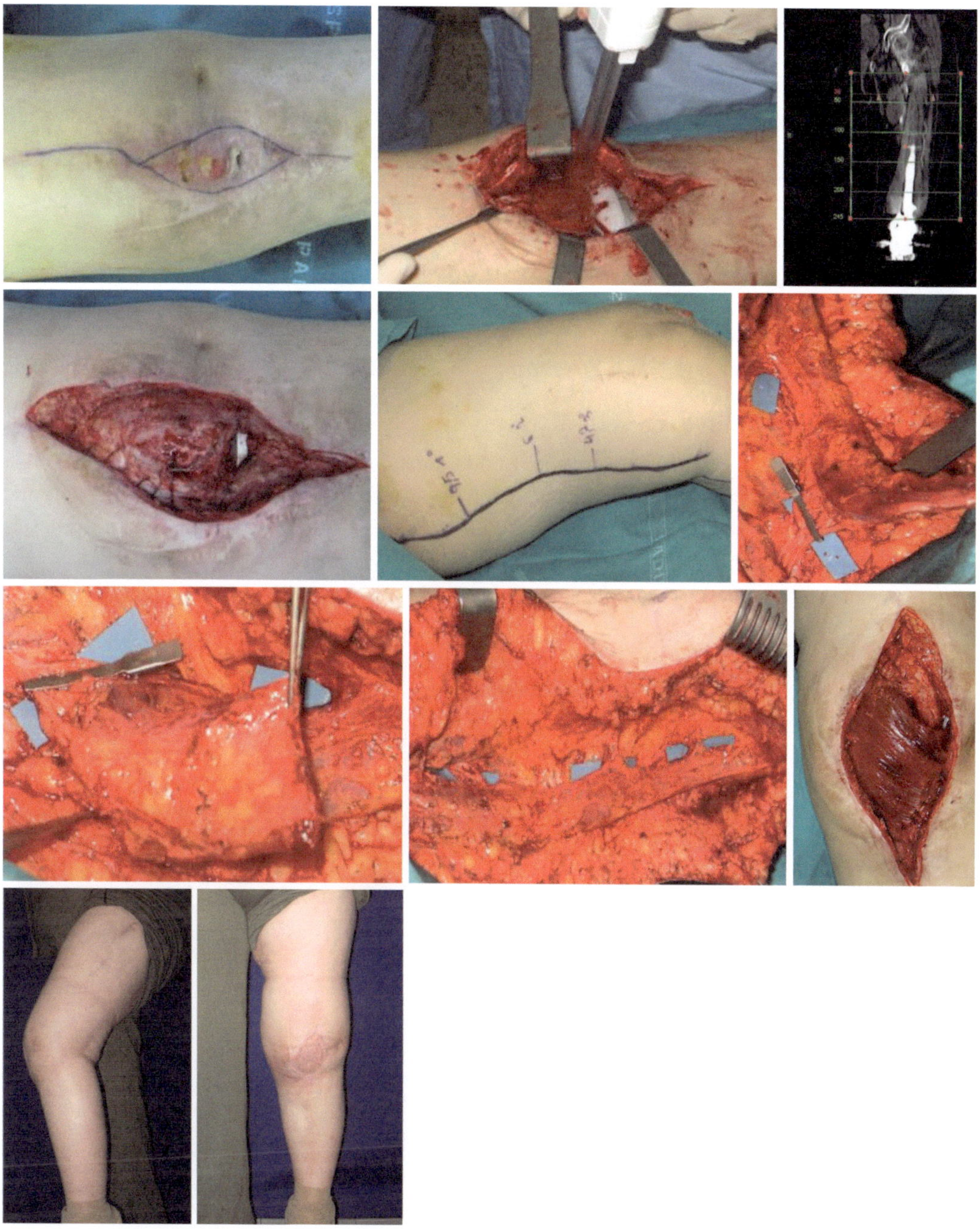

One of the most challenging problems for surgeons performing knee joint reconstructions is skin necrosis after total knee arthroplasty, which is a significant complication. The greatest approach to lower the likelihood of deep infection, prosthetic implant removal, or amputation is through early reconstructive intervention. Rather than employing local fasciocutaneous flaps or tissue expanders to cover such lesions, the presence of many scars over the knee area and the resulting poor skin vascularization sometimes need the use of a pedicled muscle flap dissected from the leg. A common and proximally based pedicled flap is the gracilis muscle, which is distantly based and fed by secondary vascular pedicles and can be an effective addition or substitute to a medial or lateral gastrocnemius flap.

### 15.2.3 Gastrocnemius Flap

The gastrocnemius flap is probably the most useful for covering the leg and knee (Figs. 15.2, 15.3, 15.4, 15.5 and 15.6). The sampling technique is simple and the blood supply is reliable. Both upper extremities of the gastrocnemius are supplied by the sural arteries which come from the popliteal artery and which are accompanied by motor nerves. Both can be mobilized on their own neurovascular peduncle. The blood supply is type 1 sec. The Mathes and Nahai classification [6].

The medial upper extremity is used more often than the lateral. The medial head is longer and its rotation arc allows easy coverage of the proximal third of the tibia and the anterior and medial aspect of the knee.

#### 15.2.3.1 Surgical Technique

*Patient positioning:* the patient is supine with an extra-rotated limb and semi-flexed knee. The incision begins in the middle of the calf, behind the posteromedial edge of the shinbone, and then curves proximally to reach the popliteal fossa.

*Incision:* the incision may be extended along the thigh. Particular care must be taken to avoid injury to the vein and saphenous nerve. The deep aponeurosis is incised on the same line as the skin incision [7]. The muscular plane is developed by inserting a finger between the soleus and the medial head [8]. The sural nerve is located on the posterior surface of the gastrocnemius, enclosed in an aponeurotic layer. The nerve is freed and separated posteriorly. The space between the two ends of the

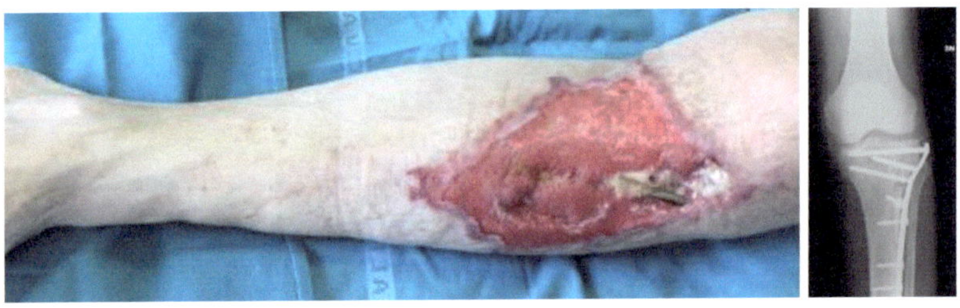

**Fig. 15.2** Clinical case of a 60-year-old man with Gustilo II fracture

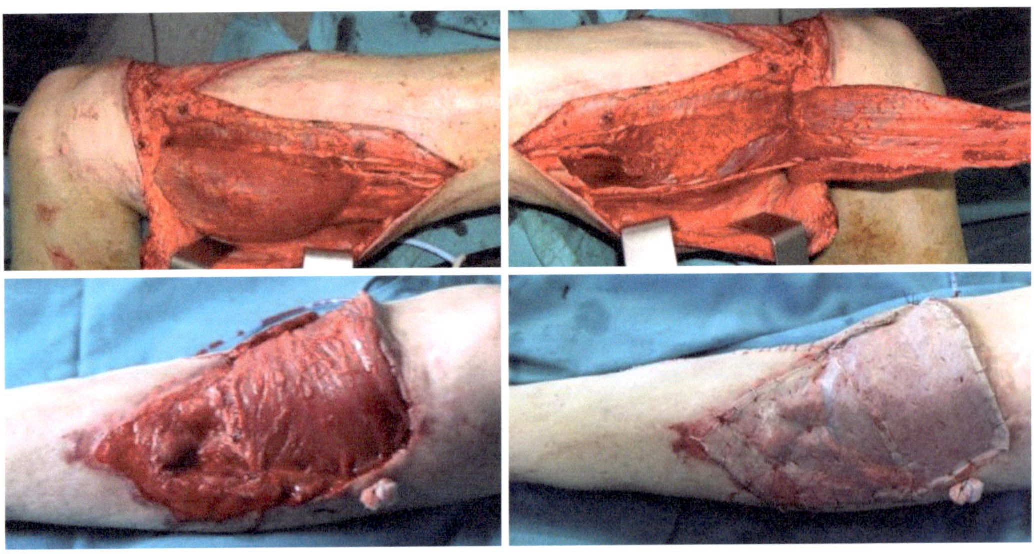

**Fig. 15.3** Sculpt of the gastrocnemius flap and its transposition to cover the bloody area and its coverage with dermo-epidermal graft

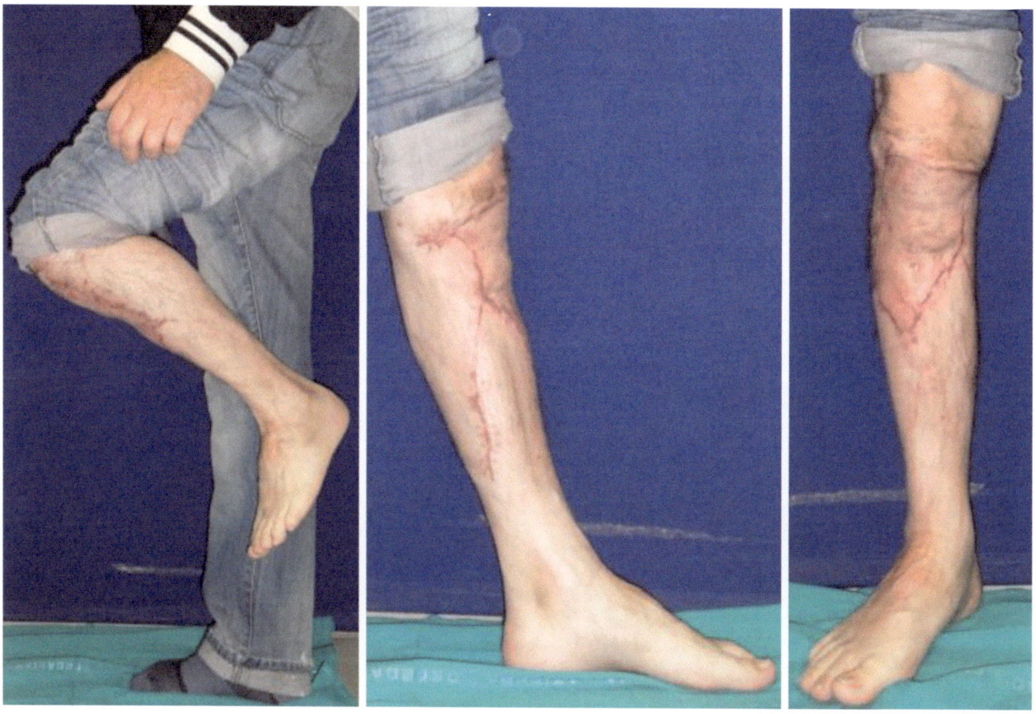

**Fig. 15.4** Fu after 1 year with good functional recovery

muscle is identified, sparing the neurovascular peduncle. The distal tendon is dissected. The muscle is gradually raised distally/proximally. The motor nerve must be interrupted to avoid postoperative pain caused by muscle contraction. The arc of rotation can be increased to free the origin of the muscle from the femur (Figs. 15.3 and 15.4). The medial head of the gastrocnemius, isolated on its vascular peduncle, must be passed underneath the semitendinosus and the gracilis, so as to reach the anterior surface of the knee [9].

### 15.2.4 Soleus Flap

The soleus is particularly useful to cover the leg's defects. It is located superficially in the posterior compartment and often it remains unharmed in open fractures of the middle third of the shinbone, also for this reason its elective is the middle third of the leg. Due to its size, often it is necessary to resort to the preparation of a medial hemisoleus which is simpler than transferring the entire muscle. The muscle is type II sec. The Mathes and Nahai classification [6]. It is vascularized by the posterior tibial and peroneal arteries which send many branches to the muscle. Each of the arteries supplies a proximal pedicle, a large median pedicle, and smaller, variable pedicles along the distal third [10]. The entire muscle can survive if supplied by the two main proximal peduncles and for this reason the muscle can be transferred without separating it from its origin [11].

#### 15.2.4.1 Surgical Technique

*Patient positioning:* the patient is placed supine with the limb extrarotated and the knee semi-flexed.

*Incision:* the incision is made halfway between the medial melleolus and the Achilles tendon. It is carried proximally up to the upper quarter of the leg posterior to the medial edge of the shinbone, taking care not to damage the vein and saphenous nerve. The plane between the soleus and gastrocnemius is identified and numerous subcutaneous peduncles are cauter-

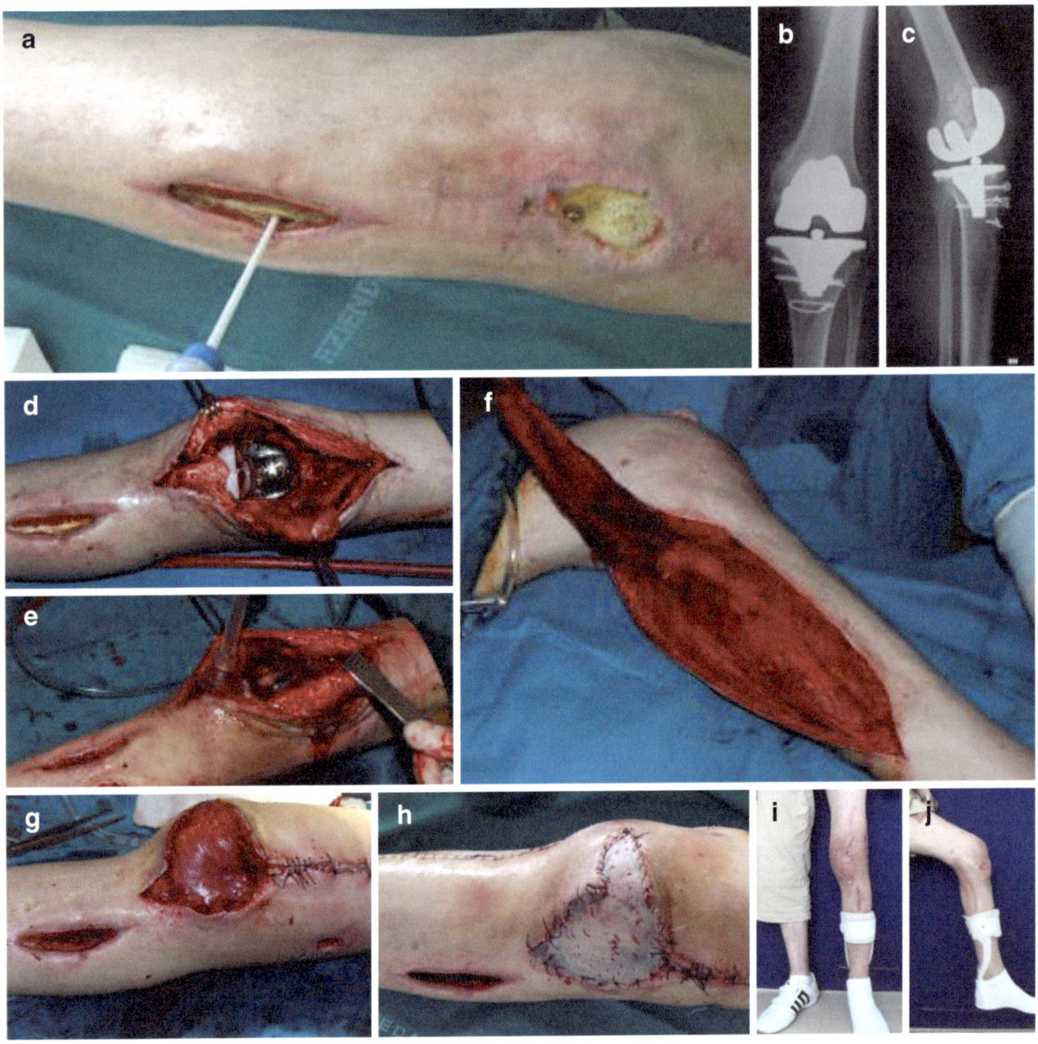


**Fig. 15.5** Clinical case of a patient with surgical fistula (**a**) after posttraumatic reconstruction with a double knee prosthesis (**b**, **c**). After pulsatile lavage of the orthopedical device (**d**, **e**) a pedicled gastrocnemius flap was elevated (**f**) and inset (**g**) to cover the soft tissue that was then covered with skin graft (**h**). Postoperative images (**i**, **j**) show 8 months outcomes

ized. It is important during the dissection to spare the intermuscular fascia that divides the two compartments in order to protect the posterior shinbone neurovascular bundle. Halfway between the medial malleolus and the knee joint there is a large peduncle that derives from the posterior shinbone vessels which must be tied to allow rotation. The distal liberation of the superficial aspect of the soleus from the gastrocnemius, with which the soleus forms the Achilles tendon, it represents another crucial point. In this case, it will be necessary to free the soleus aponeurosis from the gastrocnemius and incised to separate it completely from the Achilles tendon, saving a thin layer of aponeurosis to avoid retracting effects on the distal part of the muscle. The final phase will consist of freeing the muscle from its lateral insertions, the lateral margin must be freed as proximally as possible to allow rotation of the flap. The distal two-thirds are then mobilized and once rotated to cover defects on the anterior surface of the middle third of the shinbone.

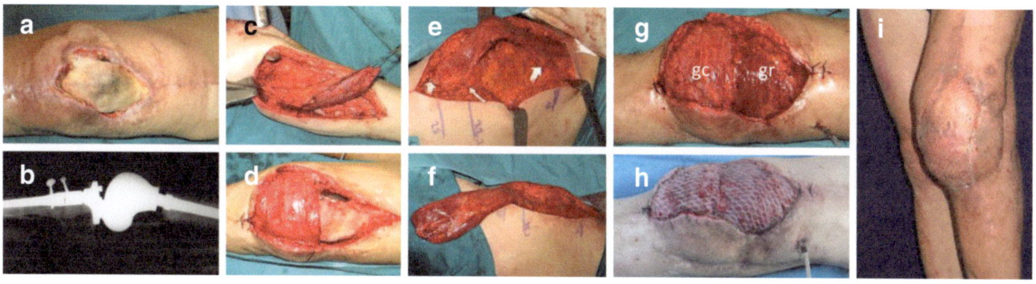


**Fig. 15.6** Case report of patellar region necrosis following double knee prosthesis (**a**, **b**). To cover the soft tissue a combination of medial gastrocnemius (**c**, **d**) and reverse gracilis (**e**, **f**) pedicled flaps was used: image g shows the two muscles inset (gc: gastrocnemius, gr: gracilis). A skin graft was then used to cover the area (**h**). Postoperative images demonstrate good esthetical outcomes (**i**)

### 15.2.5 Vascularized Fibula Flap

In limb reconstructive surgery, the vascularized fibula transplant plays a very important role. The vascularized fibula represents one of the main reconstructive flaps for the repair of long bone defects, in fact many bone areas and joints can make use of this procedure, especially in cases of serious trauma or surgery to remove tumors (Fig. 15.7). Removal of the fibula does not produce functional deficit. The main indication for use is represented by long defects of the leg, particularly useful in defects greater than 5 cm. Complex transfers benefit from the inclusion of the lateral hemisoleum or a skin package supplied by the peroneal artery in the transplant.

The fibula is supplied by the artery of the same name. The artery penetrates the bone at the junction between the proximal third and the middle third [8]. Periosteum and muscle insertions contribute to vascularization. From a hemodynamic point of view it is good to lift a muscular cuff together with the fibula, e.g., flexor hallucis longus or tibialis posterior [12]. The raised peroneal artery together with the bony tract can be useful for restoring the continuity of the main vascular axis of the recipient limb [8, 13].

#### 15.2.5.1 Surgical Technique

*Patient positioning:* the patient is supine with the limb slightly internally rotated and the knee semi-flexed, with a soft aid placed under the ipsilateral buttock. The operation is performed in the ischemic band. We proceed by incising at the level of the middle third of the leg and the aponeurosis is incised on the same line as the skin incision to identify and develop the plane between the soleus and peroneal muscles. The separation of the soleus and peroneal muscles allows the exposure of the lateral aspect of the fibula. On the front of this bone, there is the septum which separates the peroneal compartment from the extensor compartment and which is incised. Behind the fibula, the arch of the soleus is freed in its upper part. The liberation of the soleus, posteriorly, projects the posterior tibial artery and the origin of the peroneal artery [13]. The interosseous membrane is incised near the fibula. The flexor of the hallucis is freed extra-periosteally, although a small section of the flexor of the hallucis must be left inserted on the bone, in order to protect the peroneal vessels. Its divarication allows the exposure of the peroneal vessels and the posterior tibial nerve. To remember the vessels occupy a medial position with respect to the nerve. At the front, it will be necessary to include a section of the tibialis posterior muscle in the transplant. This curtailment avoids injury to the peroneal vessels and improves venous return. The periosteum is incised and separated at the two ends of the transplant. The transplant is isolated and externally rotated to expose the tibialis posterior. After ligating the vessels and sectioning distally, the graft remains connected to

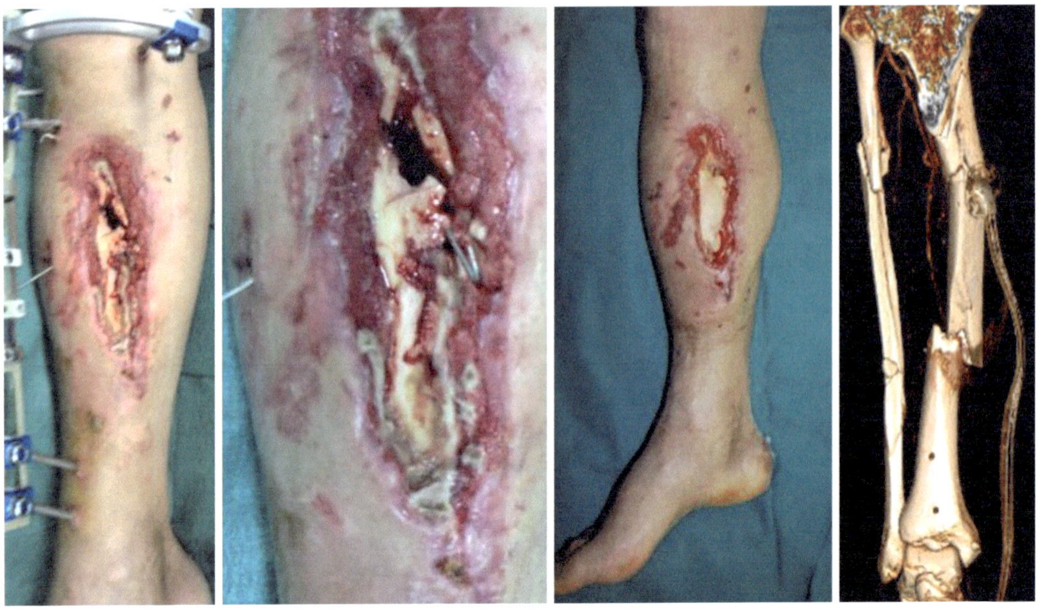

**Fig. 15.7** Clinical case: A 60-year-old woman; osteomyelitis on open fracture Gustilo IIIB

its proximal pedicle, which will be ligated and sectioned at its origin in the posterior tibial artery, or it is preserved to create a pedicled flap (Fig. 15.8). A skin island is drawn on the middle third of the leg that will be included in the transplant (Fig. 15.9).

### 15.2.6 Peroneal Artery Perforator-Based Propeller Flap

The peroneal artery perforator-based flap can be readily elevated for use as a propeller flap following dissection [14]. A localized fasciocutaneous flap that arises from a dissected perforator is an example of this type of flap. Here, the proximal leg's skin can be used for surgical reconstruction in the distal lower extremity, utilizing a propeller flap with a 180-degree perforator to reliably fill the soft tissue defect [15] (Fig. 15.10).

#### 15.2.6.1 Surgical Technique

*Patient Positioning*: The peroneal artery perforator-based propeller flaps are typically positioned along the lateral aspect of the lower leg from the lateral malleolus and can be identified preoperatively by Doppler ultrasound scanning. The propeller flap's size and form must then be planned in the vicinity of the principal perforator that is closest to the flaw. The distance between the perforator closest to the defect location plus the longitudinal length of the defect equals the longitudinal length of the flap.

*Incision:* An anterior or posterior incision is done, depending on where the defect is located.

The shape and size of the propeller flap based on a perforator are contingent upon the defect region and the perforator's limiting spatial constraint.

In order to create an isolated and mobilized fasciocutaneous flap that can be rotated 180 degrees to match the defect, the perforator is dissected to allow for rotation and mobility. The donor-site area that was opened by the flap's rotation can either be sutured directly or closed with skin grafting.

In brief, the following is a description of the specifics of the surgical procedures: Step 1: To construct the flap prior to surgery, the peroneal perforator was located and marked using a Doppler ultrasonography. Step 2: The flap was created using the perforator location that was

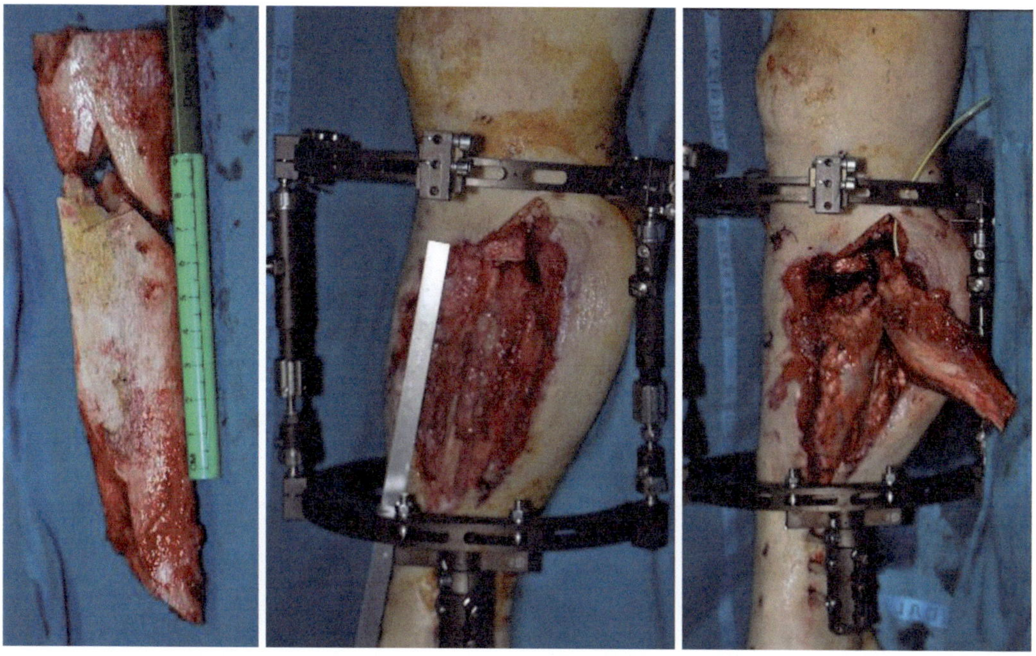

**Fig. 15.8** Tibial resection with extensive debridement; Tibial pro-gap fibula perforator bone flap

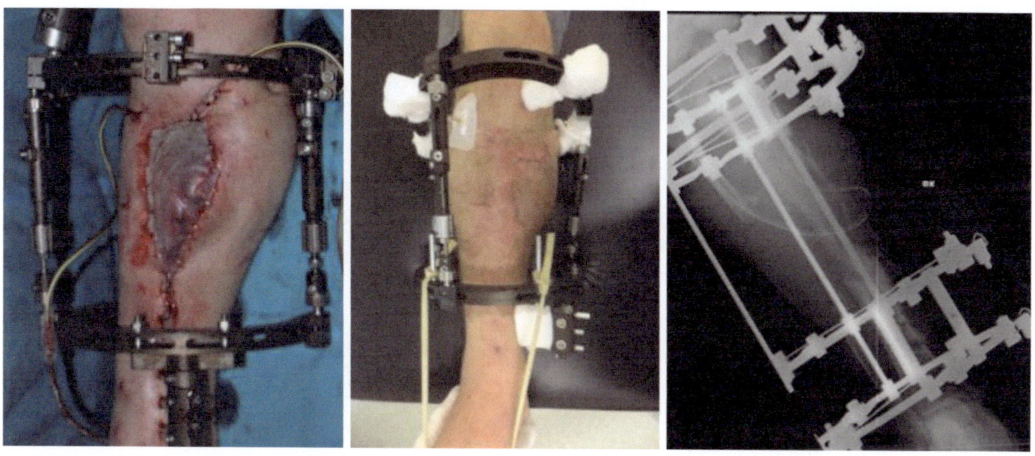

**Fig. 15.9** At 7 months full weight with extended knee brace; no pain

assessed before surgery; the perforator vessel was used as the rotational axis, and the posterolateral border of the fibula was used as an axis. The large propeller is located close to the axis. The distance between the pivot point and the distal point of the wound is less than the length of the large propeller by 0.5–1 cm. The region between the axis point and the flaw is the tiny propeller. Step 3: The anterior edge of the flap was dissected in accordance with the preoperative design. The width of the flap is 1–2 cm wider than the defect, and this size difference is determined by the thickness of the subcutaneous fat. Step 4: In order to lessen the obstruction to venous drainage caused by the compression of the vascular pedicle following rotation, the fascia tissues of the intermuscular septum surrounding it were also carefully

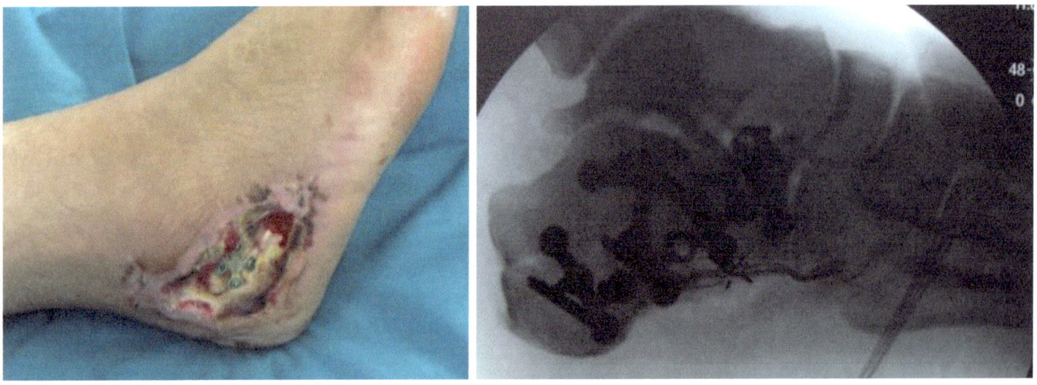

**Fig. 15.10** Clinical case: male; 40-year old; calcalnear fracture previously treated with plates and screws and primary closure

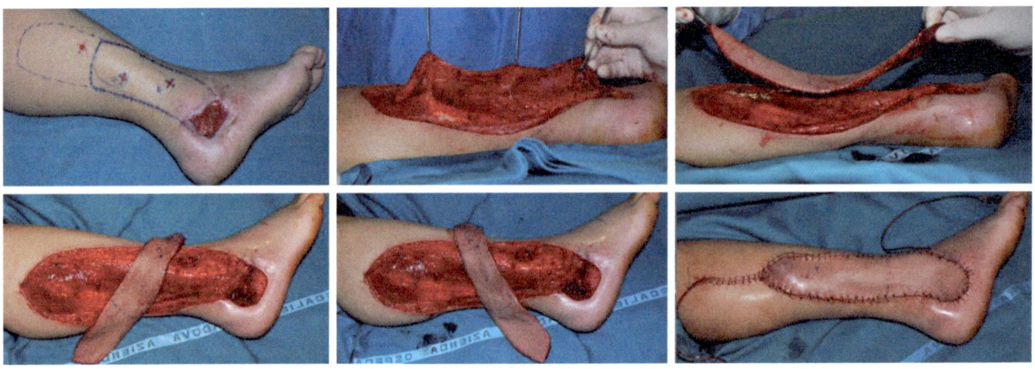

**Fig. 15.11** Dissection of the perforator enables rotation and allows sufficient mobility so that a fasciocutaneous flap can be isolated and is then rotated 180 degrees like a "propeller." The opened section due to the rotated flap being moved away from its point of origin is then repaired with direct suturing or skin grafting. The proximal point of the propeller flap and the pivot point of the flap (the position of the peroneal perforator visible in the third, fourth, and fifth figures); and (last figure) the distal point of the wound

removed. Step 5: The vascular pedicle's conditions were observed following its twisting and compression due to the 180-degree rotation. Step 6: If blood circulation was good after the rotation, the flap was sutured to the wound and the donor site of the flap was sutured directly (Figs. 15.11 and 15.12).

### 15.2.7 Sural Flap

The sural flap is a pedicled option for restoration of small defects of the Achilleal and the lateral malleolar region (Fig. 15.13). It is based on the sural artery that extends on the posterior aspect of the calf with numerous anastomosis with the peroneal artery; the most distal is found approximately three fingers above the lateral malleolus and is generally considered the pivot point. This

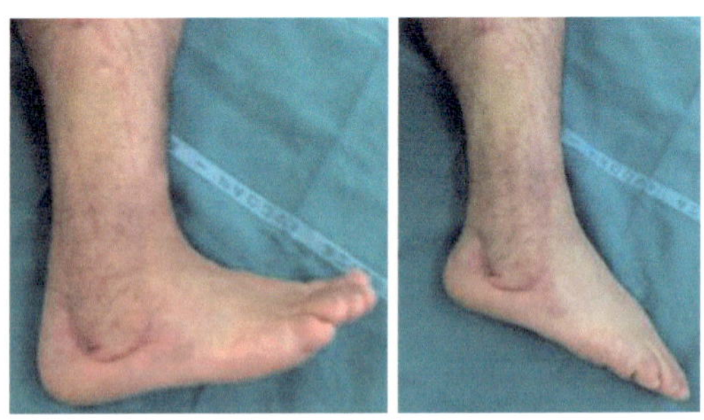

**Fig. 15.12** Eight month follow-up showing satisfactory mobility recovery and excellent functional-esthetic outcome

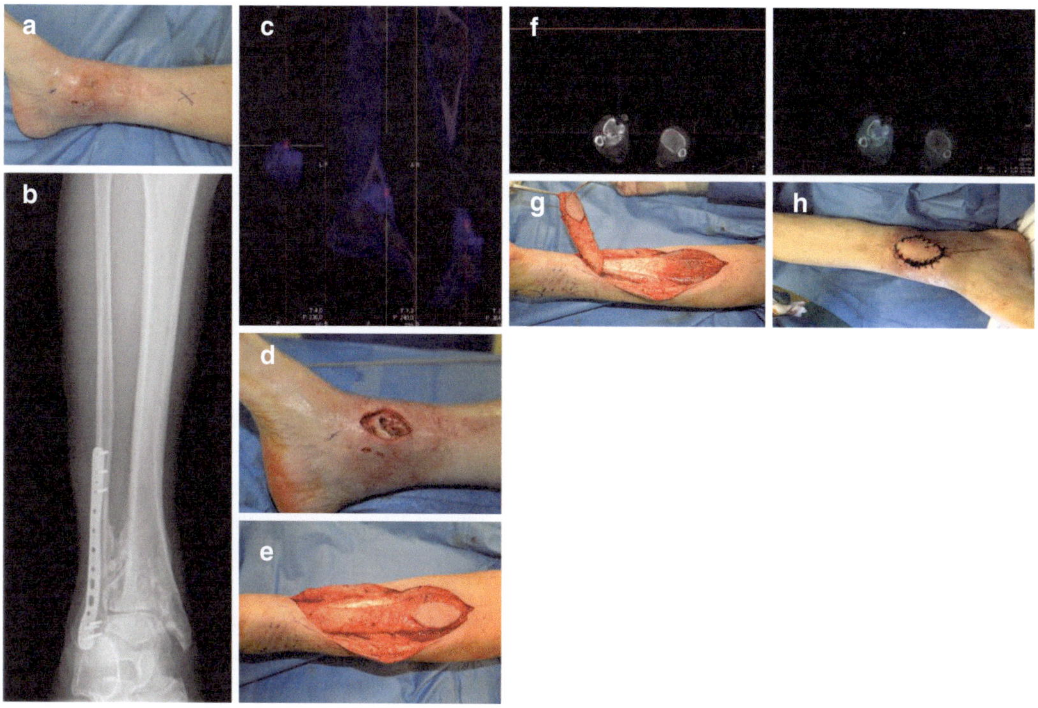


**Fig. 15.13** Case report of a 79-year-old male with chronic osteomyelitis due to posttraumatic tibial and fibular fractures, treated with plaques (**a**). Radiological findings showing delay of osteosintesis (**b**) and an augmented metabolic activity at the tibial surgical site, suggesting underlying infection (**c**, **d**). After debridement of non-vital tissue (**e**) the patient was positioned in a prone position and a sural flap was harvested and elevated (**f**, **g**). Postoperative result with inset of the flap to cover the initial tibial defect (**h**)

fasciocutaneous flap contains the sural nerve, the sural artery, and the sural vein that ensures the venous drainage [16]. It cannot be inset proximally to the junction of the two heads of the gastrocnemius muscle, as above this level nerve and artery runs beneath the fascia.

#### 15.2.7.1 Surgical Technique

*Patient Positioning*: the patient is placed in a prone position.

*Incision*: The flap is usually raised from the junction of the two heads of the gastrocnemius muscle, with the incision prolonged distally among the expected course of the sural vein and artery.

*Harvest and flap transfer*: The dissection is then performed until the aforementioned pivot point, therefore allowing isolation of the neurovascular pedicle and its aponeurosis. Small anastomosis branches from the peroneal artery must be ligated in order to isolate the desired vessel. Finally, a distal incision is performed to properly bury the pedicle.

*Closure*: A distal incision is performed to properly bury the pedicle, while the donor site can be either closed with a skin graft or primarily.

## 15.3 Microsurgical Flaps

### 15.3.1 Anterolateral Thigh Flap

The anterolateral thigh (ALT) flap is a well-known and versatile free flap that is based on the lateral circumflex femoral artery (LCFA) perforators. This branch of the profunda femoris artery originates 8–10 cm distal to the anterior superior iliac spine, and it divides into three main branches: ascending, transverse, and descending. The descending one runs on the medial side of the vastus lateralis giving off several perforator vessels to the fascia and the overlying fat and skin. This flap can be raised as fasciocutaneous, fascial, composite, including a portion of the rectus femoris muscle, or chimeric with a part of the vastus lateralis muscle (Figs. 15.9 and 15.10). Preoperative Angio–CT scan is mandatory to properly plan the flap, especially in patients where damage of the vascular system is suspected.

#### 15.3.1.1 Surgical Technique

*Patient Positioning*: The patient is placed in the supine position; if the defect is contralateral to the donor site, the lower extremities are usually parallel, otherwise there are no specific position for the unaffected lower limbs.

*Incision:* The skin island is generally taken centrally over the chosen perforator, with a variable dimension based on the defect size: skin island up to 8 cm may be closed primarily, although greater dimensions have been described [17]. The pedicle length is around 11 cm with a caliber of 2.1 mm. The venous drainage depends on a series of vessels that drains in the greater saphenous vein.

*Harvest*: The flap is raised medially to laterally, in the subfascial plan, isolating the chosen perforator.

*Vascular Pedicle Dissection*: Once identified, the perforator is carefully dissected retrogradely through the muscle to its origin from the descending branch of the LCFA. Depending on the necessity of the pedicle length, dissection of the LCFA can be continued proximally.

*Flap Transfer*: The flap is then inset to the recipient site. The vascular pedicle is anastomosed using microsurgical techniques.

*Closure*: The incision in the thigh is closed in layers, and a drain is generally used to prevent fluid accumulation.

*Postoperative Care*: The patient is closely monitored at least every two2 h for the first 72 h, both clinically and with doppler technology, in order to promptly intercept any sign of vascular compromise (Figs. 15.14 and 15.15).

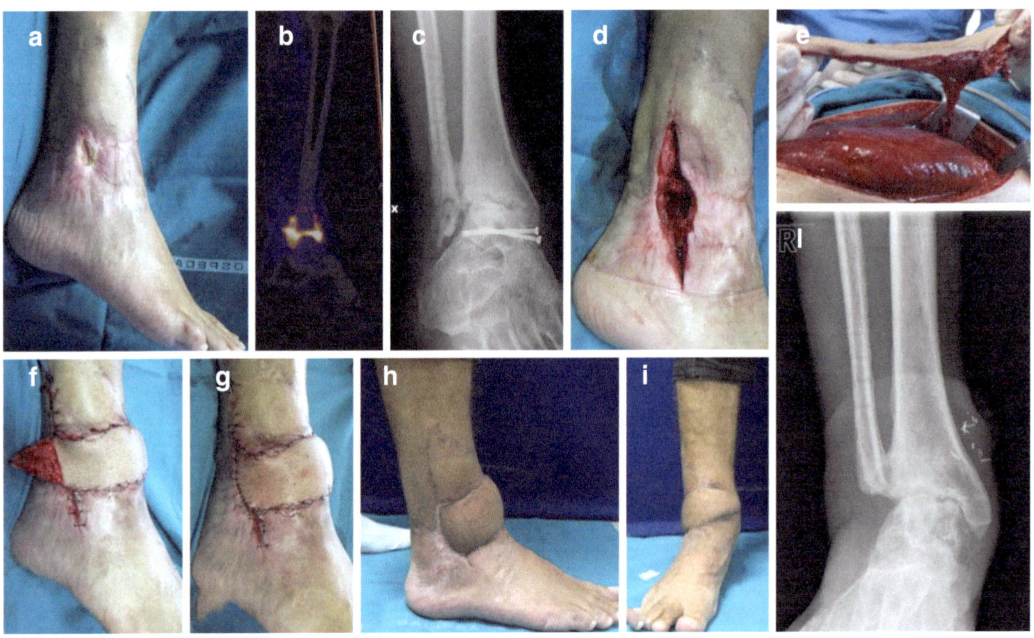


**Fig. 15.14** Management of a patient with radiographically diagnosed chronic osteomielitis (**a**–**c**). After surgical debridement of non-vital tissue (**d**), an ALT free flap was elevated (**e**) and inset in the dorsal aspect of the foot, with the lateral part disepithelized (**f**) and then buried to cover the Achilles tendon for a better gliding (**g**). Postoperative images show adequate functional outcomes (**h**, **i**) and radiographical signs of healing (**j**)

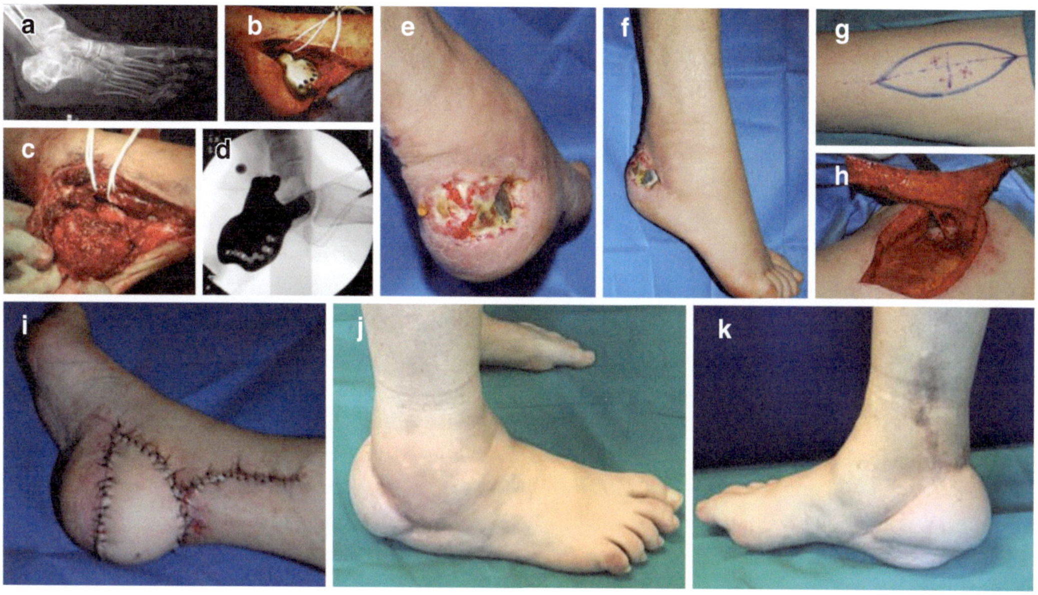


**Fig. 15.15** Clinical case of a calcaneal osteosarcoma (**a**, **b**) reconstructed with a titanium prosthesis (**c**, **d**). The orthopaedic device then suffered from local infection that caused necrosis of the soft tissue (**e**, **f**). Microsurgical reconstruction with an ALT-free flap was then performed: flap planning (**g**), pedicle isolation (**h**), and inset (**i**). Postoperative results are shown in images (**j**) and (**k**)

### 15.3.2 Latissimus Dorsi Muscle Flap

With a maximum size of 20 by 40 cm, the latissimus dorsi muscle is the biggest muscle in the body, and thus able to cover extensive soft tissue defects (Fig. 15.11). Despite its size, the removal of the muscle causes no functional impairment in the patient. It is the biggest flap that can be harvested on a single pedicle and can also be combined with the scapular, parascapular, and serratus flaps to form a chimeric flap that may cover even larger wounds. Because of the muscle thickness (<1 cm in the normal population), this flap can be placed over uneven surfaces with ease.

The muscle originates from the thoracolumbar fascia posteriorly and from the inferior iliac crest inferiorly. It inserts into the humerus where it adducts and internally rotates the arm. The posterior axillary fold is formed by the narrowing of the superior aspect of the muscle before transitioning into the tendon of insertion. Innervation is from the thoracodorsal nerve, a branch of the posterior cord of the brachial plexus that accompanies the thoracodorsal artery that is usually the second branch of the subscapular artery (after the circumflex scapular branch). From its origin on the axillary artery, the subscapular axis can provide a pedicle up to 15 cm long. The pedicle can be harvested either distally from the undersurface of the muscle or proximally from the axilla. The thoracodorsal vessels are normally split into two muscular branches, the transverse and the lateral (or vertical) branch that diverge at a 45-degree angle. Thus, the muscle can be divided longitudinally to form a bilobed or two-tongued flap, or the muscle paddle can be formed by the irroration territory of only one distal branch of the thoracodorsal artery.

#### 15.3.2.1 Surgical Technique

*Incision:* The lateral border of the latissimus is palpably identified and outlined with a marking pen. The incision is then marked from the axilla or the posterior axillary fold inferiorly and medially over the latissimus muscle, with the recipient site defect dictating the incision length. If a skin paddle is necessary, a pencil Doppler is used to identify and map out the perforators of the distal branches of the thoracodorsal artery that are then marked over the flap.

*Harvest:* Anterior and posterior skin flaps are raised to expose the muscle, with dissection proceeding to the extent of the pocket necessary for an adequate muscle size harvest. Smaller muscles can be taken if the entirety of the muscle is not needed. Vascular supply of the remaining muscle will be granted from perforators of the lumbar and intercostal arteries. The inferior angle of the scapula is where the superior edge of the latissimus is located. It is important not to dissect underneath the serratus when raising the flap from inferior to superior. Once identified, the superior edge of the latissimus is elevated and dissection then proceeds toward the midline, where the muscle is divided from its insertion. Harvest then continues inferiorly to free the medial muscle insertion and then underneath the muscle toward the axilla.

*Vascular Pedicle Dissection:* On this plane, the pedicle is identified and followed proximally up to the desired length. The branch to serratus is ligated, as well as the circumflex scapular branch if more length is necessary.

*Closure:* The donor site is closed primarily. Suction drains are usually placed and the patient is allowed to move the ipsilateral arm postoperatively.

*Postoperative Care:* The patient is closely monitored at least every 2 h for the first 72 h, both clinically and with doppler technology, in order to promptly intercept any sign of vascular compromise (Fig. 15.16).

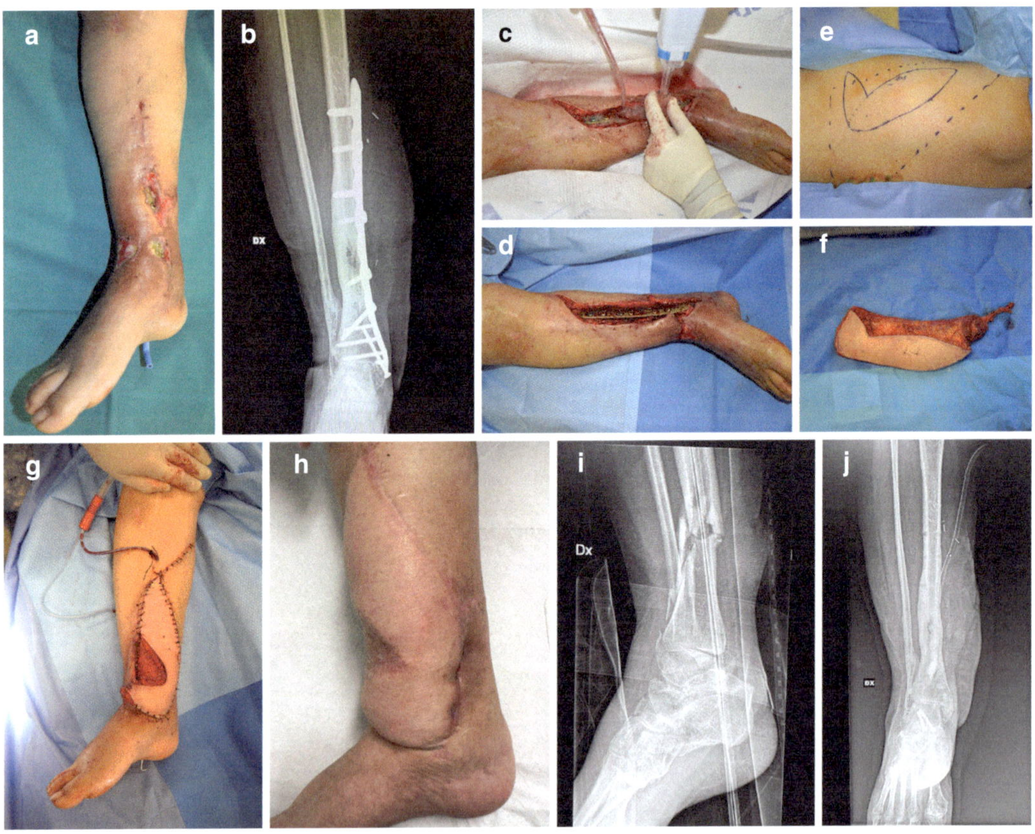


**Fig. 15.16** Management of chronic osteomyelitis after osteosynthesis of a tibial fracture with plaque (**a**, **b**). After hydrodebridement of non-vital soft tissue (**c**, **d**), a latissimus dorsi flap with a skin paddle was drawn (**e**). The flap was elevated (**f**) and inset (**g**) distally in the medial aspect of the leg, with the remaining tegmental defect covered with a skin graft. Postoperative image shows no recurrence of bone infection (**h**), while radiographic images demonstrate preoperative sign of a lack of osteosynthesis (**i**) and a follow-up with good healing of the tibia (**j**)

### 15.3.3 Gracilis Free-Flap

Both the reversed gracilis pedicle flap and the gracilis free flap offer reliable soft tissue coverage and promote wound healing in complex knee injuries. However, there are some key differences between the two techniques. The reversed gracilis pedicle flap is a simpler and less invasive procedure compared to the gracilis free flap, which requires microvascular anastomosis. The reversed gracilis pedicle flap is also associated with a lower risk of donor site morbidity, as it does not require the sacrifice of the gracilis muscle. On the other hand, the gracilis free flap allows for a greater degree of customization, as it can be harvested as a muscle-only, muscle-skin, or muscle-bone composite flap. This allows for better matching of the contour and volume of the defect. Additionally, the gracilis free flap can provide stable soft tissue coverage and promote bone healing, making it suitable for more complex cases. The reversed gracilis pedicle flap and the gracilis free flap are both valuable tools in the armamentarium of orthopedic and trauma surgeons. The choice between the two techniques depends on the specific needs of the patient and the extent of the soft tissue defect. Further research and refinement of surgical techniques will continue to enhance the role of these flaps in soft tissue reconstruction.

The gracilis free flap is a versatile surgical technique used for the reconstruction of soft tissue defects and bone defects around the knee. This procedure involves harvesting the gracilis muscle, along with its vascular pedicle, from the inner thigh and transferring it to the recipient site, where it is used to cover the defect and promote healing. The gracilis free flap is indicated for cases of soft tissue trauma, such as open fractures, degloving injuries, and extensive soft tissue loss, as well as for bone defects resulting from trauma, infection, or tumor resection. It is particularly useful in cases where local tissue is insufficient or compromised. Preoperative planning is crucial for the success of the gracilis free flap. The surgeon must carefully assess the size and location of the defect, as well as the quality of the surrounding tissue. Imaging studies, such as CT scans or MRI, may be used to evaluate the extent of the defect and the condition of the bone.

#### 15.3.3.1 Surgical Technique

*Patient Positioning*: The patient is placed in the supine position with the affected limb elevated and the thigh abducted and externally rotated to expose the inner thigh.

*Incision:* A longitudinal incision is made along the medial aspect of the thigh, starting at the pubic tubercle and extending distally to the knee. The incision is deepened through the subcutaneous tissue to expose the gracilis muscle.

*Muscle Harvest*: The gracilis muscle is identified and dissected free from its surrounding attachments, preserving its vascular pedicle. The muscle is then divided at its origin and insertion, leaving the vascular pedicle intact.

*Vascular Pedicle Dissection*: The vascular pedicle of the gracilis muscle is carefully dissected, preserving the main artery and vein. The pedicle is then ligated distally to prevent bleeding.

*Flap Transfer*: The gracilis muscle, along with its vascular pedicle, is transferred to the recipient site. The muscle is positioned over the defect and secured in place using sutures. The vascular pedicle is then anastomosed to the recipient vessels using microsurgical techniques.

*Closure*: The incision in the thigh is closed in layers, and a drain may be placed to prevent fluid accumulation.

*Postoperative Care*: The patient is closely monitored for signs of flap or vascular compromise. Physical therapy may be initiated to promote early mobilization and prevent contractures.

The gracilis free flap is a valuable technique for the reconstruction of soft tissue and bone defects around the knee. Through careful preoperative planning and meticulous surgical technique it can provide several advantages including reliable soft tissue coverage, preservation of the main artery and vein, minimal donor site morbidity, ability to provide muscle, skin, or muscle-skin composite flaps and a good esthetic outcome.

**Clinical Case** 16-year-old male, unstable open fracture of Gustilo type III B in the right lower limb. The open fracture led to the diagnosis of osteomyelitis affecting the site of the open fracture.

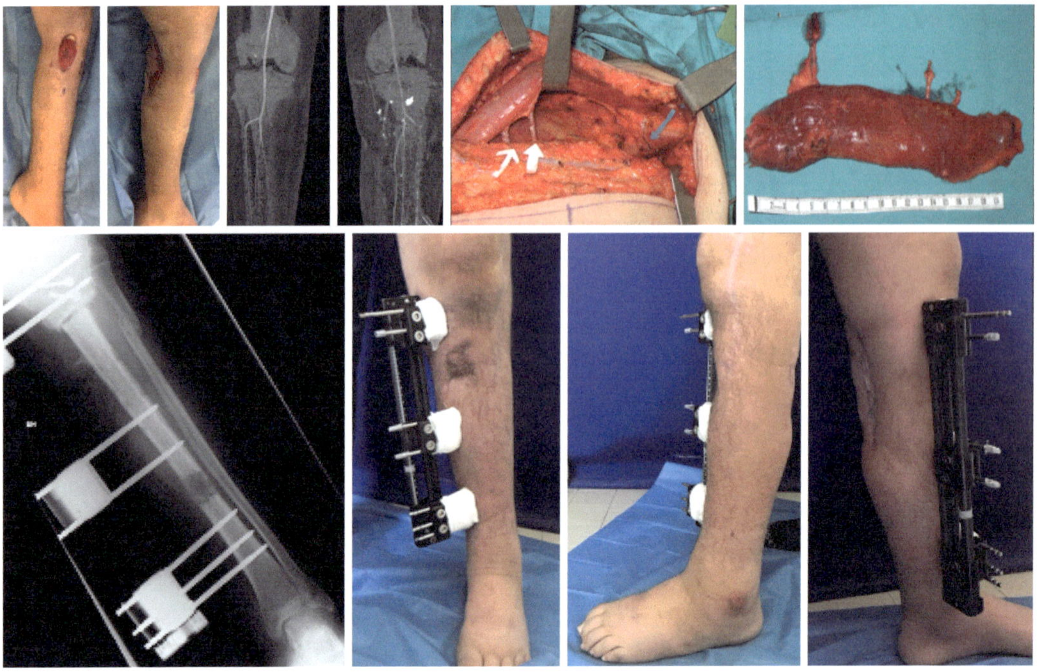

The patient was involved in a road accident that resulted in an unstable open fracture of Gustilo type III B in the right lower limb. The open fracture led to the diagnosis of osteomyelitis affecting the site of the open fracture.

The patient underwent intensive treatment, which included the application of negative pressure therapy (NPWT) for 23 days with continuous instillation. The treatment aimed at mitigating the infection and promoting healing of the unstable open fracture, while simultaneously reducing the risk of complications such as sepsis and osteomyelitis.

After the treatment, the patient showed signs of improvement, with a reduction in pain and an increase in the mobility of the affected limb. Laboratory tests confirmed a decrease in signs of infection and a better response from the immune system. The patient was then discharged with instructions for regular follow-up and oral antibiotic therapy to complete the treatment of osteomyelitis. The case illustrates the importance of timely and appropriate treatment for unstable open fractures, especially when associated with complications such as osteomyelitis. The use of NPWT with continuous instillation has proven to be effective in treating such conditions, reducing the risk of complications and promoting optimal healing.

Then, a gracilis microsurgical flap has been positioned with bone transport technique.

## 15.4 Conclusion and Possible Complications

It is essential to properly and treat possible soft tissue complications early, mainly because they can result in delay of the orthopedic operations that are sometimes necessary, especially in trauma, where external fixation is necessary.

Flap failure is the most tragic scenario in these operations, while wound dehiscence, infection, seroma, or hematoma formation are among the most common complications. Simple wound healing disorders such as dehiscences or infections are oftentimes consequential to the surgical expertise, whereas drains are effective to avoid hematoma or seroma formations that can further lead to a reduction of the blood support and ultimately lead to a failure of the procedure. Flap congestion or ischemia usually depends on the accuracy of the anastomosis and the status of the patient's vessels. In pedicled and propeller flaps, necrosis can also be caused by an improper placement of the flap itself that leads to a reduced blood flow because the pedicle is squeezed or twisted beneath the soft tissues. To promptly recognize possible suffering of the pedicle, it is mandatory that at least in the first 72 h the microsurgical flap is clinically inspected to identify early signs of venous or arterial deficiency (i.e., congested or pale skin paddle), alongside with Doppler examination of the pedicle.

The goals of surgical therapy for chronic osteomyelitis are skeletal stability restoration, dead space management, and debridement. The primary objectives are skin closure, bone union, and infection healing. The so-called radical resection of all contaminated bone and soft tissues is a crucial step in the management of osteitis, and it may lead to a very difficult restoration. Our findings and the literature suggest that one-stage surgical treatment of chronic osteomyelitis may be a useful strategy for some patients, particularly when there is a significant impairment of local soft tissue and bone exposition and when immediate bone coverage with vascularized soft tissue is required [18]. Introducing healthy blood vessels from vascularized tissues to damaged tissues protects against further tissue loss from fibrosis, infection, and desiccation and creates an ideal setting for bone mending. Based on related disorders, defect characteristics (wound location, size, and insufficient tissue components), and the patient's reconstructive needs, the right flap must be chosen.

Single-stage management has been introduced with limited indications for persistent osteomyelitis. The benefits include decreasing and shortening the patient's morbidity due to a single surgical procedure; enabling a full debridement without worrying about the size of the resulting defect because of simultaneous skin and bone reconstruction, which can eliminate the problem of filling dead spaces; and providing immediate bone reconstruction and coverage with a well-vascularized tissue that has its blood supply independent of surrounding tissue and, as a result, delivers oxygen and antibiotics to the bone.

Depending on the location and the size of the soft tissue defect, divers flaps can be used to successfully preserve the underlying osteosynthesis material and be responsible for the final treatment of the chronic osteomyelitis: for proximal small defects, a variety of local flaps are available, while distal tissue coverage, as well as open fractures (that thus usually require large debridements), free flaps are the primary options.

Vascularized fasciocutaneous or musculocutaneous flaps offer significant advantages in the healing of bone infections by providing a robust blood supply to the affected area. These flaps, though differing in volume, share the crucial characteristic of being vascularized tissues, which play a pivotal role in stabilizing bone infection. Furthermore, these flaps contribute to wound coverage and protection, minimizing the risk of further contamination and promoting a favorable environment for bone healing. Overall, the incorporation of vascularized fasciocutaneous or musculocutaneous flaps represents a valuable strategy in the management of bone infections, facilitating improved outcomes and reduced morbidity for patients.

An orthoplastic approach is then crucial to better coordinate surgical timing to obtain the best outcome for each patient that needs to be planned individually.

## References


1. Bihariesingh VJ, Stolarczyk EM, Karim RB, van Kooten EO. Plastic solutions for orthopaedic problems. Arch Orthop Trauma Surg. 2004;124(2):73–6.
2. Lima ALL, Oliveira PR, Carvalho VC, et al. Recommendations for the treatment of osteomyelitis. Braz J Infect Dis. 2014;18(5):526–34.
3. Gupta S, Gabriel A, Lantis J, Téot L. Clinical recommendations and practical guide for negative pressure wound therapy with instillation. Int Wound J. 2016;13(2):159–74.
4. Tiengo C, Macchi V, Vigato E, et al. Reversed gracilis pedicle flap for coverage of a total knee prosthesis. J Bone Joint Surg. 2010;92:1640–6. Journal of Bone and Joint Surgery Inc.
5. Tiengo C, Monticelli A, Sonda R, Angelini A, Ruggieri P, Bassetto F. Role of plastic surgery in the treatment of pelvic tumors. In: Surgery of pelvic

bone tumors. Springer International Publishing; 2021. p. 225–32.
6. Mathes SJ, Nahai F. Clinical atlas of muscle and musculocutaneous flaps. Mosby; 1979.
7. Salibian AH, Meniak FJ. Bipedicle gastrocnemius myocutaneous flap for defects of the distal one third of the leg. Plast Reconstr Surg. 1982;70:17–23.
8. McCraw JB, Fishman JH, Sharzer CA. The versatile gastrocnemius myocutaneous territories. Plast Reconstr Surg. 1977;62:15–23.
9. Barclay TL, Sharpe DT, Chisholm EM. Cross-leg fasciocutaneous flaps. Plast Reconstr Surg. 1983;72:843–6.
10. Wright JK, Watkins RP. Use of soleus muscle flap to cover part of the distal tibia. Plast Reconstr Surg. 1981;68:957–8.
11. Tobin GR. An inferiorly based soleus muscle flap. Br J Plast Surg. 1985;31:210–3.
12. Tiengo C, Macchi V, Vigato E, Porzionato A, Stecco C, Azzena B, Morra A, De Caro R. Reversed gracilis pedicle flap for coverage of a total knee prosthesis. J Bone Joint Surg Am. 2010;92(7):1640–6.
13. Beveridge J, Masquelet A, Romana M, Vinh T. Surgical-Radiologic Anatomy Anatomic basis of a fascio-cutaneous flap supplied by the perforating branch of the peroneal artery. Surg Radiol Anat. 1988;10:195–9.
14. Tolhurst DE, Haeseker B, Zeeman RJ. The development of the fascio cutaneous flap and its clinical application. Plast Reconstr Surg. 1983;71:597–606.
15. Shen L, Liu Y, Zhang C, et al. Peroneal perforator pedicle propeller flap for lower leg soft tissue defect reconstruction: Clinical applications and treatment of venous congestion. J Int Med Res. 2017;45(3):1074–89.
16. Robbins TH. Use of fascio-muscle flaps to repair defects in the leg. Plast Reconstr Surg. 1976;57:460–2.
17. Wong CH, Wei FC. Anterolateral thigh flap. Head Neck. 2010;32(4):529–40.
18. Doi K, Kawakami F, Hiura Y, Oda T, Sakai K, Kawai S. One-stage treatment of infected bone defects of the Tibia with skin loss by free vascularized osteocutaneous grafts. Microsurgery. 1995;16:704–12.

# Diabetic Foot Osteomyelitis (DFO) 16

Carlo Biz, Elisa Pagliarini, and Pietro Ruggieri

## 16.1 Introduction

### 16.1.1 Diabetic Foot Infection (DFI) and Diabetic Foot Osteomyelitis (DFO)

Osteomyelitis is a challenging condition characterized by the invasion of external microorganisms into the bone, often linked with diabetes mellitus (DM), making it difficult to treat. It is costly for healthcare, imposing a significant social burden with a substantial financial impact on healthcare resources to avoid amputation [1]. The complexity of treating osteomyelitis necessitates close collaboration among various medical specialists: surgeons, infectious disease experts, endocrinologists, and podiatrists, as patients with osteomyelitis commonly have other complicating health issues.

According to the diabetes map of the International Diabetes Federation (tenth version), there are 578 million diabetic patients (DPs) in the world [2]. With the increasing global prevalence of DM, many healthcare providers will likely encounter patients with bone infections [1]. In the long term, DM involves many complications such as retinopathy, nephropathy, neuropathy, and vasculopathy. These last two complications increase the risk of developing plantar foot ulcers that allow infections to reach the bone [2].

Diabetic foot osteomyelitis (DFO) is generally categorized as acute or chronic based on the histopathological findings or the duration of the symptoms and the infection [3]. In recent years, an increase in cases of osteomyelitis has been recorded, also linked to the increase in the prevalence of DM because bone infection is caused by the hematogenous dissemination or from the direct contamination of the bone from open wounds or adjacent soft tissue infections (Fig. 16.1) [3].

Today, there is still a lack of comprehensive assessment regarding its outcomes, such as chronic osteomyelitis, amputation, or disability [4].

According to the International Working Group on Diabetic Foot (IWGDF) report, one patient will lose a leg because of Diabetic Foot (DF) every 20 s [3]. Hence, Diabetic Foot is associated with serious financial and health-related burdens affecting patients, their families, and society.

DFO designates all infections that involve bone and joint structures below the malleoli in patients diagnosed with diabetes. The extension of a foot ulcer infection to the foot osteoarticular structures can occur between 20% and 60% of patients with a diabetic foot ulcer depending on

C. Biz · E. Pagliarini · P. Ruggieri (✉)
Department of Orthopedics and Orthopedic Oncology, University of Padova, Padova, Italy
e-mail: carlo.biz@unipd.it; elisa.pagliarini@aopd.veneto.it; pietro.ruggieri@unipd.it



P. Ruggieri et al. (eds.), *Bone and Joint Infections*, https://doi.org/10.1007/978-3-031-96383-4_16

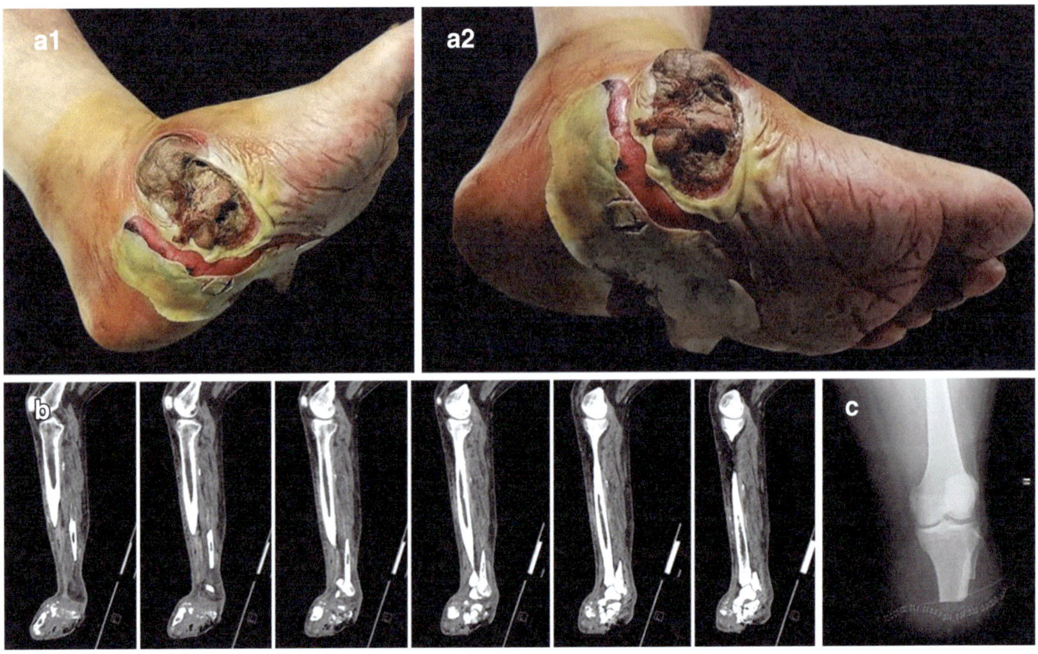


**Fig. 16.1** A 48-year-old type II diabetic man having undergone a below-knee amputation for sepsis due to severe infection of soft tissues, gangrene, and osteomyelitis of his left foot: clinical images (**a1**, **a2**), and CT sagittal plane (**b**) of his leg and foot at the time of presentation and X-ray after aggressive surgery (**c**)

the contiguous spread of any infection which may complicate an ulcer. It is exclusively the consequence of a soft-tissue infection (usually an infected DFU) that spreads to the underlying osteoarticular structures [5]. Bacteria enter from the wound and reach the cortex where they can affect the bone. For this reason, the most commonly affected sites are the phalanges, metatarsal heads, and calcaneus [6].

Currently, there is no universally accepted definition for diagnosing DFO. However, specific ulcer characteristics such as size, depth, lack of healing despite appropriate wound care, and absence of ischemia can suggest an increased likelihood of underlying DFO [7].

The treatment approach for DFO is distinct from that of skin and soft tissue infections, necessitating prolonged anti-infective therapy and carrying a significantly higher risk of amputation. Traditionally, it was believed that complete removal of infected bone was necessary. However, recent research indicates that DFO in the toe can be resolved with antibiotic therapy alone, without the need for amputation. Further studies advocate for conservative surgery, where the necrotic bone is entirely removed. Still, adjacent bone can be preserved if it appears "normal" post-operation, characterized by being hard, with healthy red bone marrow, and free of apparent purulent necrosis.

## 16.2 Epidemiology, Etiology, and Pathophysiology of DFO

Patients with diabetes have a 25% risk during their lifetimes to develop a foot complication such as soft tissue wounds and ulcers, which in more than half of cases may eventually become infected [8]. The most common DF problems are plantar infected ulcers from overloading skin or lesions. These alterations can be caused by the typical peripheral neuropathy of diabetic patients which makes ischemia asymptomatic and delays the diagnosis of a Charcot joint (Fig. 16.2).

The incidence of DFI is 35–40 per 1000 persons per year, and osteomyelitis is present in 20%–70% of diabetic foot ulcers DFUs. For dia-

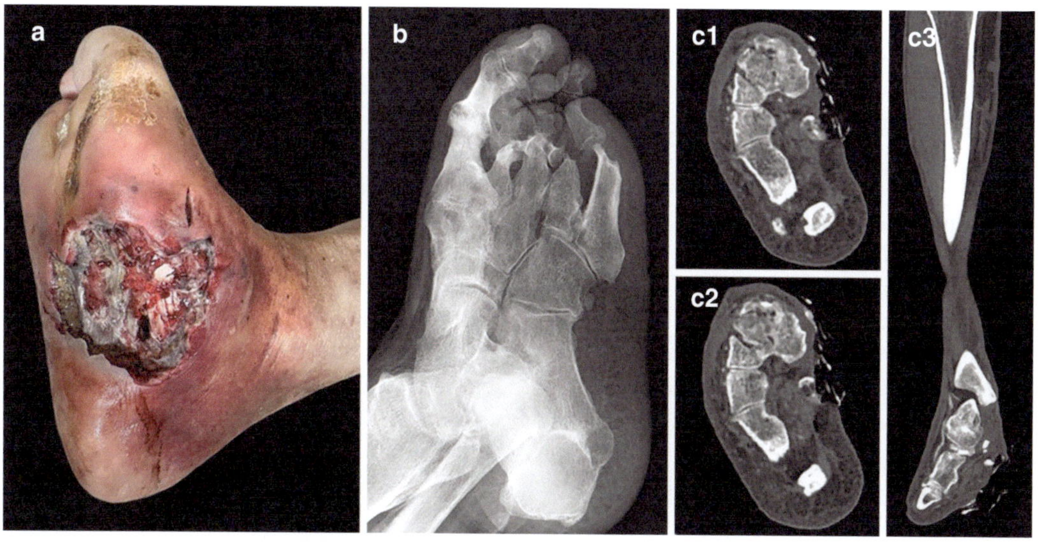


**Fig. 16.2** A 62-year-old type I diabetic man presenting a mid-foot plantar ulcer of his right Charcot foot: clinical (**a**), radiographic images (**b**) and CT axial (**c1**, **c2**) and sagittal (**c3**) views of the joint deformities

betic patients, 84% of amputations are performed because of an infected or unhealed ulcer [9]. Any foot bone can be affected by DFO, but it is more frequent in the forefoot (90%), followed by the midfoot (5%) and the hindfoot (5%). Forefoot osteomyelitis has a better prognosis than the others, and the risk of ankle amputation is significantly higher for hindfoot (50%) than midfoot (18.5%) and forefoot (0.33%) osteomyelitis.

The microbiological etiology of DFOs is like that of the contiguous soft-tissue infection, although fewer isolates are usually found in bone compared with soft-tissue infections. Bacteria are responsible for most DFOs, and the colonization is usually polymicrobial [8].

In developed countries, the most common pathogen cultured is Gram-positive bacteria, such as *Staphylococcus aureus* (up to 50% of cases), *Staphylococcus epidermidis* (approximately 25%), *Streptococci* (around 30%), and Enterobacteriaceae (up to 40%). Gram-negative bacilli (such as *Pseudomonas aeruginosa* and *Escherichia coli*, *Klebsiella pneumonia,* and *Proteus*) are more frequent in warm climate countries. Obligate anaerobes (e.g., *Finegoldia magna*, *Clostridium* spp., or *Bacteroides* spp.) are generally less frequently cultured, but this depends on how the bone fragments are sampled and transported to the laboratory. Bacteria usually considered contaminants, such as coagulase-negative staphylococci and *Corynebacterium* sp., have been documented as pathogens in DFO.

At present, the resistance to antibiotics is increasing in the diabetic population, and multiresistant organisms (MDRO) are common in DFI. Hospitalization, surgical procedures, and long antibiotic therapy induce the development of MDRO or methicillin-resistant *Staphylococcus aureus* (MRSA) and extended-spectrum beta-lactamase ESBL-producing Enterobacteriaceae [5]. Rates of antibiotic-resistant pathogens vary widely, making it necessary for prescribing clinicians to remain updated on their prevalence in their work sites.

The process of bone infection in DFO involves bacteria entering from the overlying soft tissue, penetrating the cortex, and reaching the marrow. This can lead to periostitis, osteitis, and ultimately osteomyelitis, impacting also the surrounding soft tissues. The spread of infection from soft tissue to bone can take several weeks, and pathogens adhere to the bone by expressing adhesion factors for components of the bone matrix, leading to complications in blood flow as pus spreads into vascular channels. Bone involvement in DF results from the spread of infection from soft tissue in an ongoing process that can take several weeks. Fissures in the dried skin can harbor microorganisms, and microbes may invade bone tissue, entering through the cortex before spreading to the marrow if the infection persists [10]. Pathogens adhere to bone by expressing adhesion factors for components of the bone matrix. Then, pus spreads into vascular channels, raising the intraosseous pressure, and impairing blood flow. The main risk factor for skin ulceration and secondary spread to bone is chronic wound infection. Consequently, all factors contributing to prolonging healing time will increase the risk of osteomyelitis. In addition, inefficient off-loading of a foot ulcer increases the incidence of osteomyelitis [10].

## 16.3 Diagnosis of DFO

Dealing with DFO is perhaps the most difficult and controversial aspect of the management of diabetic foot infections. Its diagnosis is based currently on clinical signs of infection supported by laboratory, microbiological, and radiological evaluation and completed by the results of the bone sample examination: positive culture and histological abnormalities consistent with the diagnosis of bone infection.

The guidelines suggest that the diagnosis of DFO includes combining different diagnostic tests, such as pulmonary tuberculosis (PTB), serum inflammatory markers, Xray, MRI, or radionuclide scanning. X-ray should always be the first imaging evaluation; when more specific imaging is required, MRI is the first choice. Severe osteomyelitis involving midfoot, hindfoot, and ankle detected by magnetic resonance imaging cell-labelled radionuclide scan, SPECT/CT, and 18F-FDG PET/CT are used only if MRI is contraindicated [11].

DFO must be considered a potential complication of any deep or extensive ulcer, especially one that is chronic or overlies a bony prominence (Fig. 16.3). Osteomyelitis should be considered when an ulcer does not heal after at least 6 weeks of appropriate care and off-loading. Any ulcer in which bone is either visible or can be easily palpated with a sterile blunt metal probe is likely to be complicated by osteomyelitis. In patients with a limb-threatening infection, positive results of a probe-to-bone test (PTB) may be taken as nearly sufficient for diagnosis, but the performance characteristics of this test have not yet been fully defined. A swollen foot in a patient with a history of foot ulceration, the classic "sausage toe" (i.e., a red, swollen digit), or an unexplained high WBC count or inflammatory markers should also arouse suspicion of osteomyelitis. Finally, radiologically evident bone destruction beneath an ulcer should be considered to represent osteomyelitis unless proven otherwise [12].

### 16.3.1 Clinical Signs and Presentation

Infected wounds usually show purulent secretions or some signs of inflammation: swelling, erythema, blood serum secretion, or simply blood with or without bone fragments. However, DFO can occur without any local sign of inflammation. Systemic symptoms such as fever and malaise are uncommon, especially in cases of chronic DFOs [13].

Physical examination is essential for the diagnosis. Osteomyelitis is unlikely when there is no clinical foot ulcer even when bone lesions are present on imaging. The most suitable clinical approach involves examining the wound with a sterile metal probe to search for positive bone contact, as described above. This indicates osteomyelitis in infected ulcers but does not rule it out if positive contact is lacking. A negative result, however, is likely to rule out bone infection in ulcers without clinical signs of infection. Combining bone contact with data from standard foot radiographs enhances the accuracy of DFO diagnosis, which should be suspected in cases of exposed bone or when bone fragments are present. The absence of local signs of inflammation does not eliminate the possibility of DFO diagnosis [5].

Most DPs present with erythema and drainage, but pain may be absent because of the associated neuropathy. Often, they are afebrile, and some present with an ulcer without evidence of surrounding inflammation. The ulcer size

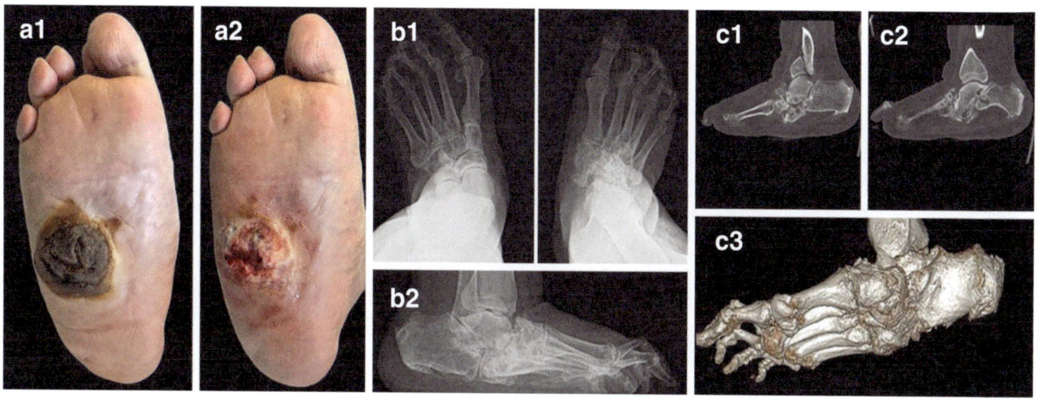


**Fig. 16.3** A 74-year-old type I diabetic woman with chronic plantar DFU of her right Charcot foot: clinical images before (**a1**) and after (**a2**) debridement; AP (**b1**) and LL (**b2**) X-ray images; and CT sagittal plane images (**c1**, **c2**) with 3D reconstruction (**c3**)

(>2 cm$^2$) and depth (>3 mm) predict the likelihood of bone involvement (Fig. 16.3).

Three specific clinical signs are predictive of osteomyelitis:

- the width and depth of the foot ulcer. An ulcer larger than 2 cm$^2$ has a sensitivity of 56% and a specificity of 92%. Deep ulcers (>3 mm) are more easily associated with underlying osteomyelitis than superficial ulcers (82% vs 33%) [14].
- the probe-to-bone test, performed by probing the ulcer area with a sterile blunt probe. If the probe reaches the bone surface, the test is considered positive. This test was found to have a sensitivity of 87%, a specificity of 91%, a positive predictive value of only 57%, and a negative predictive value of 98%. The combination of the PTB test with X-ray improves the sensitivity and specificity in the diagnosis of DFO [15].
- no ulcer healing despite appropriate nursing and off-loading, an inflammatory toe ("sausage toe"), drainage of synovial liquid, and its location over a bony prominence [9] (Fig. 16.4).

## 16.3.2 Serum Inflammatory Markers

Serum inflammatory markers such as white blood cells (WBC), C-reactive protein, erythrocyte sedimentation rate (ESR), and procalcitonin (PCT) are usually higher in DFO than in soft-tissue infections. However, WBC and procalcitonin may be negative, while ESR > 60 mm/h and/or CRP > 3.2 mg/dL in the presence of an ulcer deeper than >3 mm may significantly predict DFO. Furthermore, WBC, CRP, and PCT values return to their normal range in approximately three weeks after treatment in both soft-tissue and bone infection, while ESR usually remains high only in the case of osteomyelitis. ESR appears to be the most useful inflammatory biomarker available in daily practice for diagnosis. A high erythrocyte sedimentation rate, especially if it is over 70 mm/hour, helps make the diagnosis of osteomyelitis more likely, but a negative test is less helpful in excluding the presence of bone infection. Leukocytosis is a poor indicator of foot osteomyelitis: the white blood cell (WBC) count is normal in 50% of cases [16].

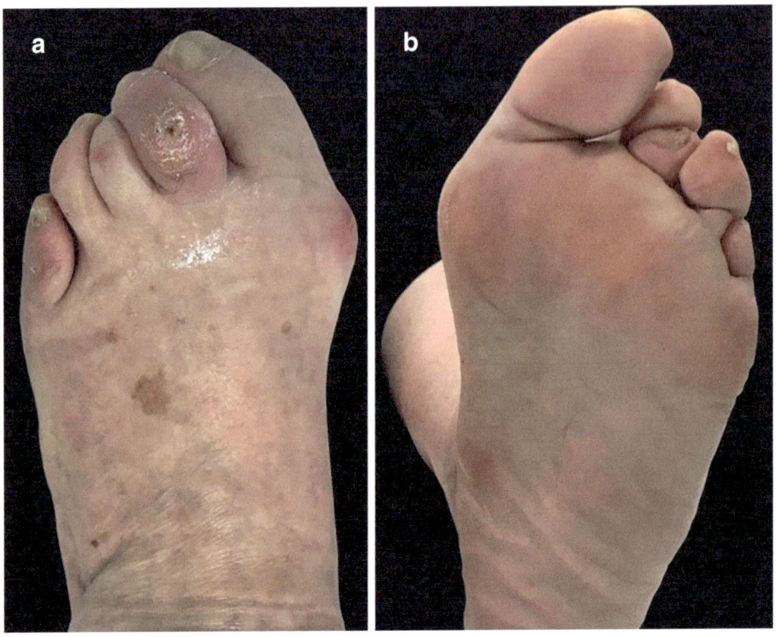


**Fig. 16.4** A 73-year-old type II diabetic woman with a history of swollen left foot, second "sausage toe, and signs of ulceration: dorsal (**a**) and plantar (**b**) clinical aspects

### 16.3.3 Radiographic Examinations

Radiographic examinations are usually required to detect bone involvement in cases of suspected osteomyelitis. Because bone destruction is usually not seen with plain radiography performed during the early stages of disease and neuro-osteoarthropathy can mimic infection, diagnosing osteomyelitis when the patient is first examined can be difficult. Characteristic progressive changes on serial plain radiographs may help in more chronic cases [17].

If the findings of radiography are only consistent with, but not characteristic of DFO, one of the following choices should be considered (Fig. 16.5):

1. *Additional imaging studies:* Magnetic resonance imaging is the preferred imaging study, with nuclear medicine scans (preferably using newer generation leukocyte or immunoglobulin techniques) being a second choice. If the results of the imaging tests are negative, osteomyelitis is unlikely; if results suggest osteomyelitis, bone biopsy should be considered [18].
2. *Empirical treatment:* antibiotic therapy should be provided for another 24 weeks, and then radiographs should be taken again to determine whether bony changes have progressed (which would suggest infection).
3. *Bone biopsy:* an appropriate procedure should be used, as described here. Collection of a sample of a bony lesion (either operatively or percutaneously) is recommended if the diagnosis remains in doubt after imaging or if osteomyelitis is likely but the etiologic agent or antibiotic susceptibilities are not predictable [19]. Some physicians would also obtain biopsy specimens of most mid- or hind-foot lesions because these are more difficult to treat and more often lead to a high-level amputation. Percutaneous biopsy should preferably be done under fluoroscopic or CT guidance, traversing uninvolved skin if possible. For DPs with sensory neuropathy, anesthesia may be unnecessary. Various types of bone-cutting needles, such as Jamshidi (Perfectum Corporation; distributed by Propper and Sons) and Ostycut (Bard Products; distributed by Angiomed), have been used. Obtain specimens if possible, sending at least one for

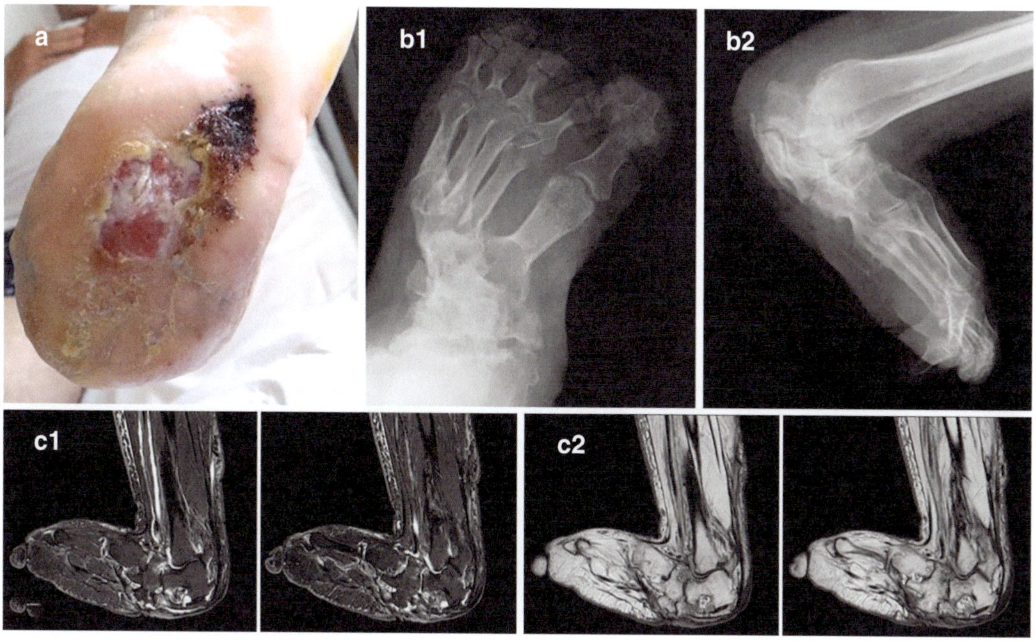


**Fig. 16.5** A 67-year-old type II diabetic man with a history of spina bifida presenting a left hind-foot plantar ulcer with radiographic signs of osteomyelitis: clinical image (**a**); X-rays (**b1**, **b2**) and MRI (**c1**, **c2**) images at the time of presentation

culture and another for histological analysis. With small toe bones, it may only be possible to aspirate a few bony spicules. Foot bone biopsy is a safe procedure, and cultures of bone specimens provide more accurate microbiologic data than those of soft-tissue specimens for DPs with osteomyelitis [19].

#### 16.3.3.1 X-ray

Plain X-rays have indisputable advantages for a first diagnostic study: they are not expensive, can be repeated and therefore can be compared, are easily performed, and are not limited by contraindications. Signs of DFO are bone erosion of cortical bone, osteopenia, cortical osteolysis, sequestration, and periosteal thickening, but they become evident after 2–3 weeks from onset (Figs. 16.2, 16.3, 16.5, and 16.6). Moreover, X-rays are useful for understanding the severity of bone involvement and the possible presence of gas (for example in gangrene), foreign bodies, and enlargement of soft tissue in cases of associated cellulitis [20].

Planar beam radiography can visualize anomalies indicative of osteitis, such as periosteal reaction, sequestrum, medulla damage, and cortical rupture. In the case of clinically suspected osteitis, it is advisable to repeat the radiographic process at least two weeks later due to delayed appearances of these anomalies.

#### 16.3.3.2 MRI

MRI is the most useful of the available imaging modalities for defining bone infections, providing the most reliable image of deep soft-tissue infections (Fig. 16.5). Its sensitivity and specificity for diagnosing DFOs are 90% and 83%, respectively [21]. The performance characteristics of all of these diagnostic tests are highly correlated with the pretest probability of osteomyelitis, and they are most useful for probable cases. However, the gold standard for diagnosing osteomyelitis is the isolation of bacteria from a reliably obtained sample of bone, concomitant with histological findings of inflammatory cells and osteonecrosis.

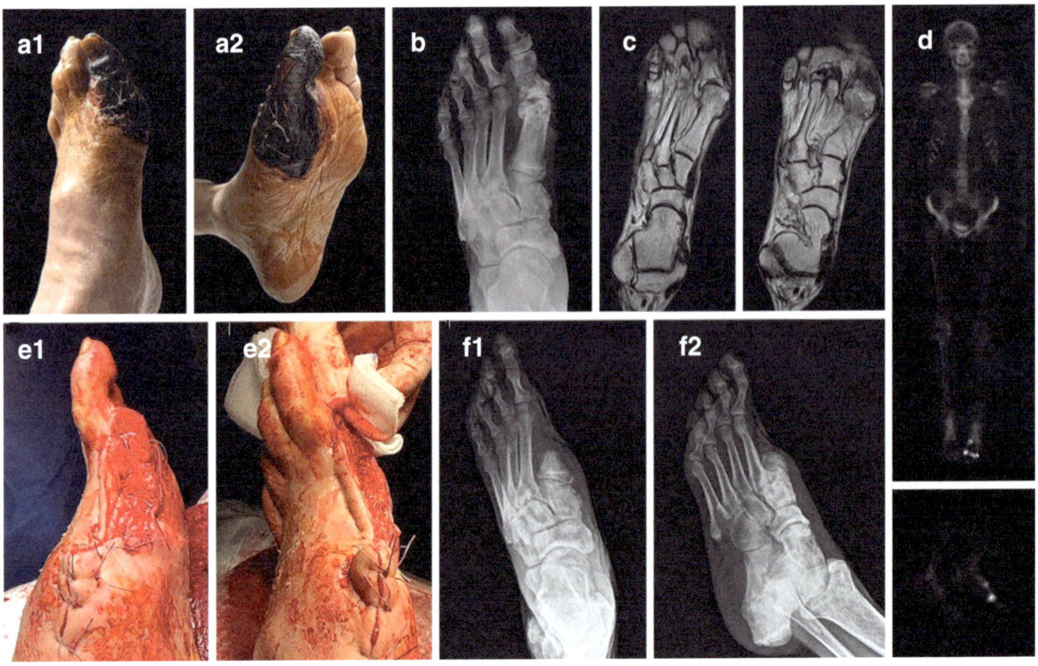


**Fig. 16.6** An 81-year-old type II diabetic man presenting ischemia and gangrene of the first ray of his left foot with signs of osteomyelitis of the first metatarsal head: clinical (**a1**, **a2**), X-ray (**b**), MRI (**c**), and Scintigraphy (**d**) images before surgery; clinical (**e1**, **e2**) and radiographic (**f1**, **f2**) images during and after surgical procedure

MRI is usually not needed as a first-line investigation in cases of DFO. When osteomyelitis is a possibility, obtaining plain radiographs often suffices. If these radiographs show no evidence of pathological findings in bone, the patient should be treated for 2 weeks for the soft-tissue infection [22]. If suspicion of osteomyelitis persists, plain radiography should be performed again 24 weeks later. If the initial X-rays show clear changes suggestive of osteomyelitis (cortical erosion, periosteal reaction, and mixed lucency and sclerosis), and if there is little likelihood of noninfectious osteoarthropathy, treatment for presumptive osteomyelitis should be carried out, preferably after obtaining appropriate specimens for culture.

#### 16.3.3.3 PET-CT

Positron Emission Tomography-Computed Tomography (PET-CT) is useful to distinguish soft tissues from bone infections as well as MRI with gadolinium. An undoubted advantage of this method is that the pathology becomes evident only 3 days after the onset, thus allowing an early diagnosis [8]. PET-CT offers exceptional spatial resolution and identifies essential anatomical details necessary for effective management. Its sensitivity and specificity in the diagnosis of DFO are 90% and 83%, respectively. Additionally, the use of SPECT-CT and labeled polynuclear scintigraphy aids in locating hyperfixation in soft tissues and bone tissues, allowing for precise determination of the extension of infectious lesions (Fig. 16.6). Moreover, 18F-FDG PET/Scan offers significant sensitivity (89%) and specificity (92%), but it does not consistently differentiate between soft tissue infection and osteitis from inflammation in acute Charcot osteoarthropathy [21].

### 16.3.4 Biopsy

The undoubted gold standard for diagnosing osteomyelitis is bone biopsy, which provides histological findings such as necrosis and the presence of inflammatory cells as well as microbiological characterization. To achieve a truthful antibiogram, it is mandatory to perform this procedure after an antibiotic-free period of at least two weeks because of the prolonged release of some antibiotics from bones [5]. When antibiotic therapy is initiated before a bone biopsy can be obtained, the bacteria may be suppressed, which can interfere with the accurate identification of the infecting organism [3]. If possible, bone biopsy should be performed without passing through an open wound to avoid contamination by colonizing organisms. In patients with profound peripheral neuropathy, bone biopsy can generally be done with little or no anesthesia.

Bone biopsy provides histological and microbiological findings characteristic of DFO [23], such as bone erosion, marrow edema, fibrosis, and necrotic inflammatory cells.

The bone can be removed by a percutaneous approach through non-infected skin or during open surgical procedures. In the case of bone infection, a superficial swab shows low sensitivity; a reliable correspondence between bacteria isolated from bone biopsy and swab culture is approximately 38%. Therefore, a superficial swab should not be used in case of DFO. Bone biopsy is the most accurate test even if in several cases it is not technically feasible. However, a recent study showed that the pathogens isolated from a culture of deep tissues (removed from the area closest to the bone) are very similar to those obtained from bone biopsy (74.3% vs 82.8%) [24].

While bone biopsy has traditionally been viewed as the primary method for diagnosing diabetic foot osteomyelitis, recent research has questioned its reliability as a standalone test. The International Working Group on the Diabetic Foot (IWGDF) suggests using a combination of clinical, radiographic, and laboratory findings, along with diagnostic categories like "definite," "probable," "possible," and "unlikely" to diagnose osteomyelitis. The term "bone biopsy" can be ambiguous, as it may refer to the physical act of removing a bone specimen rather than the specific examination conducted on the excised fragment [25].

## 16.4 Treatment of DFO

In the past, the only successful method of eradicating DFO was complete surgical resection. There are now many published case series, and at least one randomized controlled trial [17], demonstrating that for properly selected patients with DFO, antibiotic therapy without surgery can offer similar results to those with surgery. The most recent and comprehensive guidance for treating DFO is found in the 2023 update of the guidelines on infection from the International Working Group on the Diabetic Foot (IWGDF), which provides rigorously reviewed recommendations on managing all aspects of diabetic foot infections.

These guidelines broadly recommend the specific conditions for a medical approach combined with conservative surgery. Conservative surgery is usually a procedure in which only the infected bone and the nonviable soft tissues are removed without any amputation. Although an aggressive surgical approach could be mandatory under some circumstances, retrospective studies have shown that conservative treatment associated with prolonged antibiotic therapy is effective in promoting wound healing and reducing the risk of major amputation and ulcer recurrence [26].

Definitive surgical solutions to osteomyelitis, such as ray and transmetatarsal amputations, may risk architectural reorganization of the foot, resulting in altered biomechanics and additional cycles of ulceration (Fig. 16.7). Neuropathy and reduced systemic manifestations of infection may make osteomyelitis tolerable for the patient, who may thus opt for attempts at medical management. In contrast, these diabetic complications may also mask progressive bone destruction, with delayed or inadequate surgery resulting in poorly

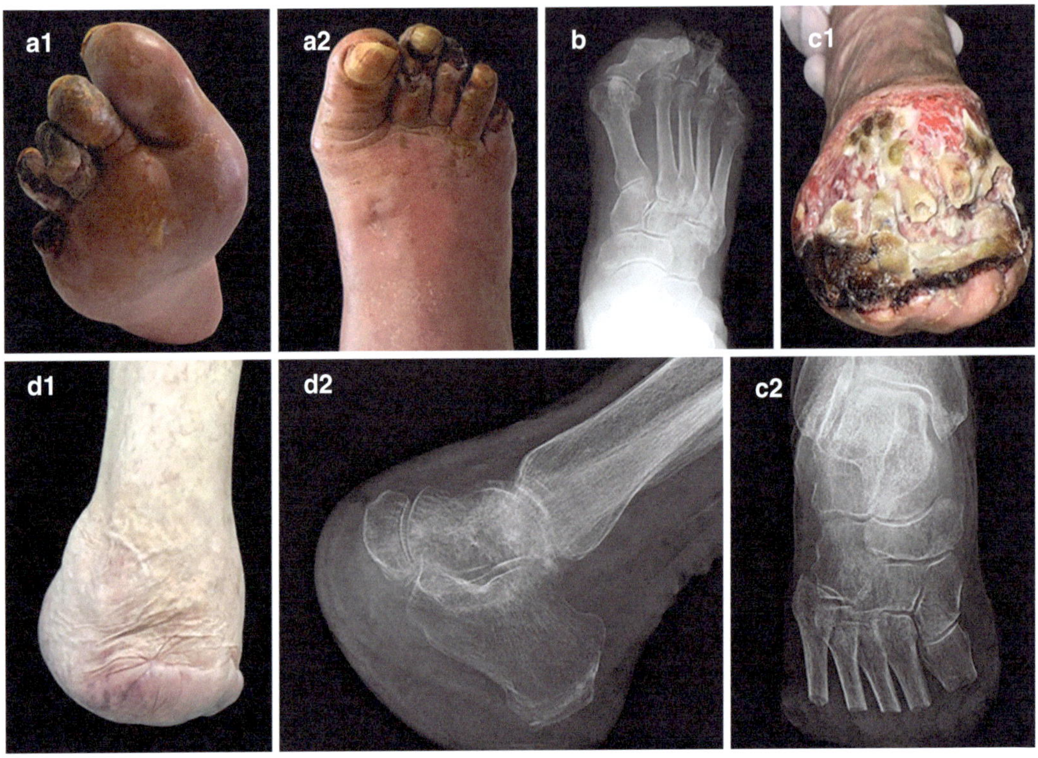


**Fig. 16.7** An 87-year-old type II diabetic woman with a history of gangrene and osteomyelitis of her right foot after severe peripheral arterial disease: clinical and radiographic images at the time of presentation (**a1**, **a2**, **b**), after failure of the transmetatarsal amputation (**c1**, **c2**) and following effective Chopart amputation (**d1**, **d2**)

controlled infection, additional bone or soft-tissue necrosis, and a nonhealing wound [27].

The determination of which patients are suitable for nonsurgical treatment, as well as what duration of antibiotic therapy is needed, are important areas for future study. There are four cases in which conservative management of osteomyelitis might be considered:

- there is no acceptable surgical target (radical cure of the infection would cause unacceptable loss of function).
- the patient has ischemia caused by unreconstructable vascular disease but desires to avoid amputation.
- infection is confined to the forefoot, and there is minimal soft tissue loss.
- the patient and health care professional agree that surgical management carries excessive risk or is otherwise inappropriate or desirable.

Medical treatment alone has shown similar scarring rates and duration compared to surgery combined with postoperative antibiotic therapy. Success rates of medical treatment range from 60% to 82%, with comparable efficacy reported for *S. Aureus* osteitis when combined with debridement or surgery.

The goals of treating a DFI remain the eradication of its clinical evidence and the avoidance of soft-tissue loss and amputations. Overall, good resolution of clinical evidence of infection is possible after appropriate therapy in 80%–90% of mild-to-moderate infections and in 60%–80% of severe infections or cases of osteomyelitis.

Factors associated with a poor outcome include signs of systemic infection, inadequate limb perfusion, osteomyelitis, necrosis or gangrene, an inexperienced surgeon, and proximal location of the infection. Relapses occur in

20%–30% of patients, especially in those with osteomyelitis, which may be difficult to differentiate from reinfection.

Hyperbaric oxygen therapy (HBOT) can be perceived as a viable, effective, and safe treatment for managing chronic refractory DFO. It can be useful for patients who have previously undergone surgical interventions and substantial antibiotic regimens, yet relentless and unyielding affliction continues to be a struggle for them. HBOT emerges as a significant contender in this scenario, increasing oxygen levels within the body, fortifying natural immune defences, enhancing the efficacy of antibiotics, and providing a strategic weapon against the infections [28].

### 16.4.1 Antibiotics Therapy

Preference should be given to those antibiotics that exhibit high diffusion into bone, such as fluoroquinolones, sulfamides, cyclines, macrolides, rifampicin, fusidic acid, and oxazolidinones. Antibiotics should be administered at high daily doses, given the limitations in the diffusion into infected bones and diminished susceptibility of bacteria involved in chronic DFOs. Nevertheless, this may be limited by the risk of adverse effects, especially for antibiotics with potential renal or liver toxicity in DPs, who are likely to have comorbidities. Regarding the method of administration, there is no difference between oral versus parenteral antibiotics for the treatment of osteomyelitis if the bacteria are sensitive to the antibiotic used. The therapy should be administered for 6–8 weeks [8].

However, the optimal duration of antibiotic therapy is not precisely defined. The Infectious Disease Society of America (IDSA) considers 4–6 weeks adequate when the infected bone is not completely removed by surgery and at least 3 months in case of antibiotic therapy alone [23]. However, the recent report of International Working Group of Diabetic Foot (IWGDF) suggested 6 weeks of antibiotic therapy if the infected bone was not removed by surgery and no more than a week if the infected bone was resected. Lately, the aim is to reduce the duration of antibiotic therapy. Prolonged use of antibiotics increases the risk of bacterial resistance, side effects, and costs.

Antibiotic therapy is widely used in association with surgery, both for minimal and extended procedures. However, some authors have reduced the role of surgery in treating bone infection, mainly in cases of chronic osteomyelitis [29].

Currently, there are no tests regarding the long-term resolution of osteomyelitis. The IWGDF suggests that decreasing serum inflammatory markers, especially erythrocyte sedimentation rate (ESR), associated with the resolution of soft tissue infection, healing, and positive evolution of radiological signs can be used to discontinue antibiotic therapy. Despite long antibiotic therapy, chronic osteomyelitis is associated with a high percentage of recurrence (rate 30%) [6].

To ensure achieving adequate bone levels of antibiotics, clinicians have therefore long assumed that high serum concentrations are needed [5]. Achieving high serum levels to treat DFO was thought to require parenteral (generally intravenous) therapy. For almost 40 years, however, evidence from case reports and case series suggested that therapy with orally administered antibiotics with high bioavailability could successfully treat DFO. Recently, strong evidence supporting this view emerged from the OVIVA study, a randomized, controlled, multicenter trial in the UK. This study demonstrated that treatment during the first 6 weeks with oral antibiotic therapy regimens (after about a week of intravenous therapy) was not inferior to entirely intravenous antibiotic therapy regimens. It was also associated with fewer intravenous catheter-related complications and lower financial costs.

Clinicians must know that antibiotic-related adverse events are frequent in all types of infections (15%–30%), mostly occurring during the first 3 weeks of therapy. Therefore, in patients with recurrent diabetic foot problems, antibiotics should not be prescribed to treat contaminated superficial wounds for which there is no proven benefit [30] and only be used in infected wounds with a clear need. However, clinicians should not always prescribe antibiotics based solely on the academic consideration of the presence of infection even if contamination is excluded according to international guidance [23]. It may be appropriate to withhold futile antibiotic therapy in some cases, such as in a patient with complete toe bone destruction who refuses to undergo surgery. It may be appropriate to administer antibiotic therapy for relatively brief periods to suppress the local worsening of infection for such a patient.

Osteomyelitis may be treated with Rifampicin, an antibiotic agent with several characteristics that make it potentially attractive for treating osteomyelitis. It is absorbed well when taken orally, has good penetration into bone, and has high activity against the biofilm organisms that often infect bone, including *S. aureus*. There has been recent interest in the potential value of adding rifampin to combination therapy for DFOs.

As part of the IWGDF's work to update the 2019 DFI guidelines, a systematic review of publications on all types of interventions used to manage DFI was conducted. The conclusion was that the main advantages to treating DFO "medically" by antibiotics are to avoid biomechanical changes after surgery, and that it may be more cost effective [31].

### 16.4.2 Conservative Surgery

For conservative surgical treatment, debridement of the infected tissue is the most common intervention. The aim is to remove the necrotic tissue, which is the pathological substratum of the chronic infection (Fig. 16.3). Surgery may be required in several situations: bone protrudes through the ulcer, imaging reveals extensive bone destruction, there is progressive bone damage in a patient undergoing antibiotic treatment, or there is gangrene or spreading soft tissue infection. Demolitive surgery may be needed to save the patient from the septic state in these cases [8]. The planned surgical approach to DFO should balance the benefits and risks of removing as much infected bone as possible against those of preserving viable tissue to aid foot function.

The presence of limb ischemia or soft tissue infection in the case of DFO is associated with a worse prognosis for successful treatment. Again, careful planning of the surgical approach is fundamental. In the hands of experienced surgeons, conservative surgery often eradicates infection and produces more acceptable anatomic outcomes.

Currently, conservative operative methods are safe and effective with overall healing rates of 80%–100%. From 1986 to the present day, in different decades, relatively few original studies regarding Minimally Invasive Metatarsal Osteotomies (MIMOs) for PDFUs have been published, and different osteotomy shapes have been proposed for the treatment of DFUs [32, 33]. A minimally invasive distal metatarsal diaphyseal osteotomy (DMDO) procedure has been described as effective for the prevention and treating complicated DFUs under lateral metatarsal bones while minimizing various surgery-related complications [7, 34].

Although 90% of osteomyelitis occurs in the forefoot, in many cases, the infection range is large because the phalangeal bone is broken, and the metatarsophalangeal joint capsule is damaged (Fig. 16.8). Hence, toe amputation is often required. The optimum approach for treatment has been controversial. If the metatarsal bone is damaged and purulent, it will be removed, but generally, the entire metatarsal bone will not be removed (unless it is entirely damaged, and the infection extends to the midfoot or even the hindfoot). Instead, it will be retained up to the residual end of the metatarsal bone that the surgeon considers "normal." However, it cannot be determined immediately whether these stumps are truly sterile based on pathology or bacteria culture. The 2023 IWGDF guidelines require the urgent study of the relationship between the true infection of these "normal" stumps and prognosis. In cases where the phalangeal bone is completely necrotic, part of the metatarsophalangeal joint capsule is involved, but the side connected with the metatarsal bone is normal. However, these conditions are not conducive to granulation growth and wound healing. To promote growth, experts have concluded that it is necessary to open the joint capsule and expose the metatarsal head to facilitate the growth of granulation tissue and accelerate wound healing [35].

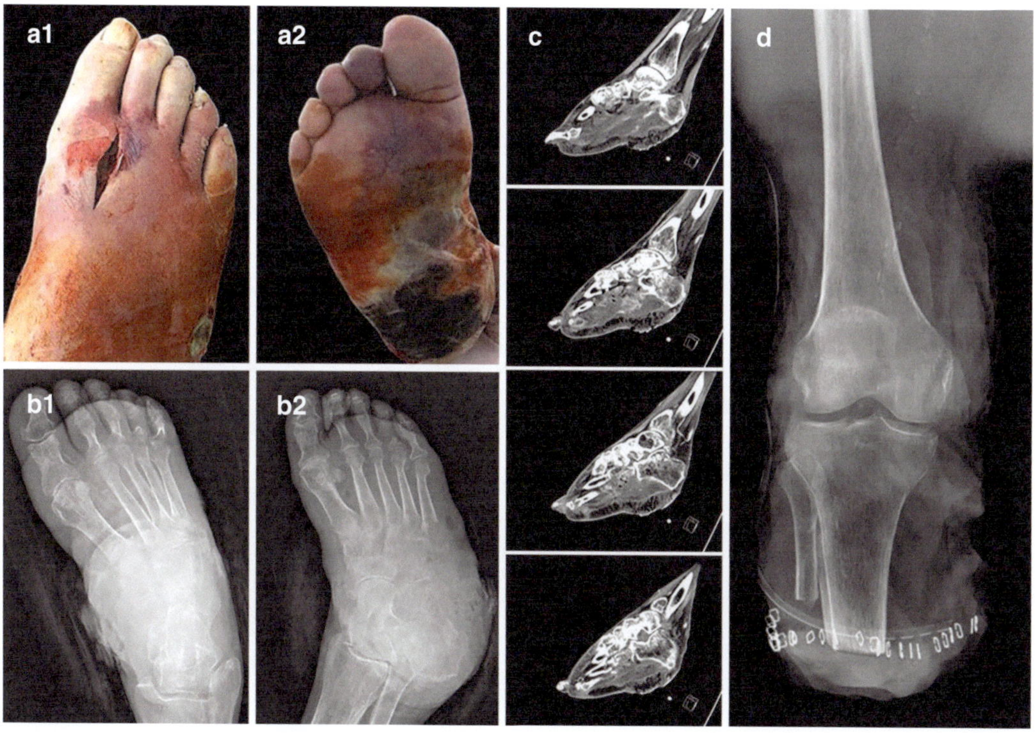


**Fig. 16.8** A 72-year-old type I diabetic woman with ischemia, gangrene, and osteomyelitis in her right foot: clinical images (**a1**, **a2**); X-ray (**b1**, **b2**) and CT sagittal plane (**c**) images before and after below-knee amputation (**d**)

When conservative surgery and medical treatments for osteomyelitis fail, consider several issues:

- the original diagnosis was incorrect.
- the residual necrotic or infected bone or surgical hardware was not resected or removed.
- the selected antibiotic regimen likely covers the causative organisms and achieves adequate levels in bone, but probably it was not administered for a sufficient duration.
- the failure to eradicate bone infection was not the real cause of the current wound problem.

Each case needs an individualized approach, usually in consultation with a knowledgeable surgeon. Selected patients may benefit from implanted antibiotics (e.g., embedded in beads or cement), HBOT, or revascularization. In contrast, others may require long-term or intermittent antibiotic suppression or, in some cases, amputation [28].

### 16.4.3 Aggressive Surgery

Amputation is often necessary in patients with diabetic foot osteomyelitis. Factors such as Grade 3 or Grade 4 Common Terminology Criteria for Adverse Events (CTCAE) infection, severe soft tissue infection, presence of deep abscess, extensive necrosis, gangrene, subcutaneous crepitation or gas bubbles on imagery, or compartment syndrome may necessitate emergency surgical consultation (Figs. 16.1, 16.8 and 16.9). In severe cases, aggressive surgical debridement to remove all necrotic tissue is crucial. Delay in surgical treatment is a major risk factor for high amputation and prolonged hospitalization.

In cases requiring amputation, the patient should be fully involved in the therapeutic decision. Since there are limited randomized studies, the choice between medical and surgical treatment should be individualized, considering sev-

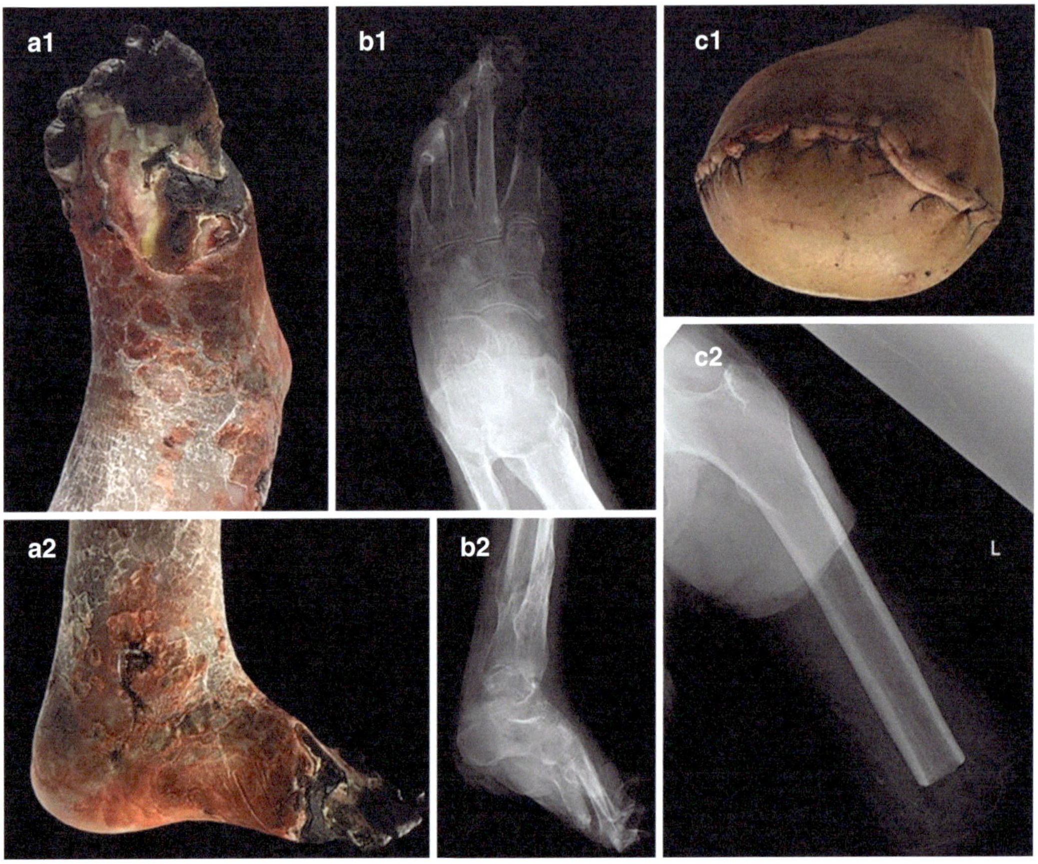


**Fig. 16.9** A 76-year-old type I diabetic man presenting dry gangrene and osteomyelitis in his left foot after severe peripheral arterial disease and infected soft tissues having undergone amputation to midthigh: clinical and radiographic images before (**a1**, **a2**; **b1**, **b2**) and after surgery (**c1**, **c2**)

eral criteria. Vascular assessment is essential before deciding on medical treatment, which may be as effective as surgery in certain cases and preserves foot anatomy and functionality [28].

Total amputation of all necrotic and infected tissue is perhaps the easiest, fastest, and surest way to achieve a rapid cure of DFO. The most appropriate level of amputation is decided by the transcutaneous oxygen pressure (TCPO2) as well as by the bone involvement and soft tissue status. While 35 mmHg is considered an acceptable threshold for uneventful stump healing, this number must be interpreted cautiously and in conjunction with other factors. Available studies in the literature often suggest there is a decisive threshold for the prediction of stump healing, or refer to the auxiliary help of $TCPO_2$ measurements, but they fail to provide strict thresholds. Many trials have also failed to determine any thresholds because, in everyday practice, multiple factors influence stump healing, including infection, surgical techniques, hematoma, and patient compliance. We believe that for foot amputations, the TCPO2 level may confirm the clinical impression but does not replace it; surgeons should avoid relying solely on this measurement to select the level of amputation [9].

Amputation is effective in preventing the spread of infection, and various studies have found that the procedure increased the life expectancy by 2 years in 50% of the diabetic subjects studied [4]. In many patients, amputation does not need to be total but only sufficient to remove infected tissue unlikely to respond to just antibiotic therapy. Then, it is mandatory to follow an appropriate course of antibiotic therapy to eradicate remaining soft tissue or bone infection [9]. However, amputation itself, especially in the absence of reversing the reasons for the patient's initial infection, does not protect against secondary surgical site infections or new DFO episodes.

Calcaneal osteomyelitis is an uncommon presentation of DFO (<15% of cases) with somewhat different epidemiology, clinical features, and approach to management. Compared to those with non-calcaneal DFI, these patients more often require special surgical techniques and off-loading approaches [36]. Undertaking any calcaneal amputation procedure requires that the patient's posterior tibial artery is patent. If patency is not present or restorable, transtibial amputation under the knee (11 cm from the knee joint) is usually indicated (Figs. 16.1 and 16.8). Partial calcanectomy, despite a high clinical failure rate, is most often indicated for calcaneal osteomyelitis and, fortunately, has a limited adverse effect on walking ability. When there are no specific restrictions to the choice of surgical procedure, a partial calcanectomy is recommended. This procedure allows the patient to be fitted with an orthopedic shoe after the surgical wound has healed, allowing nearly normal weight-bearing and walking without the compromised energy expenditure accompanying a below knee amputation. Patients undergoing total calcanectomy, however, usually require a prosthesis that is nearly the height of the type required after below-knee amputation [36]. Furthermore, we recommend the surgeon perform an Achilles tenotomy if the tendon lies within the ulcer area.

Some patients with DFO require lower extremity amputation if they have extensive bone destruction or widespread or difficult-to-control soft-tissue infection, especially if they are already non-ambulatory. Other possible indications for amputation may include progressive necrosis, severe foot deformities, recurrent foot ulcers, the presence of osteosynthetic material that requires removal, or the patients' wish to move beyond a conservative approach. Surgeons and their patients should, however, be wary of amputation of an acute bone infection that has occurred in the setting of a surgical site infection in the DF after elective surgery for any indication.

### 16.4.4 Success and Failures of the Therapies

Defining the successful resolution of DFO is even more difficult than defining its presence. Deeming the outcome of treatment, a clinical success usually requires healing of overlying soft tissue infection and wounds, with a return of any abnormally elevated inflammatory markers to normal. A retrospective 2021 study reviewed 150 patients who underwent surgery for DFI, comparing those with DFO to those with only soft tissue infection. Surprisingly, they found no significant differences in length of hospital stay, duration of antibiotic treatment, time to healing, limb salvage, or recurrence of infection.

Most clinical failures after DFO treatment occur within a few months, or signs and symptoms of infection may even persist during ongoing therapy. However, cultures of appropriate bone specimens in these clinical recurrences often yield a different bacteriological constellation than the prior episode, suggesting they may represent a reinfection on a former problematic anatomical site rather than a relapse of the original infection [37].

It is essential to recognize that surgical procedures for DFO can also yield unsatisfactory outcomes. There are no data to support the widely held belief that outcomes are better with surgery than with antibiotic therapy in the long term because the inherent problems leading to DFO (peripheral neuropathy, foot deformities, improper foot care) are rarely reversed by surgery anymore than by antibiotics. A study from Switzerland reported that, despite professional wound care, many patients needed further surgeries, e.g., proximal re-amputation (39%), of which 11% were major and 25% were minor amputations. Similarly, a retrospective review from the USA found that the risk for re-amputation after partial first-ray amputation in diabetic patients was 42% after a mean of 34 months follow-up.

The authors suggested that surgeons consider a more proximal level amputation at the initial presentation, such as transmetatarsal, to provide a more functional and reliable residual weight-bearing foot. However, a meta-analysis of re-amputations after transmetatarsal amputation showed that the major re-amputation rate was 30% (Fig. 16.7). Finally, in surgical procedures for patients with calcaneal DFO, the failure rates are higher: after partial calcanectomy, 29% of patients needed a secondary amputation. Among all patients undergoing revision surgery after total calcanectomy, 50% had to undergo secondary amputation, suggesting that this is not the best option in calcaneal osteomyelitis.

## 16.5 Prevention of DFO

The concept of preventive surgery for persons with diabetic foot complications is gaining momentum. In the presence of flexible forefoot deformities, such as claw or hammer toes, percutaneous toe flexor tenotomies effectively reduce soft tissue ulceration, with minimal risk of wound healing complications. If dorsiflexion of the ankle is limited to less than five degrees (equine deformity), this restricts the leg from rolling over the foot during the late stance phase of walking, thus placing excessive pressure on the plantar forefoot. Older clinical trials demonstrated that Achilles tendon lengthening decreased plantar pressure over the forefoot and reduced the recurrence of ulceration of the plantar aspect of the forefoot in patients with limited ankle dorsiflexion. Kim et al. recommended a plantar fascia release procedure, which could be associated with fewer complications, and advocated for this technique before considering Achilles tendon lengthening. Gastrocnemius release is another technique reported to decrease plantar pressure, which thereby helps treat ulcers in the treat ulcers in the forefoot and midfoot.

A patient who has had one-foot infection is likely to have another, which calls for preventive actions with the patient [38]. Detection of neuropathy before its complications ensue is the best method to prevent DFIs. Patients must be educated about the importance of optimizing glycemic control, always using appropriate footwear, avoiding foot trauma, performing daily self-examination of the feet, and reporting any changes to healthcare professionals. Those with severe neuropathy, substantial foot deformity, or critical ischemia should be referred to appropriate specialists to deal with these problems [37].

## References


1. Hatzenbuehler J, Pulling TJ. Diagnosis and management of osteomyelitis. Am Fam Physician. 2011;84(9):1027–33. PMID: 22046943
2. Xu J, Chen W, He L, Feng S, Zhang J, Chang B. Most postoperative reserved "normal" metatarsal stumps of diabetic foot osteomyelitis are infected but have healing potential. Front Endocrinol (Lausanne). 2023;2(14):1165305. https://doi.org/10.3389/fendo.2023.1165305. PMID: 37600693; PMCID: PMC10433740
3. Zgonis T. Surgical reconstruction of the diabetic foot and ankle. Philadelphia: Wolters Kluwer; 2018.
4. Ha Van G, Amouyal C, Bourron O, Aubert C, Carlier A, Mosbah H, Fourniols E, Cluzel P, Couture T, Hartemann A. Diabetic foot ulcer management in a multidisciplinary foot centre: one-year healing, amputation and mortality rate. J Wound Care. 2020;29(8):464–71. https://doi.org/10.12968/jowc.2020.29.8.464. PMID: 32804035
5. Senneville E, Robineau O. Treatment options for diabetic foot osteomyelitis. Expert Opin Pharmacother. 2017;18(8):759–65. https://doi.org/10.1080/14656566.2017.1316375. Epub 2017 May 19. PMID: 28406331
6. Game FL. Osteomyelitis in the diabetic foot: diagnosis and management. Med Clin North Am. 2013;97(5):947–56. https://doi.org/10.1016/j.mcna.2013.03.010. Epub 2013 May 4. PMID: 23992902
7. Biz C, Ruggieri P. Minimally invasive surgery: osteotomies for diabetic foot disease. Foot Ankle Clin. 2020;25(3):441–60. https://doi.org/10.1016/j.fcl.2020.05.006. Epub 2020 Jul 9. PMID: 32736741
8. Lipsky BA, Uçkay İ. Treating diabetic foot osteomyelitis: a practical state-of-the-art update. Medicina (Kaunas). 2021;57(4):339. https://doi.org/10.3390/medicina57040339. PMID: 33916055; PMCID: PMC8066570
9. Aicale R, Cipollaro L, Esposito S, Maffulli N. An evidence based narrative review on treatment of diabetic foot osteomyelitis. Surgeon. 2020;18(5):311–20. https://doi.org/10.1016/j.surge.2020.01.007. Epub 2020 Feb 17. PMID: 32081665
10. Molines-Barroso RJ, García-Álvarez Y, García-Klepzig JL, García-Morales E, Álvaro-Afonso FJ,

Lázaro-Martínez JL. Differences in the sub-metatarsal fat pad atrophy symptoms between patients with metatarsal head resection and those without metatarsal head resection: a cross-sectional study. J Clin Med. 2020;9(3):794. https://doi.org/10.3390/jcm9030794. PMID: 32183276; PMCID: PMC7141333
11. Lipsky BA, Aragón-Sánchez J, Diggle M, Embil J, Kono S, Lavery L, Senneville É, Urbančič-Rovan V, Van Asten S, International Working Group on the Diabetic Foot, Peters EJ. IWGDF guidance on the diagnosis and management of foot infections in persons with diabetes. Diabetes Metab Res Rev. 2016;32(Suppl 1):45–74. https://doi.org/10.1002/dmrr.2699. PMID: 26386266
12. Rajbhandari SM, Sutton M, Davies C, Tesfaye S, Ward JD. 'Sausage toe': a reliable sign of underlying osteomyelitis. Diabet Med. 2000;17(1):74–7. https://doi.org/10.1046/j.1464-5491.2000.00194.x. PMID: 10691164
13. Eneroth M, Larsson J, Apelqvist J. Deep foot infections in patients with diabetes and foot ulcer: an entity with different characteristics, treatments, and prognosis. J Diabetes Complicat. 1999;13(5-6):254–63. https://doi.org/10.1016/s1056-8727(99)00065-3. PMID: 10764999
14. Lipsky BA. Osteomyelitis of the foot in diabetic patients. Clin Infect Dis. 1997;25(6):1318–26. https://doi.org/10.1086/516148. PMID: 9431370
15. Álvaro-Afonso FJ, Lázaro-Martínez JL, Aragón-Sánchez J, García-Morales E, García-Álvarez Y, Molines-Barroso RJ. Inter-observer reproducibility of diagnosis of diabetic foot osteomyelitis based on a combination of probe-to-bone test and simple radiography. Diabetes Res Clin Pract. 2014;105(1):e3–5. https://doi.org/10.1016/j.diabres.2014.04.024. Epub 2014 Apr 28. PMID: 24857262
16. Michail M, Jude E, Liaskos C, Karamagiolis S, Makrilakis K, Dimitroulis D, Michail O, Tentolouris N. The performance of serum inflammatory markers for the diagnosis and follow-up of patients with osteomyelitis. Int J Low Extrem Wounds. 2013;12(2):94–9. https://doi.org/10.1177/1534734613486152. Epub 2013 May 9. PMID: 23667102
17. Bonham P. A critical review of the literature: part II: antibiotic treatment of osteomyelitis in patients with diabetes and foot ulcers. J Wound Ostomy Continence Nurs. 2001;28(3):141–9. https://doi.org/10.1067/mjw.2001.114892. PMID: 11337700
18. Jeffcoate WJ, Lipsky BA. Controversies in diagnosing and managing osteomyelitis of the foot in diabetes. Clin Infect Dis. 2004;39 Suppl 2:S115–22. https://doi.org/10.1086/383272. PMID: 15306989
19. Khatri G, Wagner DK, Sohnle PG. Effect of bone biopsy in guiding antimicrobial therapy for osteomyelitis complicating open wounds. Am J Med Sci. 2001;321(6):367–71. https://doi.org/10.1097/00000441-200106000-00002. PMID: 11417751
20. Senneville EM, Lipsky BA, van Asten SAV, Peters EJ. Diagnosing diabetic foot osteomyelitis. Diabetes Metab Res Rev. 2020;36 Suppl 1:e3250. https://doi.org/10.1002/dmrr.3250. Epub 2020 Jan 17. PMID: 31950555
21. Bonnet E, Maulin L, Senneville E, Castan B, Fourcade C, Loubet P, Poitrenaud D, Schuldiner S, Sotto A, Lavigne JP, Lesprit P, Individual members of the "Review group". Clinical practice recommendations for infectious disease management of diabetic foot infection (DFI) – 2023 SPILF. Infect Dis Now. 2024;54(1):104832. https://doi.org/10.1016/j.idnow.2023.104832. Epub 2023 Nov 10. PMID: 37952582
22. Wrobel JS, Connolly JE. Making the diagnosis of osteomyelitis. The role of prevalence. J Am Podiatr Med Assoc. 1998;88(7):337–43. https://doi.org/10.7547/87507315-88-7-337. PMID: 9680770
23. Lipsky BA, Berendt AR, Cornia PB, Pile JC, Peters EJ, Armstrong DG, Deery HG, Embil JM, Joseph WS, Karchmer AW, Pinzur MS, Senneville E, Infectious Diseases Society of America. 2012 Infectious Diseases Society of America clinical practice guideline for the diagnosis and treatment of diabetic foot infections. Clin Infect Dis. 2012;54(12):e132–73. https://doi.org/10.1093/cid/cis346. PMID: 22619242
24. Malone M, Bowling FL, Gannass A, Jude EB, Boulton AJ. Deep wound cultures correlate well with bone biopsy culture in diabetic foot osteomyelitis. Diabetes Metab Res Rev. 2013;29(7):546–50. https://doi.org/10.1002/dmrr.2425. PMID: 23653368
25. Weiner RD, Viselli SJ, Fulkert KA, Accetta P. Histology versus microbiology for accuracy in identification of osteomyelitis in the diabetic foot. J Foot Ankle Surg. 2011;50(2):197–200. https://doi.org/10.1053/j.jfas.2010.12.001. Epub 2011 Jan 20. PMID: 21251855
26. Pittet D, Wyssa B, Herter-Clavel C, Kursteiner K, Vaucher J, Lew PD. Outcome of diabetic foot infections treated conservatively: a retrospective cohort study with long-term follow-up. Arch Intern Med. 1999;159(8):851–6. https://doi.org/10.1001/archinte.159.8.851. PMID: 10219931
27. Lipsky BA, Berendt AR, Deery HG, Embil JM, Joseph WS, Karchmer AW, LeFrock JL, Lew DP, Mader JT, Norden C, Tan JS, Infectious Diseases Society of America. Diagnosis and treatment of diabetic foot infections. Plast Reconstr Surg. 2006;117(7 Suppl):212S–38S. https://doi.org/10.1097/01.prs.0000222737.09322.77. PMID: 16799390
28. Menekse S. Outcome of chronic foot osteomyelitis treated with hyperbaric oxygen: an observational study. Int J Low Extrem Wounds. 2024;23(1):80–5. https://doi.org/10.1177/15347346231217641. Epub 2023 Dec 10. PMID: 38073097
29. Game FL, Jeffcoate WJ. Primarily non-surgical management of osteomyelitis of the foot in diabetes. Diabetologia. 2008;51(6):962–7. https://doi.org/10.1007/s00125-008-0976-1. Epub 2008 Apr 3. PMID: 18385975
30. Abbas M, Uçkay I, Lipsky BA. In diabetic foot infections antibiotics are to treat infection, not

to heal wounds. Expert Opin Pharmacother. 2015;16(6):821–32. https://doi.org/10.1517/14656566.2015.1021780. Epub 2015 Mar 3. PMID: 25736920
31. Peters EJG, Lipsky BA, Senneville É, Abbas ZG, Aragón-Sánchez J, Diggle M, Embil JM, Kono S, Lavery LA, Malone M, Urbančič-Rovan V, Van Asten SA. Interventions in the management of infection in the foot in diabetes: a systematic review. Diabetes Metab Res Rev. 2020;36(Suppl 1):e3282. https://doi.org/10.1002/dmrr.3282. PMID: 32176437
32. Biz C, Ruggieri P. Distal metatarsal osteotomies for chronic plantar diabetic foot ulcers. Foot Ankle Clin. 2022;27(3):545–66. https://doi.org/10.1016/j.fcl.2022.02.003. Epub 2022 Aug 6. PMID: 36096551
33. Biz C, Belluzzi E, Crimì A, Bragazzi NL, Nicoletti P, Mori F, Ruggieri P. Minimally Invasive Metatarsal Osteotomies (MIMOs) for the Treatment of Plantar Diabetic Forefoot Ulcers (PDFUs): a systematic review and meta-analysis with meta-regressions. Appl Sci. 2021;11:9628. https://doi.org/10.3390/app11209628.
34. Biz C, Gastaldo S, Dalmau-Pastor M, Corradin M, Volpin A, Ruggieri P. Minimally Invasive Distal Metatarsal Diaphyseal Osteotomy (DMDO) for chronic plantar diabetic foot ulcers. Foot Ankle Int. 2018;39(1):83–92. https://doi.org/10.1177/1071100717735640. Epub 2017 Nov 7. PMID: 29110516
35. Ferreira L, Carvalho A, Carvalho R. Short-term predictors of amputation in patients with diabetic foot ulcers. Diabetes Metab Syndr. 2018;12(6):875–9. https://doi.org/10.1016/j.dsx.2018.05.007. Epub 2018 May 17. PMID: 29802073
36. Waibel FWA, Uçkay I, Sairanen K, Waibel L, Berli MC, Böni T, Gariani K, Lipsky BA. Diabetic calcaneal osteomyelitis. Infez Med. 2019;27(3):225–38. PMID: 31545766
37. Lebowitz D, Gariani K, Kressmann B, Dach EV, Huttner B, Bartolone P, Lê N, Mohamad M, Lipsky BA, Uçkay I. Are antibiotic-resistant pathogens more common in subsequent episodes of diabetic foot infection? Int J Infect Dis. 2017;59:61–4. https://doi.org/10.1016/j.ijid.2017.04.012. Epub 2017 Apr 24. PMID: 28450198
38. Lázaro-Martínez JL, García-Madrid M, García-Álvarez Y, Álvaro-Afonso FJ, Sanz-Corbalán I, García-Morales E. Conservative surgery for chronic diabetic foot osteomyelitis: procedures and recommendations. J Clin Orthop Trauma. 2020;16:86–98. https://doi.org/10.1016/j.jcot.2020.12.014. PMID: 33680830; PMCID: PMC7919928

# Osteomyelitis of the Jaws

17

Stefano Fusetti and Bacci Christian

## 17.1 Acute and Chronic Osteomyelitis

Osteomyelitis is defined as an infection of the bone marrow with a tendency to progress involving both the cortical and medullary portions related to bacterial or fungal activity. The incidence of osteomyelitis in the maxillofacial region is much higher in the mandible due to the dense poorly vascularized cortical plates and the blood supply primarily from the inferior alveolar neurovascular bundle. Diminished host defenses and infective foci (even dental in this region), both local and systemic, can contribute significantly to the emergence and clinical course of the disease. Various classification and staging systems have been adopted to describe the nature of the disease and lay down the most appropriate treatment plan. Chronic osteomyelitis evolves over months to years and is characterized by low-grade inflammation due to relapsing and persistent infection. Based on the presentation of the disease, chronic osteomyelitis can be differentiated as suppurative and a nonsuppurative type. A suppurative course is associated with an abscess or fistula formation and sequestration at some stage. Osteomyelitis may also appear as a non-suppurative chronic inflammation of the jaw with no underlying cause being identified. General features of the primary (non-suppurative) osteomyelitis are hard swelling, malaise, recurrent deep boring pain, paresthesia of the inferior alveolar nerve, trismus, and general fatigue. Various patterns include primary chronic osteomyelitis, diffuse sclerosing osteomyelitis, juvenile mandibular chronic osteomyelitis, chronic recurrent multifocal osteomyelitis, and chronic non-bacterial osteomyelitis [1, 2].

Chronic recurrent multifocal osteomyelitis (CRMO) is an aseptic inflammatory disorder of unknown cause characterized by multifocal bone lesions with pain and swelling recurring over months to years. It is supposed to be the more severe form of chronic non-bacterial osteomyelitis. A form of diffuse sclerosing osteomyelitis or recurrent multifocal osteomyelitis may have its presentation indicating the mandibular location of SAPHO (synovitis, acne, pustulosis, hyperostosis, osteitis) syndrome. It occurs because of an unknown etiology with a synchronous combination of osteoarticular and skin manifestations. Involvement of the mandible is found in almost 10% of cases. Bone manifestation is typically characterized by non-suppuration and a mixed radiographic pattern accompanied by a solid type of periosteal reaction, external bone resorption, and bone enlargement. The presence of skin diseases, such as palmoplantar pustulosis, strongly suggests SAPHO syndrome.

S. Fusetti (✉) · B. Christian
Department of Neurosciences, University of Padova, Padova, Italy
e-mail: stefano.fusetti@unipd.it; christian.bacci@unipd.it



P. Ruggieri et al. (eds.), *Bone and Joint Infections*, https://doi.org/10.1007/978-3-031-96383-4_17

The biopsy tissue consists of a fibrous tissue that replaces the bone trabeculae, and presents a phlogistic infiltrate made up of lymphocytes and granulocytes. The fibrous tissue mixes with fragments of necrotic bone tissue devoid of viable osteocytes. Radiolucency with indistinct margins containing a sequestration of the thick, bone casting that surrounds the radiolucent area is thickened and the cortical area can n Histopathology cause a periosteal reaction. Treatment of acute osteomyelitis consists of the administration of antibiotics and drainage of the abscess. In chronic forms, it is advisable to remove the bone sequestration by combining high-dose intravenous antibiotic treatment. In the case of very large lesions. It is necessary to carry out a bone resection followed by bony reconstruction. In the case of chronic osteomyelitis, hyperbaric oxygen therapy, low laser, and ozone therapy are useful [1, 2].

In the current clinical practice, in the past 20 years, the most common forms of osteomyelitis are osteoradionecrosis (ORN) and medication-related osteonecrosis of the jaws (MRONJ).

### 17.1.1 Osteoradionecrosis (ORN)

Osteoradionecrosis (ORN) of the jaw is one of the most feared complications of head and neck radiation therapy. Radiation therapy (RT) plays a key role in the management of head and neck cancers resulting in improved tumor control and increased survival rates. Despite these advances, patients treated with RT often develop radiation-associated toxicities such as osteoradionecrosis (ORN). Based on the consensus in the literature [3, 4], the clinical diagnostic criteria of ORN are as follows:

- The affected site is within the head and neck radiation field.
- Mucosal breakdown or failure to heal, resulting in bone exposure.
- The overlying bone is "dead" or necrotic.
- The bone exposure persists for at least 3 months.
- There is an absence of recurrent tumor/metastases on the affected site.

Notani's classification is a simple system to stage ORN, based on anatomical boundaries:

Stage I ORN is confined to alveolar bone.
Stage II ORN is limited to the alveolar bone and/or above the level of the inferior alveolar canal.
Stage III ORN is under the lower part of the inferior alveolar canal, with fistula or bone fracture.

A recent study [3] has applied the American Academy of Maxillofacial Surgeons classification system, commonly used for medication-related osteonecrosis of the jaw, in analyzing the severity of ORN in head-neck cancer patients. Clinical sign typically includes an area of the exposed bone area or a fistula that probes to the bone. Tooth mobility or spontaneous tooth exfoliation can also be an indication of ORN. Several cases of "radiographic" ORN with unexposed bone necrosis and intact mucosa have also been reported. Radiographic signs can range from localized osteolytic areas, extensive osteolytic areas, sequestrum, and mandibular fracture as seen on a panoramic radiograph. ORN can present as radiolucent areas surrounding the extraction sockets that remain visible for more than 12 months. Computed tomography scans can depict ORN lesions as osteolytic lesions or cortical erosions involving the buccal or lingual surface and often associated with bone fragmentation. Early stages of ORN can be asymptomatic. However, pain, with or without swelling, is a common symptom associated with ORN.

Poor oral hygiene and food impaction within the exposed bone area may also be present. Patients may present with sensory neurological symptoms such as dysesthesia, or anesthesia in the distribution of the inferior alveolar nerve in the mandible in late-stage ORN. As ORN progresses, patients may develop trismus, neuropathic pain, and other symptoms such as secondary infection resulting in chronic pus drainage, draining extra oral fistulae, or even pathological jaw fracture. ORN has a known predilection for the mandible over the maxilla.

This vulnerability may be due to its relative hypovascular nature and proximity to the primary tumor causing inevitable radiation exposure within the radiation field. The posterior mandible is more commonly affected because of its high bone density resulting in an increased absorption of radiation dose.

Many theories have been proposed regarding the etiopathogenesis of ORN [3], but the exact mechanism is complex and poorly understood. Early studies showed evidence of bacteria in tissues affected by ORN as well as microscopic tissue changes, with the classic triad sequence of pathogenesis as "radiation, trauma, and infection". ORN was thought to result from secondary infection due to local injury to the devitalized bone resulting in "radiation-induced osteomyelitis." This theory explained the role of antibiotic therapy in ORN management. Based on the evidence of ORN in the absence of trauma (extraction), a new theory was proposed, which formulated that the cause was a radiation-induced endarteritis resulting in "hypoxia, hypovascularity, and hypocellularity". Driven by his theory that persistent hypoxia can cause a chronic non-healing wound, his hypothesis formed the cornerstone for the use of hyperbaric oxygen (HBO) in the treatment of ORN. A current theory proposes that ORN occurs by a "radiation-induced fibro atrophic mechanism" whereby the activation and dysregulation of fibroblastic activity leads to atrophic tissue within a previously irradiated area. To reverse these changes, new therapeutic regimens have been developed wherein pentoxifylline and tocopherol (vitamin E) act synergistically as potent antifibrotic agents.

#### 17.1.1.1 Prevalence

The prevalence of ORN varies widely in the literature ranging from 0.4% to 56%. There is an approximately 20% decrease in the rate of ORN from earlier decades to 4–8% in the modern era. This overall reduction of ORN can be attributed to the evolution in radiation modalities from the conventional/2D RT to 3-D conformal RT to intensity-modulated radiation therapy (IMRT). Proton radiation therapy (PRT) allows further conformal treatment volumes and greater tissue-sparing capability in head and neck radiation due to its inert property of Bragg Peak. This technique includes a smaller volume of the jaw that receives high irradiation doses thus potentially decreasing the likelihood of ORN [3, 4].

#### 17.1.1.2 Time Lapse to ORN

ORN can occur at any time, even beyond 10 years following RT. The median time interval between RT and development of ORN was 13 months range, 2–122 months). However, it is most frequently noted (70–94%) in the first few years after completion of RT. The median latency period is usually reported as 12–24 months. Early onset ORN occurring within 24 months after RT is thought to be related to radiation doses higher than 60Gy; it can develop spontaneously or following dentoalveolar trauma. In contrast, late-onset ORN is thought to arise from trauma in a chronically hypoxic tissue environment.

#### 17.1.1.3 Management

The management of patients with ORN varies considerably and depends on the severity of the complication. Conservative approaches are generally reserved for asymptomatic or mildly symptomatic patients (Notani I or II). This implies close observation, strict oral hygiene maintenance, saline irrigation and chlorhexidine mouth rinses, systemic antibiotic therapy for acute infections, anti-inflammatory and analgesics, when necessary, avoidance of local irritants like tobacco and alcohol use, and discontinuation of ill-fitting dentures. Simple surgical intervention involves smoothening of sharp bony edges to prevent traumatic ulcerations to adjacent soft tissues and gentle debridement of mobile bony sequestrum if present. Fixation plates and screws are removed if they appear to be a contributing factor. Studies have shown that early intervention with minor surgical procedures combined with pharmacological methods may improve the prognosis of ORN. Surgical management is generally employed when conservative management is unsuccessful and there is progressive (Notani III) ORN resulting in pathological fractures and draining fistulae. Those with more advanced ORN may require extensive surgical resections such as segmental mandibulectomy and osteocutaneous free-flap reconstruction. Although a variety of free flaps are available for microvascular reconstructive technique, the fibula remains the workhorse for reconstruction in mandibular ORN. The literature on the use of HBO for the prevention or management of ORN is controversial. Based on a systematic review, there was no conclusive evidence to support the routine use of HBO for the prevention or management of ORN. However, adjunctive HBO may be considered for use on an individual basis in patients who failed to response to conservative management and subsequent surgical resection. There is insufficient evidence to support the use of HBO prior to dentoalveolar procedures to prevent ORN [3, 4].

### 17.1.2 Risk Prediction

One of the main strategies in mitigating ORN risk focuses on patient-related factors including dental extractions before and after RT. To prevent risk for ORN, it is generally recommended to remove dental foci of infection within the RT field before RT. All patients receiving head and neck RT should be referred to the Dental Service for pre-treatment oral and dental evaluation. The decision to perform pre-RT dental extractions is based on several factors. Knowledge of radiation dose, treatment modality, field of radiation, and tumor prognosis plays an important role in the clinical decision-making. Consideration is given to the pre-existing dental status, and extraction is indicated when there is evidence of advanced caries with poor restorative prognosis, periodontal disease, and non-functional teeth within the radiation field. An atraumatic approach in the extraction procedure with primary closure at the time of extraction is applied for soft tissue integrity and to minimize postoperative complications. Adequate time for healing of extraction sites before RT is considered essential. The current recommendation is for a healing time of 10 to 14 days between extractions and the commencement of head and neck RT. The protocol for dentate patients undergoing head and neck RT or with a history of head and neck RT also includes a prescription of neutral sodium fluoride 1.1% with 5000 parts per million (ppm) in the form of a dentifrice toothpaste. The major risk of ORN has been associated with post-RT dental extraction. Wound healing in the mandibular posterior arches is considered compromised when dental extractions are performed in the field of radiation doses above 60Gy. Because of IMRT's complex 3-dimensional dose delivery and tissue sparing favoring the major salivary glands, different dose gradients across the mandible are created. This makes it difficult to determine the dosimetric distribution to the jaws and thus, predict areas at risk for ORN. Dosimetric contouring provides an estimate of the prescribed radiation dose to specified regions of the jaws, thus allowing the clinician to make dental treatment recommendations based on predicted risk for ORN.

#### 17.1.2.1 Conclusion

ORN remains a significant oral complication of head and neck RT. Future research directions include multi-institutional studies with large sample sizes and randomized controlled trials focused on the management of established cases. Management of ORN should focus on prevention or risk mitigation. Standardized preventive protocols are the most effective way to reduce the risk for ORN. Multidisciplinary team communications, and carefully planned dentoalveolar procedures pre- and post-radiation therapy can reduce risk for ORN and maintain and improve quality of life in head and neck cancer patients [3, 4].

### 17.1.3 Medication-Related Osteonecrosis of the Jaw (MRONJ)

Medication-related osteonecrosis of the jaw (MRONJ) is a severe adverse drug reaction, consisting of progressive bone destruction in the maxillofacial region of patients. ONJ can be caused by two pharmacological agents: Antiresorptive (including bisphosphonates (BPs) and receptor activator of nuclear factor kappa-B ligand inhibitors) and antiangiogenic MRONJ pathophysiology is not completely elucidated. Several suggested hypotheses could explain its unique localization to the jaws: Inflammation or infection, microtrauma, altered bone remodeling or over suppression of bone resorption, angiogenesis inhibition, soft tissue BPs toxicity, a peculiar biofilm of the oral cavity, terminal vascularization of the mandible, suppression of immunity, or Vitamin D deficiency. Dental screening and adequate treatment are fundamental to reduce the risk of osteonecrosis in patients under antiresorptive or antiangiogenic therapy, or before initiating the administration. The treatment of MRONJ is generally difficult and the optimal therapy strategy is still to be established. For this reason, prevention is even more important. It is suggested that a multidisciplinary team approach includes a dentist, an oncologist, and a maxillofacial surgeon to evaluate and decide the best therapy for the patient. The choice between conservative treatment and surgery is not easy, and it should be made on a case-by-case basis. However, the initial approach should be as conservative as possible. The most important goals of treatment for patients with established MRONJ are primarily the control of infection, bone necrosis progression, and pain [5–7].

#### 17.1.3.1 Medications

Bisphosphonates (BPs) are antiresorptive medications that are effective in managing cancer-related conditions, including hypercalcemia of malignancy, spinal cord compression, and pathologic fractures (skeletal-related events [SREs]) associated with bone metastases in the context of solid tumors (such as breast, prostate, and lung cancers) and multiple myeloma. While the potential for BPs to improve cancer-specific survival remains controversial, these medications have had a significant positive effect on the quality of life for patients with advanced cancer involving the skeleton and reducing or preventing skeletal-related events. Bisphosphonates also are used for the prevention of osteoporosis-related fractures (fragility fractures) in patients with osteoporosis and osteopenia. BPs administered orally–including alendronate (Fosamax®), risedronate (Actonel") or parenterally (zoledronic acid [Reclast®]), and ibandronate (Boniva®) and neridronato (Nerixia®) can result in a significant reduction in vertebral and nonvertebral fractures for patients with osteoporosis. Bisphosphonate therapy also is indicated for other metabolic bone diseases such as Paget's disease of bone and osteogenesis imperfecta. However, clinical trials have not demonstrated the efficacy of bisphosphonate therapy in the management of fibrous dysplasia.

Denosumab (Xgeva®) (DMB), a receptor activator of nuclear factor kappa-B ligand (RANK-L), is an antiresorptive agent that exists as a fully humanized antibody against RANK ligand and inhibits osteoclast function and associated bone resorption. When denosumab (Prolia") is administered subcutaneously every 6 months, there is a significant reduction in the risk of vertebral, nonvertebral, and hip fractures in osteoporotic patients. Denosumab (Xgeva®) also is effective in reducing SREs related to metastatic bone disease from solid tumors when administered monthly. RANK ligand inhibitors also have proven efficacy in the treatment of giant cell tumors of bone and fibrous dysplasia. In contrast to BPs, RANK-L inhibitors do not bind to bone, and their effects on bone remodeling are mostly diminished within 6 months of treatment cessation [5–7].

#### 17.1.3.2 MRONJ Definition

MRONJ should be distinguished from other forms of osteonecrosis (ONJ) conditions and identified by history and clinical exam. The clinical criteria required to establish a diagnosis of MRONJ have remained unchanged from the previous position paper.

The case definition of MRONJ includes all the following elements:

1. Current or previous treatment with antiresorptive therapy alone or in combination with immune modulators or antiangiogenic medications.
2. Exposed bone or bone that can be probed through an intraoral or extraoral fistula(e) in the maxillofacial region that has persisted for more than 8 weeks.
3. No history of radiation therapy to the jaws or metastatic disease to the jaws.

#### 17.1.3.3 Patients At-Risk

**Staging**

No apparent necrotic bone in asymptomatic patients who have been treated with IV or oral antiresorptive therapy.

**STAGE 0 (Nonexposed Bone Variant)**

Patients with no clinical evidence of necrotic bone but who present with nonspecific symptoms or clinical and radiographic findings, such as:

**Symptoms**

- Odontalgia not explained by an odontogenic cause.
- Dull, aching bone pain in the jaw, which may radiate to the temporomandibular joint region.
- Sinus pain, which may be associated with inflammation and thickening of the maxillary sinus wall.
- Altered neurosensory function.

**Clinical Findings**

- Loosening of teeth not explained by chronic periodontal disease.
- Intraoral or extraoral swelling.

**Radiographic Findings**

- Alveolar bone loss or resorption not attributable to chronic periodontal disease.
- Changes to trabecular pattern sclerotic bone and no new bone in extraction sockets.
- Regions of osteosclerosis involving the alveolar bone and/or the surrounding basilar bone.
- Thickening/obscuring of periodontal ligament (thickening of the lamina dura, sclerosis, and decreased size of the periodontal ligament space).

These nonspecific findings, which characterize this variant of MRONJ without bone exposure, may occur in patients with a prior history of Stages 1, 2, or 3 disease who have been healed and have no clinical evidence of exposed bone. Progression to Stage 1 disease has been reported in up to 50 patients with Stage 0 disease and, therefore, AAOMS deems it prudent to consider Stage 0 disease as a potential precursor to MRONJ.

**Stage 1**

Exposed and necrotic bone or fistula that probes to the bone in patients who are asymptomatic and have no evidence of infection/inflammation. These patients also may present with radiographic findings mentioned for Stage 0 that are localized to the alveolar bone region.

**Stage 2**

Exposed and necrotic bone, or fistula that probes to the bone, with evidence of infection/inflammation. These patients are symptomatic. These patients also may present with radiographic findings mentioned for Stage 0 localized to the alveolar bone region.

**Stage 3**

Exposed and necrotic bone or fistulae that probes to the bone, with evidence of infection, and one or more of the following:

- Exposed necrotic bone extending beyond the region of alveolar bone (i.e., inferior border and ramus in the mandible, maxillary sinus, and zygoma in the maxilla)
- Pathologic fracture.
- Extraoral fistula.
- Oral antral/oral-nasal communication.
- Osteolysis extends to the inferior border of the mandible or sinus floor (Fig. 17.1).

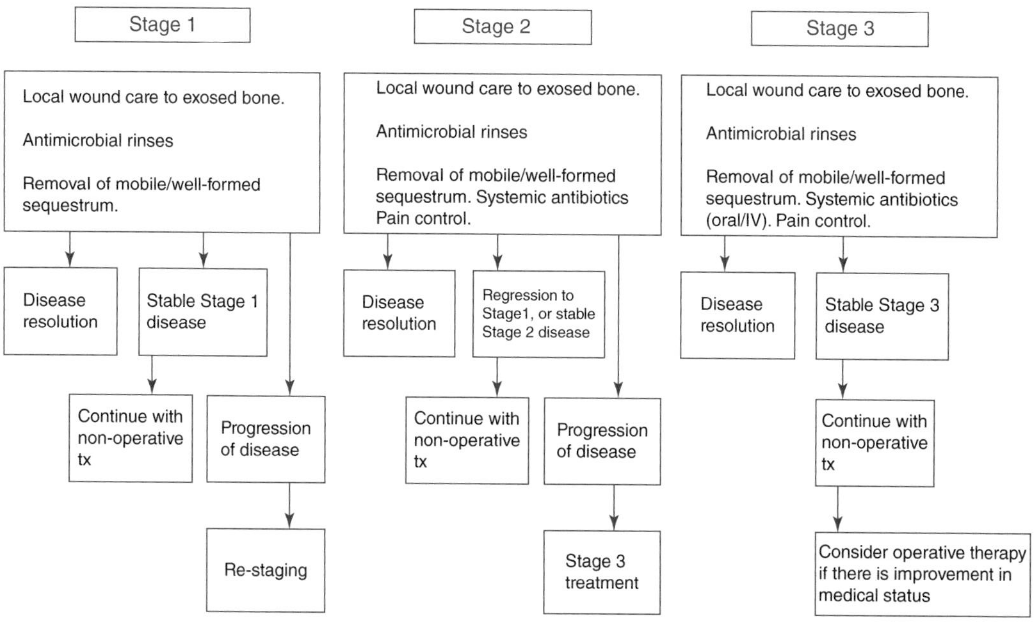


**Fig. 17.1** Non-operative therapies. (Ruggiero et al. [5]. Published with permission of Elsevier)

## 17.2 Pathophysiology

Since the AAOMS position paper in 2014, significant knowledge has been gained regarding MRONJ pathophysiology from both clinical and particularly preclinical animal studies. It should be noted that animal studies have a few limitations, are most often using supratherapeutic doses, and likely do not truly mirror the clinical environment. That said, they are critical in understanding disease mechanisms and can serve as one reference point for evidence-based clinical decision-making. Much debate persists among clinicians and researchers, contributing to the various treatment protocols utilized for patients today. Disease specificity unique to the jaws has focused leading hypotheses to include bone remodeling inhibition, inflammation or infection, angiogenesis inhibition, innate or acquired immune dysfunction, as well as genetic predisposition. Both animal and human studies suggest that an antiresorptive medication, coupled with inflammation or infection, is necessary and sufficient to induce MRONJ. However, as more knowledge is gained on the subject, it is becoming increasingly apparent that MRONJ is multifactorial, and multiple hypotheses can likely explain the overall pathophysiology of this disease [5–7].

### 17.2.1 Bone Remodeling Inhibition

The definition of MRONJ includes oral or parenteral administration of antiresorptive drugs, where suppression of bone remodeling may be the central hypothesis in its pathophysiology. Antiresorptive medications, including BPs and denosumab (DMB), have direct effects on osteoclast formation, differentiation, or function. In osteoporosis, BPs are a first-line therapy to decrease bone remodeling, increase bone mineral density, and decrease vertebral and long bone fractures. BPs, in higher doses, also are utilized in primary bone malignancy and bone metastases to decrease SREs, including hypercalcemia of malignancy, reduce severe bone pain, and improve quality of life. Although DMB has only been approved for use since 2010, its use has increased significantly for both osteoporosis and malignancy in the last decade. The prevalence of MRONJ with DMB users is at least as high as BP users, likely due to its increased potency to inhibit bone resorption. This is supported in the jaws as animal studies demonstrate absent osteoclasts around the alveolar bone of DMB-treated mice. Human bone specimens also show an increased number of non-functional osteoclasts surrounding necrotic bone in BP-treated patients, further reinforcing bone remodeling inhibition as a leading hypothesis in MRONJ pathophysiology. With the appearance of MRONJ in DMB-treated patients, it becomes increasingly apparent that the underlying pathophysiology involves dysfunctional osteoclasts. Discontinuing DMB, but not BPs, before tooth extraction successfully prevented MRONJ development in rats. Moreover, parathyroid hormone, which acts directly on osteoblasts to induce bone formation and indirectly increases osteoclastic bone resorption and overall Remodeling has been shown to prevent MRONJ and improve extraction socket healing in rodents and preliminarily in patients. This observation provides further support for the central role of osteoclast inhibition in MRONJ pathogenesis [5–7].

### 17.2.2 Inflammation or Infection?

Although most studies report tooth extraction as the major inciting event for MRONJ development, most extracted teeth had pre-existing periodontal or periapical disease. From this patient, animal models of inflammation or infection were developed to replicate clinical, radiographic, and histologic features of MRONJ. The presence of inflammatory cytokines, specifically at the site of MRONJ, also supports the strong role of inflammation. As evidence of increased systemic inflammation and its contribution to MRONJ development, mice with experimentally induced rheumatoid arthritis demonstrated more severe MRONJ with increased oral bone exposure, more pronounced radiographic features, intense local inflammatory infiltrate, and larger areas of histologic necrosis. Further support for the inflammatory etiology showed that removal of the inflammatory nidus in ligature-induced periodontitis ameliorated MRONJ development in mice, demonstrating reduced inflammation and prevention of disease progression. Moreover, transplantation of peripheral blood mononuclear cells with anti-inflammatory properties reduced MRONJ prevalence by improving soft tissue healing, decreasing inflammatory polymorphonuclear cells and inflammatory marker expression, as well as enhancing vascularity. These preclinical findings confirm the irrefutable role of inflammation or infection in MRONJ disease prevalence, severity, and resolution. The presence of bacteria on the exposed necrotic bone also contributes to disease severity, where pain and signs of infection define Stage 2 MRONJ. This is not surprising since poor oral hygiene and biofilm presence are associated with MRONJ development, and oral health maintenance and dental prophylaxis before initiating antiresorptive therapy can decrease MRONJ prevalence. Importantly, clinical treatment protocols to reduce the biofilm and eradicate infection have emerged as important alternatives to debridement and resection in patients who may not be ideal surgical candidates [5–7].

### 17.2.3 Angiogenesis Inhibition

Osteonecrosis is traditionally defined as avascular necrosis or aseptic necrosis, most characterized as osteocyte death after decreased blood flow to the femoral head. However, MRONJ is defined as necrotic bone in the maxillofacial region after exposure to either antiresorptive or antiangiogenic medications. BPs such as zoledronic acid directly inhibit angiogenesis in vitro and in vivo and animal models demonstrate decreased vascularity in sites of MRONJ and decreased micro-vessel numbers during early stages of bone healing. In addition, angiogenesis normally seen during extraction socket healing is inhibited by BPs, and both BPs and DMB have been shown to decrease arterial area, venous area, and overall vascularity of periodontal tissues during early and late MRONJ development. Importantly, antiangiogenic medications, such as VEGF inhibitors, tyrosine kinase receptor inhibitors, and immunomodulatory drugs, can be associated with MRONJ. Moreover, patients with multiple myeloma receiving both antiresorptive and antiangiogenic medications, as shown in several studies, have a higher MRONJ prevalence. Important aspects of MRONJ treatment include determining disease margins, which can be challenging as microvascular mucosal abnormalities can be seen adjacent to frank MRONJ lesions. It is important to note that the incidence of MRONJ in patients on antiangiogenics is much lower than those taking antiresorptive medications [5–7].

### 17.2.4 Acquired Immune Dysfunction

Although animal studies confirm that an antiresorptive medication—coupled with inflammation or infection—is necessary and sufficient to produce MRONJ, not all patients with dental infections develop the disease. It is well-known that patients with medical comorbidities such as diabetes or rheumatoid arthritis or immunocompromised states are at significantly higher risk for MRONJ with or without exposure to antiresorptive agents. Patients with metastatic or primary bone malignancies have a compromised immune system. This also has been confirmed with animal studies, where chemotherapy, steroids, and disease-modifying antirheumatic drugs (DMARDs), combined with antiangiogenic medications and an antiresorptive, increase MRONJ severity or prevalence. Moreover, higher rates of MRONJ occurring patients with multiple myeloma who receive multiple chemotherapeutic agents. Replenishing the area of nonhealing MRONJ lesions with mesenchymal stem cells (MSCs) to overcome immune dysfunction is a potential area of therapeutic interest, especially in patients who are immunocompromised. A recent study showed altered numbers and patterns of T-cells in human and rat MRONJ necrotic bone samples as compared to healthy patients and non-MRONJ sites. Preclinical studies also demonstrate the healing or prevention of MRONJ lesions after systemic infusion with adipose or bone marrow-derived MSCs [5–7].

## 17.3 Risk Factors for MRONJ

### 17.3.1 Medication-Related Risk Factors

To estimate the risk for medications associated with MRONJ, the primary parameter to be considered is the therapeutic indication for treatment (e.g., malignancy or osteoporosis/osteopenia). The data suggest that antiresorptive medications are associated with an increased risk for developing MRONJ. The risk of MRONJ is considerably higher in the malignancy group (<5%) than in the osteoporosis group (<0.05%). Current data are insufficient to identify other medications as risk factors for developing MRONJ.

### 17.3.2 Local Factors

#### 17.3.2.1 Dentoalveolar Procedures

Dentoalveolar procedures are the most common identifiable predisposing factor for developing MRONJ. Several studies report that among patients with MRONJ, tooth extraction is cited as a predisposing event ranging from 62% to 82%. While this information is important, it is not what most patients or clinicians want to know. Current estimates for the risk of MRONJ among osteoporotic patients exposed to BPs following tooth extraction range from 0% to 0.15%. For osteoporotic patients exposed to DMB, the risk for MRONJ following tooth extraction was 1%. For cancer patients exposed to BPs, the risk of developing MRONJ after tooth extraction ranges from 1.6% to 14.8%. While the estimates for developing MRONJ in high-risk patients undergoing tooth extraction vary, they cluster between 1% and 5%, similar to estimates of osteoradionecrosis following tooth extraction in irradiated patients. The risk of developing MRONJ among patients who have been exposed to antiresorptive medications for other dentoalveolar operations such as dental implant placement and endodontic or periodontal procedures is unknown. The risk for MRONJ after implant placement among patients treated with DMB has been reported to be 0.5%. Absent better data, AAOMS cautions against the use of these procedures in cancer patients exposed to antiresorptive therapies and recommends osteoporosis patients be informed of potential risks, albeit low, including development of MRONJ, early and late implant failure all of which have been described in case reports and clinical trials [5–7].

#### 17.3.2.2 Anatomic Factors

Limited new information regarding anatomic risk factors for MRONJ is available. MRONJ is more likely to appear in the mandible (75%) than the maxilla (25%) but can appear in both jaws (4.5%). Denture use was associated with an increased risk for MRONJ among cancer patients exposed to zoledronate%.

#### 17.3.2.3 Concomitant Oral Disease

Pre-existing inflammatory dental disease such as periodontal disease or periapical pathology is cited as a risk factor. Among cancer patients with MRONJ, the pre-existing inflammatory dental disease was a risk factor in 50% of the cases. Given that a common treatment of inflammatory dental disease is tooth extraction, pre-existing dental disease may confound the relationship between tooth extraction and risk for MRONJ. Tooth extraction may expose MRONJ as opposed to being the precipitating event. It would be valuable to see an estimate of the association between tooth extraction and MRONJ adjusted for pre-existing inflammatory dental disease. After tooth extraction and periodontal disease, the next most common risk factor is reported as "spontaneous" MRONJ with no identifiable dental risk factor.

#### 17.3.2.4 Treatment Goals

The major goals of treatment for patients at risk of developing or who have established MRONJ are:

#### 17.3.2.5 Prevention of MRONJ

Prioritization and support of continued oncologic treatment in patients receiving antiresorptive therapy alone or in combination with immune modulators or antiangiogenic medications:

- Oncology patients benefit from the therapeutic effect of antiresorptive therapy by controlling bone pain and reducing the incidence of other SREs.
- Prioritization and support of continued bone health and the prevention of fragility fractures.
- Patients with osteoporosis, osteopenia, and other metabolic bone diseases benefit from antiresorptive therapy by significantly reducing the risk of fragility fractures and other skeletal-related events.
- Preservation of quality of life through:
- Patient education and reassurance.
- Control of pain.
- Control of secondary infection.
- Prevention of extension of lesion and development of new areas of necrosis.

### 17.3.3 MRONJ Prevention Strategies

**Pretherapy (Nonmalignant Disease)**

Educate the patient about the potential risks associated with long-term ART.

Optimization of dental health can occur concurrently with ART.

**Pretherapy (Malignant Disease)**

Educate patients about the higher risk of MRONJ and the importance of regimented dental care.

Optimization of the dental health prior to the initiation of ART (extraction of non-restorable teeth.

**During Antiresorptive Therapy (Nonmalignant Disease)**

No alteration of operative plan for most patients.

Considerations include drug schedule, duration of therapy, comorbidities, other medications, degree of underlying infection/inflammation, and extent of surgery to be performed. Drug holidays are controversial.

Bone Turnover Markers are not a useful tool to assess MRONJ risk.

**During Antiresorptive Therapy/Targeted Therapies (Malignant Disease)**

Educate patients about the higher MRONJ risk in the setting of malignant disease.
Educate the patient about the importance of regimented dental care and prevention.
Avoid dentoalveolar surgery if possible.
Consider root retention techniques to avoid extractions.
Dental implants are contraindicated.
Drug holidays are controversial.

## 17.3.4 Treatment Strategies

### 17.3.4.1 Nonoperative Therapy

The efficacy of nonoperative therapies in the management of MRONJ is documented in the literature and provides a useful adjunct to the spectrum of management strategies that also include operative treatment. Nonoperative strategies can be useful in all stages, especially where significant comorbidities preclude operative treatment. They may also result in stabilization of disease or cure in earlier stages. The goal of both operative and nonoperative therapies remains the same: curative therapy and quality-of-life improvement. Nonoperative therapy heavily focuses on patient education, reassurance, control of pain, and control of secondary infection to allow for sequestration of the exposed, necrotic bone. Decisions on operative versus nonoperative therapy should be patient-specific and tailored to individual needs. The risk versus benefit ratio (including quality of life with their current symptomology), ability to perform good wound care to prevent infection and disease spread, morbidity from a major surgical procedure, as well as oral function or dental rehabilitation after marginal or segmental resection should be considered. Radiographic imaging is of utmost importance in the evaluation of MRONJ lesions. Three-dimensional imaging can identify formed or fully formed sequestrae and potentially decrease the invasiveness of a surgical procedure. Maintenance of maxillary or mandibular integrity is desirable, as the reconstruction of surgical defects in this population can be challenging.

Stage 1 patients can be managed with chlorhexidine wound care and improved oral hygiene to remove the biofilm from the necrotic bone surface. Surgery may not be indicated in the absence of disease progression, with patient adequate quality of life. Stage 2 patients may struggle with local wound care and may require antibiotics for symptom control. Those patients who remain refractory to nonoperative treatment or those patients who cannot maintain adequate hygiene may benefit from operative therapy. In the presence of developing or established bony sequestrae, nonoperative therapy may be indicated to allow for ultimate sequestrectomy. Exfoliation of the exposed, necrotic bone will often result in disease resolution. Therefore, for those patients with Stage 2 or 3 diseases who are poor surgical candidates, nonoperative therapies may be indicated. There is little evidence to suggest that the use of adjunctive therapies, such as hyperbaric oxygen or ozone therapy, can lead to MRONJ resolution. Larger studies and controlled trials have yet to demonstrate the efficacy of the treatments. Therefore, these therapies should not be recommended as a mainstay of treatment at this time. The use of vitamin E and pentoxifylline as an adjunct to standard MRONJ therapies has been reported only in case studies. A randomized, prospective, placebo-controlled trial of vitamin E and pentoxifylline is underway and will provide additional information about this treatment modality. Teriparatide, one of the few anabolic agents used for the treatment of osteoporosis, also has shown promise as an adjunct for the treatment of MRONJ in osteoporotic patients [5–7] (Fig. 17.2).

## 17.3.5 Operative Therapy

While nonoperative therapy continues to be a treatment option for MRONJ, operative therapy is increasingly reported as a viable option with high success rates for all stages of the disease. Numerous reports have identified high success

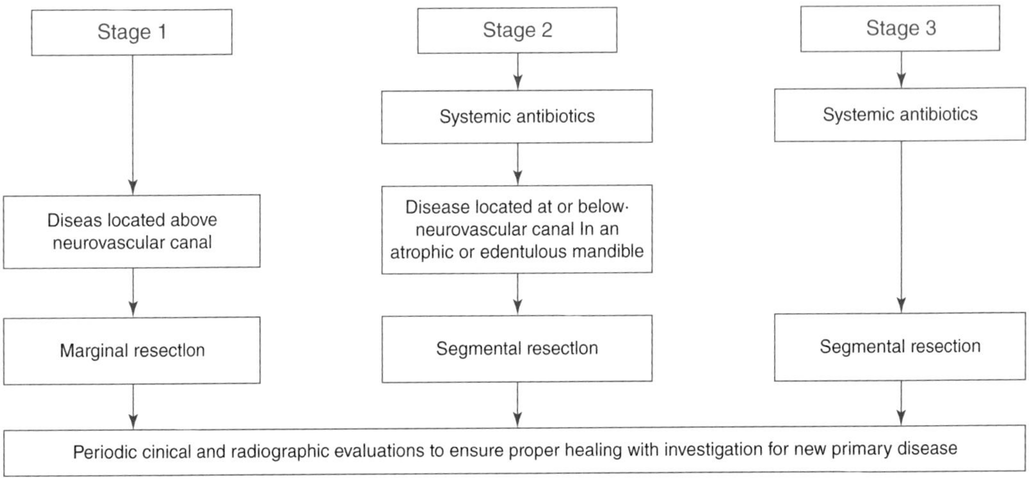


**Fig. 17.2** Operative therapies for maxillary disease. (Ruggiero et al. [5]. Published with permission of Elsevier)

rates associated with the resection of MRONJ lesions. Importantly, one must consider that MRONJ may progress over time, albeit in an unpredictable manner. Furthermore, adopting a nonoperative approach to MRONJ does not uniformly result in sequestration of the exposed necrotic bone with disease resolution. Thus, operative intervention should be explored and presented as a treatment option to reduce the progression of disease with the recognition that early surgical intervention can predict beneficial patient outcomes. Segmental or marginal resection of the mandible and partial maxillectomy are effective methods to control MRONJ. This approach can be applied to patients with all stages of MRONJ, including Stage 1 disease. These resections require margins beyond the borders of the necrotic bone to an area of vital, bleeding bone. Additional reports have identified success when surgical resection of MRONJ was performed by experienced surgeons. Consistent with surgical principles, control of comorbid conditions is paramount in managing MRONJ. Physiologically compromised patients, such as those with an increasing burden of distant metastatic disease, may not respond favorably to resection of their osteonecrotic jaw, and may occasionally develop refractory disease. Finally, surgical resection for MRONJ in patients with metastatic cancer may identify metastases in the jaw specimen, albeit in a minority of patients. Active clinical and radiographic surveillance is critical in the nonoperative management of patients with Stage 1, 2, and 3 diseases to monitor for signs of disease progression. In patients who demonstrate the failure of nonoperative therapy, early operative intervention is recommended. In patients with a progressive clinical or radiographic disease or more advanced disease at presentation, surgical resection of MRONJ should be performed without first instituting prolonged nonoperative measures. MRONJ represents a complex wound whereby operative therapy can be performed in a timely fashion. Although controversy between operative and nonoperative therapies exists, operative treatment of patients has demonstrated maintenance of mucosal coverage, improved quality of life, and expedient resumption of antiresorptive therapy for all stages of MRONJ disease. The benefit of drug holidays for the operative intervention of MRONJ has not been substantiated [5–7] (Fig. 17.3).

### 17.3.6 Odontogenic Infections Leading to Osteomyelitis

Odontogenic infections are a cause of acute and chronic osteomyelitis. The natural progression of the disease is the onset of dental pulpitis that evolves into pulp necrosis and then into a periapical abscess, then a granuloma that may evolve into a cyst.

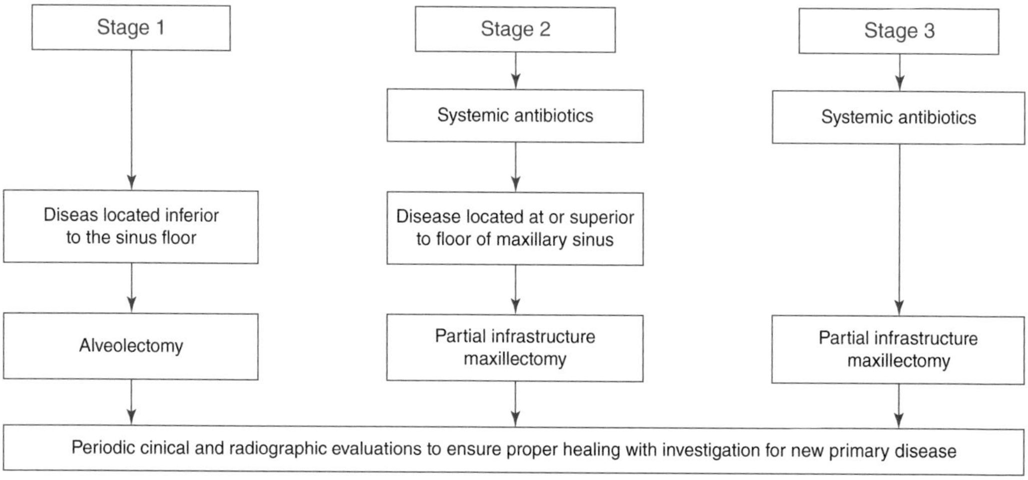


**Fig. 17.3** Operative therapies for maxillary disease. (Ruggiero et al. [5]. Published with permission of Elsevier)

#### 17.3.6.1 Pulpitis

Pulpitis is an inflammation of the dental pulp that usually occurs acutely. When the pulpitis is in an early stage it is called pulpal hyperemia or reversible pulpitis. If the causes that caused it are not eliminated, pulpal hyperemia transforms into irreversible frank pulpitis. In most cases, pulpitis represents a real dental emergency, because it is extremely painful. The most frequent cause by far is dental caries. Pulp inflammation causes edema of the capillaries with the expansion of the tissue volume and increase in pressure inside the pulp chamber. The compression on the neurovascular bundle, caused by edema in a confined space, explains the intense painful symptoms. The dental pulp progressively goes into necrosis if timely action is not taken to eliminate the causes that triggered its development.

#### 17.3.6.2 Acute Apical Periodontitis (Periapical Abscess)

Acute apical periodontitis (periapical abscess) is the consequence of pulp necrosis where the infection from the pulp chamber has spread to the tissues around the tooth apex. Other causes may be of a chemical nature following the inappropriate use of medications during endodontic treatments. Acute apical periodontitis causes intense pain in the affected tooth, which is exacerbated by the pressure exerted by chewing. In some patients, pain is associated with swelling and erythema of the tissues adjacent to the apex of the affected tooth. The tooth itself appears partially extruded from the alveolar cavity due to the pressure exerted by the exudate collected at the apex. A useful test for the diagnosis of acute apical periodontal disease is the percussion of the dental crown, an act that causes acute pain. The radiographic examination shows an enlargement of the periodontal space and a partial destruction of the lamina dura. If the abscess is of fair size, it is associated with a loss of the periapical trabeculate and the formation of a real area of radiolucency with blurred contours. Treatment of pulpitis varies depending on the clinical presentation. In reversible pulpitis, elimination of the causal factors and conservative therapy of the affected tooth are generally curative. In irreversible frank pulpitis, depending on the state of the tooth, endodontic treatment or extraction is indicated. Pulp polyps require extraction of the affected tooth in most cases.

#### 17.3.6.3 Periapical Granuloma

Periapical granuloma is a chronic inflammatory process that follows pulp necrosis. The presence of necrotic tissue in the pulp chamber and root canal triggers a chronic inflammatory reaction in the periapical area. Periapical granuloma, if not treated the area slowly grows, transforming into a periapical cyst. The periapical granuloma is in most cases asymptomatic and is discovered casually during a routine radiographic check-up. On the orthopantomogram, the periapical granuloma appears as a round or oval-shaped area of periapical radiolucency with clear contours of a few millimeters in diameter. In rare cases, radiolucency is observed on the side of the root at the level of the opening of a lateral canal. The periapical granuloma is composed of a mass of granulation tissue surrounded by a fibrous capsule. The tissue is infiltrated by granulocytes, plasma cells, lymphocytes, and macrophages. Cholesterine crystals and macrophages with the cytoplasm filled with cholesterine may be present. Treatment is strictly dependent on the state of the affected tooth. Endodontic therapy is the treatment of choice if the integrity of the tooth allows the execution of conservative therapies.

#### 17.3.6.4 Periapical Cyst

The periapical cyst develops from a long-standing periapical granuloma that has not undergone treatment. The chronic irritative stimulus, which is generally determined by pulp necrosis, causes progressive transformation of the granuloma into a cavity lined by epithelium. The cystic epithelium originates from the epithelial remnants of Malassez. Some authors base the clinical distinction between cyst and granuloma based on the dimensions observed on the radiograph. It has been stated that periapical radiolucent lesions that are no more than 10–15 mm in diameter are granulomas and not periapical cysts. This distinction is artificial and only histopathological examination can establish the definitive nature of the lesion [8].

### 17.3.7 Differential Diagnosis (Rare Entities)

#### 17.3.7.1 Condensing Osteitis (Chronic Focal Sclerosing Osteomyelitis)

This disease is characterized by areas of bone thickening localized at the apex of a non-vital tooth. Condensing osteitis is associated with a dental element affected by penetrating decay, or which has undergone conservative treatment for a large carious cavity. Condensing osteitis is observed especially in children and young adults. The characteristic appearance of condensing osteitis is a diffuse opacity in the periapical area of a non-vital tooth. Most lesions are seen on the molars and premolars. Condensing osteoarthritis must be distinguished from periapical cementum dysplasia, focal cementum dysplasia, and idiopathic osteosclerosis. Therapeutic approach consists in the elimination of the periapical infectious focus using endodontic treatment or tooth extraction if is not possible to perform endodontic treatment.

#### 17.3.7.2 Diffuse Sclerosing Osteomyelitis (CDSO)

This disease is like condensing osteitis, of which it represents a more diffuse form. Unlike condensing osteitis, it is observed in adult patients and affects the jaw exclusively. The lesions develop in contact with teeth or in edentulous mandibular areas that have been affected by long-lasting inflammatory phenomena such as periodontitis, pericoronitis, and periapical granulomas. On the orthopantomogram, single or multiple areas of radiopacity with a cottony appearance are noted. Under the microscope, the areas of bone thickening consist of mature bone tissue with poorly represented marrow. In some cases, in the areas adjacent to the inflammation, a chronic inflammatory infiltrate and necrosis of the bone lamellae may be present.

#### 17.3.7.3 Garre's Sclerosing Osteomyelitis

This disease is characterized by a periosteal reaction with thickening of the lower edge of the mandible which takes on a typical "onion skin" appearance. The use of the eponym "Garre's disease" has recently been questioned as the clinical aspects of this disease do not correspond at all to the original description made by Garrè. The periosteal reaction is triggered by an infection starting from a non-vital tooth that penetrates the bone cortex and stimulates the formation of bone by the periosteum.

Ossifying periostitis, which has a predilection for the jaw, is observed in children and adults and is associated with a periapical phlogistic process or periodontal inflammation. A significant cause is untreated mandibular fractures, pericoronitis, and impacted teeth associated with inflammation. However, in some patients, it is impossible to identify the causes. Most cases develop in the molars and premolars with the cortical reaction occurring on the lower outer edge of the mandible. In rarer cases, the periosteal reaction is localized Radiographically, a characteristic "onion skin" appearance is observed, due to humidification of the periosteum which undergoes a process of calcification and forms multiple layers of lower mandibular border. Clinical and radiographic aspects AND lingual. Clinically the periosteal reaction is highlighted as a painful swelling that has. Histopathology Under the microscope, the lesion shows a stratified proliferation of immature bone tissue and bony trabeculae oriented with the major axis perpendicular to the surface. Sometimes in the fibrous tissue between the bone trabeculae, there is a scant inflammatory infiltrate. Treatment should be aimed at eliminating the primary infection focus. Once the infectious focus has been resolved, a regression of the periostitis is observed within 6 months or a year [8].

## References


1. Kudva A, Kamath AT, Dhara V, Ravindranath V. Chronic recurrent osteomyelitis: a surgeon's enigma. J Oral Pathol Med. 2019;48(2):180–4. https://doi.org/10.1111/jop.12814. Epub 2019 Jan 4. PMID: 30565322
2. Haeffs TH, Scott CA, Campbell TH, Chen Y, August M. Acute and chronic suppurative osteomyelitis of the jaws: a 10-year review and assessment of treatment outcome. J Oral Maxillofac Surg. 2018;76(12):2551–8. https://doi.org/10.1016/j.joms.2018.05.040. Epub 2018 Jun 12. PMID: 30509394
3. Singh A, Huryn JM, Kronstadt KL, Yom SK, Randazzo JR, Estilo CL. Osteoradionecrosis of the jaw: a mini review. Front Oral Health. 2022;28(3):980786. https://doi.org/10.3389/froh.2022.980786. PMID: 35967463; PMCID: PMC9366306
4. Kün-Darbois JD, Fauvel F. Medication-related osteonecrosis and osteoradionecrosis of the jaws: update and current management. Morphologie. 2021;105(349):170–87. https://doi.org/10.1016/j.morpho.2020.11.008. Epub 2020 Dec 3. PMID: 33281055
5. Ruggiero SL, Dodson TB, Aghaloo T, Carlson ER, Ward BB, Kademani D. American Association of Oral and Maxillofacial Surgeons' position paper on medication-related osteonecrosis of the jaws-2022 update. J Oral Maxillofac Surg. 2022;80(5):920–43. https://doi.org/10.1016/j.joms.2022.02.008. Epub 2022 Feb 21. PMID: 35300956
6. Rosella D, Papi P, Giardino R, Cicalini E, Piccoli L, Pompa G. Medication-related osteonecrosis of the jaw: clinical and practical guidelines. J Int Soc Prev Community Dent. 2016;6(2):97–104. https://doi.org/10.4103/2231-0762.178742. PMID: 27114946; PMCID: PMC4820581
7. Topkan E, Kucuk A, Somay E, Yilmaz B, Pehlivan B, Selek U. Review of osteoradionecrosis of the jaw: radiotherapy modality, technique, and dose as risk factors. J Clin Med. 2023;12(8):3025. https://doi.org/10.3390/jcm12083025. PMID: 37109361; PMCID: PMC10143049
8. Ficarra G. Manuale di Patologia e Medicina Orale, 3a edizione. McGraw-Hill; 2006, ISBN 88–386–2391-0

# 18 Prevention of Postoperative Infections

Khaled M. Emara and Mohamed O. Eissa

## 18.1 Introduction

Surgical site infection (SSI) stands as the second most prevalent healthcare-associated infection, contributing to 14–16% of hospital-acquired infections [1]. The reported rates of SSI vary between 0.5% and 13%, contingent on factors such as the type of surgery and patient characteristics [2, 3]. Within orthopedic surgery, SSI remains a formidable challenge for surgeons and poses a potential threat to patients. Managing osteo-articular infections, particularly those involving multi-resistant pathogens like methicillin-resistant Staphylococcus aureus (MRSA), proves difficult and carries a lifelong recurrence risk of approximately 10–20% [1].

Given these challenges, prevention takes precedence. SSI prevention in orthopedic surgery presents specific considerations not seen in general surgery, including low inocula for implant-related foreign body infections, the pathogenicity of skin commensals, a potential hematogenous origin for some infections, and the necessity for prolonged post-discharge surveillance, with a recommended follow-up of at least 1 year for implant-related surgeries [2–5].

## 18.2 Risk Factors

The likelihood of developing a surgical site infection (SSI) in orthopedic surgery is influenced by various factors, including patient characteristics, the surgical procedure itself, and perioperative care. Notably, approximately half of these factors are endogenous and pose challenges for immediate pre- and postoperative modification. Systemic patient-related elements, such as malnutrition, diabetes mellitus, elevated serum glucose levels, anticoagulation, smoking, and iatrogenic immune suppression (due to steroid therapy or the use of tumor necrosis factor-a inhibitors), contribute to the risk of wound healing and infection in surgery in general, likely extending to orthopedic surgery [2].

While some factors are challenging to modify in the immediate pre- and postoperative phases, certain aspects can be influenced. For instance, it is advisable, when feasible, to taper preoperative high-dose corticosteroid therapy before elective orthopedic surgery and optimize glycemia and anticoagulation. Smoking cessation before and after surgery proves beneficial in reducing post-surgical complications and the potential for healthcare-associated infections [2].

K. M. Emara · M. O. Eissa (✉)
Department of Orthopedic Surgery, Ain Shams University, Cairo, Egypt



P. Ruggieri et al. (eds.), *Bone and Joint Infections*, https://doi.org/10.1007/978-3-031-96383-4_18

## 18.3 Evidence-Based Preventive Measures

Several preventive measures are currently considered as very effective with a high level of evidence according to guidelines [5, 6].

### 18.3.1 Preoperative Measures

#### 18.3.1.1 Surgical Hand Preparation

Surgical hand preparation stands out as the most crucial strategy in preventing orthopedic SSI [7]. Due to ethical considerations, conducting a randomized, controlled study to directly compare surgeries with and without prior surgical hand preparation is not feasible. However, a cluster-randomized, cross-over trial has reported the comparable effectiveness of surgical hand preparation using non-medicated soap and water versus alcohol-based hand rub in reducing postoperative SSI rates [8]. The act of hand-rubbing with an alcohol-based formulation is deemed as effective as traditional scrubbing, and although the optimal duration for both techniques remains uncertain, it is likely that a minimum duration of 2–3 minutes is adequate [7, 9].

#### 18.3.1.2 Antibiotic Perioperative Prophylaxis

Antibiotic prophylaxis plays a pivotal role in preventing surgical site infections (SSI), with its efficacy hinging on proper administration, antibiotic selection, and understanding pharmacokinetics. Inappropriately administered antibiotics not only fail to provide protection against SSI but can also lead to adverse effects such as systemic toxicity, increased antibiotic resistance, and elevated costs, exemplified by the rise in *Clostridium difficile* infections.

The choice of antibiotic is guided by the patient's presumed colonization and the prevalent pathogens in each surgical specialty. The antimicrobial agent's half-life should cover the critical time interval for SSI prevention, typically 2 hours after incision or contamination.

First- and second-generation cephalosporins are recommended for their broad-spectrum coverage against aerobic gram-positive and gram-negative bacteria, excellent bactericidal activity, favorable distribution in bony, synovial, and muscle tissues, low systemic toxicity, and reasonable cost. Identifying the target pathogen is essential for choosing the appropriate antibiotic, as most orthopedic SSIs involve coagulase-negative staphylococci, particularly S. epidermidis and S. aureus.

Guidelines suggest routine prophylaxis with first- and second-generation cephalosporins, with glycopeptides (vancomycin/teicoplanin) reserved for patients with a history of MRSA colonization/infection or those from environments with frequent MRSA infections. Glycopeptides or clindamycin are recommended for patients allergic to beta-lactams. In open fractures, the usual recommendations for second-generation cephalosporins are maintained, sometimes combined with aminoglycosides, quinolones, or regimens targeting anaerobic pathogens.

In 2016, authors responded to the isolation of gram-negative bacteria in a significant proportion of surgical site infections (SSI) following hip procedures at their institution. They adapted their standard protocol, originally based on cephazolin, by incorporating gentamicin or aztreonam exclusively for hip arthroplasty patients. This expanded prophylaxis approach proved to be effective in reducing the local SSI rate [10].

**Timing of Prophylaxis Administration**

The timing of antibiotic administration is critical, and the first dose should be given intravenously 30–60 minutes before surgical incision (at least 5–10 minutes before tourniquet application, if used). Inadequate timing increases the risk of SSI. For vancomycin, administration should start within 120 minutes before incision due to prolonged infusion times. The optimal dosing for obese patients (BMI >30 kg/m$^2$) remains uncertain, with varying expert opinions recommending higher doses.

**Antibiotic-Containing Cement for Prophylaxis**

Additionally, the use of antibiotic-loaded cement has demonstrated benefits in reducing SSI, as evidenced by studies reporting up to a 50% reduction in infection rates in cases of cost-effective antibiotic cementing [11, 12].

#### 18.3.1.3 MRSA Screening and Nasal Decolonization

Infections attributed to *Staphylococcus aureus* constitute a substantial proportion of SSI. In recent years, there has been a noticeable rise in methicillin-resistant *Staphylococcus aureus* (MRSA) infections within the field of orthopedic surgery. Numerous studies have demonstrated an elevated risk of infection in patients carrying S. aureus and have reported a decrease in SSI rates through the implementation of screening and decolonization measures, involving the use of nasal mupirocin and chlorhexidine showers. However, statistical significance was not consistently observed in all studies [13].

#### 18.3.1.4 Screening and Treatment of Asymptomatic Bacteriuria in Patients Undergoing TJA

Asymptomatic bacteriuria (ASB) is prevalent in the general population, particularly among females, the elderly, and individuals with diabetes or genitourinary abnormalities [14]. The incidence of ASB varies, ranging from 5.1% to 35.7% in patients awaiting total joint arthroplasty (TJA) [15]. It peaks at 50% in the elderly residing in long-term care facilities [14] or in non-institutional community settings [16]. However, the potential benefits of screening and treating ASB in patients undergoing major orthopedic surgery, such as total joint arthroplasty, have not been conclusively demonstrated.

Several studies have indicated the absence of postoperative hematogenous seeding to the prosthesis after implementing ASB treatment before TJA [17, 18]. Yet, the routine preoperative screening and treatment of ASB might lead to the unnecessary administration of antibiotics to a large number of patients, carrying inherent risks such as the development of diarrhea, allergies, and *C. difficile* infections. Furthermore, this practice may contribute to prolonged preadmission length and hospitalization.

#### 18.3.1.5 Preoperative Bathing or Showering

While the skin serves as an effective barrier against microbes, it also harbors numerous pathogens responsible for SSI. In fact, patient skin is considered the primary source of microbial agents implicated in orthopedic infections. Skin colonization acts as a reservoir, allowing bacteria to be introduced when the skin barrier is breached. Pathogens can directly reach the surgical site during the procedure or through hematogenous dissemination later on. Maintaining meticulous personal hygiene for both the operative staff and the patient is standard practice before any type of intervention.

Despite the skin's role in infection, there is limited evidence supporting the effectiveness of preoperative showering with an antiseptic agent in reducing SSI rates, although it has been shown to decrease skin colonization [5]. The U.S. Centers for Disease Control and Prevention (CDC) recommends that patients shower or bathe with an antiseptic agent before surgery [5]. However, a Cochrane review, which included six trials with 10,000 participants, found no conclusive evidence supporting the superiority of preoperative bathing and showering over a placebo [19].

#### 18.3.1.6 Preoperative Skin Preparation

Preoperative skin preparation in the operating theatre, conducted immediately before surgery, is a standard practice worldwide based on expert opinion [5]. However, there is currently no consensus on the best antiseptic agent to be used for this purpose [2, 20, 21]. It's worth noting that even with optimal preparation, achieving true sterilization of the skin is impossible.

Studies investigating the efficacy of different antiseptic agents have yielded conflicting results. For example, a prospective, randomized, non-blinded study suggested the superiority of 2% chlorhexidine combined with 70% isopropyl alcohol compared to 10% povidone-iodine for preventing SSI after clean-contaminated surgery. However, another study using a different design found contradictory results [22, 23]. The choice of antiseptic agent may depend on various factors, and ongoing research aims to provide more clarity on the most effective options for preoperative skin preparation.

#### 18.3.1.7 Hair Removal

The removal of hair from the intended site of surgical incision has long been a standard practice in routine preoperative preparation, aimed at reducing SSI rates. Traditionally, hair has been associated with a potential lack of cleanliness that could contribute to SSI. Furthermore, hair removal is often seen as facilitating adequate exposure, preoperative skin marking, suturing, and the application of adhesive dressings.

However, despite these perceived benefits, there is currently no evidence supporting the idea that preoperative hair removal effectively reduces SSI rates. This conclusion was drawn in a Cochrane review published in 2011 [24] and has been affirmed by subsequent studies [25, 26].

If a surgeon deems it necessary to remove hair due to concerns about interference with the operative site, it is recommended that clippers, not razors, be used for the procedure. Furthermore, if hair removal is deemed necessary, it should be performed immediately before surgery and outside the operating room (OR) [2, 24, 27–30].

#### 18.3.1.8 Glycemic Control

Hyperglycemia, whether related to diabetes or not, has been linked to an increased risk of SSI, as indicated by observational studies across various surgical specialties [31–33]. Surgical stress during and after surgery contributes to elevated blood glucose levels, putting both diabetic and non-diabetic patients at a heightened risk of hyperglycemia in the peri- and postoperative periods, consequently increasing the susceptibility to SSI.

Studies in different surgical contexts have produced conflicting results regarding the optimal perioperative target levels of blood glucose, the ideal timing and treatment for glucose control, and associated adverse effects. A systematic review conducted on behalf of the World Health Organization (WHO) demonstrated that intensive protocols with stricter blood glucose target levels ($\leq$150 mg/dL), compared to conventional protocols with higher target levels ($\leq$220 mg/dL), are associated with a reduction in the number of SSIs. However, this reduction comes with an inherent risk of hypoglycemic events, although without an increased risk of stroke or death [34].

The Centers for Disease Control and Prevention (CDC) suggests fasting blood glucose levels <200 mg/dL for all surgical patients but does not specify the optimal timing, duration, or delivery method for glucose control [35]. The Society for Healthcare Epidemiology of America (SHEA) recommends maintaining postoperative blood glucose levels <180 mg/dL and advises against levels $\leq$110 mg/dL due to the associated risk of hypoglycemic events [28]. Both the International Consensus Meeting (ICM) and SHEA recommend reducing HbA1c levels to less than 7% before surgery in diabetic patients [27]. A recent study also indicated a threshold value of 7.5% for HbA1c levels [36].

### 18.3.2 Intraoperative Measures

#### 18.3.2.1 Gloves, Gowns, Drapes, and Masks

Sterile gloves and adhesive drapes are standard in the operating theatre; however, post-use examination often reveals tiny punctures that often go unnoticed by the operating team [7]. Although practices such as double gloving or regular glove-changing may help reduce the risk of punctures, they do not guarantee their complete absence. Despite efforts to enhance barrier precautions, a Cochrane review of 26 trials examining the practice of double gloving did not provide conclusive evidence regarding its effectiveness in reducing SSI [37].

#### 18.3.2.2 Second Dose Antibiotic

In cases of prolonged surgical procedures or significant blood loss, the administration of a second dose of antibiotics is recommended. However, there is uncertainty regarding whether the repeated administration should utilize the same dosage or a reduced one. The standard guideline for redosing time is typically considered to be double the antibiotic's half-life. For instance, if cephazolin is the antibiotic of choice, redosing would be indicated if the surgical procedure extends beyond 4 hours.

**Adhesive Incise Drapes**

Among the various sterile surgical drapes available, adhesive incise drapes, whether plain or impregnated with an antimicrobial agent (often an iodophor), are typically applied to the patient's skin after completing the surgical site preparation. As these drapes adhere to the skin, the surgeon cuts through both the skin and the drape itself during the procedure. The rationale behind using such drapes is the belief that they prevent wound contamination by microorganisms present on the skin surrounding the operative site, thereby reducing the risk of SSI.

However, meta-analyses conducted by both the World Health Organization (WHO) and the Centers for Disease Control and Prevention (CDC) have concluded that the use of plastic adhesive drapes, whether with or without antimicrobial properties, is not essential for preventing SSI [35, 38]. Despite these general findings, in major orthopedic surgery, especially joint replacement procedures, the use of adhesive incise drapes may still have practical benefits in facilitating the preparation of the operating field and isolating the surgical site from potential contamination. In such applications, it is crucial to regularly check the full adhesion of the drapes throughout the surgery to ensure their effectiveness.

#### 18.3.2.3 Incisional Wound Irrigation

Intraoperative wound irrigation, commonly performed at the end of surgery just before wound closure, is a widely adopted practice aimed at reducing the risk of SSI. This procedure not only acts as a physical cleaner by removing debris, body fluids, and potential contamination but also has the potential to serve as a local antibacterial agent when an antiseptic or antibiotic is added to the irrigation solution.

However, recommendations on this practice vary among major institutions. SHEA advocates for antiseptic wound lavage, recognizing its potential benefits [28]. In contrast, ICM acknowledges the mechanical advantage of irrigation but refrains from making specific recommendations regarding the type of solution [27]. On the other hand, the National Institute for Health and Care Excellence (NICE) advises against the use of wound irrigation to reduce the risk of SSI [6].

The World Health Organization (WHO) conducted a systematic review with a meta-analysis, revealing no significant difference in the incidence of SSI between wound irrigation with saline solution and no irrigation. However, when using an aqueous povidone-iodine (PI) solution for clean and clean-contaminated wounds, a decrease in SSI risk was observed compared to saline solution [38, 39].

Importantly, wound irrigation with an antibiotic solution did not demonstrate added benefits compared to saline solution or no irrigation [39]. Therefore, major institutions do not recommend the use of antibiotic solutions for wound irrigation due to the lack of supporting evidence and the potential risk of increasing antibiotic resistance [6].

#### 18.3.2.4 Perioperative Oxygenation

The impact of perioperative oxygenation on the risk of SSI is well-documented in the literature. This practice involves providing patients with a higher fraction of inspired oxygen (FiO2), typically 80%, as compared to the usual administration of 30% FiO2. Numerous trials have investigated the use of high FiO2 concentrations during the perioperative period and their potential association with lower rates of SSI. The rationale behind this practice lies in the fact that high FiO2 increases oxygen tension in the blood, compensating for potentially inadequate perfusion at the surgical site. Additionally, higher oxygen tension is known to enhance host defense mechanisms, particularly by improving neutrophil oxidative killing [40]. This strategy aims to optimize conditions for tissue healing and reduce the likelihood of postoperative infections.

#### 18.3.2.5 Maintaining Normal Body Temperature (Normothermia)

Hypothermia, defined as a core temperature below 36 °C, is a common occurrence during and after major surgical procedures lasting more than

2 hours. Anesthetic-induced impairment of thermoregulatory control, more than exposure to a cold operating room environment, is the primary factor leading to hypothermia. Additionally, cool intravenous and irrigation fluids can contribute to directly cooling patients.

Inadvertent hypothermia is considered an adverse effect of anesthesia and is associated with adverse cardiac events [41, 42]. However, this increased risk can be reversed by maintaining normothermia [43]. Hypothermia may also lead to increased blood loss and transfusion requirements [44], prolonged hospitalization [45], and an elevated risk of SSI [46].

To combat hypothermia, various strategies are employed to maintain normothermia in patients undergoing surgery. These include the use of pre- and intraoperative warming devices and the administration of pre-warmed intravenous fluids. These measures aim to mitigate the negative effects of hypothermia and contribute to better patient outcomes during and after surgery.

#### 18.3.2.6 Laminar Flow Ventilation Systems

The ventilation system within the operating room (OR) is considered an extrinsic factor that can influence the rate of SSI. Intraoperative wound contamination can occur directly through contact with non-sterile devices or indirectly through exposure to airborne microbial agents. Traditional ventilation systems introduce air with mixed or turbulent flow into the OR, creating irregular movement of aerosols and particles within the room. In contrast, laminar flow (LF) systems aim to pass air unidirectionally, driving air, aerosols, and particles out of the room, potentially reducing the risk of SSI.

Historically, evidence in the 1970s and 1980s supported the implementation of LF in total joint arthroplasty (TJA) [47, 48]. However, more recent studies have failed to demonstrate a clear benefit in terms of reducing SSI. A systematic review conducted in 2017 on behalf of the World Health Organization (WHO) evaluated whether LF is more effective in decreasing SSI risk compared to conventional ventilation systems. The review found no advantage for LF over conventional ventilation in reducing the risk of SSI and recommended against installing LF equipment in new ORs. Consequently, WHO suggests that LF should not be employed to reduce the risk of SSI for patients undergoing TJA [38].

#### 18.3.2.7 Traffic in OR

Traffic within the operating room (OR), measured by the number of people present and the frequency of door openings during surgery, constitutes another extrinsic factor that may contribute to an increased rate of SSI. People are a significant source of environmental contamination in the OR [49], and the rationale behind restricting personnel and movement is to minimize the shedding of pathogens from personnel's skin and prevent air contamination resulting from external air entering the room [50].

During total joint arthroplasty (TJA) procedures, the traffic in the OR is notably high, and it tends to be even higher in revision cases [51]. A systematic review conducted in 2015 identified a correlation between the number of people in the OR and the SSI rate or airborne contaminants. Additionally, the review found a correlation between the number of door openings and airborne bacterial counts.

Based on this evidence, various guidelines and recommendations emphasize the importance of minimizing OR traffic [6]. The International Consensus Meeting (ICM) strongly recommends, with a 100% consensus, that OR traffic should be kept to a minimum [27]. The Society for Healthcare Epidemiology of America (SHEA) recommends implementing policies to reduce unnecessary traffic in the OR [28]. The National Institute for Health and Care Excellence (NICE) advises staff wearing non-sterile theater wear to limit their movements in and out of the OR [6]. These measures are aimed at reducing the risk of SSI by minimizing potential sources of contamination within the operating environment.

#### 18.3.2.8 Behavioral Aspects

An emerging area of research in the field of surgery involves investigating changes in routine and behavioral aspects within the operating theatre, often in collaboration with nurses [52, 53]. This interdisciplinary approach aims to enhance various aspects of surgical practices and outcomes. Notably, epidemiological studies have identified noise generated by the operating staff as an independent risk factor for SSI [54]. Recognizing and addressing factors such as noise pollution within the operating room may contribute to a better understanding of the dynamics influencing SSI rates and lead to improved strategies for infection prevention.

### 18.3.3 Postoperative Measures

#### 18.3.3.1 Postsurgical Wound Care

The literature on surgical wound care and SSI prevention currently faces a paucity of information. Specifically, there is a lack of data regarding the proportion of SSIs acquired postoperatively on the ward through direct inoculation. While experts suggest that this proportion may be as high as 10%, there is currently no empirical evidence to support this estimate.

A Cochrane review aimed to assess the effectiveness of various dressings and topical agents on surgical wound healing and infection prevention. However, the review concluded that the quality of the available trials was insufficient to determine any superiority of one protocol or topical agent over another [55]. Similarly, other randomized studies comparing occlusive dressings versus gauze dressings also failed to detect superiority in terms of reducing SSIs or promoting wound healing [56–58]. This lack of conclusive evidence underscores the need for further research and robust clinical trials to better understand and improve surgical wound care practices for SSI prevention.

#### 18.3.3.2 Postoperative Antibiotics

Prolonging antibiotic prophylaxis beyond 24 hours is deemed ineffective in reducing the rate of SSI. Additionally, this practice carries various drawbacks, including increased hospital costs, heightened risk of systemic toxicity and colitis caused by *C. difficile*, and negative effects on both individual and community microflora, thereby promoting the development of pharmacological resistance.

In orthopedic trauma cases, the general consensus is that antibiotic medication should not be administered for more than 24 hours for grade I and II fractures [59]. The recommended minimum duration for grade III fractures varies, ranging from 1 day to several weeks. However, guidelines based on expert opinion and common sense typically recommend a maximum duration of 48 hours or 72 hours in such cases [60, 61].

## References

1. Teterycz D, Ferry T, Lew D, Stern R, Assal M, Hoffmeyer P, et al. Outcome of orthopedic implant infections due to different staphylococci. Int J Infect Dis. 2010;14:e913–8.
2. Uçkay I, Harbarth S, Peter R, Lew D, Hoffmeyer P, Pittet D. Preventing surgical site infections. Expert Rev Anti-Infect Ther. 2010;8:657–70.
3. Uckay I, Pittet D, Vaudaux P, Sax H, Lew D, Waldvogel F. Foreign body infections due to Staphylococcus epidermidis. Ann Med. 2009;41:109–19. Available from: https://www.tandfonline.com/doi/abs/10.1080/07853890802337045.
4. Uçkay I, Lübbeke A, Emonet S, Tovmirzaeva L, Stern R, Ferry T, et al. Low incidence of haematogenous seeding to total hip and knee prostheses in patients with remote infections. J Infect. 2009;59:337–45.
5. Mangram AJ, Horan TC, Pearson ML, Silver LC, Jarvis WR. Guideline for prevention of surgical site infection, 1999. Hospital Infection Control Practices Advisory Committee. Infect Control Hosp Epidemiol. 1999;20:250–80.
6. Overview | Surgical site infections: prevention and treatment | Guidance | NICE.
7. Widmer AF, Rotter M, Voss A, Nthumba P, Allegranzi B, Boyce J, et al. Surgical hand preparation: state-of-the-art. J Hosp Infect. 2010;74:112–22.
8. Tanner J, Dumville JC, Norman G, Fortnam M. Surgical hand antisepsis to reduce surgical site infection. Cochrane Database Syst Rev. 2016;2016:CD004288.
9. Dharan S, Pittet D. Environmental controls in operating theatres. J Hosp Infect. 2002;51:79–84.
10. Bosco JA, Tejada PRR, Catanzano AJ, Stachel AG, Phillips MS. Expanded gram-negative antimicrobial prophylaxis reduces surgical site infections in hip arthroplasty. J Arthroplast. 2016;31:616–21.
11. Jämsen E, Huhtala H, Puolakka T, Moilanen T. Risk factors for infection after knee arthroplasty. A register-based analysis of 43,149 cases. J Bone Joint Surg Am. 2009;91:38–47.

12. Parvizi J, Saleh KJ, Ragland PS, Pour AE, Mont MA. Efficacy of antibiotic-impregnated cement in total hip replacement. Acta Orthop. 2008;79:335–41.
13. Kim DH, Spencer M, Davidson SM, Li L, Shaw JD, Gulczynski D, et al. Institutional prescreening for detection and eradication of methicillin-resistant Staphylococcus aureus in patients undergoing elective orthopaedic surgery. J Bone Joint Surg Am. 2010;92:1820–6.
14. Nicolle LE, Bradley S, Colgan R, Rice JC, Schaeffer A, Hooton TM. Infectious Diseases Society of America guidelines for the diagnosis and treatment of asymptomatic bacteriuria in adults. Clin Infect Dis. 2005;40:643–54.
15. Zhang Q, Liu L, Sun W, Gao F, Cheng L, Li Z. Research progress of asymptomatic bacteriuria before arthroplasty: a systematic review. Medicine. 2018;97:e9810.
16. Rodhe N, Mölstad S, Englund L, Svärdsudd K. Asymptomatic bacteriuria in a population of elderly residents living in a community setting: prevalence, characteristics and associated factors. Fam Pract. 2006;23:303–7.
17. Donovan TL, Gordon RO, Nagel DA. Urinary infections in total hip arthroplasty. Influences of prophylactic cephalosporins and catheterization. J Bone Joint Surg Am. 1976;58:1134–7.
18. Glynn MK, Sheehan JM. The significance of asymptomatic bacteriuria in patients undergoing hip/knee arthroplasty. Clin Orthop Relat Res. 1984;(185):151–4. Available from: http://europepmc.org/abstract/MED/6705373.
19. Webster J, Osborne S. Preoperative bathing or showering with skin antiseptics to prevent surgical site infection. Cochrane Database Syst Rev. 2015;2015:CD004985.
20. Saltzman MD, Nuber GW, Gryzlo SM, Marecek GS, Koh JL. Efficacy of surgical preparation solutions in shoulder surgery. J Bone Joint Surg Am. 2009;91:1949–53.
21. Ostrander RV, Botte MJ, Brage ME. Efficacy of surgical preparation solutions in foot and ankle surgery. J Bone Joint Surg Am. 2005;87:980–5.
22. Darouiche RO, Wall MJ, Itani KMF, Otterson MF, Webb AL, Carrick MM, et al. Chlorhexidine–alcohol versus povidone–iodine for surgical-site antisepsis. N Engl J Med. 2010;362:18–26. Available from: https://www.nejm.org/doi/full/10.1056/NEJMoa0810988.
23. Swenson BR, Hedrick TL, Metzger R, Bonatti H, Pruett TL, Sawyer RG. Effects of preoperative skin preparation on postoperative wound infection rates a prospective study of 3 skin preparation protocols. Infect Control Hosp Epidemiol. 2009;30:964–71. Available from: https://www.cambridge.org/core/journals/infection-control-and-hospital-epidemiology/article/abs/effects-of-preoperative-skin-preparation-on-postoperative-wound-infection-rates-a-prospective-study-of-3-skin-preparation-protocols/6F29B56567C4F539BF2C2C5E1AC5C677.
24. Tanner J, Melen K. Preoperative hair removal to reduce surgical site infection. Cochrane Database Syst Rev. 2021;8:CD004122.
25. Shi D, Yao Y, Yu W. Comparison of preoperative hair removal methods for the reduction of surgical site infections: a meta-analysis. J Clin Nurs. 2017;26:2907–14.
26. Kowalski TJ, Kothari SN, Mathiason MA, Borgert AJ. Impact of hair removal on surgical site infection rates: a prospective randomized noninferiority trial. J Am Coll Surg. 2016;223:704–11.
27. Parvizi J, Gehrke T, Chen AF. Proceedings of the international consensus on periprosthetic joint infection. Bone Joint J. 2013;95-B:1450–2.
28. Calderwood MS, Anderson DJ, Bratzler DW, Dellinger EP, Garcia-Houchins S, Maragakis LL, et al. Strategies to prevent surgical site infections in acute-care hospitals: 2022 Update. Infect Control Hosp Epidemiol. 2023;44:695–720.
29. Niël-Weise BS, Wille JC, van den Broek PJ. Hair removal policies in clean surgery: systematic review of randomized, controlled trials. Infect Control Hosp Epidemiol. 2005;26:923–8. Available from: https://www.researchgate.net/publication/7355485_Hair_Removal_Policies_in_Clean_Surgery_Systematic_Review_of_Randomized_Controlled_Trials.
30. Maksimović J, Marković-Denić L, Bumbasirević M, Marinković J, Vlajinac H. Surgical site infections in orthopedic patients: prospective cohort study. Croat Med J. 2008;49:58–65.
31. Ata A, Lee J, Bestle SL, Desemone J, Stain SC. Postoperative hyperglycemia and surgical site infection in general surgery patients. Arch Surg. 2010;145:858–64. Available from: https://jamanetwork.com/journals/jamasurgery/fullarticle/406267.
32. Jämsen E, Nevalainen P, Kalliovalkama J, Moilanen T. Preoperative hyperglycemia predicts infected total knee replacement. Eur J Intern Med. 2010;21:196–201.
33. Richards JE, Hutchinson J, Mukherjee K, Jahangir AA, Mir HR, Evans JM, et al. Stress hyperglycemia and surgical site infection in stable nondiabetic adults with orthopedic injuries. J Trauma Acute Care Surg. 2014;76:1070–5.
34. de Vries FEE, Gans SL, Solomkin JS, Allegranzi B, Egger M, Dellinger EP, et al. Meta-analysis of lower perioperative blood glucose target levels for reduction of surgical-site infection. Br J Surg. 2017;104:e95–105.
35. Berriós-Torres SI, Umscheid CA, Bratzler DW, Leas B, Stone EC, Kelz RR, et al. Centers for disease control and prevention guideline for the prevention of surgical site infection, 2017. JAMA Surg. 2019;152:784–91.
36. Cancienne JM, Werner BC, Browne JA. Is there a threshold value of hemoglobin A1c that predicts risk of infection following primary total hip arthroplasty? J Arthroplast. 2017;32:S236–40.
37. Tanner J. Double gloving to reduce surgical cross-infection. J Perioper Pract. 2006;16:571.

38. Global guidelines for the prevention of surgical site infection [Internet]. [cited 2024 Jan 3]. Available from: https://www.who.int/publications/i/item/9789241550475.
39. de Jonge SW, Boldingh QJJ, Solomkin JS, Allegranzi B, Egger M, Dellinger EP, et al. Systematic review and meta-analysis of randomized controlled trials evaluating prophylactic intra-operative wound irrigation for the prevention of surgical site infections. Surg Infect. 2017;18:508–19.
40. Allen DB, Maguire JJ, Mahdavian M, Wicke C, Marcocci L, Scheuenstuhl H, et al. Wound hypoxia and acidosis limit neutrophil bacterial killing mechanisms. Arch Surg. 1997;132:991–6.
41. Frank SM, Beattie C, Christopherson R, Norris EJ, Perler BA, Williams GM, et al. Unintentional Hypothermia Is Associated with Postoperative Myocardial Ischemia. Anesthesiology. 1993;78:468–76. https://doi.org/10.1097/00000542-199303000-00010.
42. Frank SM, Cattaneo CG, Wieneke-Brady MB, El-Rahmany H, Gupta N, Lima JAC, et al. Threshold for adrenomedullary activation and increased cardiac work during mild core hypothermia. Clin Sci (Lond). 2002;102:119–25.
43. Frank SM, Fleisher LA, Breslow MJ, Higgins MS, Olson KF, Kelly S, et al. Perioperative maintenance of normothermia reduces the incidence of morbid cardiac events. A randomized clinical trial. JAMA. 1997;277:1127–34.
44. Rajagopalan S, Mascha E, Na J, Sessler DI. The effects of mild perioperative hypothermia on blood loss and transfusion requirement. Anesthesiology. 2008;108:71–7. https://doi.org/10.1097/01.anes.0000296719.73450.52.
45. Kurz A, Sessler DI, Lenhardt R. Perioperative normothermia to reduce the incidence of surgical-wound infection and shorten hospitalization. Study of Wound Infection and Temperature Group. N Engl J Med. 1996;334:1209–15.
46. Melling AC, Ali B, Scott EM, Leaper DJ. Effects of preoperative warming on the incidence of wound infection after clean surgery: a randomised controlled trial. Lancet. 2001;358:876–80. Available from: http://www.thelancet.com/article/S0140673601060718/fulltext.
47. Charnley J. Postoperative infection after total hip replacement with special reference to air contamination in the operating room. Clin Orthop Relat Res. 1972;87:167–87.
48. Lidwell OM, Lowbury EJ, Whyte W, Blowers R, Stanley SJ, Lowe D. Effect of ultraclean air in operating rooms on deep sepsis in the joint after total hip or knee replacement: a randomised study. Br Med J (Clin Res Ed). 1982;285:10–4.
49. Ritter MA, Eitzen H, French ML, Hart JB. The operating room environment as affected by people and the surgical face mask. Clin Orthop Relat Res. 1975;(111):147–50.
50. Parvizi J, Shohat N, Gehrke T. Prevention of periprosthetic joint infection: new guidelines. Bone Joint J. 2017;99-B:3–10.
51. Panahi P, Stroh M, Casper DS, Parvizi J, Austin MS. Operating room traffic is a major concern during total joint arthroplasty hip. Clin Orthop Relat Res. 2012;470:2690–4. Available from: https://journals.lww.com/clinorthop/fulltext/2012/10000/operating_room_traffic_is_a_major_concern_during.9.aspx.
52. Lee-Smith J. Can the orthopaedic team reduce the risk of infection? J Orthop Nurs. 1999;3:95–8.
53. Woodhead K, Taylor EW, Bannister G, Chesworth T, Hoffman P, Humphreys H. Behaviours and rituals in the operating theatre. A report from the Hospital Infection Society Working Party on Infection Control in Operating Theatres. J Hosp Infect. 2002;51:241–55.
54. Beldi G, Bisch-Knaden S, Banz V, Mühlemann K, Candinas D. Impact of intraoperative behavior on surgical site infections. Am J Surg. 2009;198:157–62.
55. Vermeulen H, Ubbink D, Goossens A, de Vos R, Legemate D. Dressings and topical agents for surgical wounds healing by secondary intention. Cochrane Database Syst Rev. 2004;2004:CD003554.
56. Shinohara T, Yamashita Y, Satoh K, Mikami K, Yamauchi Y, Hoshino S, et al. Prospective evaluation of occlusive hydrocolloid dressing versus conventional gauze dressing regarding the healing effect after abdominal operations: randomized controlled trial. Asian J Surg. 2008;31:1–5.
57. Ubbink DT, Vermeulen H, Goossens A, Kelner RB, Schreuder SM, Lubbers MJ. Occlusive vs gauze dressings for local wound care in surgical patients: a randomized clinical trial. Arch Surg. 2008;143:950–5.
58. Wynne R, Botti M, Stedman H, Holsworth L, Harinos M, Flavell O, et al. Effect of three wound dressings on infection, healing comfort, and cost in patients with sternotomy wounds: a randomized trial. Chest. 2004;125:43–9.
59. Gustilo RB, Anderson JT. Prevention of infection in the treatment of one thousand and twenty five open fractures of long bones: retrospective and prospective analyses. J Bone Joint Surg Series A. 1976;58:453–8. Available from: https://www.researchgate.net/publication/297815279_Prevention_of_Infection_in_the_treatment_of_one_thousand_and_twenty-five_open_fractures_of_long_bones_retrospective_and_prospective_analyses_J.
60. Hauser CJ, Adams CAJ, Eachempati SR. Surgical Infection Society guideline: prophylactic antibiotic use in open fractures: an evidence-based guideline. Surg Infect. 2006;7:379–405.
61. Barie PS. Breaking with tradition: evidence-based antibiotic prophylaxis of open fractures. Surg Infect (Larchmt). 2006;7(4):327–9.

# Periprosthetic Joint Infection: General Aspects

# 19

Ferdinando Da Rin de Lorenzo and Javad Parvizi

Periprosthetic joint infections (PJI) represent one of the most important surgical complications, so much so that in America, and specifically in Philadelphia, scientific meetings organized by Dr. Parvizi and Dr. Gerhke were held in 2013 and 2018, to try to create guidelines to address this issue [1] The first meeting addresses the issue of periprosthetic infections of the hip and knee while in the following meeting, all other subspecialties in orthopedics were included. Both meetings was attended by the world's leading experts and discussions centered around prevention, diagnosis, and treatment of orthopedic infections. The issue of PJI continues to take center stage as the number of arthroplasties being performed around the world continues to increase (Fig. 19.1) [2] It is estimated that more than 1.5 million hip arthroplasties are performed per year, of which 300,000 are done in the United States. Italy is among the European countries where the highest number of hip replacements are carried out, out of approximately 700,000 THA performed every year in Europe, over 100,000 are done in Italy, which is surpassed only by Germany (250,000) and France (130,000) and precedes the United Kingdom (90,000) and Spain (70,000) [3] The number of implants increases by 5% every year and that expenditure of one billion three hundred million euros corresponds to 1% of the National Health Fund. To this figure must be added the over 500 million euros spent on rehabilitation following the intervention (Figs. 19.1b and 19.2a, b) [2] It is now not uncommon to operate on 30 or 40-year-olds and every year 20,000 prostheses are implanted in people under 65, 5000 are inserted in people under 50.

The new ceramics can therefore guarantee superior durability and resistance, at a relatively higher cost, we are talking about a few hundred euros more on implants that normally cost between 3000 and 4000 euros. The data regarding prosthetics of the knee are based on approximately 500,000 implants per year in Europe and with a trend of greater increase in the hip, of 6–8% per year. The infection rates of a prosthesis are variable as can be seen from (diagram 1) [2] Va also considers that in the case of a PJI, these are mostly elderly patients with frequently associated other pathologies (diabetes, heart disease, etc.) [4, 5] Furthermore, the prolonged use of antibiotics produces side effects, such as kidney disease and liver disease. The patient falls on the family and on volunteers, as the children have little time to dedicate to their elderly parents. In 65% of cases, hip replacement concerns women, and the percentage rises to 75% if the implant is subsequent to an osteoporotic fracture. Patients

F. Da Rin de Lorenzo (✉)
National Reference Center for the Diagnosis and Treatment of Bone Infections, Codivilla-Putti Institutes, Cortina d'Ampezzo, Italy

J. Parvizi
Orthopedic Surgery, Acibadem University, Istanbul, Turkey



P. Ruggieri et al. (eds.), *Bone and Joint Infections*, https://doi.org/10.1007/978-3-031-96383-4_19

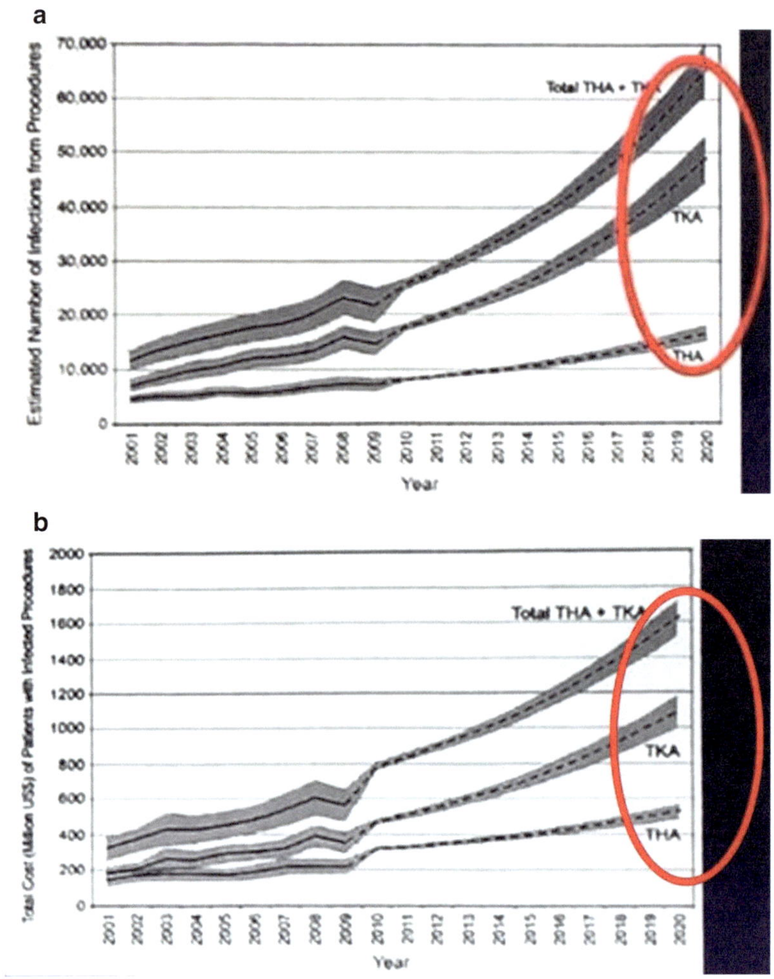


**Fig. 19.1** (**a**) The projected increase in infections in hip and knee replacements [2]. (**b**) The proportional increase in costs [3]

carrying a periprosthetic infection undergo many operations and sometimes with a resurgence of the pathology, therefore mistrust in the healthcare system. It should be considered that even after many operations, amputation can result and the patient himself and himself are at risk, as in all chronic illnesses, requires psychological support.

For the healthcare system, commitment is very important, as these are patients with long stays, there are no safety areas, and there may be contamination of other patients. This surgery requires protected surgical, resuscitation, and hospitalization areas. Furthermore, the purely surgical situation presents considerable technical-decision-making difficulties given the chronicity of the disease, the general conditions of the patient and the condition of the local bone stock. Now, as you can well imagine, these data led the specialists to the meeting described which led, for the first time, to give indications on the basis of the evaluations made.

We report the percentage of infections in America and Europe (Scheme 19.1) [6, 7].

Therefore, based on the data reported, the prevention of these pathologies becomes fundamental. Before delving into the preventive aspects, it is useful to try to give a definition of what is diagnosed as PJI (Periprosthetic Joint Infection). The Philadelphia Consensus has defined parameters within which we can say that we are faced with a periprosthetic infection [7]. The European School (EBJIS) has given another definition, both similar [8]. Other working groups have given a

**a**

| | **Primary Arthroplasty (*n* = 459)** | **Aseptic Revisions (*n* = 13)** | **DAIR (*n* = 8)** | **Two-stage Revision (*n* = 8)** |
|---|---|---|---|---|
| **Total costs** | **3,168** | **7,985** | **4,009** | **13,793** |
| **Total *hospital stay*** | **1,024** | **1,289** | **2,677** | **4,388** |
| Staff | 521 | 405 | 1,120 | 1,944 |
| Ward costs | 262 | 151 | 135 | 1,141 |
| Materials | 78 | 409 | 661 | 252 |
| Diagnostic tests | 62 | 126 | 78 | 433 |
| Medication *(excluding antibiotics)* | 83 | 94 | 78 | 108 |
| Antibiotics | 4 | 19 | 553 | 239 |
| ICU stay | 14 | 85 | 52 | 271 |
| ***Total operating room*** | **2,594** | **6,696** | **1,332** | **9,405** |
| Staff | 277 | 306 | 204 | 621 |
| OR costs | 237 | 413 | 334 | 451 |
| Clinical materials *(including prosthesis)* | 2,080 | 5,977 | 794 | 8,333 |

DAIR - Debridement, Antibiotics and Implant Retention

**b**

| | **Primary Arthroplasty (*n* = 256)** | **Aseptic Revisions (*n* = 22 [4*])** | **DAIR (*n* = 8)** | **Two-stage Revision (*n* = 7)** |
|---|---|---|---|---|
| **Total costs** | **3,230** | **6,089** *[7,840*]* | **5,528** | **11,415** |
| **Total *hospital stay*** | **1,307** | **1,728** *[1,739*]* | **3,923** | **4,584** |
| Staff | 624 | 773 | 1,802 | 1,772 |
| Ward costs | 407 | 151 *[162*]* | 291 | 1,026 |
| Materials | 94 | 404 | 1,028 | 274 |
| Diagnostic tests | 95 | 248 | 317 | 703 |
| Medication *(excluding antibiotics)* | 36 | 48 | 99 | 293 |
| Antibiotics | 6 | 10 | 287 | 243 |
| ICU stay | 45 | 94 | 87 | 273 |
| ***Total operating room*** | **1,923** | **4,361** *[6,101*]* | **1,605** | **6,831** |
| Staff | 238 | 305 *[351*]* | 304 | 464 |
| OR costs | 292 | 392 | 208 | 719 |
| Clinical materials *(including the prosthesis)* | 1393 | 3,664 *[5,358*]* | 1,093 | 5,648 |

**Fig. 19.2** (**a**) Economic Data on 488 TKA cases (average cost per patient in euros) [3]. (**b**) Economic Data on 293 THA cases (average cost per patient in euros) [3]

**Scheme 19.1** Periprosthetic infection rate

| Periprosthetic infection rates are hovering: | | | | |
|---|---|---|---|---|
| In America: | Hip | 1.99–2.18% | } | *[2] |
| | Knee | 2.05–2.18% | | |
| In Europe: | Hip | 2.05–2.48% | } | ** |
| | Knee | 2.30–3.18% | | |
| In Europe: | | | | |
| Revision prosthesis | | 5–20% | (***) | |
| Shoulder | | 0.8–1.5% | (****) | |
| Elbow | | 3.3% | (*****) | |

*Kurtz SM, Lau E, Watson H, Schmier JK, Parvizi J. Economic burden of periprosthetic joint infection in the United States. J Arthroplasty. 2012;27:61–65.e61. https://doi.org/10.1016/j.arth.2012.02.022
**Nordic Arthroplasty Register Association
***Tandea AJ, Patel R. Prosthetic Joint Infection. Clin Microbiol Rev. 2014;27(2):302–45
****Singh JA, Sperling JW, Schleck C, Harmsen W, Cofield RH. Periprosthetic infections after shoulder hemi-arthroplasty. J Shoulder Elbow Surg. 2012;21:1304–9
*****Voloshin I, Schippert DW, Kakar S, Kaye EK, Morrey BF. Complications of total elbow replacement: a systematic review. J Shoulder Elbow Surg. 2011;20:158–68
The percentage of periprosthetic hip infections is 1.5–4%. Periprosthetic infections represent from 0.5% to 3% of all implanted prostheses and of those revised it can even reach 20%

definition and in the following diagram the set of all these definitions reported by the WAIOT scientific society (Fig. 19.3) [9].

"**Prevention**" As can be seen, it is necessary to ensure that periprosthetic infections are, in percentage, reduced to a minimum. Studies on the prevention of infections mainly concern two sectors:

A. The patient's risk factors and all the aspects that can be modified during the pre-intra and post-operative process, to avoid an infection [10–17].
B. The characteristics of the prostheses to be implanted. On the latter, multiple operations were carried out considering the defensive properties of the prostheses against any bacterial load, let's say "possible" because the infection is not yet underway but everything would serve to prevent it. First of all, the patient must be evaluated when a prosthesis is to be performed, in fact, some conditions must lead to using more restrictive measures before accessing a prosthesis, for the modifiable risk factors, while for others it is a matter of applying them routinely. All conditions are evaluated in depth in relation to a probable infection. Furthermore, knowledge of risk factors also allows for a greater relationship between doctor and patient [9] Both oncological orthopedic prosthesis and traumatology are excluded but can be included, at least for their general characteristics, which however have peculiar situations not covered in this chapter.

| Definition Source | MSIS 2011 [1] | IDSA 2013 [4] | ICM 2013 [5] | ICM 2018 [7] | Proposed EBJIS 2018 [8] |
|---|---|---|---|---|---|
| Scoring system | 1 of the 2 Major Criteria<br>OR<br>≥4 of 6 Minor Criteria* | ≥1 Positive Criteria* | 1 of the 2 Major Criteria<br>OR<br>≥3 of 5 Minor Criteria* | 1 of the 2 Major Criteria<br>OR<br>Minor criteria scoring ≥6 Infected<br>3–5 Possibly infected<br>("Consider further molecular diagnostics such as next-generation sequencing")<br><3 Not infected* | ≥1 Positive Criteria |
| | *"PJI may be present if fewer than four of these criteria are met" | *"The presence of PJI is possible even if the above criteria are not met ( .. .)" | *"PJI may be present without meeting these criteria,( ... )." | *"Proceed with caution in: adverse local tissue reaction, crystal deposition disease, slow growing oranisms"" | |
| Criteria | Major:<br>1. Sinus tract communicating with the prosthesis;<br>2. A pathogen is isolated by culture from at least two separate tissue or fluid samples obtained from the affected prosthetic joint<br><br>Minor:<br>(a) Elevated ESR (>30 mm/hr) and CRP (>10 mg/L) concentration<br>(b) Elevated synovial leukocyte count<br>(c) Elevated PMN%<br>(d) Purulence in the affected joint<br>(e) Isolation of a microorganism in one culture of periprosthetic tissue or fluid<br>(f) Greater than five neutrophils per high-power field in five high-power fields observed from histologic analysis of periprosthetic tissue at ×400 magnification | 1. Sinus tract communicating with the prosthesis<br>2. Purulence without other etiology surrounding the prosthesis<br>3. Acute inflammation seen on histopathological examination of the periprosthetic tissue<br>4. ≥2 intraoperative cultures or combination of preoperative aspiration and intraoperative cultures yielding an indistinguishable organism (the growth of a virulent microorganism (e.g., Staphylococcus aureus) in a single specimen of a tissue biopsy or synovial fluid is also considered as indicative of a PJI] | Major<br>1. A sinus tract communicating with the joint<br>2. Two positive periprosthetic cultures with phenotypically identical organisms,<br><br>Minor:<br>(a) Elevated ESR (>30 mm/hr) and CRP (> 100 mg/L for acute infections; >10 mg/L for chronic infections)<br>(b) Elevated synovial fluid WBC count (>10,000 cells/mL for acute infections; >3,000 cells/mL for chronic infections) or ++ change on leukocyte esterase test strip<br>(c) Elevated PMN% (>90% for acute infections; >80% for chronic infections)<br>(d) Positive histological analysis of periprosthetic tissue (> 5 neutrophils per high-power field in five high-power fields observed on periprosthetic tissue at ×400 magnification)<br>(e) A single positive culture | Major:<br>1. Sinus tract with evidence of communication to the joint or visualization of the prosthesis<br>2. Two positive growths of the same organism using standard culture methods<br><br>Minor:<br>(a) Elevated CRP (>100 mg/L for acute infections; >10 mg/L.. for chronic infections) or D-Dimer (unknown threshold for acute infection; >860 ug/L for chronic infection) (score 2)<br>(b) Elevated ESR (no role for acute infections; >30 mm/hr for chronic infections) (score 1)<br>(c) Elevated synovial WBC count (>10,000 cells/mL for acute infections; >3,000 cells/mL for chronic infections) OR Leukocyte Esterase (++ for acute and chronic infections) OR Positive alphadefensin (score 3)<br>(d) Elevated synovial PMN% (>90% for acute infections; >70% for chronic infections) (score 2)<br>(e) Single positive culture (score 2)<br>(f) Positive histology (score 3)<br>(g) Positive intraoperative purulence (score 3) | 1. Purulence around the prosthesis or sinus tract<br>2. Increase synovial fluid leukocyte count (>2,000 cells/mL or >70 % granulocytes)<br>3. Positive histopathology<br>4. Confirmatory microbial growth in synovial fluid, periprosthetic tissue, or sonication culture<br><br>("Confirmatory microbial growth in periprosthetic tissue: if positive in ≥1 specimen in highly virulent organisms or ≥2 in low vilulent pathogens; sonication culture considered positive if >50 colony-forming units/mL of sonication fluid.") |

**Fig. 19.3** Comparison of the diagnostic criteria, adopted in five peri-prosthetic joint infection (PJI) definitions, in the differents guidelines, published from 2011 to 2018. (Reproduced from Romanò et al. [9] under the terms and conditions of the Open Access Creative Commons Attribution (CC BY) license (http://creativecommons.org/licenses/by/4.0/))

## 19.1 "General" Patient Risk Factors [11, 13, 14, 16, 18–21]

- History of previous surgical interventions [18, 22, 23].
- The age of the patient.
- Poorly controlled diabetes mellitus (blood sugar >200 mg/L or HbA1C > 7%) [4, 5].
- Malnutrition [24, 25].
- Obesity (BMI > 40/m$^2$) [26].
- An active liver disease [27, 28].
- A chronic kidney disease [29, 30].
- Excessive smoking (>1 pack per day) [31, 32].
- Excessive alcohol consumption (>40 units per week) [33].
- Intravenous drug abuse [34].
- A recent hospitalization.
- An extended stay in a rehabilitation center.
- A severe immunodeficiency [34].
- Previous transfusions.

## 19.2 "Local" Patient Risk Factors

- History of previous surgical interventions at the site of surgery.
- Associated extra-osseous structure lesions.
- The diagnosis of a previous post-traumatic arthritis.
- An inflammatory arthropathy (AR).
- A previous surgical procedure in the joint to be operated on.*
- Skin lesions such as furunculosis or impetigo.

(*) such as infiltration [35–38].

## 19.3 Risk Factors Related to the Perioperative Phase and Surgery

In addition to the patient's risk factors, other risk factors that are outside the patient but which affect the patient himself must be evaluated. We have divided all those aspects that can intervene in creating a periprosthetic infection if we do not pay due attention and do not correct the modifiable risk factors. These considerations generally apply to all major surgery such as traumatology, for example, or pelvic and spinal surgery. Furthermore, they are reported without a logical sense because there is no standard scheme in evaluating these factors but it would be good for this to happen to be careful not to forget any of them, a protocol must be made which must be followed to the letter.

## 19.4 The Factors That Concern the Risks That Can Be Controlled and Applied Have Been Divided into Factors

- *Presurgical*
- *Intra-surgical*
- *Postsurgical*

### 19.4.1 Presurgical

For suspicion of a *urinary infection* [39–41], more typical in women, the attitude varies:

| Treatment before prosthetic surgery if: | No treatment if: |
|---|---|
| Acute urinary infection | Asymptomatic |
| Bacterial count >1 × 10/ml | |
| Symptomatic infection | |

Therefore, only symptomatic forms should be treated and In the case of a full-blown form, it will also be necessary to consider the germ and the antibiogram of the urinary infection that will be treated.

Another factor to consider is the suspension of an *immunological treatment* in place before the operation (Fig. 19.4) [42, 43].

Another factor to be evaluated is the *decolonization of the nasal site* [44] if both methicillin-resistant and methicillin-susceptible *Staphylococcus aureus* are found, it should be done, with nasal application, in the short term,

**Fig. 19.4** Table listing medications, their half-lives, and recommendations for discontinuation before surgery

| **Medication** | **Half Life *** | **Recommendation** |
|---|---|---|
| Nonsteroidal Anti-inflammatory Drugs (NSAIDs) | 2–17 hours | Discontinue therapy within 1 week prior to surgery |
| Methotrexate | 0.7–5.8 hours | Discontinue therapy within 1 week prior to surgery<br>Continue therapy 2 weeks after surgery<br>(Patients with renal dysfunction, hold 2 weeks prior to surgery) |
| Sulfasalazine<br>Azathioprine | 5 hours<br>7.6 hours | Discontinue therapy prior to 1 week before surgery |
| Leflunomide | ~2 weeks | Hold for 6 weeks prior to surgery |
| Hydroxychloroqine | 1–2 months | Continue therapy up to and including the day of surgery |
| **Biological Response Modifiers** | | |
| Etanercept | 4.3 days | Hold for at least 1.5 weeks prior to surgery |
| Infliximab | 8–10 days | Hold for 3 weeks prior to surgery |
| Golimumab<br>Tocilizumab<br>Abatacept<br>Adalimumab<br>Certolizumab | 12–14 days | Hold for 1 month prior to surgery |
| Rituximab | 21 days | Hold for 2 months prior to surgery |
| **Gout agents** | | |
| Allopurinol<br>Colchicine<br>Probenecid | 1–2 hours<br>26–32 hours<br>26–32 hours | Discontinue therapy within 1 week prior to surgery |

with mupirocin, but not all authors are agreement, perhaps due to the lack of uniformity in study designs (retrospective vs prospective) [45–47].

*Preoperative skin cleansing* should be done with chlorhexidine gluconate (CHG). If CHG sensitivity is present, or when CHG is not available, an antiseptic soap is appropriate. It is recommended to start cleansing the skin at least the night before a prosthesis operation. Furthermore, after bathing, patients are advised to sleep in clean clothes and clean bed linen, without the application of any topical products. It would be useful for the patient to be hospitalized the day before the operation to be able to clean the body properly [48–50].

Another very important step is *shaving* [51–53], not recommended by hand (clipping), but better with the motorized one (shaving). It must be performed close to the operation and the skin incisions must take into account the presence of eczema, psoriasis, furunculosis, or previous traumatic scars. The guidelines for trichotomy are as follows:

- Shaving should only be carried out by expert personnel
- Wear gloves to carry out this procedure
- Make sure that the lighting is sufficient
- Never undress the patient for no reason
- Set up an environment in which privacy is maintained
- Shaving must not take place more than twice hours before the procedure This ensures that

bacterial development, due to the loss of skin integrity, is reduced to a minimum

- The skin must be wet and soapy before shaving Wet hairs cut better than dry ones and do not fly away everywhere, moreover, skin lesions are prevented
- The areas defined by the protocols or requested by the surgeon must be shaved. If there are no indications in this regard, a broad shave is applied which includes the area to be operated on
- Shave the hair in the direction of growth, not against it
- Don't rush to complete the procedure, so as not to create skin lesions.
- While shaving, pull and flatten the skin in accordance with the direction of shaving and not against it
- When shaving is complete, rinse the skin gently Do not rub the skin vigorously so as not to further, abrade the skin
- Only disposable razors must be used
- Always report skin lesions caused by trichotomy
- Always wash your hands after the procedure

Another very important preventative point is *antibacterial prophylaxis* [54–59] which must be done upon anesthetic induction: A first or second-generation cephalosporin (cefazolin or cefuroxime) must be administered for routine surgical preoperative prophylaxis. Semi-synthetic penicillin, such as cloxacillin or oxacillin may be used as an appropriate alternative.

*Vancomycin* should be considered for patients who are current MRSA carriers or have anaphylactic allergy to penicillins. It should be taken into consideration in the case of high-risk patients, such as:

- Patients in regions with a high prevalence of MRSA
- Institutionalized patients (nursing home residents, dialysis patients, and those who have been in intensive care).
- Health workers.
- Patients with a high probability of contamination.

In other cases, its use as prophylaxis must be absolutely avoided. The preoperative dose of antibiotics must be administered within an hour of the surgical incision; this can be extended to 2 hours for vancomycin and fluoroquinolones, because, especially for vancomycin, the infusion must occur slowly.

Post-operative antibiotics should not be administered for more than 24 hours after surgery. Routine prophylactic use of double administration is not recommended unless the duration of the intervention exceeds the 2 half-lives of the antibiotic (.g., if an antibiotic has a life of 4 hours, a dose must be added after 2 hours). Preoperative antibiotics have different pharmacokinetics based on patient weight and therefore the dose must be adapted to weight. The type of pre-operative antibiotic given to a patient with a previous infection should also cover the previous infecting organism.

In *thromboembolic prophylaxis* [60, 61]. The type, dose, and duration of administration of anticoagulant drugs for prophylaxis against venous thromboembolism influence the incidence of infection (SSI). In Italy, most orthopedic centers begin subcutaneous anticoagulant treatment 12 hours before surgery. In America, it starts 6–12 hours after surgery.

In both cases, they continue for about 40 days.

*Hand washing* is a step that must be respected as Ignác Semmelweis said *"Hand washing remains one of the most important steps in avoiding infections"* [62].

The surgeon and operating room staff should mechanically wash their hands with an antiseptic agent for a minimum of 2 minutes for the first surgery. A shorter period may be appropriate for subsequent cases, paying particular attention to the interdigital spaces and the periungual area. There is no clear difference between various antiseptic handwashing agents [62, 63].

### 19.4.2 Intraoperative

*The preparation of the surgical field* [64–66] is very important and must be done very carefully.

*Chlorhexidine–alcoholic* is more protective than povidone-iodine against both superficial and deep incisional infections.

There is enough evidence to enforce the universal use of *space-type suits* [67, 68] with air exhaust during prostheses, although some authors do not consider the use of this procedure routine.

We acknowledge the presence of studies showing *iodine-impregnated drapes* adhered to the skin [69–71] which tend to decrease bacterial counts, but no correlation has been established with PJI. Furthermore, the application of the adhesive sheet must remain for the entire duration of the operation without coming off and the incision passes through the sheet and then the skin on the surface.

*Laminar flow operating rooms* [72, 73] We believe that prosthetic surgery can be performed in operating rooms without laminar flow. Laminar flow chambers and other strategies that can reduce particles in operating rooms would be expected to reduce this burden but studies have not shown reduced SSI in laminar flow chambers and, in some cases, are associated with increased rates of SSI. These are complex technologies that must operate in strict adherence to maintenance protocols.

*Operating rooms with ultraviolet light* [74, 75] With UV one would expect to lower the bacterial load in operating rooms, but the technology has not been studied for this application. It could be considered an adjuvant, but not a substitute for conventional cleaning. There are potential risks to staff who inadvertently left UVs running at the start of the work day.

*Movement in the operating room* [76–78] Traffic in the operating room should be kept to a minimum. The room must be prepared with all the elements required before the intervention. It is forbidden to enter once the intervention has begun. The passage of the material occurs through "clean" routes. Use of electronic devices and other contaminating objects in the operating room. Portable electronic devices can be contaminated with bacteria, therefore it is recommended that the use of portable electronic devices be limited to what is necessary for patient care.

Use of *sterile gloves and mask* [79, 80] We recommend double gloving. We recognize the benefit of changing gloves at least every 90 minutes or more frequently and the need to change punctured gloves. Permeability appears to be affected by exposure to methacrylate cement and gloves should be changed after any cementation.

Use of the *"mother" table* [81, 82]. It is recommended that the opening times of the trays should occur as close as possible to the start of the surgical procedure the prevent of any delays between the opening of the tray and the start of a surgical procedure. We recognize a theoretical advantage of covering trays when not in use for long periods, and that larger covers may be disadvantageous if containers are moved from contaminated areas across the sterile field.

#### 19.4.2.1 Aspects of Surgical Management [83, 84]

- High rates of contamination have been recognized in studies of *scalpel blades* that have been used for skin incision and it is recommended to change the scalpel blade after skin incision [85, 86]
- It is recommended to replace *the suction* every 60 minutes based on studies showing high contamination rates. The cannulae can be introduced into the femoral canal for the time necessary to evacuate the fluids, but must not be left in the canal, where they circulate large quantities of ambient air and particles that can contaminate the surgical procedure [87]
- The theoretical basis for *irrigation* useful for diluting contamination and removing nonviable tissue is recognized and a greater volume of irrigation leads to greater dilution We recognize the advantages and disadvantages of different methods of fluid irrigation, but we do not recommend one method over another [88–91]

- The use of *containers filled with liquids* that are open during the surgery
- The surgical *checklist* protocol is supported as beneficial to patient safety, in particular as it applies to the correct administration of antibiotic prophylaxis and gauze counts [92, 93]
- There is no evidence to demonstrate that the Use of *closed drains* increases the risk of PJI
- *Surgical time* [94, 95] It is recognized that rates of PJI increase directly with the duration of surgery We recognize that some surgeries have a significant level and unavoidable complexity which will take longer for technicians of the procedure
- The exaggerated detachment of the *tissues devitalizes* the tissues and creates areas of necrosis, a source of possible infections as well as the presence of *hematomas.*
- The administration of *tranexamic acid (TA)* [96, 97] both intravenously and topically, reduces the amount of blood loss and allogeneic blood transfusions in prosthesis. Topical administration of TA has no obvious advantage over intravenous administration of the drug and both are safe. However, the topical use of TA can be used in a certain group of patients where the intravenous use of TA is considered inappropriate
- The use of *"disposable" material* ensures better asepticity [98]
- *Wound dressing at the end of surgery* [99, 100]:—The use of occlusive dressings with Hydrofiber alginate, Aquacell, when available, is highly recommended. The acute infection ratio between aquacell dressing is 0.44% and standard gauze 1.7%.
- *Silver-impregnated dressings* have not been shown to reduce PJIs
- In the absence of conclusive data and the wide variability in surgical practice, no recommendation is made regarding the type of *specific suture* to prevent infection, but one fact is certainly important that is, do not suture tense tissues. There are sutures added with antibiotics on the market but to date, there are no recognized EBMs.

### 19.4.3 Post-operative

#### 19.4.3.1 "Mechanical" Thromboembolic Prophylaxis [101, 102]

- *Elastic stockings with graduated compression* antithrombus at the pelvis height for hip prostheses, thigh height for knee prostheses, with compression at the ankle of approximately 18 mmHg; kept in place until the patient resumes effective walking; They are available in different sizes.
- *Intermittent pneumatic compression (IPC)* device composed of leg warmers and compressor, which exerts intermittent sequential compression from the calf to the thighs; it must be used postoperatively; requires careful positioning. The two systems are complementary and can be used in a combined manner (elastic stockings / intermittent pneumatic compression).
- *Lift and move the patient as soon as possible.*

*Post-operative transfusions* [103, 104], predisposing factors for allogeneic blood transfusions:

- A low preoperative hemoglobin level (7–8 g/dL) is the strongest predictor for the potential need for allogeneic transfusions.
- The use of general anesthesia.
- A higher Charlson comorbidity index (> 3).
- Female sex.
- The duration of the operation.

Allogeneic blood transfusions are associated with an increased risk of SSI / HAI The role of autologous transfusions in the risk of SSI/HAI remains inconclusive.

When to remove *drains* [105, 106]: There is no conclusive evidence for the optimal time for drain removal (recommended, however, no later than 24 hours).

Another important point, for which many surgeons and companies are working, is to put the prosthesis that is implanted in a defense condition against the germ. This position arises from the fact that having seen that the biofilm forms in the first hours after the operation it was thought that at that moment in the bone-prosthesis contact, there must be something that fights the infection at a high concentration in the case of antibiotics. Instead in other cases, it is the product, such as silver which cannot be in directly contact with the bone to act as an antibacterial or bone added with antibiotic Or, as in the case of the Japanese experience, a disinfectant such as iodine added to the prosthesis. And finally, a gel is added with a targeted antibiotic, for staphylococcus or for any germ responsible for other outbreaks which is spread directly on the prosthesis at the time of implantation. Obviously, all these systems can also be used in the treatment of periprosthetic infections in the two stages, not only as prevention in the first installation.

#### 19.4.3.2 Prostheses Cemented with the Use of Cement Added with Antibiotics [107–115]

Polymethylmethacrylate (PMMA) has been known since the 1930s and is better known by the commercial name of "Plexiglass or Perspex®". In the beginning, the material was used mainly for the construction of safety glass but in the 1930s both an English company, ICI, and a German researcher, *Otto Roehm*, proposed its use for the creation of dental prostheses. In 1941 after the Battle of Britain (August-September 1940), RAF doctors noticed that plexiglass inclusions in the skin and eyes of pilots did not induce granulomas In 1941 PMMA was used to fill bone defects in the skull *J Charnley* He began using PMMA to fix the femoral prosthetic component (in its experience, at a follow up of 15 years, a survival of the prosthetic implants equal to 85%) was observed and began the modern history of "bone cement" [116]. The use of cement (PMMA) was later resumed to fix knee prostheses (*Mc Keever, Guston*). The characteristics seen can create some problems such as the high temperature during the polymerization phase which can create necrosis of the bone tissue, at the bone-cement interface. Furthermore, a fall in arterial pressure and an increase in central venous pressure have been demonstrated, not due to embolic phenomena. No evident allergic phenomena, at least until the compound is stable.

The use of antibiotic cement was introduced in 1970 by *Buchholtz and Engelbrecht* [110] Using gentamicin sulphate. But why use cement with antibiotics in the first implant? Bone cement in the Australian Arthroplasty Registry had a lower rate of revision due to infection when antibiotic cement was used (0.67%) than when cement was used (0.91%) without antibiotics (AOANJRR 2009) The effect of antibiotic-treated cement has been studied most thoroughly in primary hip replacement, where there was convincing evidence of a reduced number of infections compared to antibiotic-free cement (Figs. 19.5 and 19.6) [112, 113] The microbiology in infected knee in previous reports from the SKAR, the cumulative revision rate (CRR) due to infection has been shown to have decreased from 27% during 1976–1985 to 11% during 1986–2000 [117]. Microbiology in infected knee arthroplasties in previous SKAR reports has shown that the cumulative revision rate (CRR) decreased from 2.7% in 1976–1985 to 1.1% during 1986–2000 due to infection.

The release time of the antibiotic (Fig. 19.3) and the biomechanical capacity of antibiotic-admixed industrial cement (Fig. 19.7).

Another element to consider is the porosity of the cement after the elimination of the antibiotic but the new pre-packaged cement already added with antibiotic have overcome this problem by giving a mechanical sealing capacity equal to cement without antibiotic (around 800 hectopascal). It is useful for the composition of the cement itself and for its porosity that the preparation takes place under vacuum in such a way as to eliminate all the possible air (Fig. 19.8).

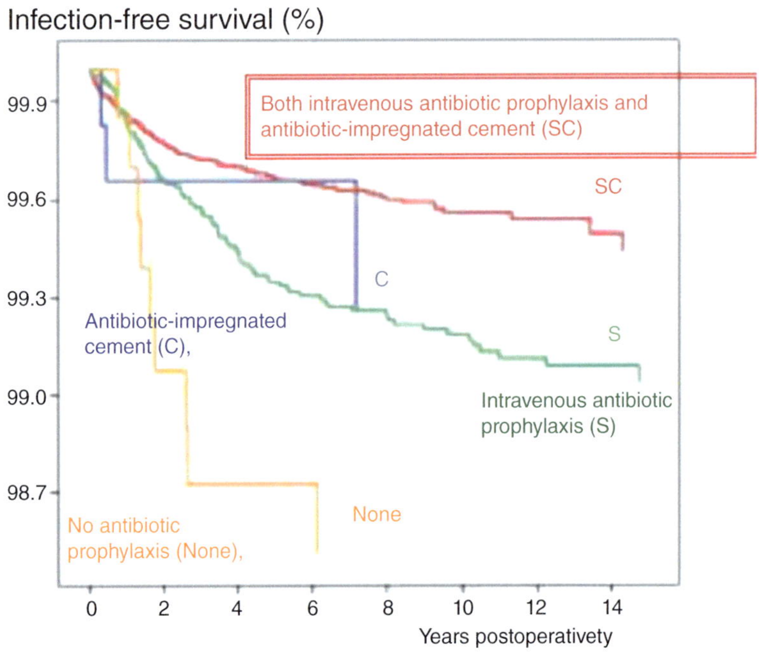


**Fig. 19.5** A study conducted on 42,250 patients who underwent total hip and knee replacement surgery from 1987 to 2007 in Norway demonstrated that the combination of venous antibiotics and antibiotic-treated cement significantly reduced the incidence of infection in primary prostheses [112]

### 19.4.4 Characteristics of Antibiotics to Be Associated with Cement (Fig. 19.9)

- Stable at heat from 50 to 150 °C
- Prolonged stability at 37 °C
- Soluble in water
- Available in powder
- Non-toxic or allergic
- Must not attach to molecules of cement
- Small volume
- Low influence on the mechanical properties of the cement
- Maximum spectrum of action
- Bactericidal action
- Activity at small doses (low MIC and MBC)

Finally, *the cost* of each single pack of antibiotic cement varies from $284 to $349; each TKA requires at least two packs. Considering approximately 250,000 cases per year of TKA, the routine use of ABLC for prophylactic purposes in primary implant prostheses in this country is expected to add a cost of approximately $75 million per year.

This price justifies it by lowering the infection rate given the costs of an infected prosthesis.

At this point, it is useless to make a comparison with how much it costs to treat an infected prosthesis where in addition to the real cost already quantified at the beginning of the chapter there are all the social costs, the prolonged use of antibiotics.

All this serves to clearly reduce the possibility of an infection.

### 19.4.5 Bone Chips Impregnated with Antibiotics (Figs. 19.10, 19.11, and 19.12) [118]

In the first implants with bone loss, bone granules impregnated with antibiotics can be used as filling.

Bone allograft as an antibiotic carrier.

Vancomycin 10 times more concentrated than cement.

High local concentration and prolonged release. Bone granules of an average size of 5 mm impregnated with antibiotic (Osteomyin®).

Refrigerated homo-bone grafts immersed in rifampicin release antibiotic, on site, at therapeutic levels for 3 weeks.

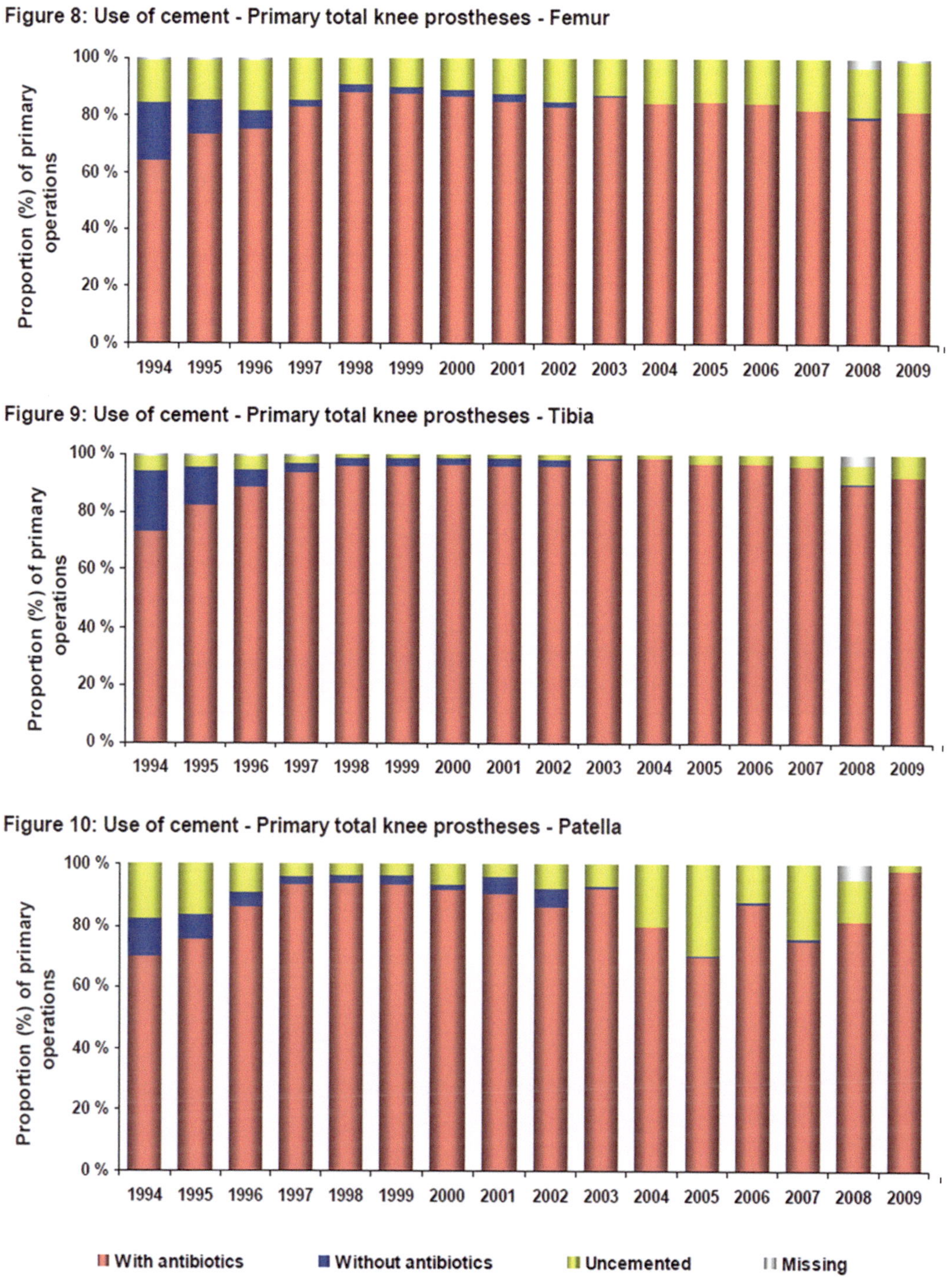


**Fig. 19.6** Use of cement in first implant prosthesis with or without antibiotics (Norwegian registry) by site (femur, tibia and patella) from 1994 to 2009. Furthermore, we know that the biofilm begins to form in the first few hours and therefore the release of antibiotics must occur in the first 24 hours [112]

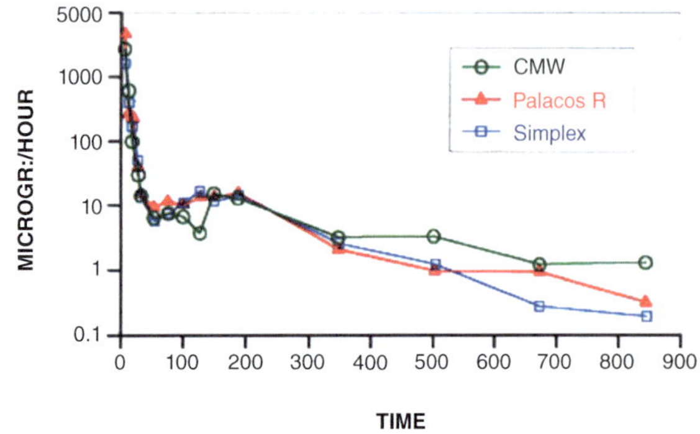


**Fig. 19.7** Release time, in hours, of the antibiotic. In the first 24 hours there is a peak with the maximum concentration of antibiotic which then gradually decreases

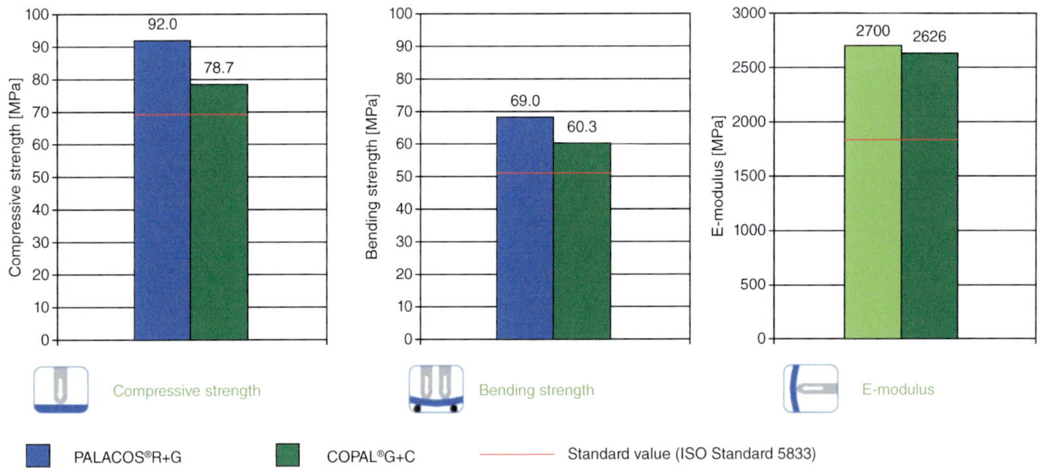


**Fig. 19.8** COPAL® G*C: (gentamycin and clindamycin), PALACOS (R) R+G (gentamycin): mechanical properties (compressive strength, bending strength and e-modolus). A red line indicates the standard value according to ISO Standard 5833

| Antibiotic group | Type of antibiotic | Activity | Dose per 40 g cement (in grams) |
|---|---|---|---|
| Aminoglvcoside | Tobramycin | Gram-negative bacteria, such as *pseudomonas* | 1–4,8 |
| Aminoglvcoside | Gentamicin | Gram-negative bacteria, such as *Escherichia coli, Klebsiella,* in particular *Pseudomonas aerogynous,* Also aerobic bacteria (not mandatory/optioanl anaerobic) | 0,25–4,8 |
| Cephalosporin, 1st gen. | Cefazolin | Gram-positive, gram-negative infections limited coverage | 1–2 |
| Cephalosporin, 2nd gen. | Cefuroxime | Reduced gram positive coverage, better gram negative coverage | 1,5–2 |
| Cephalosporin, 3rd gen. | Ceftazidime | Gram-negative bacteria, especially *pseudomonas* | 2 |
| Cephalosporin, 4th gen. | Cefotaxime | Gram-negative bacteria, no activity against *pseudomonas* | 2 |
| Cephalosporin, 5th gen. | Ceftaroline | Gram-negative bacteria, no activity against *pseudomonas* | 2–4 |
| Fluorquinolone | Ciprofloxacin | Gram-negative organisms, including activity against *Enterobactericiae* | 02–3 |
| Glycopeptide | Vancomvcin | Gram-positive bacteria, including methicillin-resistant organisms | 05–4 |
| Lincosamide | Clindamvcin | Gram-positive, anaerobic cocci | 1–2 |
| Macrolide | Erythromvcin | Cocci and aerobic gram-positive bacilli | 05–1 |
| Polymyvin | Colistin | Gram-negative | 0,24 |
| β-lactams | Piperacillin | Gram-negative bacteria (particularly *Pseudomonas*), entrobacteria and anaerobes | 4–8 |
| β-lactamase | Aztreonam | Only gram-negative bacteria | 4 |
| β-lactamase inhibitor | Tazobactam | Gram-negative bacteria (especially *Pseudomonas*), entrobacteria and anaerobes in combination with piperacillin | 0,5 |
| Oxazolidinones | Linelozid | Multiresistant gram-positive cocci, such as MRSA | 1,2 |
| Carbapenem | Meropenem | Gram-positive and gram-negative bacteria, anaerobes, *Pseudomonas* | 0,5–4 |
| Lipopeptide | Daptomvcin | Gram-positive organisms only | 2 |
| Antifungal | Amphotericin | Most fungi | 200 |
| Antifungal | Voricanazole | Most fungi | 300–600 mg |

**Fig. 19.9** The concentration of antibiotics in 40 g of cement powder and the action capabilities of the antibiotics against various germs

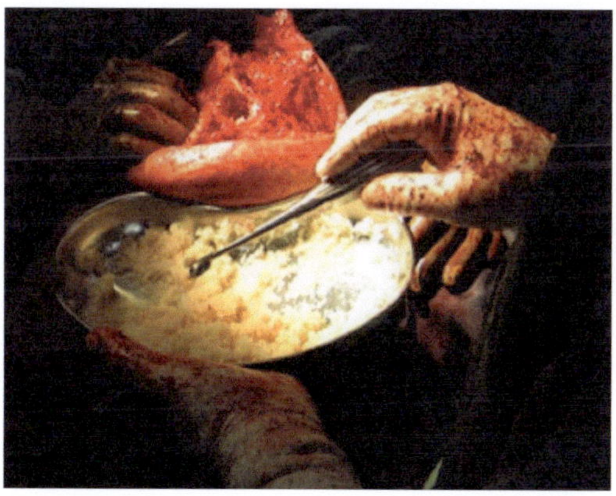

**Fig. 19.10** Mixing of bone chips, from donor, with antibiotic (commercial material) but it can also be done self-made. (© Ivyspring International Publisher. Reproduced under the terms of the Creative Commons Attribution (CC BY-NC) license (https://creativecommons.org/licenses/by-nc/4.0/). See http://ivyspring.com/terms for full terms and conditions)

**Advantages:**

- No risk of damaging the bone in the search for press-fit
- Presence of local antibiotics at high doses
- Greater adherence to the antibiotic in the cleaned bone areas

**Disadvantages:**

- Delayed direct loading while waiting for osteointegration
- Possibility to add only some antibiotics

AB loaded bone graft
versus
AB loaded cement

| AB Carrier | Purified Bone | PMMA |
|---|---|---|
| Storage capacity/10cc | 1g | 0.1g |
| Availability | >90% | >10% |
| Release 1.day | 10.000–20.000mg/l | 40–400mg/l |
| Release 6.day | 60–130mg/l | Traces |
| Release 100.day | 0 | Traces |

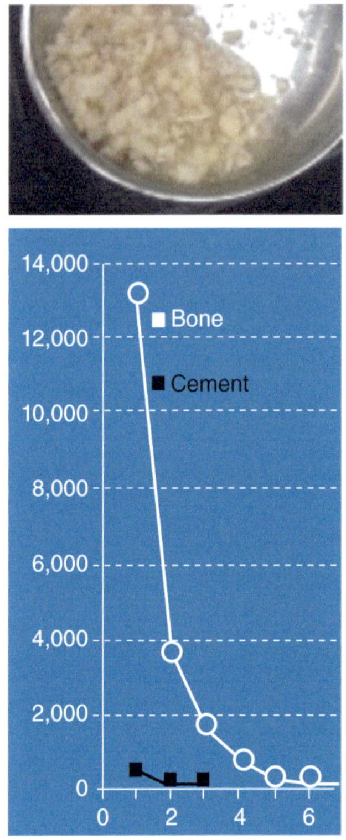


**Fig. 19.11** Demonstration of the different behavior between antibiotic-loaded bone compared to antibiotic-loaded cement. 

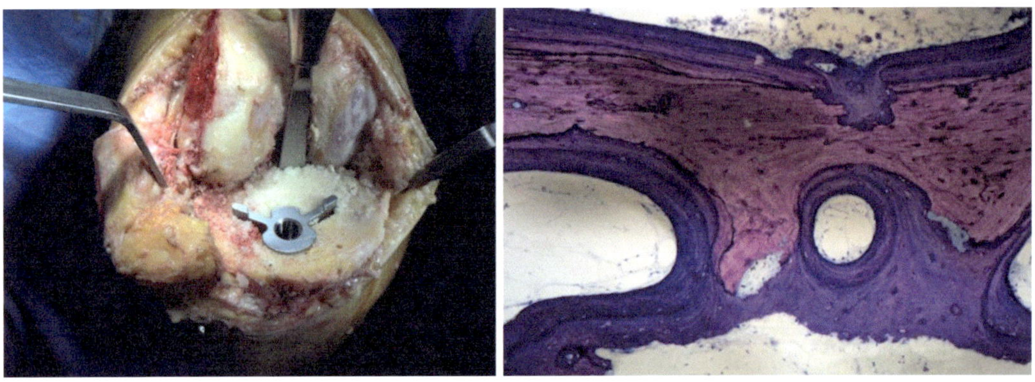

**Fig. 19.12** Osteointegration 6 months after removal of an infection (creeping substitution) with resorption of the graft and deposition of new bone. 

## 19.5 Coatings of the Prostheses During the Operation

The coating is carried out in the operating room as in the case of *DAC® (Defensive Antibacterial Coating)* (Figs. 19.13, 19.14, and 19.15) [119–123].

It consists of a gel that can be added with the targeted antibiotic in the implantation of cementless prostheses. It is applied directly to the prosthesis and allows the elimination of the antibiotic during the possible formation of the biofilm. The experiments conducted have highlighted that its introduction does not create a detachment of the same, thus avoiding its protective function, as can be seen from the example reported on a corpse where in the end the entire contact area between the bone and the prosthesis was covered by the gel. Furthermore, it has a reabsorption of approximately 24 hours.

**Advantages:**

- Possibility of adding any antibiotic not only in powder form
- Greater search for press-fit
- Presence of local antibiotics in high doses
- Direct contact between bone—gel (absorbable)—prosthesis

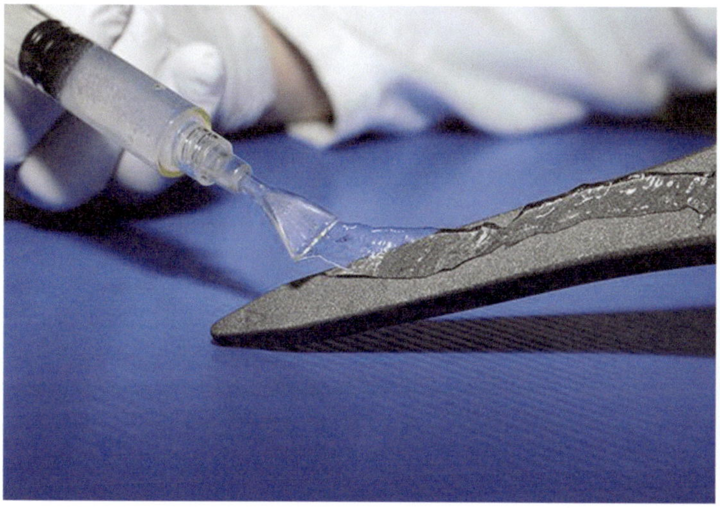
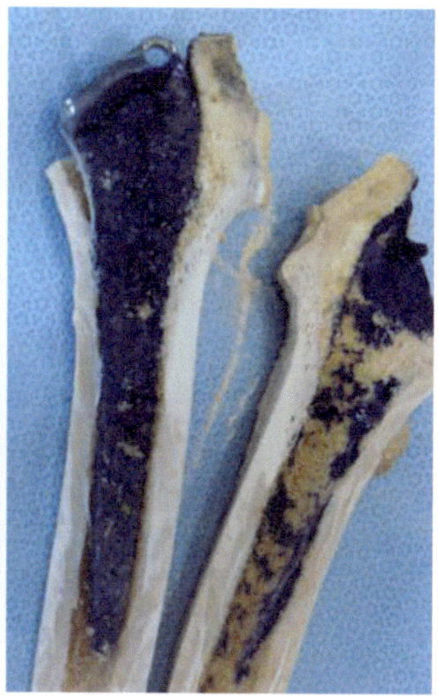

**Figs. 19.13 and 19.14** The application of the covering material can be supplemented with various antibiotics based on the sensitivity of the germs. If an antibiogram is not available, broad-spectrum antibiotics can be applied. Reproduced with permission of SAGE from Ref. (courtesy C. Romanò [120]

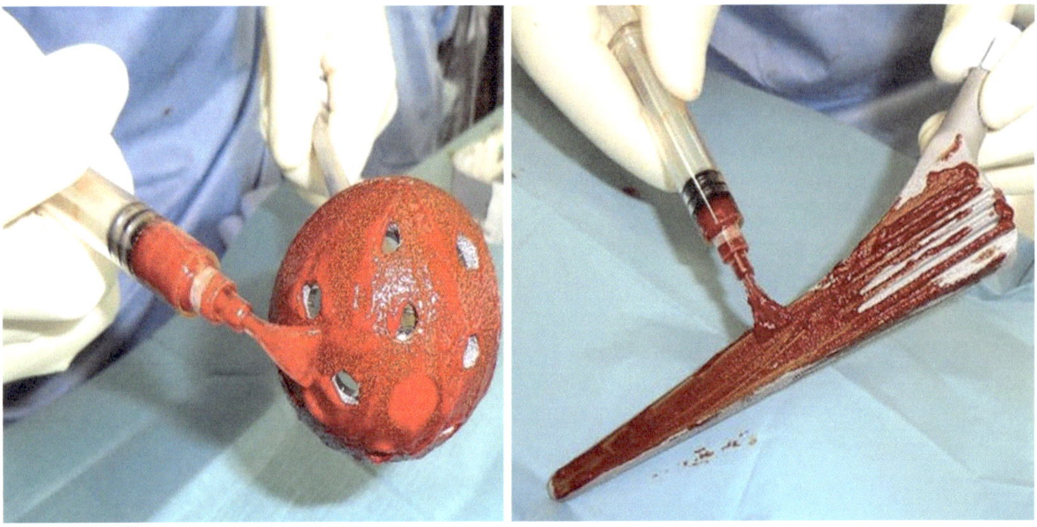

**Fig. 19.15** Coverage with gel mixed with rifampicin in one stage with sensitivity to rifampicin. (Reproduced with permission of Sage from Ref. [119])

**Disadvantages:**

- Delayed direct loading in waiting for osseointegration
- The release time of the antibiotic is not evident

Even today it is not known what the duration of the DAC is even if the Authors report that the greatest concentration must occur in the first 48 hours, i.e. the time necessary for the formation of the biofilm, and that in the following time, it can be eliminated having finished its task.

## 19.6 Prostheses Already Packaged by the Companies

### 19.6.1 Covering with Silver (PorAg® Surface) (Figs. 19.16 and 19.17) [124–132]

Silver has always been used as an antimicrobial. In 4000 BC the Egyptians used silver-coated water tanks and in 1200 BC the Phoenicians used silver-coated amphorae to transport food. In 78 AD Pliny the Elder began treating wounds with silver, in 950 BC Haian As Sufis used honey and silver, in powder form, to treat tonsillitis and in 1881 AD Dr. Cari Crede used silver nitrate eye drops for eye infections. Thus the silver coating increases surface resistance to abrasion, a decreases the elimination of Co, Cr, Ti ions, and also has a demonstrated antibacterial effect Together with mercury it represents two effective natural elements for killing bacteria *Henry Crookes* (1910) [125] demonstrated that B Coli communis was killed in 2 minutes using mercury and in 6 using silver colloid. Another study from these early years is that of *Simpson and Hewlett* [126] published in "The Lancet" in 1914. They used the suspension of colloidal silver to kill the typhoid bacillus in 15 minutes at 500 ppm and in 2 hours at 5 ppm. This was the first time in which low concentrations of colloidal silver proved effective. An important consideration by *Simpson and Hewlett* was to state that the great advantage of colloidal elements, used in such low concentrations, is that they are completely harmless to patients.

Research has confirmed that no organism capable of causing disease (bacteria, viruses and fungi) can live more than a few minutes in the presence of a trace, albeit tiny, of metallic silver, which appears to be one of the most powerful natural antibacterials without side effects.

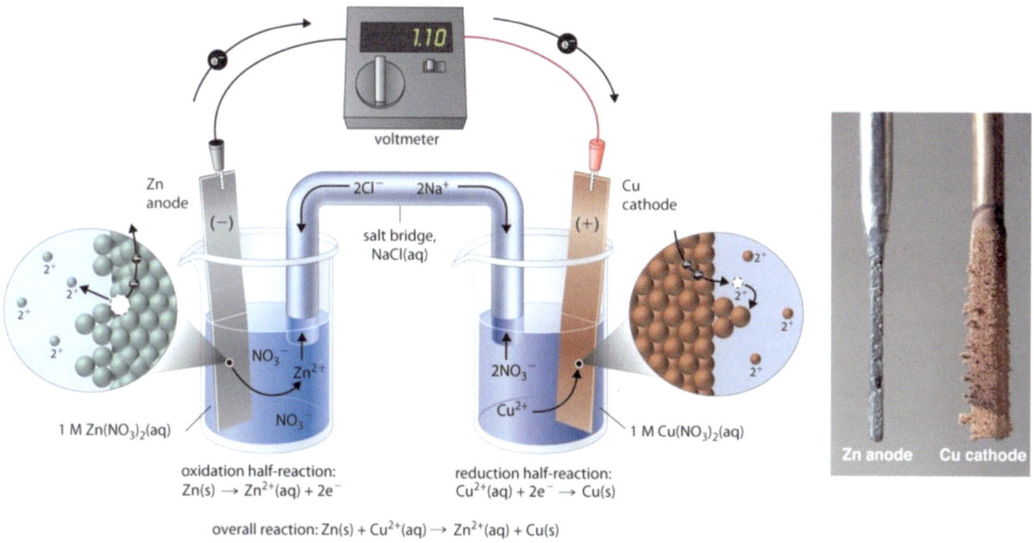


**Fig. 19.16** This example shows a galvanic reaction between zinc and copper where zinc is eliminated (Zn anode) and copper is added (Cu cathode)

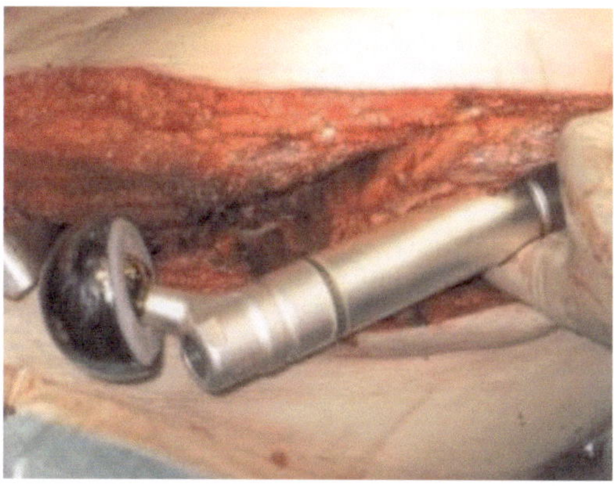

**Fig. 19.17** A silver megaprosthesis. (Courtesy R. Capanna)

Multiple tests, in different districts such as urology, neurosurgery, cardiology, skin lesions, have demonstrated the validity of silver as an antiseptic:

- *Hsu*. Biomaterials 2010
- *Khalipour*, J Biomed Mater Res B 2010
- *Juan*. Int J Nanomedicine 2010
- *Song*. J Biomed Mater Res A 2009
- *Chen*, J Biomed Mater Res A 2007
- *Furno*. J Antimictob Chemother 2004
- *Sheehan*. J Orthop Res 2004
- *Blaker*. Biomaterials 2004

*RO Becker* [133], from his research on the use of silver in medicine, deduced that the deficiency of silver in the organism is responsible for the improper functioning of the immune system and that silver is not only a powerful antibacterial. Colloidal silver is non-toxic to mammals, reptiles and all life forms that are not single-celled. Silver, however, like the most powerful chemical disinfectants, is toxic to primitive life forms such as microorganisms. Single-celled life forms use different chemical processes. For oxygen metabolism. The presence of silver, especially in the form of colloid nanoparticles, interrupts the enzymatic metabolic cycle and causes suffocation and death within six minutes; at that point, the immune, lymphatic and purifying systems will take care of their expulsion. The action of colloidal silver is so fast that the pathogen does not have time to mutate into a resistant strain. The fixation of silver to titanium occurs galvanically, like all prosthesis coating formations.

There are four types of silver:

1. Ionic silver
2. Ionic silver with the addition of proteins for stabilizing purposes
3. True colloidal silver, made up almost exclusively of nanoparticles, industrially produced

4. Silver salts sold as drugs or medical aids surgical.

The silver used is colloidal as it does not precipitate forming a salt and silver colloids are used with particles of an average size of 10–15 nm practically free of ionic silver. It is added through the industrial process of electrolysis In a work review done on 23 studies, by *Hua Li and other authors* [129] demonstrated some cases of Argyria while no cases with gentamicin coating and only one case of anaphylactic reaction to iodine-coated prosthesis. For silver, the greatest effort has been made in dressings, especially in burns because it is antiseptic and stimulates granulation, while in the orthopedic field, it has been used in megaprostheses after the removal of a bone tumor where both local and general conditions (just think of the antiblastic) are very at risk of infection with an average of 7–23% *Capanna* [127, 128] brought his work to 516 megaprostheses made from 2000 to 2015 (427 oncological and 89 non-oncological) where he demonstrated a lowering of the percentages of infection A work by *Handrik Hardes* [132, 134] compared 74 megaprostheses made only of titanium with 51 megaprostheses made of titanium with a silver covering and highlighted that in the first case there were 17.6% infections and 38% amputations In the second group there were 5–6% infections and no amputations.

A study comparing DAC and silver highlighted the longer duration of the antibacterial effect of silver compared to DAC. Even today it is not known what the duration of the DAC effect is, even if the Authors report that the greatest concentration must occur in the first 48 hours of biofilm formation time and which can be eliminated in the following time having finished its task.

A study comparing titanium megaprostheses (74 cases) and titanium Ag megaprostheses (51 cases) had the following result:

| 74 Cases Megaprosthesis in titanium | 51 Cases Megaprosthesis in titanium Silver |
|---|---|
| 17.6% infection | 5.9% infection |
| 38.5% amputation | No amputation |

### 19.6.2 Prosthesis Cover with Iodine (Figs. 19.18 and 19.19) [135–138]

Other studies involve the application of a coating *with Gentamicin or vancomycin* [139–141].

Below the Figs. 19.20 and 19.21, representing the various elements currently used as prosthetic coverings.

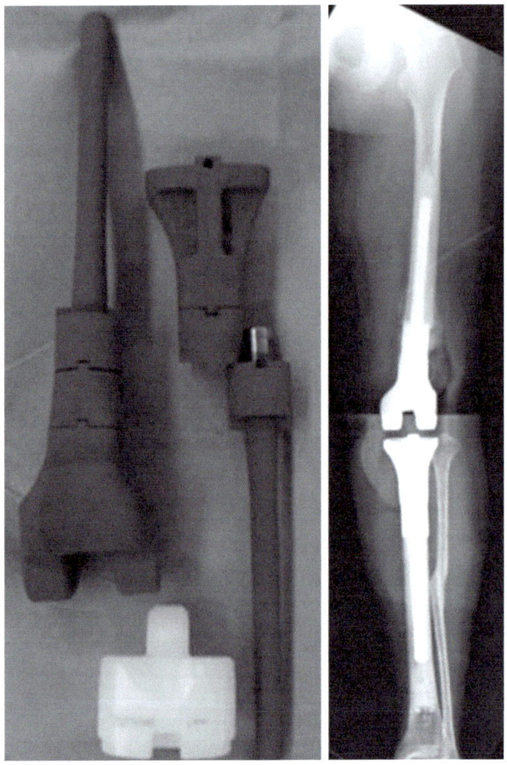

**Fig. 19.18** Iodine-coated prosthesis. (Courtesy Hiroyuki Tsuchiya)

**Advantages**
Iodine vs Silver

| Iodine | Silver |
|---|---|
| ① no systemic toxicity (Iodine is excreted from the kidney.) | ① anxious for toxicity (Metabolism is not clear) |
| ② essential trace element (thyroid hormone) | ② foreign substance in the body |
| ③ osteoconductive | ③ disturbed osteoconduction |
| ④ shelf-life: more than 10 years | ④ no continuous release (highest concentration on a few days) |
| ⑤ reasonable cost | ⑤ expensive |

**Fig. 19.19** A comparison between the silver-coated prosthesis and the iodine-coated prosthesis [135–138]

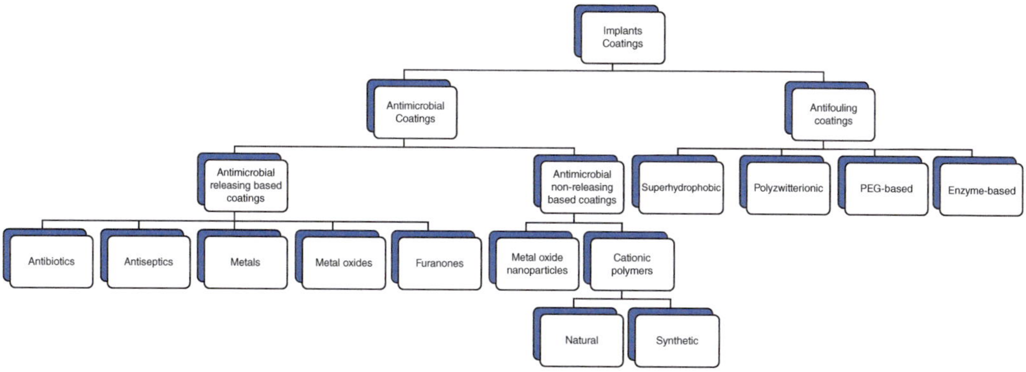


**Fig. 19.20** Shows the various coatings. (Reproduced with permission from [141] under the terms of the Creative Commons Attribution-NonCommercial 4.0 License (https://creativecommons.org/licenses/by-nc/4.0/) which permits non-commercial use, reproduction and distribution of the work without further permission provided the original work is attributed as specified on the SAGE and Open Access pages (https://us.sagepub.com/en-us/nam/open-access-at-sage))

**Fig. 19.21** Examples of anti-infective strategies proposed for the antibacterial treatment of implantable surfaces used in orthopedic surgery. (Reproduced from Gallo et al. [142] under the terms of Creative Commons Attribution (CC BY) license)

| Strategy | Features | Examples |
|---|---|---|
| Prevention in adhesion and adsoiption | | Anti-adhesive polymers<br>Albumin<br>Super-hydrophobic surfaces<br>Nano-patterned surface<br>Hydrogels |
| Methods to kill bacteria | Inorganic | Silver nanopruticles<br>Titanium dioxide<br>Selenium ion<br>Copper ion<br>Zinc ion |
| | Organic | Coated or covalently linked antibiotics<br>Chitosan derivatives |
| | | Signaling, inhibiting and antimicrobial peptides |
| | | Cytokines<br>Enzymes |
| | Other | Non-antibiotic bactericidal substances |
| | Combined | Multilayer coating<br>Synergy material intensification<br>Positively charged polymers |
| Multi-functional and smart coating | Passive | Nanostructured "smart" material |
| | Active | Concept: sensors conjoined to nanocontainers |
| Alternative approach | | Lytic bacteriophages |

At the conclusion of this chapter, it seems important to underline another big problem, the *antibiotic resistance* that we have in Italy according to the European antibiotic resistance surveillance report (2015) [143]. In Fig. 19.22 the antibiotic resistance of *K. pneumoniae* to carbapenems in Europe. In Fig. 19.23 the resistance, again in Europe, of methicillin-resistant Staphylococcus aureus. Finally, in Fig. 19.24 the evolution over time of various germs to antibiotic resistance. Note the Italian situation.

Tuberculosis should also be remembered which in Italy, after the landings of immigrants, is increasing with an extrapulmonary—bone localization of 10% (Fig. 19.25) [144, 145].

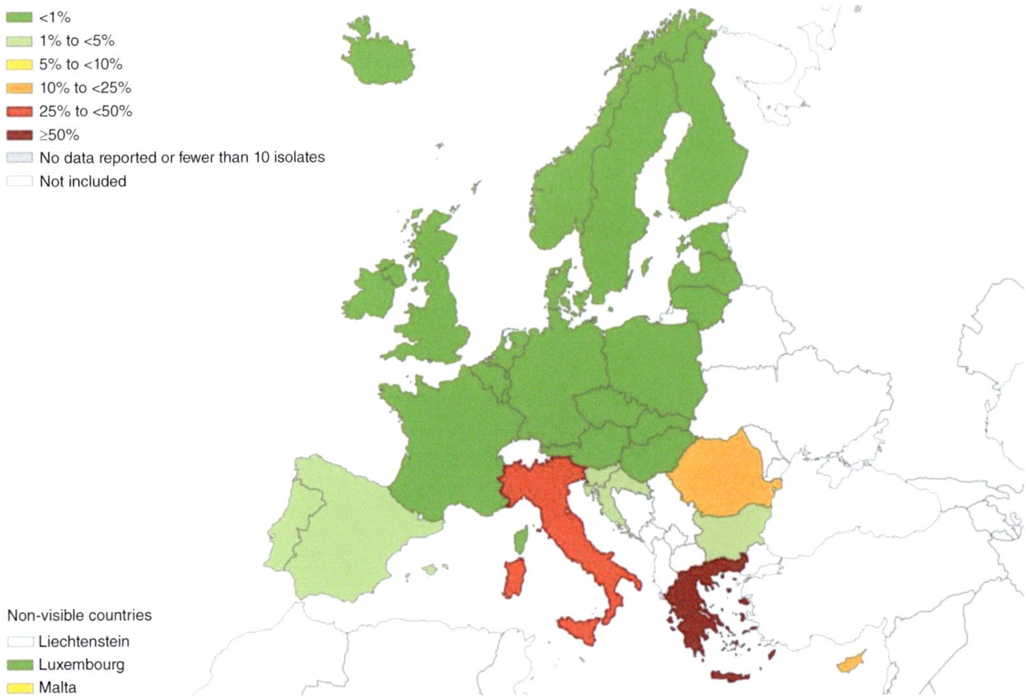


**Fig. 19.22** *K. pneumoniae*: percentage of isolates resistant to carbapenems by country and Italy, as you can see, has among the highest resistances EU/EAA area—2015 data

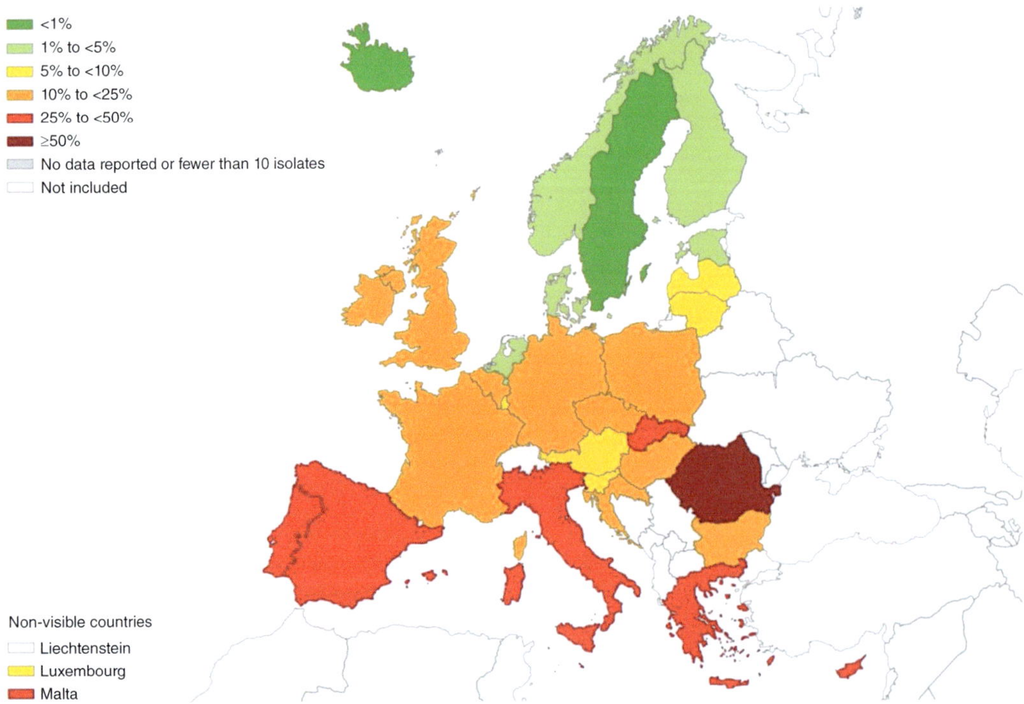


**Fig. 19.23** *For the S. aureus*, same situation of resistance in Italy. Here you see the percentage of isolated methicillin-resistant strains (MRSA), by country, EU/EAA area—2015 data

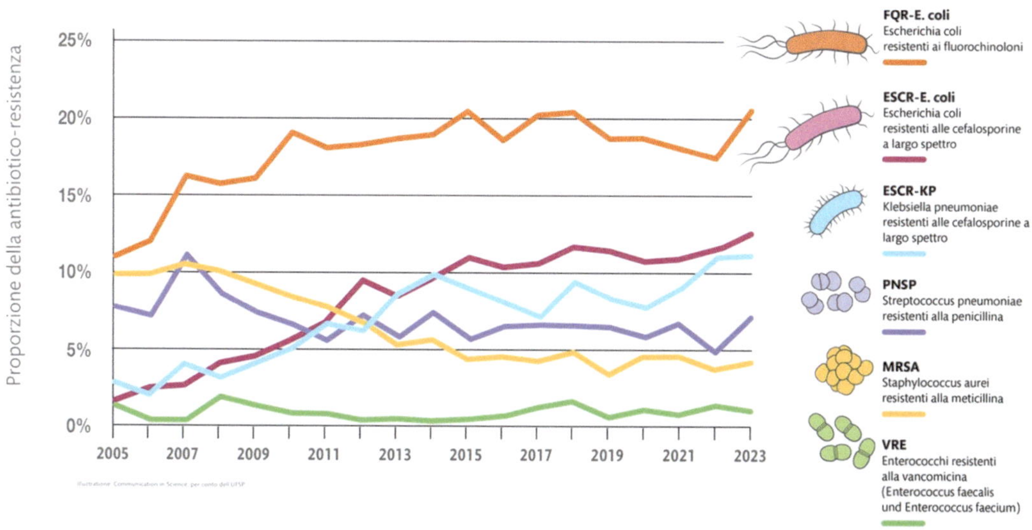


**Fig. 19.24** Evolution of the main bacterial resistance over time. *Courtesy of dell Ufficio Federale della Sanità Pubblica (UFSP) in Italian - Bundesamt für Gesundheit (BAG) in German - is the center for public health of the Swiss federal government and is part of the Federal Department of Home Affairs*

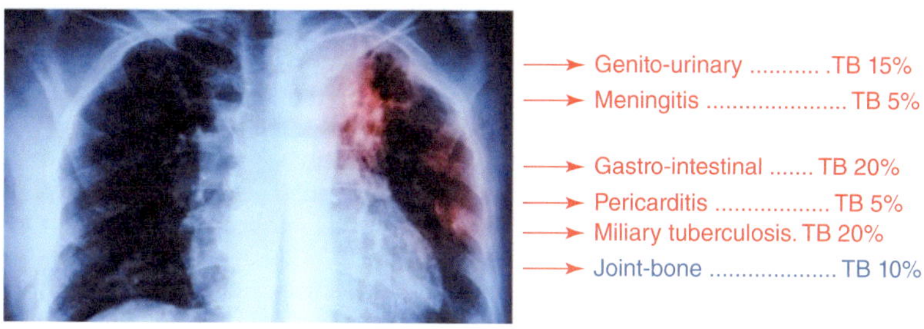


**Fig. 19.25** Percentages of extra-pulmonary tuberculosis localizations

Therefore, based on the data reported, the prevention of these pathologies becomes fundamental and all scientific and industrial efforts must go in this direction.

## References

1. Parvizi J, Gehrke T, Chen AF. Proceedings of the International consensus on periprosthetic joint infection. Bone Joint J. 2013;95-B:1450–2.
2. Kurtz S, Ong K, Lau E, Mowat F, Halpern M. Projections of primary and revision hip and knee arthroplasty in the United States from 2005 to 2030. J Bone Joint Surg Am. 2007;89:780–5.
3. Kurtz SM, Lau E, Watson H, Schmier JK, Parvizi J. Economic burden of periprosthetic joint infection in the United States. J Arthroplast. 2012; 27(8 Suppl. 1):61–5.e1.
4. American Diabetes Association. Standards of care in diabetes—2023 Abridged for primary care providers. Clin Diabetes. 2023;41:4–31.
5. Marchant MH Jr, Viens NA, Cook C, Vail TP, Bolognesi MP. The impact of glycemic control and diabetes mellitus on perioperative outcomes after total joint arthroplasty. J Bone Joint Surg Am. 2009;91(7):1621–9.
6. Ong KL, Kurtz SM, Lau E, Bozic KJ, Berry DJ, Parvizi J. Prosthetic joint infection risk after total hip arthroplasty in the Medicare population. J Arthroplast. 2009;24:105–9.
7. Parvizi J, Gehrke T, International Consensus Group on Periprosthetic Joint Infection. Definition

of periprosthetic joint infection. J Arthroplast. 2014;29:1331.
8. Corvec S, Portillo ME, Pasticci BM, Borens O, Trampuz A. Epidemiology and new developments in the diagnosis of prosthetic joint infection. Int J Artif Organs. 2012;35:923–34.
9. Romanò CL, Al Khawashki H, Benzakour T, Bozhkova S, Del Sel H, Hafez M, Johari A, Lob G, Sharma HK, Hirouchi T, Drago L, World Association against Infection in Orthopaedics and Trama (W.A.I.O.T.) Study Group on Bone and Joint Infection Definitions. The W.A.I.O.T. definition of high-grade and low-grade peri-prosthetic joint infection. J Clin Med. 2019;8(5):650.
10. Kunutsor SK, Whitehouse MR, Blom AW, et al. Systematic review of risk prediction scores for surgical site infection or periprosthetic joint infection following joint arthroplasty. Epidemiol Infect. 2017;145:1738–49.
11. Dale H, Fenstad AM, Hallan G, et al. Increasing risk of prosthetic joint infection after total hip arthroplasty. Acta Orthop. 2012;83:449–58.
12. Bozic KJ, Lau E, Kurtz S, et al. Patient-related risk factorsfor periprosthetic joint infection and postoperative mortalityfollowing total hip arthroplasty in medicare patients. J Bone Joint Surg Am. 2012;94:794–800.
13. Namba RS, Inacio MCS, Paxton EW. Risk factors associated with surgical site infection in 30491 primary total hip replacements. J Bone Joint Surg Br. 2012;94B:1330–8.
14. Maoz G, Phillips M, Bosco J, et al. The Otto Aufranc award: modifiable versus nonmodifiable risk factors for infection after hip arthroplasty. Clin Orthop Relat Res. 2015;473:453–9.
15. Zhu Y, Zhang F, Chen W, et al. Risk factors for periprosthetic joint infection after total joint arthroplasty: a systematic reviewand meta-analysis. J Hosp Infect. 2015;89:82–9.
16. Kong L, Cao J, Meng F, et al. Incidence and risk factors for surgical site infection following total knee arthroplasty: a systematic review and meta-analysis. Int J Clin Exp Med. 2016;9:20642–50.
17. Kunutsor SK, Whitehouse MR, Blom AW, INFORM Team, et al. Patient-related risk factors for periprosthetic joint infection after total joint arthroplasty: a systematic review andmeta-analysis. PLoS One. 2016;11:e0150866.
18. George DA, Drago L, Scarponi S, et al. Predicting lower limb periprosthetic joint infections: a review of risk factors and their classification. World J Orthop. 2017;8:400–11.
19. Bozic KJ, Lau E, Kurtz S, et al. Patient-related risk factors for periprosthetic joint infection and postoperative mortality following total hip arthroplasty in medicare patients. J Bone Joint Surg Am. 2012;94:794–800.
20. Zhu Y, Zhang F, Chen W, et al. Risk factors for periprosthetic joint infection after total joint arthroplasty: a systematic review and meta-analysis. J Hosp Infect. 2015;89:82–9.
21. Kunutsor SK, Whitehouse MR, Blom AW, INFORM Team, et al. Patient-related risk factors for periprosthetic joint infection after total joint arthroplasty: a systematic review and meta-analysis. PLoS One. 2016;11:e0150866.
22. Hansen AD, Osmon DR, Nelson CL. Prevention of deep peroprosthetic joint infection. Instr Course Lect. 1997;46:555–67.
23. Peersman G, Laskin R, Davis J, Peterson M. Infection in total knee replacement: a retrospective review of 6489 total knee replacements. Clin Orthop Relat Res. 2001;392:15–23.
24. Del Savio GC, Zelicof SB, Wexler LM, et al. Preoperative nutritional status and outcome of elective total hip replacement. Clin Orthop Relat Res. 1996;(326):153–61.
25. Lavernia CJ, Sierra RJ, Baerga L. Nutritional parameters and short term outcome in arthroplasty. J Am Coll Nutr. 1999;18(3):274–8.
26. Kerkhoffs GM, Servien E, Dunn W, et al. The influence of obesity on the complication rate and outcome of total kneearthroplasty. A meta-analysis and systematic literature review. J Bone Joint Surg Am. 2012;94:1839–44.
27. Pour AE, Matar WY, Jafari SM, Purtill JJ, Austin MS, Parvizi J. Total Joint arthroplasty in patient with hepatitis C. J Bone Joint Surg Am. 2011;93(15):1448–54.
28. Hsieh PH, Chen LH, Lee MS, Chen CH, Yang WE, Shin CH. Hip arthroplasty in patients with cirrhosis of the liver. J Bone Joint Surg Br. 2003;85(6):818–21.
29. Sunday JM, Guille JT, Torg JS. Vomplications of joint arthroplasty in patients with end-stage renal disease on hemodialysis. Clin Orthop Relat Res. 2002;397:350–5.
30. Lieberman JR, Fuchs MD, Haas SB, et al. Hip arthroplasty in patients with chronic renal failure. J Arthroplast. 1955;10(2):191–5.
31. Singh JA, Houston TK, Ponce BA, et al. Smoking as a risk factor for short-term outcomes following primary total hip and total knee replacement in veterans. Arthritis Care Res (Hoboken). 2011;63(10):1365–74.
32. Mills E, Eyawo O, Lockhart I, Kelly S, Wu P, Ebbert JO. Smoking cessation reduces postoperative complications: a systematic review and meta-analysis. Am J Med. 2011;124(2):144–154.e8.
33. Harris AH, Reeder R, Ellerbe L, Bradley KA, Rubinsky AD, Giori NJ. Preoperative alcohol screening scores: associayion with complications in men undergoing total joint arthroplasty. J Bone Joint Surg Am. 2011;93(à4):321–7.
34. Lehman CR, Ries MD, Paiement GD, Davidson AB. Infection after total joint arthroplasty in patient with human immunodeficiency vers or intravenous drug use. J Arthroplast. 2001;16(3):330–5.
35. Nie F, Li W. Impact of prior intra-articular injections on the risk of prosthetic joint infection following total joint arthroplasty: a systematic review and meta-analysis. Front Surg. 2021;8:737529. https://

doi.org/10.3389/fsurg.2021.737529. eCollection 2021
36. Avila A, Acuña AJ, Do MT, Samuel LT, Kamath AF. Intra-articular injection receipt within 3 months prior to primary total knee arthroplasty is associated with increased periprosthetic joint infection risk. Knee Surg Sports Traumatol Arthrosc. 2022;30(12):4088–97. https://doi.org/10.1007/s00167-022-06942-3. Epub 2022 Mar 24
37. Lai Q, Cai K, Lin T, Zhou C, Chen Z, Zhang Q. Prior intra-articular corticosteroid injection within 3 months may increase the risk of deep infection in subsequent joint arthroplasty: a meta-analysis. Clin Orthop Relat Res. 2022;480(5):971–9. https://doi.org/10.1097/CORR.0000000000002055. Epub 2021 Dec 17
38. Yang X, Li L, Ren X, Nie L. Do preoperative intra-articular injections of corticosteroids or hyaluronic acid increase the risk of infection after total knee arthroplasty? A meta-analysis. Bone Joint Res. 2022;11(3):171–9. https://doi.org/10.1302/2046-3758.113.BJR-2021-0350.R1.
39. Parvizi J, Koo K-H. Should a urinary tract infection be treated before a total joint arthroplasty? Hip Pelvis. 2019;31(1):1–3.
40. Nicolle LE, Bradley S, Colgan R, Rice JC, Schaeffer A, Hooton TM. Infectious Diseases Society of America guidelines for the diagnosis and treatment of asymptomatic bacteriuria in adults. Clin Infect Dis. 2005;40:643–54.
41. Wilson MG, Kelley K, Thornhill TS. Infection as a complication of total knee-replacement arthroplasty. Risk factors and treatment in sixty-seven cases. J Bone Joint Surg Am. 1990;72:878–83.
42. George MD, Baker FJ. Perioperative management of immunosuppression in patients with rheumatoid arthritis. Curr Opin Rheumatol. 2019;31(3):300–6.
43. Goodman SM, Springer B, Guyatt G, Abdel MP, Dasa V, George M, Gewurz-Singer O, Giles JT, Johnson B, Lee S, Mandl LA, Mont MA, Sculco P, Sporer S, Stryker L, Turgunbaev M, Brause B, Chen AF, Gililland J, Goodman M, Hurley-Rosenblatt A, Kirou K, Losina E, MacKenzie R, Michaud K, Mikuls T, Russell L, Sah A, Miller AS, Singh JA, Yates A. 2017 American College of Rheumatology/American Association of Hip and Knee Surgeons guideline for the perioperative management of antirheumatic medication in patients with rheumatic diseases undergoing elective total hip or total knee arthroplasty. Arthritis Rheumatol. 2017;69(8):1538–51.
44. Bode LG, Kluytmans JA, Wertheim HF, et al. Preventing surgical-site infections in nasal carriers of Staphylococcus aureus. N Engl J Med. 2010;362:9–17.
45. Lepelletier D, Lucet JC. Controlling meticillin-susceptible Staphylococcus aureus: not simply meticillin-resistant S. aureus revisited. J Hosp Infect. 2013;84:13–21.
46. Levy PY, Ollivier LM, Drancourt M, et al. Relation between nasal carriage of Staphylococcus aureus and surgical site infection in orthopedic surgery: the role of nasal contamination. A vancosystematic literature review and meta-analysis. Orthop Traumatol Surg Res. 2013;99:645–51.
47. Sporer SM, Rogers T, Abella L. Methicillin-resistant and methicillin-sensitive Staphylococcus aureus screening and decolonization to reduce surgical site infection in elective total joint arthroplasty. J Arthroplast. 2016;31(Suppl 9):144–7.
48. Garibaldi R. Prevention of intraoperative wound contamination with chlorhexidine shower and scrub. J Hosp Infect. 1988;11(Suppl B):5–9.
49. Swenson BR, Hedrick TL, Metzger R, et al. Effects of preoperative skin preparation on postoperative wound infection rates: a prospective study of 3 skin preparation protocols. Infect Control Hosp Epidemiol. 2009;30:964–71.
50. Webster J, Osborne S. Preoperative bathing or showering with skin antiseptics to prevent surgical site infection. Cochrane Database Syst Rev. 2007;2007(2):CD004985.
51. Tanner J, Norrie P, Melen K. Preoperative hair removal to reduce surgical site infection. Cochrane Database Syst Rev. 2011;2011(11):CD004122.
52. Shi D, Yai Y, Yu W. Comparison on preoperative hair removal methods for the reduction of surgical site infection: a meta-analysis. J Clin Nurs. 2017;26(19–20):2907–14.
53. Kowalski TJ, Kothari SN, Mathiason MA, et al. Impact of hair removal on surgical site infection rates: a prospective randomized noninferiority trial. J Am Coll Surg. 2016;223:704–11.
54. LG GLOBE/SIOT. Profilassi antibiotica perioperatoria nella chirurgia protesica dell'anca e del ginocchio. GIOT; 2011. p. 4–17.
55. Glenny AM, Song F. Antimicrobial prophylaxis in total hip replacement: a systematic review. Health Technol Assess. 1999;3:21.
56. Al Buhairan B, Hind D, Hutchinson A. Antibiotic prophylaxis for wound infections in total joint arthroplasty: a systematic review. J Bone Joint Surg Br. 2008;90:915–9.
57. Bull AN, Worth LJ, Richards MJ. Impact of vancomycin surgical antibiotic prophylaxis on the development of methicillin-sensitive Staphylococcus aureus surgical site infections. Report from Australian surveillance data (VICNISS). Ann Surg. 2012;256:1089–92.
58. Courtney PM, Melnic CM, Zimmer Z, et al. Addition of vancomycin to cefazolin prophylaxis is associated with acute kidney injury after primary joint arthroplasty. Clin Orthop Relat Res. 2015;473:2197–203.
59. Branch-Elliman W, Ripollone JE, O'Brien WJ, et al. Risk of surgical site infection, acute kidney injury, and clostridium difficile infection following antibiotic prophylaxis with vancomycin plus a beta-lactam versus either drug alone: a national propensity-score-adjusted retrospective cohort study. PLoS Med. 2017;14:e1002340.

60. Osmon DR, Berbari EF, Berendt AR, et al. Diagnosis and management of prosthetic joint infection: clinical practice guidelines by the Infectious Diseases Society of America. Clin Infect Dis. 2013;56:e1–25.
61. Jaffer AK, Barsoum WK, Krebs V, Hurbanek JG, Morra N, Brotman DJ. Duration of anesthesia and venous thromboembolism after hip and knee arthroplasty. Mayo Clin Proc. 2005;80(6):732–8.
62. Britannica. Ignaz Semmelweis | Biography & Facts. In Encyclopedia Britannica. https://www.britannica.com/EBchecked/topic/534198/Ignaz-Philipp-Semmelweis.
63. Parienti JJ, et al. Handrubbing with an aqueous alcoholic solution vs. traditional surgical hand. scrubbing and 30. day surgical site infection rates. JAMA. 2002;288:722–7.
64. George J, Klika AK, Higuera CA. Use of chlorexidine preparations in total joint arthroplasty. J Bone Joint Infect. 2017;2:15–22.
65. Mackenzie I. Preoperative skin preparation and surgical outcome. J Hosp Infect. 1988;11(Suppl B):27–32.
66. Jeng DK, Severin JE. Povidone iodine gel alcohol: a 30-second, one time application preoperative skin preparation. Am J Infect Control. 1998;26:488–94.
67. Hooper GJ, Rothwell AG, Frampton C, Wyatt MC. Does the use of laminar flow and space suits reduce early deep infection after total hip and kneereplacement? The ten–year results of the New Zealand Joint Registry. J Bone Joint Surg Br. 2011;93:85–90. https://doi.org/10.1302/0301-620X.93B1.24862.
68. Young SW, Chisholm C, Zhu M. Intraoperative contamination and space suits: a potential mechanism. Eur J Orthop Surg Traumatol. 2014;24:409–13. https://doi.org/10.1007/s00590-013-1178-1.
69. Webster J, Alghamdi AA. Use of plastic adhesive drapes during surgery for preventing surgical site infection. Cochrane Database Syst Rev. 2007;4:CD006353.
70. Webster J, Alghamdi A. Use of plastic adhesive drapes during surgery for preventing surgical site infection. Cochrane Database Syst Rev. 2013;1:CD006353.
71. Webster J, Alghamdi A. Use of plastic adhesive drapes during surgery for preventing surgical site infection. Cochrane Database Syst Rev. 2015;4:CD006353.
72. Charnley J. Postoperative infection after total hip replacement with special reference to air contamination in the operating room. Clin Orthop Relat Res. 1972;87:167–87.
73. Lidwell OM, Lowbury EJ, Whyte W, et al. Effect of ultraclean air in operating rooms on deep sepsis in the joint after total hip or knee replacement: a randomised study. Br Med J (Clin Res Ed). 1982;285:10–4.
74. Taylor GJ, Bannister GC, Leeming JP. Wound disinfection with ultraviolet radiation. J Hosp Infect. 1995;30(2):85–93.
75. Berg M, Bergman BR, Hoborn J. Ultraviolet radiation compared to an ultra-clean air enclosure. Comparison of air bacteria counts in operating rooms. J Bone Joint Surg Br. 1991;73(5):811–5.
76. Sehulster L, Chinn RY, CDC, HICPAC. Guidelines for environmental infection control in healthcare facilities. Recommendations of CDC and the Healthcare Infection Control Practices Advisory Committee (HICPAC). MMWR Recomm Rep. 2003;52(RR-10):1–42.
77. Panahi P, Stroh M, Casper DS, et al. Operating room traffic is a major concern during total joint arthroplasty. Clin Orthop Relat Res. 2012;470:2690–4.
78. Ritter MA, Eitzen H, French ML, et al. The operating room environment as affected by people and the surgical face mask. Clin Orthop Relat Res. 1975;111:147–50.
79. Bahli ZM. Does evidence based medicine support the eff ectiveness of surgical facemasks in preventing postoperative wound infections in elective surgery? J Ayub Med Coll Abbottabad. 2009;21:166–70.
80. Beldame J, Lagrave B, Lievain L, Lefebvre B, Frebourg N, Dujardin F. Surgical glove bacterial contamination and perforation during total hip arthroplasty implantation: when gloves should be changed. Orthop Traumatol Surg Res. 2012;98:432–40. https://doi.org/10.1016/j.otsr.2011.10.015.
81. Altemeier WA, Culbertson WR, Hummel RP. Surgical considerations of endogenous infections—sources, types, and methods of control. Surg Clin N Am. 1968;48(1):227–40. https://doi.org/10.1016/S0039-6109(16)38448-1.
82. Block SS. Definition of terms. Disinfection, sterilization, and preservation. Philadelphia: Lippincott Williams & Wilkins; 2001. p. 19–28.
83. Parvizi J, Gehrke T, Chen AF. Proceedings of the international consensus on periprosthetic joint infections. Bone Joint J. 2013;95B:1450–2.
84. Anderson DJ, Podgorny K, Berrıos-Torres SI, et al. Strategies to prevent surgical site infections in acute care hospitals: 2014 update. Infect Control Hosp Epidemiol. 2014;35:S66–88.
85. Mont MA, Johnson AJ, Issa K, Pivec R, Blasser KE, McQueen D, et al. Single–use instrumentation, cutt ing blocks, and trials decrease contamination during total knee arthroplasty: a prospective comparison of navigated and nonnavigated cases. J Knee Surg. 2013;26:285–90.
86. Barrack RL, Ruh EL, William BM, Ford AD, Foreman K, Nunley RM. Patient specific cutting blocks are currently of no proven value. J Bone Joint Surg Br. 2012;94(11Suppl A):95–9.
87. Meagher AP, Hugh TB, Li B, Montano SR. Physics and function of operating room suction. Aust N Z J Surg. 1991;61(9):687–91. https://doi.org/10.1111/j.1445-2197.1991.tb00321.x.
88. De Jonge SW, Boldingh QJJ, Solomkin JS, et al. Systematic review and meta-analysis of random-

ized controlled trials evaluating prophylactic intraoperative wound irrigation for the prevention of surgical site infections. Surg Infect. 2017;18:508–19. Epub 2017
89. van Meurs SJ, Gawlitta D, Heemstra KA, et al. Selection of an optimal antiseptic solution for intraoperative irrigation: an in vitro study. J Bone Joint Surg Am. 2014;96:285–91.
90. Insull PJ, Hudson J. Suction tip: a potential source of infection in clean orthopaedic procedures. ANZ J Surg. 2012;82(3):185–6.
91. Meals RA, Knoke L. The surgical suction top a contaminated instrument. J Bone Joint Surg Am. 1978;3:409–10.
92. Chhabra A, Singh A, Kuka PS, Kaur H, Kuka AS, Chahal H. Role of perioperative surgical safety checklist in reducing morbidity and mortality among patients: an observational study. Niger J Surg. 2019;25(2):192–7. https://doi.org/10.4103/njs.NJS_45_18.
93. Bratzler DW, Hunt DR. The surgical infection prevention and surgical care improvement projects: national initiatives to improve outcomes for patients having surgery. Clin Infect Dis. 2006;43:322–30.
94. Scigliano NM, Carender CN, Glass NA, Deberg J, Bedard NA. Operative time and risk of surgical site infection and periprosthetic joint infection: a systematic review and meta-analysis. Iowa Orthop J. 2022;42(1):155–61.
95. Anis HK, Sodhi N, Klika AK, Mont MA, Barsoum WK, Higuera CA, et al. Is operative time a predictor for post-operative infection in primary total knee arthroplasty? J Arthroplast. 2019;34(7s):S331–s6. https://doi.org/10.1016/j.arth.2018.11.022. Epub 2018/12/14. PubMed PMID: 30545655
96. Molloy DO, Archbold HA, Ogonda L, McConway J, Wilson RK, Beverland DE. Caomparison of topical fibrin spray and tranexamic acid on blood loss after total knee replacement: a prospective, ramdomised controlled trial. J Bone Joint Surg Br. 2007;89(3):306–9.
97. Dunn CJ, Goa KL. Tranexamic acid: a review of its use in surgery and other indications. Drugs. 1999;57(6):1005–32.
98. Davidson DJ, Spratt D, Liddle AD. Implant materials and prosthetic joint infection: the battle with the biofilm. EFORT Open Rev. 2019;4(11):633–9. https://doi.org/10.1302/2058-5241.4.180095. eCollection 2019 Nov.
99. Grosso MJ, Berg A, LaRussa S, Murtaugh T, Trofa DP, Geller JA. Silver-impregnated occlusive dressing reduces rates of acute periprosthetic joint infection after total joint arthroplasty. J Arthroplast. 2017;32(3):929–32. https://doi.org/10.1016/j.arth.2016.08.039. Epub 2016 Sep 28
100. Beele H, Van Overschelde P, Olivecrona C, Smet S. A prospective randomized controlled clinical investigation comparing two post-operative wound dressings used after elective hip and knee replacement; Mepilex® Border Post-Op versus Aquacel® surgical. Int J Orthop Trauma Nurs. 2020;38:100772. https://doi.org/10.1016/j.ijotn.2020.100772.
101. Parvizi J, et al. Deep venous thrombosis prophylaxis for total joint arthroplasty: American Academy of Orthopaedic Surgeons guidelines. J Arthroplast. 2008;23(7 Suppl):2–5.
102. Pierce TP, Cherian JJ, Jauregui J, Elmallah RK, Lieberman J, Mont MA. A current review of mechanical compression and its role in venous thromboembolic prophylaxis in total knee and total hip arthroplasty. J Arthroplast. 2015;30(12):2279–84.
103. Innerhofer P, Klinger A, Klimmer C, Fries D, Nussbaumer W. Risk for postoperative infection after transfusion of white blood cell-filtered allogenic or autologous blood components in orthopedic undergoing primary arthroplasty. Transfusion. 2005;45(1):103–10.
104. Herbert PC, Wells G, Blajchmann MA, et al. A multicenter, randomized, controlled clinical trial of transfusion requirements in critical care. Transfusion Requirements in Critical Care Investigators, Canadian Critical Care Trials Group. N Engl J Med. 1999;340(6):409–17.
105. Parker MJ, Livingstone V, Clifton R, McKee A. Closed suction surgical wound drainage after orthopaedic surgery. Cochrane Database Syst Rev. 2007;2007(3):CD001825.
106. Parker MJ, Roberts CP, Hay D. Closed suction drainage for hip and knee arthroplasty. A meta-analysis. J Bone Joint Surg Am. 2004;86-A(6):1146–52.
107. Cerulli G, Tranquilli Leali P, Moriconi F, Paoletti GC. Advancements in the cement technique of THR. In: International Orthop. Meeting, Ed. Aulo Gaggi, Bologna. 1982.
108. Parvizi J, Saleh KJ, Ragland PS, et al. Efficacy of antibiotic-impregnated cement in total hip replacement. Acta Orthop. 2008;79:335–41.
109. Wang J, Zhu C, Cheng T, et al. A systematic review and meta-analysis of antibiotic-impregnated bone cement use in primary total hip or knee arthroplasty. PLoS One. 2013;8:e82745.
110. Buchholz HW, Engelbrecht H. Depot effects of various antibiotics mixed with Palacos resins. Chirurg. 1970;41:511–5.
111. Pellegrini A, Suardi V. Antibiotics and cement: what I need to know? Hip Int. 2020;30(1_suppl):48–53. https://doi.org/10.1177/1120700020915463. Epub 2020 Apr 14
112. Engesaeter LB, Lie SA, Espehaug B, et al. Antibiotic prophylaxis in total hip arthroplasty: effects of antibiotic prophylaxis systemically and in bone cement on the revision rate of 22,170 primary hip replacements followed 0–14 years in the Norwegian Arthroplasty Register. Acta Orthop Scand. 2003;74(6):644–51.
113. Parvizi J, Saleh KJ, Ragland PS, Pour AE, Mont MA. Efficacy of antibiotic-impreg-

nated cement in total hip replacement. Acta Orthop. 2008b;79:335–41. https://doi.org/10.1080/17453670710015229.
114. Ghisellini F, Ceffa R. Trattamento delle infezioni di protesi articolari. Mediprint s.r.l. Corso Trieste 61 Roma, Italy. 1997. ISBN 2021070172822.
115. Registro Scandinavo, Registro Australiano, Registro dati regione Emilia Romagna. Scandinavian Register, Australian Register, Emilia Romagna Region Data Register.
116. Charnley L. Anchorage of the femoral head prostheses to the shaft of the femur. J Bone Joint Surg. 1960;42-B:28–30.
117. Stefánsdóttir A. The infected knee arthroplasty. Doctoral thesis, Department of Orthopaedics, Clinical Sciences, Lund University, Lund, Sweden. 2010.
118. Winkler H, Haiden P. Allograft bone as antibiotic carrier. J Bone Joint Infect. 2017;2:52–62.
119. Franceschini M, Sandiford NM, Cerbone V, Cappelli Toledo de Araujo L, Kendoff D. Defensive antibacterial coating in revision total hip arthroplasty: new concept and early experience. Hip Int. 2020;30(1S):7–11.
120. Romanò CL, Malizos K, Capuano N, et al. Does an anti-biotic-loaded hydrogel coating reduce early post-surgical infection after joint arthroplasty? J Bone Jt Infect. 2016;1:34–41.
121. Romanò CL, De Vecchi E, Bortolin M, et al. Hyaluronicacid and its composites as a local antimicrobial/antiadhesive barrier. J Bone Jt Infect. 2017;2:63–72.
122. Romanò CL, Malizos K, Capuano N, et al. Does an antibiotic-loaded hydrogel coating reduce early post-surgical infection after joint arthroplasty? J Bone Jt Infect. 2016;1:34–41.
123. Giavaresi G, Meani E, Sartori M, et al. Efficacy of antibac-terial-loaded coating in an in vivo model of acutely highly contaminated implant. Int Orthop. 2014;38:1505–12.
124. Racano A, Pazionis T, Farrokhyar F, Deheshi B, Ghert M. High infections rate outcomes in long-bone tumor surgery with endoprosthetic reconstruction in adults. Clin Orthop Relat Res. 2013;471(6):2017–27. https://doi.org/10.1007/s11999-013-2842-9. Epub 2013 Feb 12
125. Edwards D. Timeline history of colloidal silver. HistoWiki, February 16, 2023.
126. Simpson WJ, Hewlett RT. Experiments on the germicidal action of colloidal silver. Lancet. 1914;184:1359. https://doi.org/10.1016/S0140-6736(00)96700-X.
127. Fiore M, Sambri A, Zucchini R, Giannini C, Donati DM, De Paolis M. Silver-coated megaprosthesis in prevention and treatment of peri-prosthetic infections: a systematic review and meta-analysis about efficacy and toxicity in primary and revision surgery. Eur J Orthop Surg Traumatol. 2021;31(2):201–20. https://doi.org/10.1007/s00590-020-02779-z. Epub 2020 Sep 5. PMID: 32889672
128. Sambri A, Zucchini R, Giannini C, Zamparini E, Viale P, Donati DM, De Paolis M. Silver-coated (PorAg®) endoprosthesis can be protective against reinfection in the treatment of tumor prostheses infection. Eur J Orthop Surg Traumatol Orthop Traumatol. 2020;30(8):1345–53.
129. Hua L, Daofeng W, Wupeng Z, Gaoxiang X, Cheng X, Wanheng L, Jiantao L. Potential side effects of antibacterial coatings in orthopaedic implants: a systematic review of clinical studies. Front Bioeng Biotechnol. 2023;11:1111386.
130. Croes M, Bakhshandeh S, van Hengel IAJ, Lietaert K, van Kessel KPM, Pouran B, van der Wal BCH, Vogely HC, Van Hecke W, Fluit AC, Boel CHE, Alblas J, Zadpoor AA, Weinans H, Amin YS. Antibacterial and immunogenic behavior of silver coatings on additively manufactured porous titanium. Acta Biomater. 2018;81:315–27. https://doi.org/10.1016/j.actbio.2018.09.051. Epub 2018 Sep 28. PMID: 30268917
131. Diez-Escudero A, Hailer NP. The role of silver coating for arthroplasty components. Bone Joint J. 2021;103-B(3):423–9. https://doi.org/10.1302/0301-620X.103B3.BJJ-2020-1370.R1. PMID: 33641432
132. Hardes J, Henrichs MP, Hauschild G, et al. Silver-coated megaprosthesis of the proximal tibia in patients with sarcoma. J Arthroplast. 2017;32:2208–13.
133. Becker RO. Effects of electrically generated silver ions on human cells and wound healing. Electro-Magnetobiol. 2000;19:1–19.
134. Hardes J, Hardes J, von Eiff C, Streitbuerger A, Balke M, Budny T, Henrichs MP, Hauschild G, Ahrens H. Reduction of periprosthetic infection with silver-coated megaprostheses in patients with bone sarcoma. J Surg Oncol. 2010;101(5):389–95. https://doi.org/10.1002/jso.21498.
135. Shirai T, Tsuchiya H, Terauchi R, et al. The outcomes of reconstruction using frozen autograft combined with iodine-coated implants for malignant bone tumors: compared with non-coated implants. Jpn J Clin Oncol. 2016;46:735–40.
136. Tsuchiya H, Shirai T, Nishida H, et al. Innovative antimicrobial coating of titanium implants with iodine. J Orthop Sci. 2012;17:595–604.
137. Shirai T, Tsuchiya H, Terauchi R, Tsuchida S, Mizoshiri N, Mori Y, Takeuchi A, Hayashi K, Yamamoto N, Ikoma K, Kubo T. A retrospective study of antibacterial iodine-coated implants for postoperative infection. Medicine. 2019;98(45):e17932.
138. Ma PX, Zhang R. Synthetic nano-scale fibrous extracellular matrix J Biomed Mater Res.

1999;46(1):60–72. https://doi.org/10.1002/(sici)1097-4636(199907)46:160::aid-jbm73.0.co;2-h.
139. Pan C, Zhou Z, Yu X. Coatings as the useful drug delivery system for the prevention of implant-related infections. J Orthop Surg Res. 2018;13:220.
140. McLaren J, White L, Cox H, et al. A biodegradable antibiotic-impregnated scaffold to prevent osteomyelitis in a contaminated in vivo bone defect model. Eur Cell Mater. 2014;27:332–49.
141. Shahid A, Aslam B, Khurshid M. The prospects of antimicrobial coated medical implants. J Appl Biomater Funct Mater. 2021;19:22808000211040304.
142. Gallo J, Holinka M, Moucha CS. Antibacterial surface treatment for orthopaedic implants. Int J Mol Sci. 2014;15:13849–80.
143. Antibiotic resistance www.epicentro.iss.it.
144. Mazza-Stalder J, Nicod L, Janssens J-P. Extrapulmonary tuberculosis. Rev Mal Respir. 2012;29(4):566–78. https://doi.org/10.1016/j.rmr.2011.05.021. Epub 2012 Mar 29.
145. Golden MP, Vikram HR. Extrapulmonary tuberculosis: an overview. Am Fam Physician. 2005;72(9):1761–8.

# 20 Low-Grade Periprosthetic Infections

Tomas Zamora, Ianiv Klaber, and Eduardo Botello

Periprosthetic joint infection (PJI) is a complex pathology with variable clinical presentation. Acute, chronic, and/or severe clinical manifestations of infection can be present in up to 1–4% of primary joint replacements, and it's one of the leading causes of overall revision [1, 2]. However, growing awareness has gained the possibility of a "low grade" PJI. Such infections can be challenging to diagnose as their symptoms are not severe, and laboratory results may not be completely abnormal [3, 4]. Low-grade infections can still lead to procedure failure despite an otherwise successful initial clinical, radiographic outcome.

Beswick et al. conducted a systematic review of prospective studies involving patients who had undergone total hip or knee replacement for osteoarthritis. The review found that a significant proportion of people experienced long-term pain of unknown origin after the surgery, ranging from about 7%–23% after total hip joint replacement and from 10% to 34% after knee replacement [5]. Other studies have shown that between 4% and 13% of patients with a preoperative diagnosis of aseptic loosening and chronic pain were infected when the retrieved implants were analyzed using genomic identification methods [6]. All of this has raised suspicion and awareness of low-grade subclinical infections as a cause of early or late failure after joint replacement surgery.

Over the past 15 years, several definitions of periprosthetic joint infection have been suggested by different organizations or consensus groups, each with variations in their criteria. Examples of these are the Musculoskeletal Infection Society criteria (MSIS) [7], the International Consensus Meeting (ICM—2013 and 2018 criteria) [8, 9], the World Association against Infection in Orthopedics and Trauma (WAIOT) [10], and European Bone and Joints Infection Society (EBJIS) [11]. However, despite these criteria and abundant literature on the topic, there is no clear and widely accepted definition of low versus high-grade infections.

Some authors use the term "low-grade infection" to refer to an infection caused by low-virulence microorganisms, such as Methicillin-sensitive *Staphylococci epidermidis*, streptococci, anaerobic cocci, and *Cutibacterium acnes*. On the contrary, bacteria that are intrinsically resistant to antimicrobial agents and antibiotics, such as methicillin-resistant staphylococci, enterococci, and gram-negative organisms, are considered to be of high virulence [12]. These low-grade infections may present a challenge as classical serum markers of infection may not be reliable in this setting [13, 14]. For example, Choe et al. found that almost 20% of their patients with Periprosthetic Joint Infection (PJI), diagnosed using the 2018 ICM criteria, had a level of

T. Zamora · I. Klaber · E. Botello (✉)
Orthopaedic Surgery Department, Pontificia Universidad Católica de Chile, Santiago, Chile
e-mail: tezamora@uc.cl; ebotello@med.puc.cl



P. Ruggieri et al. (eds.), *Bone and Joint Infections*, https://doi.org/10.1007/978-3-031-96383-4_20

C-reactive protein (CRP) less than 10 mg/L [15]. This cutoff level is commonly used for infection screening in most institutions. Similarly, Akgun et al. [14] reported that low-virulence organisms were found in 86% of PJIs with normal CRP levels, reinforcing that typical parameters for infection screening may not always be reliable in this setting.

Other authors classify infections based on their severity and duration of symptoms. Those that do not produce systemic illness are then referred to as low-grade infections [16]. These are characterized by subclinical and slow-evolving symptoms. Typically, a low-grade infection is only observed as a painful prosthetic joint with little to no alteration in inflammatory parameters. There is no draining sinus, fever, or other systemic manifestations. Occasionally, mildly elevated inflammatory parameters may be present in an otherwise healthy, asymptomatic patient, but most commonly, only a painful joint or loosening is observed.

Factors such as medical conditions, medications, and treatments can weaken the immune system and alter the course of an infection. Examples include autoimmune diseases, chemotherapy, and radiation therapy. Awareness of these factors and their potential impact on the immune system is essential. Several authors, including McPherson and Wimmer, have suggested a staging system for PJIs based on the host's quality. McPherson et al. found a correlation between declining host grade, limb score, and poorer outcomes in total hip and knee arthroplasties [17, 18]. Immunosuppression is a clear risk factor for overall infection. Still, it is crucial in this setting since it has the highest correlation with fungal infections and other microorganisms because of its close association with the innate immune response and can manifest as low-grade indolent infections [19, 20].

The WAIOT Study Group on Bone and Joint Infections recently proposed a new definition for PJI. The definition is based on available tests to confirm or exclude this condition. The new definition includes the possibility of different clinical presentations. Patients with "otherwise unexplained pain, swelling, and/or reduced range of motion or functional impairment" and "lack of acute local inflammatory signs and in the absence of an alternative explanation" are considered at risk of having a low-grade infection. This is confirmed with a defined balance (more or equal to zero) of specific tests, which allows for post-analysis confirmation [10].

## 20.1 Diagnosis

Low-grade infections can be challenging to diagnose in an otherwise healthy patient who experiences chronic symptoms but not acute signs of infection. Sometimes, these infections are only detected during preoperative work-up for joint revision or after a theoretically "aseptic" revision with positive cultures (known as type 1 infection as classified by Tsukayama et al. [21]). In the same way, there may be conflicting laboratory results, with false-negative and low values of serum biomarkers often present, highlighting the need for an organized and systematic diagnostic process.

Standard radiographs should always be obtained as part of the work-up of a symptomatic joint replacement. However, they may not be instrumental in the diagnosis of a low-grade infection, especially in the acute setting, as they may usually appear normal. In the chronic setting, scattered foci of osteolysis, periosteal reaction, or bone resorption may be present and can mimic a conventional aseptic loosening (Fig. 20.1).

Serologic biomarkers, including erythrocyte sedimentation rate (ESR) and C-reactive protein (CRP), remain helpful for laboratory investigations. However, their sensitivity may be significantly reduced in this context [16, 22]. For example, Pérez-Prieto et al. [22] showed that in almost one-third of culture-positive PJIs, most with low-grade bacteria, CRP levels could be normal and be missed in the initial diagnosis. Similar findings have been observed with the isolated use of ESR [23]. On the other hand, serum interleukin-6 (IL-6) [24] and D-dimer [25] could represent more reliable markers of periprosthetic low-grade infection. Both tests have shown

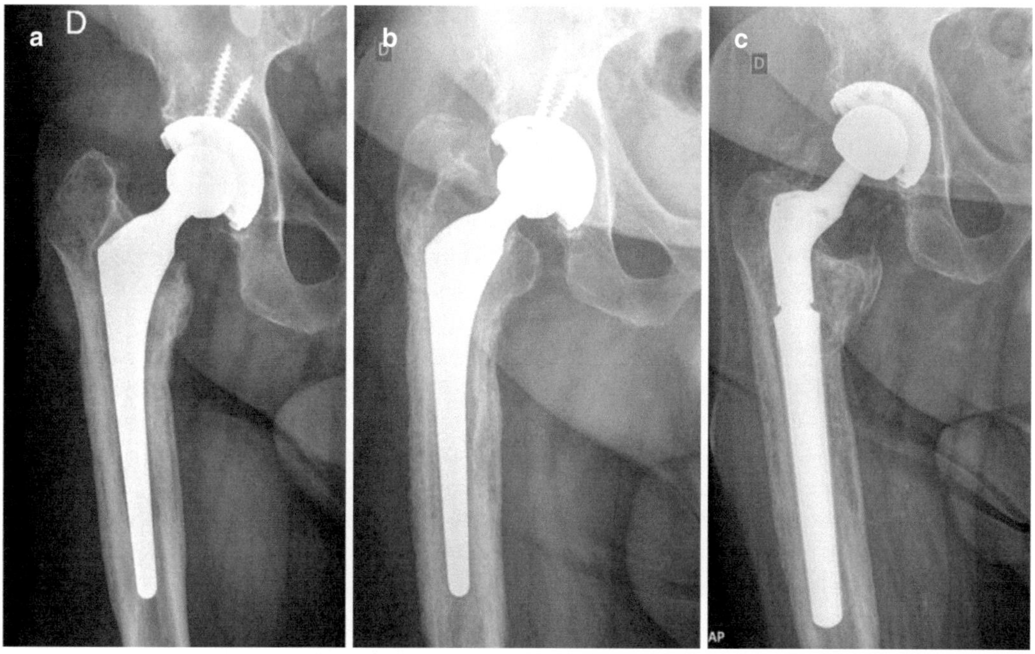


**Fig. 20.1** A 65-year-old man with a right total hip arthroplasty. The initial procedure was performed without any complications. Three years post-surgery, there was evidence of periosteal reaction and cortical thickening, with only mild pain during weight-bearing (**a**). After a year, femoral loosening and significant femoral subsidence (**b**) were observed. Laboratory results were normal. During femoral revision (**c**), two positive cultures were obtained for Methicillin-sensitive staphylococcus epidermidis, confirming a type I infection, according to Tsukayama. (Source: Based on [10], reproduce under the terms and conditions of the Creative Commons Attribution (CC BY) license (http://creativecommons.org/licenses/by/4.0/))

higher diagnostic properties and are an essential aid in the decision of reimplantation, with a threshold of more than 10 pg/mL for serum IL-6 and > 850 ng/mL for D-Dimer. However, less evidence is available regarding both studies compared to other classic serum biomarkers.

Nuclear medicine studies have been widely used for diagnosing joint infections. Their role has not been clearly established, especially in the acute setting. The conventional Technetium-99 bone scan has been shown to be sensitive but with a low specificity. However, a combination of leukocyte and bone marrow scintigraphy (in the form of Technetium-99 bisphosphonate scan in conjunction with indium-111-labeled leukocyte scan) has been found to have better specificity according to a recent systematic review and meta-analysis [26] and could help in the differentiation of an aseptic loosening and low-grade infection.

Joint aspiration is a crucial diagnostic tool for detecting PJIs before surgery. Synovial markers can be useful in detecting infections. Still, their effectiveness can be compromised in low-grade infections due to low bacterial load and weak inflammatory response, similar to serum markers. In both acute and chronic settings, an increase in synovial white blood cell count (WBC) and the percentage of neutrophils can point toward an underlying infection. In traditional settings, diagnostic cutoffs can vary between 1500 and 4000 cells/μL for WBC and from 65% to 80% for the percentage of neutrophils. The WAIOT and EBJIS [10, 11] definitions of periprosthetic joint infection include a WBC count of over 1500 cells/μL and a neutrophil percentage of over 65% to suspect an infection among their criteria [27]. Therefore, these parameters and cutoff values could be helpful in detecting low-grade infections but with lower specificity than MSIS, ICM

2013, and 2018 cutoffs for chronic infections. In the same way, cutoff values for settings other than the hip and knee are less defined.

Promising results have been shown for Alpha defensin, Leukocyte esterase, and synovial CRP in the context of PJI evaluation and have been added to the previously mentioned PJI diagnostic criteria. Recent research has demonstrated that Alpha defensin and synovial CRP may present >80% discrimination of suspected low-grade infections against aseptic loosening [28].

The identification and detection of the causative microorganisms are crucial for appropriate management. Antibiotics should be suspended for at least 2 weeks before aspiration and culture analysis to avoid false negative results. The aspirate should be sent for aerobic, anaerobic, and fungal cultures. Cultures should be kept for at least 14 days in case of revision surgery or a preoperative joint aspirate for suspected infection, which is especially relevant in low-grade infections, which commonly take longer than 5 days to retrieve; however, antibiotic prophylaxis should not be withheld and should be given prior to surgical incision [29].

When performing revision surgery, it is essential to obtain at least five reliable tissue samples, in addition to synovial fluid, using separate instruments and transfer them immediately to the laboratory. The tissue samples should be anatomically representative, especially those from the bone-implant interface membrane. These cultures should also be processed for at least 14 days to allow retrieving slow-growing microorganisms.

Detection of bacterial genetic material could be helpful in low-grade infections in which bacterial load is low and should be unaffected by antibiotic administration. Multiplex Polymerase chain reaction (PCR) on joint fluid aspirate has shown good diagnostic accuracy for low-grade prosthetic joint infections in small series, even better than classic cultures [27, 28]. Next-generation sequencing (NGS) with microbial DNA amplification may also play a role in this setting. Still, molecular techniques cannot distinguish between live and dead organisms. They may generate false-positive results, are not widely available, and their clinical utility has yet to be proven in extensive comparative studies.

It is important to be cautious when interpreting a single positive culture, whether from preoperative aspiration or tissue culture. An infection is likely present if uncommon contaminants or virulent organisms, such as Staphylococcus aureus or Gram-negative rods, are detected. On the other hand, a single positive culture of a common contaminant or low-grade microorganism, like coagulase-negative staphylococci or *Cutibacterium acnes* (previously referred to as *P. acnes*), should prompt further investigation and a complete analysis of all available tests to confirm or rule out an infection versus contamination [30]. It is advisable to avoid swab cultures as there is a high possibility of skin contamination.

Recently, it has been discovered that *C. acnes* is a hidden cause of pain after shoulder prosthesis and a major cause of shoulder PJI [31, 32]. However, the culture time for *C. acnes* is long, with a mean delay of 6 days to show positivity, reinforcing the need for prolonged cultures [28, 33]. Lutz and his colleagues [34] have proposed a three-grade classification to determine the likelihood of *C. acnes* infection. If a patient shows clinical signs of infection and has more than two positive samples, they are considered to have a certain *C. acnes* PJI. Patients who exhibit clinical signs of infection but have only one positive sample for *C. acnes* are classified as having a probable infection. Patients who do not show any clinical signs of infection and have any number of *C. acnes* cultures will only present the possibility of infection; however, contamination should also be ruled out in such cases.

Fungal PJI is another entity that can manifest as a low-grade indolent infection with nonspecific symptoms such as chronic pain, often without erythema, swelling, or effusion. Fungal organisms usually develop a robust biofilm and avoid the immune response; therefore, systemic symptoms are generally not present [20]. Similarly, laboratory affection is typically mild, adding to their difficult diagnosis. A high level of awareness is essential in patients with negative cultures, multiple revisions for infection, or loosening with no other explanation, especially in the immunocompromised patient. Prolonged fungal cultures in the adequate medium remain the most critical step for fungal PJI diagnosis. Candida species are the predominant pathogen [35]; however, a high risk of concomitant bacterial PJI exists.

Culture of samples obtained by sonication of the removed prosthesis has been shown to be more sensitive than conventional tissue cultures, especially in patients with low-virulence microorganisms or treated with antibiotics before surgery [16]. Sonication dislodges adherent bacteria from prostheses using ultrasound technology and has been long studied as an adjuvant to conventional culture analysis [36, 37]. Similarly, histopathological analysis obtained during surgery via a frozen section of periprosthetic tissue could add to previous diagnostic methods and has been included in all diagnostic definitions. More than five neutrophils per high-power field in at least five fields is considered consistent with infection. However, surgeon and pathologist experience plays a crucial role in histological diagnosis, and threshold values for the presence of neutrophils may have variability.

Nowadays, no single test can accurately diagnose a PJI, even less a low-grade infection, with adequate sensitivity and specificity. The most accurate and comprehensive method for detecting low-grade infections is the combination of a high clinical suspicion with an ordered set of diagnostic investigations with postoperative confirmation. The development of the middle groups "infection likely" in the EBJIS definition and "Low-Grade PJI" in the WAIOT definition (Tables 20.1 and 20.2) is a reflection of this elevated awareness necessity with a more "flexible" approach to detect this pathologies; however, independent and large series validation is still needed for this approach.

**Table 20.1** WAIOT definition tests

| Rule IN tests (each negative scores 0; positive scores +1) | Rule OUT tests (each negative scores −1; positive scores 0) |
|---|---|
| 1. Purulence or draining sinus or exposed joint prosthesis | 1. ESR >30 mm/hr |
| 2. Serum IL-6 > 10 pg/mL | 2. CRP >10 mg/L |
| 3. Serum Procalcitonin >0.5 ng/mL | 3. WBC count >1500/μL |
| 4. Serum D-Dimer >850 ng/mL | 4. Leukocyte esterase strip (++) |
| 5. Synovial WBC >3000/mL | 5. Alpha-defensin immunoassay (>5.2 mg/L) |
| 6. Leukocyte esterase strip (++) | 6. Tc99 bone scan |
| 7. Alpha-defensin immunoassay (>5.2 mg/L) or lateral flow test | |
| 8. Positive cultural examination | |
| 9. Positive histology—Frozen section (5 neutrophils in at least 3 HPFs) | |
| 10. Combined leukocyte and bone marrow scintigraphy | |

*ESR* erythrocyte sedimentation rate, *CRP* C-reactive protein, *IL-6* interleukin-6, *HPFs* high power fields, *WBC* white blood cell count

**Table 20.2** WAIOT definition of periprosthetic joint infection (PJI) and conditions

| Conditions | Score | Confirmation |
|---|---|---|
| No Infection | <0 | Negative culture |
| Contamination | <0 | One positive culture, negative histology |
| Biofilm-related implant malfunction | <0 | Positive culture and/or histology |
| Low-grade periprosthetic joint infection | 0 or more | Positive culture and/or histology |
| High-grade periprosthetic joint infection | 1 or more | Positive culture and/or histology |

## 20.2 Treatment of Low-grade PJI

The management principles for PJI do not differ significantly between low-grade and other PJIs. Numerous treatment options have been proposed, but the goal remains the same for all: infection eradication and maintenance of a painless and functional joint. The definitive surgical treatment can be performed in either one or two stages, provided the causative agent was identified before the operation.

In cases of low-grade infections, debridement, antibiotics, and implant retention (DAIR) may be suitable for healthy patients affected by acute gram-positive infections, provided they have a stable and well-functioning implant; however, ensuring debridement and prompt antibiotic treatment before biofilm accumulation is crucial for a successful outcome. Another scenario where DAIR (with or without chronic antibiotic suppression) could be appealing is in the elderly, frail, or challenging cases where resection and eventual reconstruction may not be feasible. Since these agents are usually more receptive to antibiotic treatments and less frequently resistant, less invasive alternatives may be considered.

A two-stage exchange is considered the gold standard for PJI in all conditions, with success rates as high as 79–96%, depending on the severity of the infection and host [38–40]. However, if certain conditions are met, such as the identification of a non-resistant pathogen prior to revision, the absence of a sinus tract or significant soft tissue damage, and an adequate host, a one-stage exchange may provide similar infection eradication with the added benefit of better functionality and shorter overall treatment duration [41]. Even more, in cases of a low-grade bacterial infection with low virulence, the single-stage approach of explantation of all components and cement, followed by debridement and implantation of new components with antibiotic cement, has shown good results [42]. This should be followed by systemic antibiotic therapy or antifungals, depending on the isolated microorganism.

## 20.3 Outcomes

The success rate for different treatment modalities for low-grade infections is predominantly based on a global series with mixed etiologies and grades of infection. The debridement, antibiotics, and implant retention (DAIR) approach has shown variable success rates, ranging from 11% to 100% [43]. Still, as previously mentioned, it could be an alternative in the acute setting or in the frail patient where a less morbid approach is warranted. Nevertheless, more data is required to determine which patients would benefit from this approach [44].

Singer et al. [42] reported a 95% success rate in a selected low-grade infection series with a single-stage approach where methicillin-resistant organisms and culture-negative infections were excluded from the analysis. Other studies have shown equivalent outcomes for selected cases with a one-stage exchange.

Two-stage exchange procedures have been found to have high success rates in treating infections, regardless of their cause or when they occur [38–40]. In fact, this approach may be even more effective when utilized for low-grade infections compared to those caused by resistant microorganisms, as reported by several authors [45–47].

According to a systematic review of 30 articles on shoulder PJI, the isolation of *C. acnes* was found to be an independent risk factor for failed treatment. However, the review also found that there was no significant difference in success rates among 1-stage, 2-stage, or resection arthroplasty revision, with each having a success rate of over 90% [48].

## 20.4 Conclusion

Low-grade PJI can be a challenging diagnosis to make. A high suspicion is necessary when a patient has persistent pain in an otherwise healthy arthroplasty. A thorough laboratory workup and synovial fluid analysis are essential, and prolonged cultures and additional techniques such as molecular analysis and signification of the retrieved implants should be considered. In some cases, the diagnosis will only be confirmed retrospectively after an assumed aseptic revision. These cases should be handled with a multidisciplinary approach involving orthopedic surgeons and infectious disease specialists, among other specialists.

## References


1. Delanois RE, Mistry JB, Gwam CU, Mohamed NS, Choksi US, Mont MA. Current epidemiology of revision total knee arthroplasty in the United States. J Arthroplasty. 2017;32(9):2663–8.
2. Bozic KJ, Kurtz SM, Lau E, Ong K, Vail DTP, Berry DJ. The epidemiology of revision total hip arthroplasty in the United States. J Bone Joint Surg. 2009;91(1):128–33.
3. Berbari EF, Marculescu C, Sia I, Lahr BD, Hanssen AD, Steckelberg JM, et al. Culture-negative prosthetic joint infection. Clin Infect Dis. 2007;45(9):1113–9.
4. Parvizi J, Suh DH, Jafari SM, Mullan A, Purtill JJ. Aseptic loosening of total hip arthroplasty: infection always should be ruled out. Clin Orthop Relat Res. 2011;469(5):1401–5. Available from: https://pubmed.ncbi.nlm.nih.gov/21365337/.
5. Beswick AD, Wylde V, Gooberman-Hill R, Blom A, Dieppe P. What proportion of patients report long-term pain after total hip or knee replacement for osteoarthritis? A systematic review of prospective studies in unselected patients. BMJ Open. 2012;2(1). Available from: https://pubmed.ncbi.nlm.nih.gov/22357571/.
6. Moojen DJF, Van Hellemondt G, Vogely HC, Burger BJ, Walenkamp GHIM, Tulp NJA, et al. Incidence of low-grade infection in aseptic loosening of total hip arthroplasty. Acta Orthop. 2010;81(6):667–73. Available from: https://pubmed.ncbi.nlm.nih.gov/20919816/.
7. Parvizi J, Zmistowski B, Berbari EF, Bauer TW, Springer BD, Della Valle CJ, et al. New definition for periprosthetic joint infection: from the Workgroup of the Musculoskeletal Infection Society. Clin Orthop Relat Res. 2011;469(11):2992–4. Available from: https://pubmed.ncbi.nlm.nih.gov/21938532/.
8. Parvizi J, Tan TL, Goswami K, Higuera C, Della Valle C, Chen AF, et al. The 2018 definition of periprosthetic hip and knee infection: an evidence-based and validated criteria. J Arthroplasty. 2018;33(5):1309–1314. e2. Available from: https://pubmed.ncbi.nlm.nih.gov/29551303/.
9. Parvizi J, Gehrke T, Chen AF. Proceedings of the international consensus on periprosthetic joint infection. Bone Joint J. 2013;95-B(11):1450–2. Available from: https://pubmed.ncbi.nlm.nih.gov/24151261/
10. Romanò CL, Al Khawashki H, Benzakour T, Bozhkova S, del Sel H, Hafez M, et al. The W.A.I.O.T. definition of high-grade and low-grade peri-prosthetic joint infection. J Clin Med. 2019;8(5). Available from: https://pubmed.ncbi.nlm.nih.gov/31083439/.
11. McNally M, Sousa R, Wouthuyzen-Bakker M, Chen AF, Soriano A, Vogely HC, et al. The EBJIS definition of periprosthetic joint infection. Bone Joint J. 2021;103-B(1):18–25. Available from: https://pubmed.ncbi.nlm.nih.gov/33380199/
12. Fehring TK, Odum SM, Berend KR, Jiranek WA, Parvizi J, Bozic KJ, et al. Failure of irrigation and débridement for early postoperative periprosthetic infection. Clin Orthop Relat Res. 2013;471(1):250–7. Available from: https://pubmed.ncbi.nlm.nih.gov/22552768/.
13. Kheir MM, Tan TL, Shohat N, Foltz C, Parvizi J. Routine diagnostic tests for periprosthetic joint infection demonstrate a high false-negative rate and are influenced by the infecting organism. J Bone Joint Surg (Am Vol). 2018;100(23):2057–65.
14. Akgün D, Müller M, Perka C, Winkler T. The serum level of C-reactive protein alone cannot be used for the diagnosis of prosthetic joint infections, especially in those caused by organisms of low virulence. Bone Joint J. 2018;100-B(11):1482–6. Available from: https://pubmed.ncbi.nlm.nih.gov/30418061/
15. Choe H, Kobayashi N, Abe K, Hieda Y, Tezuka T, Inaba Y. Evaluation of serum albumin and globulin in combination with C-reactive protein improves serum diagnostic accuracy for low-grade periprosthetic joint infection. J Arthroplasty. 2023;38(3):555–61. Available from: https://pubmed.ncbi.nlm.nih.gov/36115535/.
16. Vasso M, Schiavone Panni A. Low-grade periprosthetic knee infection: diagnosis and management. J Orthop Traumatol. 2015;16(1). Available from: https://pubmed.ncbi.nlm.nih.gov/24821631/.
17. McPherson EJ, Woodson C, Holtom P, Roidis N, Shufelt C, Patzakis M. Periprosthetic total hip infection: outcomes using a staging system. Clin Orthop Relat Res. 2002;(403):8–15.
18. Wimmer MD, Randau TM, Friedrich MJ, Ploeger MM, Schmolder J, Strauss AC, et al. Outcome predictors in prosthetic joint infections – validation of a risk stratification score for prosthetic joint infections in 120 cases. Acta Orthop Belg. 2016;82(1):143–8.
19. Garcia-Vidal C, Viasus D, Carratalà J. Pathogenesis of invasive fungal infections. Curr Opin Infect Dis. 2013;26(3):270–6. Available from: https://pubmed.ncbi.nlm.nih.gov/23449139/.
20. Nace J, Siddiqi A, Talmo CT, Chen AF. Diagnosis and management of fungal periprosthetic joint infections. J Am Acad Orthop Surg. 2019;27(18):e804–18. Available from: https://pubmed.ncbi.nlm.nih.gov/30520804/.
21. Tsukayama DT, Estrada R, Gustilo RB. Infection after total hip arthroplasty. A study of the treatment of one hundred and six infections. J Bone Joint Surg Am.

1996;78(4):512–23. Available from: https://pubmed.ncbi.nlm.nih.gov/8609130/.
22. Pérez-Prieto D, Portillo ME, Puig-Verdié L, Alier A, Martínez S, Sorlí L, et al. C-reactive protein may misdiagnose prosthetic joint infections, particularly chronic and low-grade infections. Int Orthop. 2017;41(7):1315–9. Available from: https://pubmed.ncbi.nlm.nih.gov/28321490/
23. Berbari E, Mabry T, Tsaras G, Spangehl M, Erwin PJ, Murad MH, et al. Inflammatory blood laboratory levels as markers of prosthetic joint infection: a systematic review and meta-analysis. J Bone Joint Surg Am. 2010;92(11):2102–9. Available from: https://pubmed.ncbi.nlm.nih.gov/20810860/
24. Yoon JR, Yang SH, Shin YS. Diagnostic accuracy of interleukin-6 and procalcitonin in patients with periprosthetic joint infection: a systematic review and meta-analysis. Int Orthop. 2018;42(6):1213–26. Available from: https://pubmed.ncbi.nlm.nih.gov/29294147/
25. Shahi A, Kheir MM, Tarabichi M, Hosseinzadeh HRS, Tan TL, Parvizi J. Serum D-Dimer test is promising for the diagnosis of periprosthetic joint infection and timing of reimplantation. J Bone Joint Surg Am. 2017;99(17):1419–27. Available from: https://pubmed.ncbi.nlm.nih.gov/28872523/
26. Verberne SJ, Sonnega RJA, Temmerman OPP, Raijmakers PG. What is the accuracy of nuclear imaging in the assessment of periprosthetic knee infection? A meta-analysis. Clin Orthop Relat Res. 2017;475(5):1395–410. Available from: https://pubmed.ncbi.nlm.nih.gov/28050818/
27. Lee YS, Koo KH, Kim HJ, Tian S, Kim TY, Maltenfort MG, et al. Synovial fluid biomarkers for the diagnosis of periprosthetic joint infection: a systematic review and meta-analysis. J Bone Joint Surg Am. 2017;99(24):2077–84. Available from: https://pubmed.ncbi.nlm.nih.gov/29257013/
28. Ettinger M, Savov P, Calliess T, Windhagen H, Lichtinghagen R, Lukasz A, et al. Improved diagnostic accuracy with the classification tree method for diagnosing low-grade periprosthetic joint infections by quantitative measurement of synovial fluid alpha-defensin and C-reactive protein. Int Orthop. 2020;44(1):31–8. Available from: https://pubmed.ncbi.nlm.nih.gov/31127365/.
29. Wouthuyzen-Bakker M, Benito N, Soriano A. The effect of preoperative antimicrobial prophylaxis on intraoperative culture results in patients with a suspected or confirmed prosthetic joint infection: a systematic review. J Clin Microbiol. 2017;55(9):2765–74. Available from: https://pubmed.ncbi.nlm.nih.gov/28659322/.
30. Schwarze J, Moellenbeck B, Gosheger G, Puetzler J, Deventer N, Kalisch T, et al. The role of single positive cultures in presumed aseptic total hip and knee revision surgery-a systematic review of the literature. Diagnostics (Basel). 2023;13(9). Available from: https://pubmed.ncbi.nlm.nih.gov/37175046/.
31. Millett PJ, Yen YM, Price CS, Horan MP, Van Der Meijden OA, Elser F. Propionibacterium acnes infection as an occult cause of postoperative shoulder pain: a case series. Clin Orthop Relat Res. 2011;469(10):2824–30. Available from: https://pubmed.ncbi.nlm.nih.gov/21240577/.
32. Hsu JE, Bumgarner RE, Matsen FA. Propionibacterium in shoulder arthroplasty: what we think we know today. J Bone Joint Surg Am. 2016;98(7):597–606. Available from: https://pubmed.ncbi.nlm.nih.gov/27053589/.
33. Boisrenoult P. Cutibacterium acnes prosthetic joint infection: diagnosis and treatment. Orthop Traumatol Surg Res. 2018;104(1):S19–24.
34. Lutz MF, Berthelot P, Fresard A, Cazorla C, Carricajo A, Vautrin AC, et al. Arthroplastic and osteosynthetic infections due to Propionibacterium acnes: a retrospective study of 52 cases, 1995-2002. Eur J Clin Microbiol Infect Dis. 2005;24(11):739–44.
35. Schoof B, Jakobs O, Schmidl S, Klatte TO, Frommelt L, Gehrke T, et al. Fungal periprosthetic joint infection of the hip: a systematic review. Orthop Rev (Pavia). 2015;7(1):18–22. Available from: https://pubmed.ncbi.nlm.nih.gov/25874063/.
36. Trampuz A, Piper KE, Jacobson MJ, Hanssen AD, Unni KK, Osmon DR, et al. Sonication of removed hip and knee prostheses for diagnosis of infection. N Engl J Med. 2007;357(7):654–63. Available from: https://pubmed.ncbi.nlm.nih.gov/17699815/.
37. Li C, Renz N, Thies CO, Trampuz A. Meta-analysis of sonicate fluid in blood culture bottles for diagnosing periprosthetic joint infection. J Bone Jt Infect. 2018;3(5):273. Available from: /pmc/articles/PMC6328302/
38. Biring GS, Kostamo T, Garbuz DS, Masri BA, Duncan CP. Two-stage revision arthroplasty of the hip for infection using an interim articulated Prostalac hip spacer: a 10- to 15-year follow-up study. J Bone Joint Surg Series B. 2009;91(11):1431–7.
39. Leung F, Richards CJ, Garbuz DS, Masri BA, Duncan CP. Two-stage total hip arthroplasty: how often does it control methicillin-resistant infection? Clin Orthop Relat Res. 2011;469(4):1009. Available from: /pmc/articles/PMC3048283/.
40. Zamora T, Garbuz DS, Greidanus NV, Masri BA. An articulated spacer made of new primary implants in two-stage exchange for infected total knee arthroplasty may provide durable results. Bone Joint J. 2020;102-B(7):852–60. Available from: https://pubmed.ncbi.nlm.nih.gov/32600135/.
41. Zahar A, Klaber I, Gerken AM, Gehrke T, Gebauer M, Lausmann C, et al. Ten-year results following one-stage septic hip exchange in the management of periprosthetic joint infection. J Arthroplasty. 2019;34(6):1221–6. Available from: https://pubmed.ncbi.nlm.nih.gov/30857953/
42. Singer J, Merz A, Frommelt L, Fink B. High rate of infection control with one-stage revision of septic knee prostheses excluding MRSA and MRSE. Clin

Orthop Relat Res. 2012;470(5):1461–71. Available from: https://pubmed.ncbi.nlm.nih.gov/22081299/.
43. Kunutsor SK, Beswick AD, Whitehouse MR, Wylde V, Blom AW. Debridement, antibiotics and implant retention for periprosthetic joint infections: a systematic review and meta-analysis of treatment outcomes. J Infect. 2018;77(6):479–88. Available from: https://pubmed.ncbi.nlm.nih.gov/30205122/.
44. Malahias MA, Gu A, Harris EC, Adriani M, Miller AO, Westrich GH, et al. The role of long-term antibiotic suppression in the management of peri-prosthetic joint infections treated with debridement, antibiotics, and implant retention: a systematic review. J Arthroplasty. 2020;35(4):1154–60. Available from: https://pubmed.ncbi.nlm.nih.gov/31955984/.
45. Kurd MF, Ghanem E, Steinbrecher J, Parvizi J. Two-stage exchange knee arthroplasty: does resistance of the infecting organism influence the outcome? Clin Orthop Relat Res. 2010;468(8):2060–6. Available from: https://pubmed.ncbi.nlm.nih.gov/20300903/.
46. Darwich A, Dally FJ, Olba KA, Mohs E, Gravius S, Hetjens S, et al. Superinfection with difficult-to-treat pathogens significantly reduces the outcome of periprosthetic joint infections. Antibiotics (Basel). 2021;10(10). Available from: https://pubmed.ncbi.nlm.nih.gov/34680726/
47. Cordero-Ampuero J, Esteban J, García-Rey E. Results after late polymicrobial, gram-negative, and methicillin-resistant infections in knee arthroplasty. Clin Orthop Relat Res. 2010;468(5):1229–36. Available from: https://pubmed.ncbi.nlm.nih.gov/20087702/.
48. Nelson GN, Davis DE, Namdari S. Outcomes in the treatment of periprosthetic joint infection after shoulder arthroplasty: a systematic review. J Shoulder Elbow Surg. 2016;25(8):1337–45. Available from: https://pubmed.ncbi.nlm.nih.gov/27012542/.

# What Is New in Periprosthetic Joint Infection After Hip and Knee Arthroplasty

21

Shayan Hosseinzadeh, Jesus Villa, and Carlos Higuera

## 21.1 Introduction

Periprosthetic joint infection (PJI) is a devastating complication following hip and knee arthroplasty, causing significant morbidity and mortality. Despite advances, PJI remains a challenging problem in orthopedics mainly due to the lack of understanding of physiopathology [1]. This chapter discusses recent developments in PJI's understanding and management.

PJI's clinical significance stems from increasing joint replacements, an aging population, and related comorbidities like obesity and diabetes. It poses serious health and economic challenges, with projected annual hospital costs of $1.85 billion by 2030 in the USA. Urgent preventive strategies are needed to address this issue and combat antibiotic-resistant pathogens [2, 3].

To address healthcare-associated infections, research has explored antiseptics, antimicrobial sutures, and extended oral antibiotic prophylaxis [4, 5]. Intraosseous regional administration of antibiotics has also shown potential for enhancing prevention, and treatment outcomes [6].

Advances in PJI diagnosis involve next-generation sequencing, metagenomic sequencing, and various biomarkers like leucocyte esterase, calprotectin, serum D-dimer, and immune checkpoint molecules, leading to faster and more accurate identification of pathogens [7–16].

Treatment approaches include debridement and antibiotics with implant retention (DAIR), two-stage, one-stage, and one-and-a-half-stage revision arthroplasty, with each having benefits and considerations [17, 18].

In summary, recent developments emphasize a comprehensive approach to PJI, focusing on prevention, improved diagnostics, and customized treatments to enhance patient outcomes [19].

S. Hosseinzadeh · J. Villa · C. Higuera (✉)
Levitetz Department of Orthopaedic Surgery, Cleveland Clinic Florida. 2950 Cleveland Clinic Blvd, Weston, FL, USA
e-mail: higuerc@ccf.org

## 21.2 Etiology and Risk Factors

### 21.2.1 Novel Insights into PJI Microbiology

Recent research has expanded our understanding of PJI, traditionally linked to bacterial pathogens like *Staph aureus* and coagulase-negative staphylococci. New evidence suggests the involvement of previously overlooked microorganisms, including fungi and mycobacteria, broadening the understanding of PJI's etiology. Polymicrobial infections and anaerobic bacteria are sometimes associated with atypical presentations and diagnostic challenges. A study comparing PJI organisms in different nations revealed variations in the type of microorganisms and increased overall



P. Ruggieri et al. (eds.), *Bone and Joint Infections*, https://doi.org/10.1007/978-3-031-96383-4_21

incidence of resistant bacteria. Next-generation sequencing techniques have significantly enhanced the detection of bacterial lineages within clinical specimens, particularly in the context of polymicrobial infections, where *E. coli*, *C. acnes*, *S. epidermidis*, and *S. aureus* are commonly identified as the predominant organisms. However, the sensitivity of next-generation sequencing for bacterial detection may lead to the identification of contaminants, necessitating careful interpretation of the results. Investigating the baseline microbial signal enhances clinical translation and understanding of PJI's microbial changes during joint infections or prosthesis failure [20–22].

### 21.2.2 Advancements in Identifying Host Risk Factors

Recent studies have shed light on host risk factors associated with PJI, providing a deeper understanding of the risks faced by joint arthroplasty patients. Obesity has been identified as an independent risk factor due to its impact on inflammatory responses and increased adipose tissue, with patients having a BMI greater than 40 facing a three-fold higher risk of PJI compared to those with lower BMI values. Various techniques have been developed to assess local adiposity in the knee joint, including the ratio of the prepatellar thickness (PPT) to the thickness of the patella, the measurement of both PPT and pretubercular thickness, and the determination of the soft tissue-to-bone ratio in lateral knee radiographs. These specific assessments of local knee adiposity have demonstrated associations with the risk of PJI following TKA. Nevertheless, the collective evidence indicates that BMI serves as a superior predictor of PJI occurrence after TKA when compared to localized measurements of knee adipose tissue [23].

Additionally, systemic conditions, such as diabetes mellitus, rheumatoid arthritis, and chronic kidney disease, have shown an elevated likelihood of PJI following joint arthroplasty, with patients with diabetes carrying a 1.7-fold greater risk. Elevated HbA1c levels have demonstrated a clear association with an increased risk of PJI. Notably, a threshold of 7.7% appears to provide a more accurate indicator of infection risk compared to the commonly utilized 7%. Therefore, it may be prudent to set 7.7% as the target HbA1c level during preoperative patient optimization [24]. In addition to HbA1c, fructosamine emerges as another valuable predictor of complications following TKA. Fructosamine offers several advantages, including a more precise reflection of glycemic control, enhanced predictive capacity for adverse events, and quicker responsiveness to treatment when compared to HbA1c. Recent research findings strongly endorse the inclusion of fructosamine screening for all patients undergoing TKA. For individuals with fructosamine levels exceeding 293 μmol/l, it is imperative to conduct a comprehensive risk-benefit analysis prior to considering surgery. Optimizing glycemic control becomes paramount as a prerequisite for proceeding with the surgical intervention [25].

Immunocompromised individuals receiving long-term corticosteroid therapy, immunotherapy, or chemotherapy face heightened risks due to compromised immune defenses, highlighting the need for vigilant monitoring and additional optimization in these cases. Both the American College of Rheumatology and the American Association of Hip and Knee Surgeons guidelines provide recommendations for managing these patients [26].

Furthermore, smoking and malnutrition are increasingly recognized as modifiable risk factors, with smoking contributing to a 3.5-fold higher risk of PJI in patients with obesity. It has also been shown that individuals who currently smoke face a markedly heightened risk of requiring reoperation for infection within 90 days following a surgical procedure when compared to their non-smoking counterparts. Additionally, it has been proven that the cumulative lifetime consumption of cigarettes, irrespective of one's present smoking status, substantially contributes to an elevated risk of nonoperative readmission [27]. As a result, it is advisable for patients to try to cease smoking at least 2–3 weeks before the scheduled procedure.

## 21.3 Prevention of PJI: Recent Advancements and Novel Strategies

Healthcare-associated infections, particularly surgical site infections (SSIs), continue to pose significant challenges despite efforts to combat antibiotic-resistant pathogens and enforce guidelines. In response to this concern, studies have investigated innovative approaches to preventing SSI without solely relying on antibiotics. Its discussions have centered around the use of antiseptics and antimicrobial sutures in surgical practice. A broader implementation of antiseptics has also been proposed to reduce the reliance on antibiotics for infection prevention, encompassing preoperative measures such as showering, hand hygiene, and skin preparation, along with postoperative wound management. Additionally, there is growing support for the use of antimicrobial sutures in high-risk procedures and cases where SSI could be life-threatening despite low occurrence rates [4].

The introduction of chlorhexidine-impregnated wipes or soap in the presurgical environment has had mixed results in the reduction of SSI incidence [28, 29], however, in our practice, we have noted an effect on SSI reduction, and for that reason, we continue its use. We usually prescribe a chlorhexidine solution to be used at least the day before and the day of the procedure, mainly in the surgical area. It has also been demonstrated that both single and 24-h antibiotic dosages are equally effective in preventing PJI in TJA. Therefore, the use of a single antibiotic dose can be safely considered for patients undergoing routine primary TJA [30]. Furthermore, studies indicate that administering additional antibiotics after skin closure may not be necessary for primary TJA, irrespective of the patient's preoperative risk of PJI [31].

Recent research studies have investigated the effects of extended oral antibiotic prophylaxis (EOA) on infection-related outcomes following primary and revision surgeries for TKA and THA. The findings of these investigations suggest that employing EOA prophylaxis can effectively reduce the incidence of PJI among high-risk primary and revision THA and TKA patients [32–34].

Meanwhile, the use of intraosseous regional administration (IORA) of antibiotics has emerged as a novel technique for delivering antibiotics directly to the surgical site in patients undergoing TKA and THA. This approach involves administering antibiotics into the bone leading to higher local tissue concentrations of antibiotics [6, 35].

A comprehensive analysis was undertaken to evaluate the efficacy of IORA, focusing on studies reporting on perioperative prophylaxis during TKA. The analysis included eight studies, with four of them being randomized controlled trials comparing local tissue antibiotic concentrations between patients receiving IORA and those receiving intravenous (IV) antibiotics. Additionally, six studies assessed the rate of PJI among patients receiving IORA versus IV antibiotics [6]. The combined findings from these studies consistently indicated a significant increase in antibiotic concentration in femoral bone and fat samples among patients treated with IORA. Notably, the tissue concentrations achieved with IORA were, on average, 10 times higher than those achieved with IV administration alone. For example, after the administration of 500 mg of intraosseous vancomycin, the antibiotic concentrations in fat and bone samples were 44.04 μg/g and 49.3 μg/g, respectively, compared to 3.5 μg/g (fat) and 5.2 μg/g (bone) following 1 g IV of vancomycin [6].

Moreover, the results of two adequately powered studies demonstrated a statistically significant decrease in the rate of PJI among patients receiving IORA compared to those receiving IV antibiotics. The overall incidence of PJI in patients treated with IORA was only 0.3%, while it was 1.1% in patients receiving IV antibiotics across all studies [6].

The use of topical vancomycin powder (VP) in joint replacement surgeries has become popular due to positive outcomes in spinal surgery [36] and open fracture treatment [37]. However, it can contribute to antibiotic resistance. Understanding VP's behavior in synovial fluid is limited [38], particularly its potential to create wear between joint components. Yet, VP does not seem to affect wear between ultra-high-molecular-weight polyethylene (UHMWP) and cobalt-chrome alloy (CoCr) [39]. Reviews on VP in hip and knee arthroplasty yield conflicting results, mostly based on lower-level evidence with confounding factors. Currently, there's insufficient data to recommend routine VP use in these surgeries [40]. A well-powered randomized trial is needed to clarify its role. VP seems safe in terms of systemic side effects, and if its efficacy can be established, it could offer cost-effective benefits [40].

Povidone-iodine (PI) effectively eliminates methicillin-resistant Staphylococcus aureus (MRSA) within 30 s [41]. In primary TKA and THA, a diluted 0.35% PI lavage before wound closure reduced postoperative prosthetic infections from 0.97% to 0.15% [42]. However, not all studies support PI's use [43, 44]. While efficacy reports vary, it's a cost-effective, low-risk option. Several organizations, including the 2017 International Consensus Meeting Clinical Practice Guidelines, endorse PI lavage before closure to prevent infection [45–47].

In a recently updated randomized clinical trial involving patients who underwent knee or hip arthroplasty, researchers found that aspirin prophylaxis demonstrated comparable efficacy and safety outcomes when compared to other anticoagulants. Furthermore, when compared to a placebo, aspirin prophylaxis showed a significant reduction in venous thromboembolism (VTE) risk while maintaining a similar safety outcome [48]. There is newer evidence that the use of aspirin instead of other anticoagulants to prevent VTE is correlated with a lower incidence of SSI [49].

In a comprehensive meta-analysis, the Grading of Recommendations, Assessment, Development, and Evaluations (GRADE) revealed high-certainty evidence supporting the prophylactic application of negative pressure wound therapy on primary closed incisional wounds for the prevention of surgical site infections. Furthermore, this analysis suggested reduced uncertainty compared to earlier meta-analyses. Additionally, the trial sequential analysis performed suggested that additional trials are unlikely to alter the estimated effect of incisional negative pressure wound therapy on the prevention of surgical site infections [50]. A multicenter randomized study showed that the risk of reoperations is also lower when this technology is used in high-risk patients [51].

Anti-glucosaminidase (GMD) immunization: A recent study indicated higher levels of endogenous anti-Gmd antibodies in patients' sera correlate with better infection control rates and lower adverse outcomes in *S. aureus* bone infections. This suggests the potential benefit of exploring GMD immunization as a strategy for improving treatment outcomes in osteomyelitis [52]. It is a probability that in the future we may have vaccines available to prevent PJI.

In a recent cohort study involving 9427 cases of late prosthetic joint infections, no compelling evidence was discovered to establish a temporal link between invasive dental procedures and PJIs. Consequently, these findings challenged the prevailing recommendations advocating for antibiotic prophylaxis administration to patients with prosthetic joints before undergoing invasive dental procedures. This challenge stemmed from cost concerns, the potential for adverse drug reactions, and the associated risk of inducing antibiotic resistance, all of which are linked to antibiotic prophylaxis [53].

In a comparable scenario, research has also indicated that administering antibiotic prophylaxis does not reduce the risk of PJI in individuals who have undergone TJA when they undergo colonoscopy. When adjusting for established risk factors, it was observed that TJA recipients undergoing colonoscopy, both with and without antibiotic prophylaxis, exhibited similar PJI risks in comparison to a control group that did not undergo colonoscopy. However, it is important to note that individuals with a history of alcohol abuse, diabetes, or rheumatoid arthritis experienced a greater risk of PJI when undergoing colonoscopy after TJA compared to those who did not have colonoscopies. Therefore, the findings suggest that for most TJA patients undergoing colonoscopy, the use of antibiotics may not be necessary, except for those individuals with these high-risk factors [54].

## 21.4 Diagnosis of PJI: Recent Advances and Approaches

The diagnosis of PJI relies on a combination of clinical criteria and diagnostic markers. Elevated serum C-reactive protein (CRP), D-dimer, and erythrocyte sedimentation rate (ESR), along with various synovial fluid parameters, are commonly investigated. Intraoperative findings, such as frozen section analysis, the presence of purulence, and pathogen isolation by culture, also play a crucial role in confirming the diagnosis.

To establish infection status, a scoring system is employed based on the diagnostic markers. An elevated serum CRP (>1 mg/dL), D-dimer (>860 ng/mL), and ESR (>30 mm/h) receive assigned points of 2, 2, and 1, respectively. Similarly, elevated synovial fluid white blood cell count (>3000 cells/μL), alpha-defensin (signal-to-cutoff ratio > 1), leukocyte esterase (++), polymorphonuclear percentage (>80%), and synovial CRP (>6.9 mg/L) are assigned points of 3, 3, 3, 2, and 1, respectively. A total aggregate score of 6 or higher indicates a PJI diagnosis, while scores between 2 and 5 necessitate consideration of intraoperative findings for confirmation or refutation. Intraoperative findings such as positive histology, presence of purulence, and single positive culture are assigned points of 3, 3, and 2, respectively. When combined with the preoperative score, a total score of 6 or higher confirms infection, a score between 4 and 5 remains inconclusive, and a score of 3 or less rules out infection. This updated evidence-based approach for diagnosing hip and knee PJI demonstrates higher sensitivity (97.7%) compared to the older MSIS (79.3%) and International Consensus Meeting definitions (86.9%), while maintaining a similar specificity of 99.5%. These refined diagnostic criteria enable more accurate identification of PJI, facilitating timely and targeted treatment interventions [7].

The reported incidence of culture-negative PJI in the hip or knee varies between 7% and 42%, yielding an overall estimated incidence rate of 11% utilizing a random-effects model [55]. Recent findings indicate that the semiautomated periprosthetic tissue culture method using blood culture bottles exhibits greater sensitivity and comparable specificity when compared to agar and thioglycolate broth cultures, while also delivering faster results [56].

The leucocyte esterase (LE) strip test has gained recognition as a valuable biomarker for PJI diagnosis. This test detects the presence of leukocyte esterase, an enzyme released by white blood cells, in synovial fluid. It offers convenience, speed, and immediate results, making it a promising option in the diagnostic workup for PJI. However, the LE strip test has limitations, such as imprecision and susceptibility to interference mainly on bloody aspirations. To address these limitations, new technologies, including machine reading, quantitative detection, and artificial intelligence, are being applied to enhance the accuracy of the LE strips test. These advancements aim to improve its precision and minimize potential sources of interference, ultimately improving its diagnostic accuracy [10]. Alpha-defensin is another promising synovial biomarker with encouraging results. Its utilization as a diagnostic marker alongside synovial white cell count, culture bacteriology, and other biomarkers is particularly valuable, especially in complex PJI diagnostic scenarios [11]. Another biomarker that has shown promise in PJI diagnosis is calprotectin. The calprotectin point-of-care (POC) test has demonstrated excellent diagnostic characteristics, including high sensitivity and specificity, particularly in patients undergoing revision TKA. The calprotectin POC test can effectively serve as a rule-out test, helping to exclude PJI when the results are negative. With its rapid and reliable results, the calprotectin POC test contributes to more efficient management of patients where PJI is suspected [12].

Furthermore, recent research has evaluated immune checkpoint molecules as potential predictors of PJI. Periprosthetic joint infections induce an immunosuppressive cytokine profile through an unknown mechanism. Immune checkpoints, like programmed cell death 1 (PD-1) and its ligand (PD-L1), initiate innate immunosuppressive pathways essential for self-tolerance. Several malignancies and chronic infections co-opt these pathways to derive a survival advantage.

In a study evaluating PD-1/PD-L1 expression in periprosthetic tissue from patients undergoing revision hip or knee arthroplasty for PJI versus aseptic failure, PD-1/PD-L1 expression was analyzed using immunohistochemistry. The results of this study supported immune checkpoint upregulation as a mechanism of PJI-induced local immune dysfunction. Further studies are needed to confirm PD-L1 as a risk factor for reinfection in larger cohorts [13, 14].

In parallel, the effectiveness of the D-Dimer as a new diagnostic tool for PJI has been explored through two distinct studies, each offering unique insights into its diagnostic performance. These studies, conducted by Pannu et al. [15] and Tarabichi et al. [16], contribute to the ongoing discussions surrounding the utility of D-Dimer in distinguishing between septic and aseptic revisions in patients undergoing revision total hip and knee arthroplasty.

In the retrospective review undertaken by Pannu et al., the researchers analyzed a cohort of 143 patients who had undergone revision total hip and knee arthroplasties with preoperative D-Dimer orders. The central focus was on differentiating cases with low-virulence (LV) and high-virulence (HV) organisms. The results revealed that despite its potential sensitivity in detecting PJI cases with LV organisms—cases that are often difficult to diagnose using conventional methods—the overall accuracy of D-Dimer was disappointingly low, at around 57%. This suggests that while D-Dimer might excel in identifying certain specific cases of PJI, its general diagnostic performance in distinguishing septic from aseptic revisions fell short of expectations. Nonetheless, the study highlights the potential of D-Dimer as a viable option for cases that tend to be overlooked by traditional diagnostic techniques [15].

On the other hand, the prospective study led by Tarabichi et al. involved a larger sample size of 502 patients who were undergoing revision hip or knee arthroplasty. Their findings painted a more optimistic picture of D-Dimer's diagnostic capabilities. In this study, D-Dimer's diagnostic utility for PJI was compared to other commonly used biomarkers, such as serum CRP and ESR. The results suggested that plasma D-Dimer demonstrated diagnostic performance on par with these established biomarkers. This points to the potential of D-Dimer to serve as a valuable adjunct in the screening process for patients undergoing revision total joint arthroplasty. By demonstrating comparable diagnostic efficacy to established markers, D-Dimer's inclusion in the diagnostic toolkit could potentially enhance the accuracy of identifying PJI cases [16].

Next-generation sequencing (NGS) is a powerful molecular technique that has emerged as a valuable tool in the diagnosis of PJI. It involves the parallel sequencing of DNA fragments in a sample, allowing for the identification of various microorganisms. Recent advancements in NGS have made it more routine and cost-effective especially in cases where the cultures have been negative [8]. Metagenomic next-generation sequencing (mNGS) is a specific application of NGS that has revolutionized the field of infectious disease diagnostics. It detects the entire DNA or RNA sequence in a sample, enabling the identification of pathogens, including bacteria, viruses, fungi, and parasites, within 24–48 h. This is significantly faster compared to traditional bacterial culture methods, which can take several days to identify bacteria in synovial fluid. mNGS is particularly valuable in cases where there is a strong suspicion of PJI but conventional diagnostic tests, such as cultures, yield negative results [9].

New evidence on MRI sequences such as MAVRIC has demonstrated that magnetic resonance imaging using MAVRIC is a highly specific diagnostic tool for detecting PJI with a minimal false-positive rate. This suggests that when healthcare providers encounter an MRI result that unexpectedly indicates infection, it warrants a formal assessment for the presence of infection. In cases where diagnostic results are inconclusive, MRI may serve as a valuable tool to support the diagnosis and potentially the treatment of PJI, although it may not definitively rule it out [57].

Lastly, combining labeled-leucocyte imaging (e.g., leucocytes labeled with indium-111) with bone marrow imaging utilizing technetium-99 m-labeled sulfur colloid proves to be more accurate in detecting infections associated with prosthetic joints than technetium-99 imaging alone, a combination of bone and gallium-67 imaging, or labeled-leucocyte and bone imaging. When compared directly, this combination stands as the preferred choice for an imaging scan when infection assessment is necessary [58].

## 21.5 Treatment of PJI: Recent Advances and Strategies

### 21.5.1 Multidisciplinary Approach

The management of PJI requires a multidisciplinary approach involving orthopedic surgeons, infectious disease specialists, microbiologists, and other healthcare professionals. Collaboration between these experts is crucial to developing an individualized treatment plan tailored to the patient's specific circumstances [19, 59].

### 21.5.2 Surgical Strategies

Recent advancements have focused on refining surgical strategies to improve outcomes in PJI treatment.

#### 21.5.2.1 Debridement and Antibiotics and Implant Retention (DAIR)

DAIR is an effective treatment for acute postoperative or hematogenous PJI in an appropriately selected patient with well-fixed implants. Over the last two decades, significant progress has been made in this field. While definitively determining which of these improvements has been the most efficacious remains a challenge, one of the most notable advancements has been the recognition of the critical importance of meticulous and aggressive debridement techniques. Furthermore, there has been a growing adoption of antimicrobial irrigation, which may also contribute to reducing infection risk, though the available evidence is somewhat mixed [60].

Another substantial innovation has been the introduction of intraosseous vancomycin [61]. This method has proven to be both safe and effective in providing antibiotic prophylaxis while minimizing the systemic side effects associated with vancomycin. Emerging evidence has demonstrated safety along with enhanced outcomes when contrasted with earlier studies utilizing conventional DAIR methods without intraosseous antibiotic delivery, although further data is still needed for confirmation [62].

Additionally, a more recent technique known as "Double DAIR" has emerged, offering improved solutions to address the limitations of a single-stage DAIR procedure. Initial results from "Double DAIR" procedures have shown promising success in managing infections [63].

#### 21.5.2.2 Two-Stage Revision Arthroplasty

Two-stage exchange arthroplasty is the preferred treatment for chronic PJI in the United States. It involves two surgeries with a time interval between them. In the first stage, the prosthesis is removed, the area is thoroughly cleaned and treated with antibiotics, and an antibiotic-eluting cement spacer is inserted to maintain joint space and motion. Articulating spacers generally offer better outcomes, while static spacers are preferred for certain conditions like ligamentous instability, widespread bone loss, or significant soft tissue defects. Cultures and preoperative work-ups are crucial, and prophylactic antibiotics are given before incision. The duration of antibiotic therapy for patients with PJI is primarily based on expert recommendations rather than evidence. Patients usually receive long courses of antibiotic therapy, which can take up to 6 months for staph infections [17]. Several studies suggest that shorter courses may be adequate for most cases of PJI and that they may be associated with shorter hospital stays, fewer side effects, and the establishment of microbiologic resistance. However, recent prospective randomized noninferiority research compared a 6-week course of antibiotic treatment to a 12-week course and found that antibiotic therapy for 6 weeks resulted in a larger percentage of patients with poor outcomes [64]. There's also debate about the need for a 2-week antibiotic-free period before reimplantation [17].

Confirming infection control before reimplantation is vital, but the available criteria have limitations. The decision for reimplantation is complex and may involve various tests, including cultures. Unfortunately, there is no definitive marker that establishes absolute infection control [65]. It is also worth mentioning that plasma D-dimer levels paradoxically increase prior to reimplantation, while other inflammatory markers such as ESR and CRP decrease, which emphasizes the importance of exercising caution when incorporating D-dimer into clinical decision-making by surgeons [66]. Moreover, there is a lack of consensus regarding the necessity of aspiration prior to reimplantation, with conflicting data on this matter.

After confirming infection control, the second stage involves removing the cement spacer and reimplanting the new prosthesis. Two-stage revision is suitable for patients with more challenging infections and bone deficiencies. It has drawbacks like increased cost and higher morbidity. In some cases, patients may choose to retain the spacer instead of proceeding with the second stage, which has shown acceptable results in selected cases [17].

#### 21.5.2.3 One-Stage Revision Arthroplasty

One-stage revision arthroplasty is an alternative to two-stage revision for PJI. While two-stage revision is standard, it has a 26% mortality rate at 5 years [67]. In contrast, one-stage revision offers comparable reinfection rates and better functional outcomes.

Strict selection criteria include moderate bone loss, no immunocompromising conditions, healthy soft tissues, known organisms with antibiotic sensitivities, and favorable immune status. Notably, while 6.7% of two-stage patients experienced reinfection 3 years postoperatively in a study by Haddal et al., not a single one-stage patient experienced recurrent infection [68]. One-stage revision showed high success rates for both hip and knee revisions [17].

Choosing the right procedure at presentation is crucial, as the success of repeated revisions decreases over time [68]. One-stage revision should be considered for PJI patients meeting such strict criteria.

#### 21.5.2.4 One-and-a-Half Stage Revision Arthroplasty

The 1.5-stage revision TKA is a promising alternative that involves the use of a prosthetic articulating spacer, preserving knee function, and potentially delaying the need for a second surgery indefinitely. This technique has shown an 85% infection-free survival rate after nearly 3 years [69]. The procedure involves the resection of infected TKA components, thorough debridement, and implantation of revision components in a single surgery.

Key surgical considerations include meticulous debridement with a focus on preserving collateral ligaments, assessing techniques for restoring the joint line, and ensuring precise placement of the femoral component. It is crucial to properly evaluate bone loss, use augmentations when necessary, and be meticulous during the cementing process, and avoid common pitfalls such as rushing component removal [70].

Overall, the 1.5-stage revision TKA is a viable option for treating chronic PJI in TKA, offering advantages such as reduced costs and improved patient outcomes. Further studies are needed to determine its broader applicability and indications, but it has been successful in providing excellent knee function and avoiding the urgency of planning for the next revision surgery. If ever needed in the future, this procedure can be scheduled more electively, providing patients with greater flexibility and peace of mind [71–74].

### 21.5.3 Other Therapeutic Strategies

In one study, researchers explored whether a 3-month course of oral antibiotics could reduce the risk of infection-related failure following a two-stage joint replacement procedure. Results showed that patients treated with oral antibiotics experienced a significantly lower failure rate due to infection compared to those without antibiotics (5% vs. 19%). However, some patients encountered adverse reactions to antibiotics, and issues related to adherence were observed. Further follow-up is necessary to confirm the long-term efficacy and safety of this approach [5].

Recent research demonstrated that PlySs2, a bacteriophage-derived lysin, is more effective than vancomycin in reducing *S. aureus* biofilm and colony-forming units on orthopedic implants. When combined with vancomycin, PlySs2 significantly reduces the bacterial load on implant surfaces and in periprosthetic tissue. This highlights the potential of lysins to enhance the treatment of prosthetic joint infections caused by *S. aureus* biofilms [75, 76].

Other recent studies emphasize the potential of phage therapy as a promising approach to treating prosthetic joint infections. Phages have the ability to degrade biofilms and target bacterial cells, working synergistically with antibiotics. They can be personalized to target specific bacterial strains. However, more research is needed to optimize delivery methods and understand phage-host interactions to ensure successful translation into clinical practice [77–79].

WLBU2, an engineered peptide, demonstrates effectiveness in removing *S. aureus* biofilms on surgical implants. It effectively treats biofilms formed by various clinical strains and leads to culture-negative implants. WLBU2 shows rapid elimination of implants in vitro and has sufficient efficacy in vivo with minimal systemic toxicity [80, 81].

TRL1068, a fully human antibody, also shows potential for disrupting biofilms formed by gram-positive and gram-negative bacteria. It targets a conserved epitope on DNABII proteins, which are crucial for biofilm formation. The absence of similar counterparts in human proteins enhances their therapeutic potential [82–86].

## References

1. Mian HM, Lyons JG, Perrin J, Froehle AW, Krishnamurthy AB. A review of current practices in periprosthetic joint infection debridement and revision arthroplasty. Arthroplasty. 2022 Sep 1;4(1):31.
2. Premkumar A, Kolin DA, Farley KX, Wilson JM, McLawhorn AS, Cross MB, Sculco PK. Projected economic burden of Periprosthetic joint infection of the hip and knee in the United States. J Arthroplast. 2021 May;36(5):1484–1489.e3.
3. Urban-Chmiel R, Marek A, Stępień-Pyśniak D, Wieczorek K, Dec M, Nowaczek A, Osek J. Antibiotic resistance in bacteria-a review. Antibiotics (Basel). 2022 Aug 9;11(8):1079.
4. Leaper D, Wilson P, Assadian O, Edmiston C, Kiernan M, Miller A, Bond-Smith G, Yap J. The role of antimicrobial sutures in preventing surgical site infection. Ann R Coll Surg Engl. 2017 Jul;99(6):439–43.
5. Frank JM, Kayupov E, Moric M, Segreti J, Hansen E, Hartman C, Okroj K, Belden K, Roslund B, Silibovsky R, Parvizi J, Della Valle CJ, Knee Society Research Group. The Mark Coventry, MD, award: oral antibiotics reduce reinfection after two-stage exchange: a multicenter, randomized controlled trial. Clin Orthop Relat Res. 2017 Jan;475(1):56–61.
6. Miltenberg B, Ludwick L, Masood R, Menendez ME, Moverman MA, Pagani NR, Puzzitiello RN, Smith EL. Intraosseous regional administration of antibiotic prophylaxis for total knee arthroplasty: a systematic review. J Arthroplast. 2023 Apr;38(4):769–74.
7. Parvizi J, Tan TL, Goswami K, Higuera C, Della Valle C, Chen AF, Shohat N. The 2018 definition of Periprosthetic hip and knee infection: an evidence-based and validated criteria. J Arthroplast. 2018 May;33(5):1309–1314.e2.
8. Yin H, Xu D, Wang D. Diagnostic value of next-generation sequencing to detect periprosthetic joint infection. BMC Musculoskelet Disord. 2021 Mar 6;22(1):252.
9. Indelli PF, Ghirardelli S, Violante B, Amanatullah DF. Next generation sequencing for pathogen detection in periprosthetic joint infections. I Open Rev. 2021 Apr 1;6(4):236–44.
10. Chisari E, Yacovelli S, Goswami K, Shohat N, Woloszyn P, Parvizi J. Leukocyte esterase versus ICM 2018 criteria in the diagnosis of Periprosthetic joint infection. J Arthroplast. 2021 Aug;36(8):2942–2945.e1.
11. Bonanzinga T, Ferrari MC, Tanzi G, Vandenbulcke F, Zahar A, Marcacci M. The role of alpha defensin in prosthetic joint infection (PJI) diagnosis: a literature review. I Open Rev. 2019 Jan 23;4(1):10–3.
12. Bottagisio M, Viganò M, Pellegrini A, Logoluso N, Zagra L, Prina A, de Girolamo L, De Vecchi E. Evaluation of synovial calprotectin by using a lateral flow test for the diagnosis of prosthetic joint infections. Diagnostics (Basel). 2023 Feb 15;13(4):741.
13. Maimaiti Z, Li Z, Xu C, Fu J, Hao LB, Chen JY, Chai W. Host immune regulation in implant-associated infection (IAI): what does the current evidence provide us to prevent or treat IAI? Bioengineering (Basel). 2023 Mar 13;10(3):356.
14. Warren SI, Charville GW, Manasherob R, Amanatullah DF. Immune checkpoint upregulation

in periprosthetic joint infection. J Orthop Res. 2022 Nov;40(11):2663–9.
15. Pannu TS, Villa JM, Riesgo AM, Patel PD, Barsoum WK, Higuera-Rueda CA. Serum D-dimer in the diagnosis of Periprosthetic knee infection: where are we today? J Knee Surg. 2020 Feb;33(2):106–10.
16. Tarabichi S, Goh GS, Baker CM, Chisari E, Shahi A, Parvizi J. Plasma D-dimer is noninferior to serum C-reactive protein in the diagnosis of Periprosthetic joint infection. J Bone Joint Surg Am. 2023 Apr 5;105(7):501–8.
17. Pannu TS, Villa JM, Higuera CA. Diagnosis and management of infected arthroplasty. SICOT J. 2021;7:54.
18. Siddiqi A, Mahmoud Y, Forte SA, Novack TA, Nace J. One and a half-stage revision with prosthetic articulating spacer for definitive management of Knee Periprosthetic joint infection. Arthroplast Today. 2022 Dec;5(19):100993.
19. Carlson VR, Dekeyser GJ, Certain L, Pupaibool J, Gililland JM, Anderson LA. Clinical experience with a coordinated multidisciplinary approach to treating prosthetic joint infection. Arthroplast Today. 2020 Jun 12;6(3):360–2.
20. Rottier W, Seidelman J, Wouthuyzen-Bakker M. Antimicrobial treatment of patients with a periprosthetic joint infection: basic principles. Arthroplasty. 2023 Mar 2;5(1):10.
21. Villa JM, Pannu TS, Theeb I, Buttaro MA, Oñativia JI, Carbo L, Rienzi DH, Fregeiro JI, Kornilov NN, Bozhkova SA, Sandiford NA, Piuzzi NS, Higuera CA, Kendoff DO. International organism profile of Periprosthetic total hip and knee infections. J Arthroplast. 2021 Jan;36(1):274–8.
22. Goswami K, Clarkson S, Phillips CD, Dennis DA, Klatt BA, O'Malley MJ, Smith EL, Gililland JM, Pelt CE, Peters CL, Malkani AL, Palumbo BT, Lyons ST, Bernasek TL, Minter J, Goyal N, McDonald JF 3rd, Cross MB, Prieto HA, Lee GC, Hansen EN, Bini SA, Ward DT, Shohat N, Higuera CA, Nam D, Della Valle CJ, Parvizi J. Orthopedic genomics workgroup. An enhanced understanding of culture-negative Periprosthetic joint infection with next-generation sequencing: a multicenter study. J Bone Joint Surg Am. 2022 Sep 7;104(17):1523–9.
23. Shearer J, Agius L, Burke N, Rahardja R, Young SW. BMI is a better predictor of Periprosthetic joint infection risk than local measures of adipose tissue after TKA. J Arthroplast. 2020 Jun;35(6S):S313–8.
24. Tarabichi M, Shohat N, Kheir MM, Adelani M, Brigati D, Kearns SM, Patel P, Clohisy JC, Higuera CA, Levine BR, Schwarzkopf R, Parvizi J, Jiranek WA. Determining the threshold for HbA1c as a predictor for adverse outcomes after Total joint arthroplasty: a multicenter, retrospective study. J Arthroplast. 2017 Sep;32(9S):S263–S267.e1.
25. Shohat N, Tarabichi M, Tan TL, Goswami K, Kheir M, Malkani AL, Shah RP, Schwarzkopf R, Parvizi J. 2019 John Insall award: Fructosamine is a better glycaemic marker compared with glycated haemoglobin (HbA1C) in predicting adverse outcomes following total knee arthroplasty: a prospective multicentre study. Bone Joint J. 2019 Jul;101-B(7_Supple_C):3–9.
26. Ji B, Zhang X, Xu B, Ren J, Guo W, Mu W, Cao L. The fate of immunocompromised patients in the treatment of chronic periprosthetic joint infection: a single-Centre experience. Int Orthop. 2018 Mar;42(3):487–98.
27. Tischler EH, Matsen Ko L, Chen AF, Maltenfort MG, Schroeder J, Austin MS. Smoking increases the rate of reoperation for infection within 90 days after primary Total joint arthroplasty. J Bone Joint Surg Am. 2017 Feb 15;99(4):295–304.
28. Farber NJ, Chen AF, Bartsch SM, Feigel JL, Klatt BA. No infection reduction using chlorhexidine wipes in total joint arthroplasty. Clin Orthop Relat Res. 2013 Oct;471(10):3120–5.
29. Kapadia BH, Elmallah RK, Mont MA. A randomized, clinical trial of preadmission chlorhexidine skin preparation for lower extremity Total joint arthroplasty. J Arthroplast. 2016 Dec;31(12):2856–61.
30. Christensen DD, Moschetti WE, Brown MG, Lucas AP, Jevsevar DS, Fillingham YA, Dartmouth Hitchcock Medical Center. Perioperative antibiotic prophylaxis: single and 24-hour antibiotic dosages are equally effective at preventing Periprosthetic joint infection in Total joint arthroplasty. J Arthroplast. 2021 Jul;36(7S):S308–13.
31. Tan TL, Shohat N, Rondon AJ, Foltz C, Goswami K, Ryan SP, Seyler TM, Parvizi J. Perioperative antibiotic prophylaxis in Total joint arthroplasty: a single dose is as effective as multiple doses. J Bone Joint Surg Am. 2019 Mar 6;101(5):429–37.
32. Bukowski BR, Owen AR, Turner TW, Fruth KM, Osmon DR, Pagnano MW, Berry DJ, Abdel MP. Extended Oral antibiotic prophylaxis after aseptic revision Total hip arthroplasty: does it decrease infection risk? J Arthroplast. 2022 Dec;37(12):2460–5.
33. Inabathula A, Dilley JE, Ziemba-Davis M, Warth LC, Azzam KA, Ireland PH, Meneghini RM. Extended Oral antibiotic prophylaxis in high-risk patients substantially reduces primary Total hip and knee arthroplasty 90-day infection rate. J Bone Joint Surg Am. 2018 Dec 19;100(24):2103–9.
34. Villa JM, Pannu TS, Braaksma W, Higuera CA, Riesgo AM. Extended Oral antibiotic prophylaxis after aseptic Total hip or knee arthroplasty revisions: a preliminary report. J Arthroplast. 2023 Jan;38(1):141–5.
35. Harper KD, Park KJ, Brozovich AA, Sullivan TC, Serpelloni S, Taraballi F, Incavo SJ, Clyburn TA. Otto Aufranc award: intraosseous vancomycin in Total hip arthroplasty–superior tissue concentrations and improved efficiency. J Arthroplast. 2023 Jul;38(7S):S11–5.
36. Oktay K, Özsoy KM, Çetinalp NE, Erman T, Güzel A. Efficacy of prophylactic application of vancomycin powder in preventing surgical site infections after instrumented spinal surgery: a retrospective analysis of patients with high-risk conditions. Acta Orthop Traumatol Turc. 2021 Jan;55(1):48–52.

37. Marchand LS, Sprague S, O'Hara NN, Li CS, O'Toole RV, Joshi M, Viskontas D, Romeo N, Hymes RA, Obremskey WT, Higgins TF, Potter GD, Bergin PF, Gage M, Gary JL, Bhandari M, Slobogean GP. Local administration of vancomycin powder in orthopaedic fracture surgery: current practice and trends. OTA Int. 2023 Feb 21;6(1):e223.
38. Mancino F, Gant V, Meek DRM, Haddad FS. Vancomycin powder in total joint replacement. Bone Joint J. 2023 Aug 1;105-B(8):833–6.
39. Qadir R, Ochsner JL, Chimento GF, Meyer MS, Waddell B, Zavatsky JM. Establishing a role for vancomycin powder application for prosthetic joint infection prevention-results of a wear simulation study. J Arthroplast. 2014 Jul;29(7):1449–56.
40. Mancino F, Yates PJ, Clark B, Jones CW. Use of topical vancomycin powder in total joint arthroplasty: why the current literature is inconsistent? World J Orthop. 2023 Aug 18;14(8):589–97.
41. Goldenheim PD. In vitro efficacy of povidone-iodine solution and cream against methicillin-resistant Staphylococcus aureus. Postgrad Med J. 1993;69(Suppl 3):S62–5.
42. Brown NM, Cipriano CA, Moric M, Sporer SM, Della Valle CJ. Dilute betadine lavage before closure for the prevention of acute postoperative deep periprosthetic joint infection. J Arthroplast. 2012 Jan;27(1):27–30.
43. Hernandez NM, Hart A, Taunton MJ, Osmon DR, Mabry TM, Abdel MP, Perry KI. Use of povidone-iodine irrigation prior to wound closure in primary Total hip and knee arthroplasty: an analysis of 11,738 cases. J Bone Joint Surg Am. 2019 Jul 3;101(13):1144–50.
44. Hart A, Hernandez NM, Abdel MP, Mabry TM, Hanssen AD, Perry KI. Povidone-iodine wound lavage to prevent infection after revision Total hip and knee arthroplasty: an analysis of 2,884 cases. J Bone Joint Surg Am. 2019 Jul 3;101(13):1151–9.
45. Blom A, Cho J, Fleischman A, Goswami K, Ketonis C, Kunutsor SK, Makar G, Meeker DG, Morgan-Jones R, Ortega-Peña S, Parvizi J, Smeltzer M, Stambough JB, Urish K, Ziliotto G. General assembly, prevention, antiseptic irrigation solution: proceedings of international consensus on orthopedic infections. J Arthroplast. 2019 Feb;34(2S):S131–8.
46. Allegranzi B, Bischoff P, de Jonge S, Kubilay NZ, Zayed B, Gomes SM, Abbas M, Atema JJ, Gans S, van Rijen M, Boermeester MA, Egger M, Kluytmans J, Pittet D, Solomkin JS, WHO Guidelines Development Group. New WHO recommendations on preoperative measures for surgical site infection prevention: an evidence-based global perspective. Lancet Infect Dis. 2016 Dec;16(12):e276–87.
47. Berríos-Torres SI, Umscheid CA, Bratzler DW, Leas B, Stone EC, Kelz RR, Reinke CE, Morgan S, Solomkin JS, Mazuski JE, Dellinger EP, Itani KMF, Berbari EF, Segreti J, Parvizi J, Blanchard J, Allen G, Kluytmans JAJW, Donlan R. Schecter WP; healthcare infection control practices advisory committee. Centers for Disease Control and Prevention guideline for the prevention of surgical site infection, 2017. JAMA Surg. 2017 Aug 1;152(8):784–91.
48. Haykal T, Kheiri B, Zayed Y, Barbarawi M, Miran MS, Chahine A, Katato K, Bachuwa G. Aspirin for venous thromboembolism prophylaxis after hip or knee arthroplasty: an updated meta-analysis of randomized controlled trials. J Orthop. 2019 Mar 21;16(4):294–302.
49. Tarabichi S, Parvizi J. Prevention of surgical site infection: a ten-step approach. Arthroplasty. 2023 Apr 8;5(1):21.
50. Groenen H, Jalalzadeh H, Buis DR, Dreissen YEM, Goosen JHM, Griekspoor M, Harmsen WJ, Ijpma FFA, van der Laan MJ, Schaad RR, Segers P, van der Zwet WC, de Jonge SW, Orsini RG, Eskes AM, Wolfhagen N, Boermeester MA. Incisional negative pressure wound therapy for the prevention of surgical site infection: an up-to-date meta-analysis and trial sequential analysis. Eclin Med. 2023 Jul;24(62):102105.
51. Higuera-Rueda CA, Emara AK, Nieves-Malloure Y, Klika AK, Cooper HJ, Cross MB, Guild GN, Nam D, Nett MP, Scuderi GR, Cushner FD, Piuzzi NS, Silverman RP. The effectiveness of closed-incision negative-pressure therapy versus silver-impregnated dressings in mitigating surgical site complications in high-risk patients after revision knee arthroplasty: the PROMISES randomized controlled trial. J Arthroplast. 2021 Jul;36(7S):S295–S302.e14.
52. Kates SL, Owen JR, Beck CA, Xie C, Muthukrishnan G, Daiss JL, Schwarz EM. Lack of humoral immunity against Glucosaminidase is associated with postoperative complications in Staphylococcus aureus osteomyelitis. J Bone Joint Surg Am. 2020 Nov 4;102(21):1842–8.
53. Thornhill MH, Crum A, Rex S, Stone T, Campbell R, Bradburn M, Fibisan V, Lockhart PB, Springer B, Baddour LM, Nicholl J. Analysis of prosthetic joint infections following invasive dental procedures in England. JAMA Netw Open. 2022 Jan 4;5(1):e2142987.
54. Bains SS, Sax OC, Chen Z, Gilson GA, Nace J, Mont MA, Delanois RE. Antibiotic prophylaxis is often unnecessary for screening colonoscopies following total knee arthroplasty. J Arthroplast. 2023 Jun;38(6S):S331–6.
55. Reisener M, Perka C. Do culture-negative Periprosthetic joint infections have a worse outcome than culture-positive Periprosthetic joint infections? A systematic review and meta-analysis. Biomed Res Int. 2018 Jul;12(2018):6278012.
56. Peel TN, Dylla BL, Hughes JG, Lynch DT, Greenwood-Quaintance KE, Cheng AC, Mandrekar JN, Patel R. Improved diagnosis of prosthetic joint infection by culturing Periprosthetic tissue specimens in blood culture bottles. MBio. 2016 Jan 5;7(1):e01776–15.
57. Levack AE, Koch C, Moore HG, Cross MB. The utility of MRI with multiacquisition variable-resonance image combination (MAVRIC) in diagnosing

deep Total hip arthroplasty infection. HSS J. 2022 May;18(2):277–83.
58. Del Arco A, Bertrand ML. The diagnosis of periprosthetic infection. Open Orthop J. 2013 Jun;14(7):178–83.
59. Sires JD, Pham K, Daniel S, Inglis M, Wilson CJ. A multi-disciplinary approach for the management of prosthetic joint infections: an Australian perspective. Malays Orthop J. 2022 Jul;16(2):41–5.
60. Deckey DG, Christopher ZK, Bingham JS, Spangehl MJ. Principles of mechanical and chemical debridement with implant retention. Arthroplasty. 2023 Apr 6;5(1):16.
61. Young SW, Zhang M, Moore GA, Pitto RP, Clarke HD, Spangehl MJ. The John N. Insall award: higher tissue concentrations of vancomycin achieved with intraosseous regional prophylaxis in revision TKA: a randomized controlled trial. Clin Orthop Relat Res. 2018 Jan;476(1):66–74.
62. Kildow BJ, Patel SP, Otero JE, Fehring KA, Curtin BM, Springer BD, Fehring TK. Results of debridement, antibiotics, and implant retention for periprosthetic knee joint infection supplemented with the use of intraosseous antibiotics. Bone Joint J. 2021 Jun;103-B(6 Supple A):185–90.
63. McQuivey KS, Bingham J, Chung A, Clarke H, Schwartz A, Pollock JR, Beauchamp C, Spangehl MJ. The Double DAIR: a 2-stage debridement with prosthesis-retention protocol for acute Periprosthetic joint infections. JBJS Essent Surg Tech. 2021;11(1):e19.00071.
64. Bernard L, Arvieux C, Brunschweiler B, Touchais S, Ansart S, Bru JP, Oziol E, Boeri C, Gras G, Druon J, Rosset P, Senneville E, Bentayeb H, Bouhour D, Le Moal G, Michon J, Aumaître H, Forestier E, Laffosse JM, Begué T, Chirouze C, Dauchy FA, Devaud E, Martha B, Burgot D, Boutoille D, Stindel E, Dinh A, Bemer P, Giraudeau B, Issartel B, Caille A. Antibiotic therapy for 6 or 12 weeks for prosthetic joint infection. N Engl J Med. 2021 May 27;384(21):1991–2001.
65. George J, Kwiecien G, Klika AK, Ramanathan D, Bauer TW, Barsoum WK, Higuera CA. Are frozen sections and MSIS criteria reliable at the time of Reimplantation of two-stage revision arthroplasty? Clin Orthop Relat Res. 2016 Jul;474(7):1619–26.
66. Pannu TS, Villa JM, Manrique J, Higuera CA, Riesgo AM. Paradoxical behavior of plasma d-dimer from Explantation to Reimplantation in a two-stage revision for Periprosthetic joint infection. J Arthroplast. 2022 Aug;37(8S):S977–82.
67. Zmistowski B, Tetreault MW, Alijanipour P, Chen AF, Della Valle CJ, Parvizi J. Recurrent periprosthetic joint infection: persistent or new infection? J Arthroplast. 2013 Oct;28(9):1486–9.
68. Haddad FS, Sukeik M, Alazzawi S. Is single-stage revision according to a strict protocol effective in treatment of chronic knee arthroplasty infections? Clin Orthop Relat Res. 2015 Jan;473(1):8–14.
69. Nabet A, Sax OC, Shanoada R, Conway JD, Mont MA, Delanois RE, Nace J. Survival and outcomes of 1.5-stage vs 2-stage exchange Total knee arthroplasty following prosthetic joint infection. J Arthroplast. 2022 May;37(5):936–41.
70. Nace J, Chen Z, Bains SS, Kahan ME, Gilson GA, Mont MA, Delanois RE. 1.5-stage versus 2-stage exchange Total hip arthroplasty for chronic Periprosthetic joint infections: a comparison of survivorships, reinfections, and patient-reported outcomes. J Arthroplast. 2023 Jul;38(7S):S235–41.
71. Hernandez NM, Buchanan MW, Seyler TM, Wellman SS, Seidelman J, Jiranek WA. 1.5-stage exchange arthroplasty for Total knee arthroplasty Periprosthetic joint infections. J Arthroplast. 2021 Mar;36(3):1114–9.
72. Zamora T, Garbuz DS, Greidanus NV, Masri BA. An articulated spacer made of new primary implants in two-stage exchange for infected total knee arthroplasty may provide durable results. Bone Joint J. 2020 Jul;102-B(7):852–60.
73. Danoff JR, Heimroth J, Willinger M, Trout S, Sodhi N. Surgical technique: robotic-assisted 1.5-stage exchange Total knee arthroplasty for Periprosthetic joint infection. Arthroplast Today. 2023 May;15(21):101126.
74. Song SJ, Hwang SH, Baek HJ, Park CH. Aseptic survival of the 1.5-stage exchange arthroplasty for periprosthetic joint infection was acceptable when using an autoclaved femoral component and a new polyethylene insert. Knee Surg Sports Traumatol Arthrosc. 2023 Aug 29;31:4996.
75. Łusiak-Szelachowska M, Weber-Dąbrowska B, Górski A. Bacteriophages and Lysins in biofilm control. Virol Sin. 2020 Apr;35(2):125–33.
76. Sosa BR, Niu Y, Turajane K, Staats K, Suhardi V, Carli A, Fischetti V, Bostrom M, Yang X. 2020 John Charnley award: the antimicrobial potential of bacteriophage-derived lysin in a murine debridement, antibiotics, and implant retention model of prosthetic joint infection. Bone Joint J. 2020 Jul;102-B(7_Supple_B):3–10.
77. Akanda ZZ, Taha M, Abdelbary H. Current review-the rise of bacteriophage as a unique therapeutic platform in treating periprosthetic joint infections. J Orthop Res. 2018 Apr;36(4):1051–60.
78. Cano EJ, Caflisch KM, Bollyky PL, Van Belleghem JD, Patel R, Fackler J, Brownstein MJ, Horne B, Biswas B, Henry M, Malagon F, Lewallen DG, Suh GA. Phage therapy for limb-threatening prosthetic knee Klebsiella pneumoniae infection: case report and in vitro characterization of anti-biofilm activity. Clin Infect Dis. 2021 Jul 1;73(1):e144–51.
79. Khalifa AA, Hussien SM. The promising role of bacteriophage therapy in managing total hip and knee arthroplasty related periprosthetic joint infection, a systematic review. J Exp Orthop. 2023 Feb 14;10(1):18.
80. Mandell JB, Koch JA, Deslouches B, Urish KL. Direct antimicrobial activity of cationic amphipathic peptide WLBU2 against Staphylococcus aureus biofilms is

enhanced in physiological buffered saline. J Orthop Res. 2020 Dec;38(12):2657–63.
81. Elsalem L, Khasawneh A, Al SS. WLBU2 antimicrobial peptide as a potential therapeutic for treatment of resistant bacterial. Turk J Pharm Sci. 2022 Feb 28;19(1):110–6.
82. Estellés A, Woischnig AK, Liu K, Stephenson R, Lomongsod E, Nguyen D, Zhang J, Heidecker M, Yang Y, Simon RJ, Tenorio E, Ellsworth S, Leighton A, Ryser S, Gremmelmaier NK, Kauvar LM. A high-affinity native human antibody disrupts biofilm from Staphylococcus aureus bacteria and potentiates antibiotic efficacy in a mouse implant infection model. Antimicrob Agents Chemother. 2016 Mar 25;60(4):2292–301.
83. Visperas A, Santana D, Klika AK, Higuera-Rueda CA, Piu-zzi NS. Current treatments for biofilm-associated periprosthetic joint infection and new potential strategies. J Orthop Res. 2022 Jul;40(7):1477–91.
84. Raafat D, Otto M, Reppschläger K, Iqbal J, Holtfreter S. Fighting Staphylococcus aureus biofilms with monoclonal antibodies. Trends Microbiol. 2019 Apr;27(4):303–22.
85. Ryser S, Tenorio E, Estellés A, Kauvar LM. Human antibody repertoire frequently includes antibodies to a bacterial biofilm associated protein. PLoS One. 2019 Jul 9;14(7):e0219256.
86. Xiong YQ, Estellés A, Li L, Abdelhady W, Gonzales R, Bayer AS, Tenorio E, Leighton A, Ryser S, Kauvar LM. A human biofilm-disrupting monoclonal antibody potentiates antibiotic efficacy in rodent models of both Staphylococcus aureus and Acinetobacter baumannii infections. Antimicrob Agents Chemother. 2017 Sep 22;61(10):e00904–17.

# PJI After Shoulder and Elbow Arthroplasty

# 22

Georg Hauer, Sebastian M. Klim, and Andreas Leithner

## 22.1 PJI After Shoulder and Elbow Arthroplasty

### 22.1.1 Introduction

Shoulder and elbow arthroplasty is proving to be an effective treatment for people suffering from painful shoulder or elbow arthritis [11, 30, 75]. Periprosthetic joint infection (PJI) after total shoulder arthroplasty (TSA) and total elbow arthroplasty (TEA) is rare but can have serious consequences, potentially resulting in significant damage to soft tissues, bone loss, and impaired functional outcomes [11, 44]. Prompt diagnosis and appropriate treatment are critical to cure the infection and minimize extensive damage to bone and soft tissue.

While a significant number of knee and hip replacement operations were performed in England and Wales in 2021, there were far fewer shoulder and elbow replacements. According to the National Joint Registry for England, Wales, Northern Ireland, and the Isle of Man, approximately 80,000 procedures were performed for hip and knee joints, respectively. In contrast, the number of shoulder and elbow replacement surgeries was notably lower, with roughly 5500 and 760 procedures, respectively [42]. Interestingly, although shoulder PJI is less common [14], affecting about 1% of patients [5], the treatment of PJI in the shoulder is particularly more demanding compared to PJI in other joints [32]. It is associated with higher morbidity and higher costs [4, 39]. In addition, the incidence of elbow PJI is higher than for hip or knee arthroplasty, with reported rates ranging from 1% to 19% [32, 48, 54].

Historically, much of the guidance and expertise related to PJI has been derived from research and guidelines developed in the field of lower limb arthroplasty [49]. Little attention has been paid to shoulder and elbow PJI, primarily because TSA and TEA are used less frequently and the incidence of acute fulminant PJI is relatively low [21, 81]. To effectively diagnose and assess PJI in the shoulder and elbow, it is essential to begin the process with a standardized, and universally accepted definition. This is particularly important because of the microbiological differences and the difficulties arising from the increased rates of positive intraoperative cultures in revision cases that do not appear to have an infection [2, 21, 29, 36]. Fortunately, in recent years there has been a marked increase in research efforts focusing on the complexities and unique factors in this particular area, suggesting that there is increasing recognition of the particular challenges associated with shoulder and elbow PJI [17].

G. Hauer · S. M. Klim (✉) · A. Leithner
Department of Orthopaedics and Trauma, Medical University of Graz, Graz, Austria
e-mail: georg.hauer@medunigraz.at; Sebastian.klim@medunigraz.at; Andreas.leithner@medunigraz.at



P. Ruggieri et al. (eds.), *Bone and Joint Infections*, https://doi.org/10.1007/978-3-031-96383-4_22

## 22.2 PJI After Shoulder Arthroplasty

### 22.2.1 Epidemiology

The epidemiology of shoulder PJI has been thoroughly investigated, with data collected from various sources including observational studies and meta-analyses. In a recent systematic meta-analysis using 105 articles, the pooled PJI incidence following TSA was 0.61% (0.34–0.93) over a follow-up period of 1.1 years [32]. The authors also found that the PJI incidence was higher following inverse TSA compared with anatomical TSA. In an arthroplasty register analysis, the authors described a 1.4% (95% CI 1.2 to 1.6) ten-year cumulative revision rate due to infection [38]. The adjusted relative risk of revision surgery due to infection was about 2.5 times higher for inverse TSA compared to anatomical TSA. Shah and colleagues could demonstrate a 2.4% shoulder PJI rate at a mean follow-up of 4.3 years for primary inverse TSA [61]. There was also a tendency for increased infection rates in the revision surgery groups compared to the primary arthroplasty groups, i.e., in line with other studies [67, 71]. Zumstein et al. published a systematic review and found that the incidence of PJI after inverse TSA was 3.8%, a figure comparable to that of anatomical arthroplasty. Again, the revision group had a higher infection rate compared to the primary group (5.8% versus 2.9%) [82].

The available studies used a wide range of follow-up periods and different diagnostic criteria to identify PJI cases. Because of these different approaches, it is difficult to determine the exact incidence of shoulder PJI based on the available data. Conducting more comprehensive studies using generally accepted diagnostic criteria would provide a more reliable estimate of shoulder PJI incidence.

### 22.2.2 Risk Factors

The evidence in the present literature lacks uniform consistency, as the studies used different diagnostic criteria for shoulder PJI, the follow-up time varied and the number of participants varied. This variety of factors makes it difficult to reach reliable conclusions about the risk factors associated with PJI. The likelihood of infection occurring after any type of arthroplasty depends on several factors related to the patient, the surgical procedures, and the indication [33]. Regarding the influence of patient characteristics, there is strong evidence that men show an increased risk of needing revision surgery due to PJI [32, 40, 56, 63] and that older age is associated with a decreased risk of joint infection [12, 32, 56, 63]. With each additional year of life, the risk of infection decreases by 5% [40]. The increased risk of shoulder PJI in younger patients remains uncertain [38], while in men it is associated with a higher bacterial load of *Cutibacterium acnes* [56].

There is no robust evidence of associations of other patient characteristics or comorbidities such as heart failure, obesity, peripheral vascular disease, chronic lung disease, diabetes mellitus, liver disease, renal failure, or smoking status with the risk of PJI following TSR. While some studies indicate a correlation with an elevated risk associated with these factors [3, 26, 40, 46, 64, 67], others suggest no significant influence [32, 40, 62, 63].

Studies demonstrated that revision arthroplasties had significantly higher infection rates than primary arthroplasties [12, 67, 71, 82]. In addition, inverse TSA was associated with higher infection rates compared to conventional shoulder arthroplasty [56, 82]. Studies also found that previous treatments such as steroid injections given within 3 months prior to arthroplasty and patients with a history of non-arthroplasty shoulder surgery were associated with an increased risk of shoulder PJI [12, 76, 77].

The risk of shoulder PJI is complex and influenced by several factors. Particular attention should be paid to those at higher risk of PJI after primary TSR, including younger men and those with previous shoulder surgery. These patients should receive appropriate advice and guidance [32].

## 22.2.3 Definition and Diagnosis

### 22.2.3.1 Definition

With the number of TSA increasing every year, the incidence of complications requiring revision surgery has also increased [42]. The COVID-19 pandemic did lead to a decrease in the number of implantations. However, the numbers are now expected to exceed those of the previous year again on an annual basis [42]. It is expected that the demand for shoulder prostheses will increase sevenfold in the next 15 years [9]. Among the complications after TSA, PJI is one of the main causes of implant failure [8, 46, 60]. In the past, it was challenging to measure the consequences of shoulder PJI, due to the absence of a precise and unambiguous definition. In order to create uniform standards for clinical decision-making and research reporting, a precise definition of shoulder PJI was established at the 2018 International Consensus Meeting on Orthopaedic Infections [21].

An exact and universally accepted definition of shoulder PJI is of great importance. This definition helps in clinical decision-making and provides a consistent basis for future research reports. In addition, the adoption of a recognized definition is the first fundamental step toward a rigorously tested diagnostic method [21]. The use of different PJI definitions among researchers dealing with shoulder problems has probably led to different and contradictory conclusions regarding both diagnosis and treatment [27].

When defining infections after prosthetic joint replacement, there is agreement that a combination of clinical, laboratory, and radiological features should be used to confirm or exclude an infection [50]. This approach is also appropriate for shoulder PJI. It has been recognized that certain features of shoulder PJI can be considered as definite indicators of infection and should be given more importance in the definition. On the other hand, some less specific features may indicate infection but may also be present in patients without infection. As a result, two levels of certainty have been introduced for these diagnostic features. The criteria can be classified as either confirmatory (indicating definite infection if fulfilled) or suggestive (indicating features suggestive of possible infection and warranting further investigation) [21].

### 22.2.3.2 Diagnostic Criteria

Despite ongoing debates and uncertainties regarding the definition and treatment of PJI of the shoulder, there are cases where the presence of infection is undeniable. To address this, a subgroup known as "definite PJI" of the shoulder has been introduced to categorically identify such cases [21].

Confirmatory Criteria for Shoulder PJI

1. Presence of a sinus tract from the skin surface to the prosthesis.
2. Gross intra-articular pus.
3. Two positive tissue cultures with phenotypically identical virulent organisms.

Suggestive Criteria for Shoulder PJI.

In cases where there are no confirmatory signs of infection, the diagnosis of shoulder PJI can be difficult. To avoid this, a system was introduced with three categories: probable PJI, possible PJI, and unlikely PJI. To categorize these cases, minor criteria with different weights were introduced (Table 22.1) [21].

A score of 6 or higher with an identified organism is considered an indicator of *probable* shoulder PJI. A score of 6 without an identified organism indicates *possible* PJI. Fewer than 6 with one positive culture with a virulent organism or two positive cultures with a low-virulence organism indicates *possible* PJI. Shoulder PJI is considered *unlikely* if the cultures are negative or there is only one positive culture with a low-virulence organism.

### 22.2.3.3 Clinical Presentation

The most common initial symptom is pain (86%), followed by a draining sinus (44%), stiffness (35%), redness (35%), swelling (32%), fever (21%), night sweats (9%) and chills (9%) [7]. Non-specific symptoms such as pain and impaired function play an important role, especially in cases of late shoulder PJI, when the postoperative function was normal until that point. In the case of painful shoulder arthroplasty, confirming a diagnosis of infection is often difficult and

**Table 22.1** Minor criteria for definition of shoulder PJI

| Minor criteria | Weight |
|---|---|
| Unexpected wound drainage | 4 |
| Single positive tissue culture with virulent organism | 3 |
| Single positive tissue culture with low-virulence organism | 1 |
| Second positive tissue culture (identical low-virulence organism) | 3 |
| Humeral loosening | 3 |
| Positive frozen section (5 PMNs in ≥5 high-power fields) | 3 |
| Positive preoperative aspirate culture (low or high virulence) | 3 |
| Elevated synovial neutrophil percentage (>80%)[a] | 2 |
| Elevated synovial WBC count (>3000 cells/μL)[a] | 2 |
| Elevated ESR (>30 mm/h)[a] | 2 |
| Elevated CRP level (>10 mg/L) | 2 |
| Elevated synovial α-defensin level | 2 |
| Cloudy fluid | 2 |

*PJI* periprosthetic joint infection, *PMN* polymorphonuclear leukocyte, *WBC* white blood cell, *ESR* erythrocyte sedimentation rate, *CRP* C-reactive protein

[a] Beyond 6 weeks from recent surgery

requires additional investigations. However, in such cases, it is important to consider the possibility of infection [18].

Erythema and swelling may indicate infection, but these indicators are usually not specific enough to definitively diagnose infection. The presence of fever as a systemic sign of infection associated with PJI of the shoulder indicates a more aggressive course of the disease. Nevertheless, it is noteworthy that fever is rare in PJI of the shoulder [7].

The only clinical sign that is confirmatory for shoulder PJI is the presence of a sinus tract even without other clinical, laboratory, or microbiological findings. A strong indication of PJI of the shoulder is also the development of unexpected wound drainage from a previously dry, healing wound [18].

#### 22.2.3.4 Radiology

Plain radiographs may be helpful in diagnosing PJI. Radiographic findings of concern for PJI of the shoulder include loosening or migration of components, radiolucent lines, osteolysis, endosteal scalloping, and new bone formation [11, 13, 18]. However, these findings are often absent in indolent or low-grade infections. Especially if humeral loosening is found, this should significantly increase the suspicion of PJI of the shoulder. In their research, Pottinger et al. [53] showed that loosening of the humeral component and humeral osteolysis, as seen on plain radiographs, were associated with a threefold and tenfold increase in the likelihood of a positive *Cutibacterium acnes* culture, respectively. Computed tomography (CT) can be useful in assessing bone stock and the current implant configuration, while magnetic resonance imaging (MRI) can help in assessing possible osteomyelitis or an abscess in the area [18]. Various nuclear imaging techniques have been introduced to improve the accuracy of infection diagnosis, however, they have a limited role in the workup for shoulder PJI. Three-phase bone scintigraphy is one of the most frequently used imaging techniques used in the diagnosis of PJI, especially for evaluating late PJI [25].

#### 22.2.3.5 Inflammatory Markers

Limited research is available regarding the use of serum erythrocyte sedimentation rate (ESR), C-reactive protein (CRP), or white blood count (WBC) for assessing shoulder PJI [41, 70]. Serum ESR, CRP, and WBC have low sensitivity in the diagnosis of shoulder PJI [18]. Despite their inclusion in a standard infection investigation, normal values should not be used to definitively exclude infection [18]. Piper et al. [51] have published thresholds for CRP and ESR associated with PJI in the shoulder. The optimized ESR cut-off for shoulder arthroplasty has been set at 26 mm/h. This specific ESR cut-off has shown a sensitivity of 32% and a specificity of 93% in the diagnosis of shoulder PJI. Similarly, the optimized CRP cut-off is 7 mg/L, with this value showing a sensitivity of 63% and a specificity of 73% for the detection of shoulder PJI.

#### 22.2.3.6 Synovial Aspirate

A standard examination for the diagnosis of shoulder PJI is synovial aspiration and analysis.

Aspiration of synovial fluid is mandatory if a distinct fluid collection is identified, however, "dry taps" are often observed in *Cutibacterium acnes* infections [6, 7]. Due to the lower virulence of *Cutibacterium acnes*, the threshold for an increased number of leukocytes in the context of a shoulder, PJI remains unknown and may be lower than accepted values for other PJIs. Consequently, the currently accepted leukocyte count thresholds of >1100–3000 cells/ml with a polymorphonuclear neutrophils (PMN) differentiation of >80% for chronic hip and knee PJI are unlikely to be appropriate for the diagnosis of shoulder PJI, as the bacterial pathogens in the shoulder usually produce a less severe inflammatory response [18].

#### 22.2.3.7 Microbiological Profile

The uniqueness of shoulder PJI lies in the underlying processes, which are primarily due to the specific microorganisms that colonize the shoulder. The predominant pathogens of surgical site infections (SSI) and shoulder PJI surgery are usually coagulase-negative Staphylococcus species, *Cutibacterium acnes* and *Staphylococcus aureus* [24, 31, 56, 63]. *Cutibacterium acnes*, in particular, has recently emerged as the predominant cause of PJI in the shoulder [18]. However, *Cutibacterium acnes* infection can be particularly challenging because of its slow and gradual progression, and confirming positive cultures often necessitates longer incubation periods for samples [10]. A potential disadvantage associated with the increased sensitivity of prolonged cultures for *Cutibacterium acnes* is the fact that this may also carry an increased risk of contamination and false-positive results [16]. Unexpected positive cultures (UPCs) without clinical or radiographic signs of infections are a dilemma. However, the exact definition and management of UPCs in the context of shoulder arthroplasty revisions remains unclear, as does the role of *Cutibacterium acnes* [18]. *Cutibacterium acnes* is the predominant microorganism identified in most positive UPC cases, however, it remains uncertain whether the significance of UPC caused by one bacterium differs from that of UPC with another bacterium. Providing semi-quantitative and quantitative reports of bacterial culture results (eg, density of bacteria, Cuti [Propi] score) could be of clinical value in diagnosing PJI in the shoulder and in assessing the significance of UPCs [18]. Nevertheless, the lack of adequately designed studies addressing this issue makes it difficult to draw definitive conclusions.

### 22.2.4 Management

#### 22.2.4.1 Prevention

Targeting the microorganisms most likely to cause shoulder PJI is an important aspect of prophylactic measures. Patients scheduled for TSA should be prescribed intravenous antibiotics that are effective against both Gram-positive and Gram-negative microorganisms [18]. Cefazolin is the standard antibiotic to be administered. Patients who are intolerant to beta-lactam antibiotics should be further investigated to determine if they are eligible for treatment with cefazolin. In patients with a true hypersensitivity reaction or side effects that make cefazolin treatment impossible, alternative options such as vancomycin or clindamycin should be considered [20].

#### 22.2.4.2 Treatment

Treatment strategies for shoulder PJI include chronic antibiotic treatment, irrigation, and debridement with or without the exchange of components, one- or two-stage revision procedures, the use of antibiotic spacers, and resection arthroplasty. These approaches are based on the collective knowledge and literature on hip and knee arthroplasty [20]. The choice of the most suitable antibiotic, the method of administration, and the duration of treatment depend on the surgical therapy concept chosen and the pathogen detection and should be determined individually after consultation with infectious disease experts [19].

##### Implant Retention

In acute shoulder PJI, the choice of irrigation and debridement with retention of components or replacement of modular components is often considered practical. It is recommended that debridement, antibiotics, and implant retention (DAIR) be considered for shoulder arthroplasty when infection is confirmed within a 30-day window of symptom onset [7, 20]. However, it is noteworthy that this strategy is associated with a reported failure rate of 42% to 63% and less favourable functional outcomes [7, 19]. Given these results, the surgeon must carefully weigh the potential for recurrent infection against the morbidity associated with implant removal.

#### One-Stage Revision Arthroplasty

Utilizing the knowledge acquired from managing knee and hip infections, the concept of single-stage replacement is presented as a viable solution when the responsible microorganism is clearly identified [19]. This approach offers advantages such as shorter hospital stays, cost efficiency, shorter antibiotic treatment duration, and the potential to optimize clinical outcomes [5]. The criteria for choosing between a one-stage and a two-stage exchange are currently unclear [19]. While the pooled data suggest a potential superiority of the one-stage exchange over the two-stage approach, it is important to recognize that this observation could be influenced by selection bias and other variables such as the specific pathogen, the antibiotic resistance pattern, the timing of the infection or diagnostic elements such as obvious clinical signs of infection [19].

#### Two-Stage Revision Arthroplasty

A two-stage replacement arthroplasty, which includes removal of the implant, irrigation, and debridement, followed by insertion of an antibiotic spacer and delayed re-implantation, has been suggested as the "gold standard" for shoulder PJI [19, 22]. If the microorganism responsible for the infection is not known, this is strongly recommended. The first step is to eradicate the infection after removal of the prosthesis. Usually, a cement spacer loaded with antibiotics is implanted and general antibiotics are administered, adjusted according to the microorganism identified later. In case of persistent infection, an additive irrigation and debridement procedure may be proposed. In the re-implantation phase, inverse TSA has become the implant of choice in recent years. It offers several advantages, including the ability to perform more extensive debridement in the initial phase with less consideration for soft tissue preservation [5, 19].

#### Antibiotic Spacer

In two-stage revision arthroplasty, an antibiotic-loaded cement spacer can be used to provide localized, highly concentrated antibiotic administration. In certain cases, an antibiotic-loaded cement spacer may also serve as a definitive and permanent treatment option [7, 19]. The aim is to eliminate the infection while maintaining a functional, pain-free joint shoulder. Complications of permanent spacer, however, include erosion of the glenoid and humeral components, as well as potential problems associated with spacer fracture and rotation [35].

#### Resection Arthroplasty

In cases where the patient's medical comorbidities or technical complexity make revision with a definitive implant too risky, resection arthroplasty serves as an acceptable salvage procedure to eradicate shoulder PJI [17]. Although it achieves a remarkable infection eradication rate of over 90%, it is usually chosen for patients with lower functional requirements as it provides less favourable functional outcomes [5, 57–59].

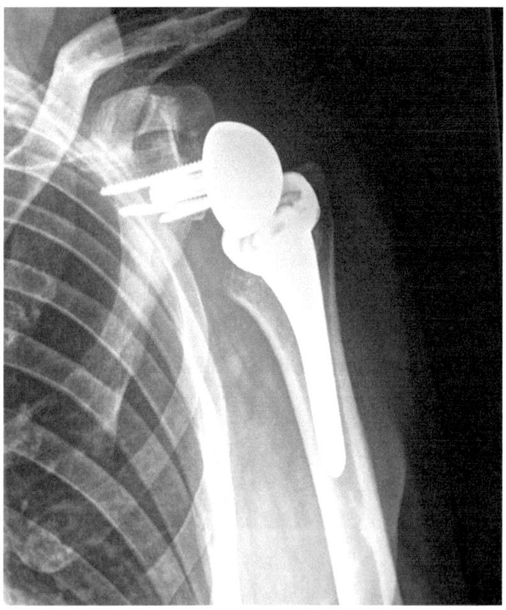

06/2021 inverse shoulder prosthesis

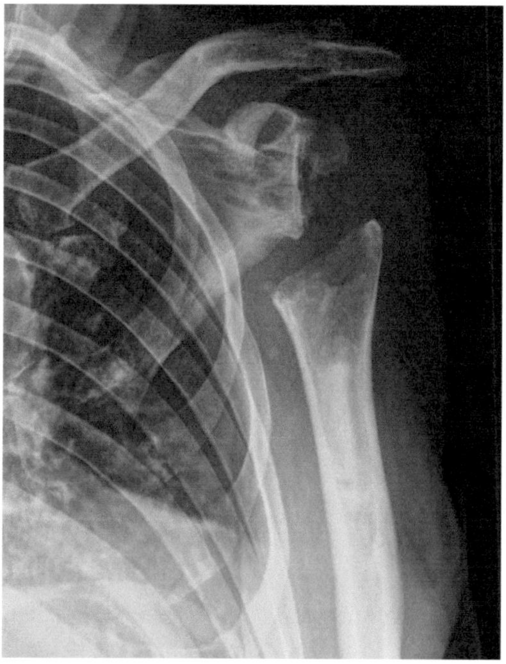

01/2022 first stage: prosthesis removal with intramedullary antibiotic carrier due to PJI

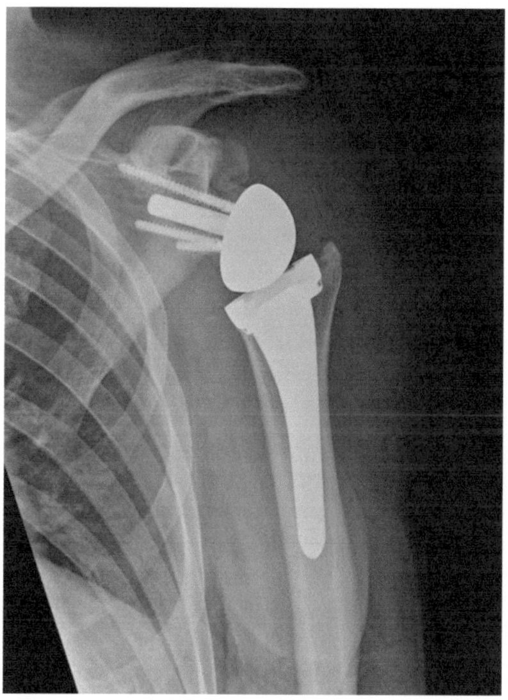

03/2022 second stage: reimplantation inverse shoulder prosthesis

## 22.3 PJI after Elbow Arthroplasty

### 22.3.1 Introduction and Epidemiology

Following the first successful implantation of a total elbow prosthesis in the 1970s, the TEA procedure became an orthopaedic standard operation with steadily increasing numbers [80]. The indications for TEA include primary and post-traumatic osteoarthritis, rheumatoid arthritis, and cases of non-reconstructible joint fractures. However, implantation numbers and functional outcomes lag behind those of total hip and knee prostheses, despite the past and ongoing developments of new prosthesis designs. This indirectly affects the available data on periprosthetic elbow infections and their treatment. Available implants can be sub-classified into hinged and non-hinged designs with marginal outcome differences following primary TEA [75]. Following aseptic component loosening, PJI is the main cause of revision surgery after TEA with a median rate of 3.3% and a range of 2.5 to 12% in the literature [37, 74].

### 22.3.2 Risk Factors

Evidence on specific risk factors for PJI following TEA is rare compared to other arthroplasty procedures. Nevertheless, it seems safe to say that most patient-related risk factors for PJI such as young age at the time of surgery, duration of the surgery, immunosuppression, malnutrition, number of revisions as well as prolonged surgical time and prior local infections play a negative role in TEA.

Obesity, a common risk factor in total joint arthroplasty, also has a negative impact on the PJI rate following TEA. A study including 7580 cases indicated that patients with a BMI under 30 exhibited an infection rate of 2.1%, whereas those with a BMI ranging from 30 to 40 experienced a rate of 4.7%. For individuals with a BMI of 40 or higher, the infection rate rose to 7% [23].

A database analysis of 13,698 individuals who underwent TEA, with 2270 patients (16.5%) having diabetes, revealed elevated rates of wound infections (1.6% compared to 0.83%), consequently influencing the susceptibility to PJI. Diabetes also has a negative effect on length of stay, blood transfusion rates, and the overall number of perioperative complications [52].

A specific risk factor for PJI following TEA which is commonly discussed is the poor local soft tissue coverage. This is further exacerbated by existing rheumatoid arthritis, as this patient group tends to have impaired wound healing, resulting in an increased risk for PJI [28]. A higher overall revision rate for patients with rheumatoid arthritis was also reported by a systematic review including 1253 cases of primary TEA (compared to post-traumatic osteoarthritis and trauma), however, the PJI rate was not significantly different [54]. This is in contrast to the results of another study including 1452 patients, reporting rheumatoid arthritis to be a significant risk factor for PJI after TEA (odds ratio (OR) = 3.31; $p < 0.001$) [65].

This study also reported that hypothyroidism (OR = 2.04; $p = 0.045$) and smoking (OR = 3.39; p = 0.003) represent significant risk factors for PJI following TEA. Preoperative optimization of thyroid function, smoking reduction, or complete abstinence as well as management of rheumatoid disease is recommended [65]. Further, surgical procedures prior to the index arthroplasty seem to increase the risk of subsequent PJI. This is displayed by the mean PJI rate of 11% in 6 studies, whereas 69% (201/291) of patients were reported to have had prior surgery before TEA [73].

### 22.3.3 Diagnosis

The diagnosis of PJI can be challenging, especially in low-grade cases in the absence of the classic clinical criteria (warmth, swelling, pain, redness). Systemic symptoms are reportedly less commonly observed in infected elbow prostheses compared to hip and knee endoprostheses. Assessing potential current risk factors for PJI (see above), as well as the medical history following TEA implantation (i.e. wound drainage, multiple revision surgeries), provides crucial information regarding the likelihood of an existing PJI [78].

Studies investigating serum biomarkers in PJI following TEA are rare, and transferring study results from hip and knee PJI research must be done with caution. Especially when considering that many patients with TEA may suffer from an underlying inflammatory condition and may have a different baseline level of inflammatory markers [66]. Experts therefore recommend considering the classic inflammatory markers over time, in conjunction with clinical symptoms and other diagnostic tests. It is advised not to make diagnostic decisions solely based on elevated serum biomarkers, especially following TEA [49]. No specific studies investigating alternative serum markers (i.e. fibrinogen, procalcitonin, interleukin-6) in PJI following TEA were found.

While joint aspiration as a diagnostic tool in TEA has not been extensively studied, its value has been extensively proven in hip and knee arthroplasty cases. While joint aspiration is useful as a rule-in test (purulence around the joint, positive culture), a negative result cannot exclude an underlying PJI following TEA [74]. Elevated synovial fluid white blood cell count, especially with a high percentage of polymorphonuclear neutrophils, strongly suggests PJI. In cases of suspected PJI, joint aspiration is recommended, as it allows different subsequent analyses including routine culture, white blood cell count, neutrophil percentage determination, and potentially molecular analyses for pathogen identification [49].

A 2013 study involving 227 procedures was conducted to explore intraoperative histology and compare it to the gold standard of intraoperative cultures [1]. The results revealed that histology indicated acute inflammation in 33 procedures (14.5%), whereas cultures tested positive in 39 procedures (17.2%). The study found intraoperative histology to be accurate in 85.9% of cases, with a sensitivity of 51.3% and a specificity of 93.1%. While intraoperative histology in revision elbow arthroplasty exhibits high specificity and negative predictive value, it demonstrates lower sensitivity and positive predictive value for PJI. The combination with other diagnostic methods is necessary to ensure an accurate PJI diagnosis.

Biofilm sonication of removed implants in revision TEA showed no statistically significant diagnostic advantage compared to tissue culture in a study from 2011 including 36 patients [72]. Based on this study, in 2018, expert recommendations were published against the routine use of sonication for explanted elbow prosthesis components. However, the severely limited data compared to hip and knee PJI cases was criticized [49]. A more recent study conducted by the group led by Robin Patel presented different results in a larger cohort. In a retrospective analysis of 112 sonicate fluid cultures and tissue cultures from patients who underwent TEA revision between 2007 and 2019, the study identified 49 PJI cases and 63 aseptic cases. The sensitivity of sonicate fluid culture was 76%, surpassing the 63% sensitivity of tissue culture alone. When combined with tissue culture, sonicate fluid culture demonstrated an even higher sensitivity of 84%, indicating an improved microbiologic diagnosis of PJI after TEA using sonication [15].

### 22.3.4 Treatment

#### 22.3.4.1 Implant Retention

No randomized, controlled trials or prospective studies have been conducted regarding the surgical management of PJI after TEA. The debate over which procedure effectively eliminates the infection, while also yielding improved functional outcomes and reduced complications, remains ongoing. The treatment options include DAIR, one-stage exchange, two-stage exchange, and various salvage procedures. For optimal infection eradication rates, functional outcomes, and patient quality of life, choosing the right therapy for the right patient is crucial.

A DAIR procedure can be performed if:

1. Biofilm has not yet reached its mature form.

The duration of this time window, starting with the onset of clinical symptoms, is currently being discussed. The authors recommend a maximum of 4 weeks, where each day of treatment delay shows a trend towards worse outcomes [69].

2. Soft tissue coverage intact, no sinus tract present.
3. Targeted biofilm-active antibiotics available.

A DAIR procedure, even though it may appear straightforward, should be conducted by an experienced team for optimal results. If all the abovementioned criteria are met and a radical debridement is performed, infection eradication rates range between 11.1% and 85.7% (mean 57.7%) [37]. DAIR procedures in PJI cases caused by S. epidermidis seem to have less favourable outcomes in some published papers, however, further research is necessary on this topic [74]. A small cohort series with 26 included cases investigated the infection eradication rate after DAIR and the reasons for failure. The DAIR procedure was successful in nine cases (35%) with a median time to failure of 43 days. All DAIR procedures performed with an existing sinus tract or negative cultures failed. Short symptom duration and monomicrobial infections showed a trend towards a better outcome without statistical significance [69].

#### 22.3.4.2 One-Stage Revision Arthroplasty

The removal of a prosthesis and the implantation of a revision TEA in a single operation is a rarely executed procedure. This rarity is evident in a recent review article, which included a small case series of only nine cases from four different studies. Among these cases, just three papers documented instances of a single-stage exchange. Due to the limited number of cases, it is challenging to draw definitive conclusions about eradication rates, with an average of 66.7% and a wide range spanning from 0% to 100% [37].

#### 22.3.4.3 Two-Stage Revision Arthroplasty

Two-stage revision surgery for PJI has long been the gold standard in all PJI procedures of the upper and lower limbs. This seems slowly changing in total hip and knee replacements based on recently published, excellent infection eradication rates in both, one and two-stage exchanges. Taking the favourable outcomes regarding, function, bone loss, patient comfort, and cost into account, arguments in favour of one-stage exchange seem increasingly convincing [47, 68].

In contrast, the available literature on revision procedures in PJI following TEA indicates that two-stage exchange remains the undisputed gold standard. A recent review article identified 11 articles on the subject including 121 patients treated with a two-stage exchange for PJI following TEA. The mean infection eradication rate was 76% (range 44.4% to 100%). This was significantly higher compared to the infection eradication rates for the DAIR procedure, but not significantly different compared to other procedures [37].

A recent study including 52 elbows undergoing two-stage exchange for PJI following TEA reports an infection eradication rate of 69% at a mean follow-up of 6 years. The risk for treatment failure, determined as recurrent infection, was 3.3 times higher in elbows with residual bone cement (p = 0.04), and 3.5 times higher in PJI cases due to *Staphylococcus epidermidis* (p = 0.06) [34].

#### 22.3.4.4 Salvage Procedures

Resection arthroplasty, arthrodesis/fusion and antibiotic suppression are considered possible salvage procedures in cases where a complete PJI eradication cannot be achieved. Currently, there is very limited data available in the literature to support a treatment recommendation.

In cases of extensive bone loss, a resection arthroplasty with or without a temporary spacer may be considered. A study including 49 elbows reported frequently encountered complications comprised of infections in 24 elbows (47%), intraoperative fractures in eighteen (35%), and lasting nerve damage in nine elbows (18%). Improved stability post-resection demonstrated a significant association with higher long-term Mayo Elbow Performance Scores ($p < 0.05$) [79]. A different study presented the results of resection arthroplasty in ten elbows belonging to nine patients, with an average follow-up duration of 52 months. One elbow had to be re-revised due to recurrent infection. The mean Disabilities of the Arm, Shoulder, and Hand (DASH) score changed significantly from 46.5 (range, 29–67) preoperatively to 53.0 (range, 33–65) at the last follow-up. The authors considered the procedure suitable for low-demand patients where both columns of the distal humerus can be retained during implant removal [55].

Generally, an elbow arthrodesis leads to poor functional results due to the inability to compensate for shoulder motion [43]. A case series involving four patients who underwent arthrodesis following the failure of staged reimplantation for infection at the site of a total elbow arthroplasty showed discouraging results. Despite thorough debridement and the use of an antibiotic cement spacer, none of the four elbows achieved bone healing after a minimum follow-up of 12 months [45].

If further surgery is technically not possible or not feasible due to the patient's health condition, an antibiotic suppression therapy may be employed. However, there is not enough data available to justify specific therapy recommendations in PJI following TEA.

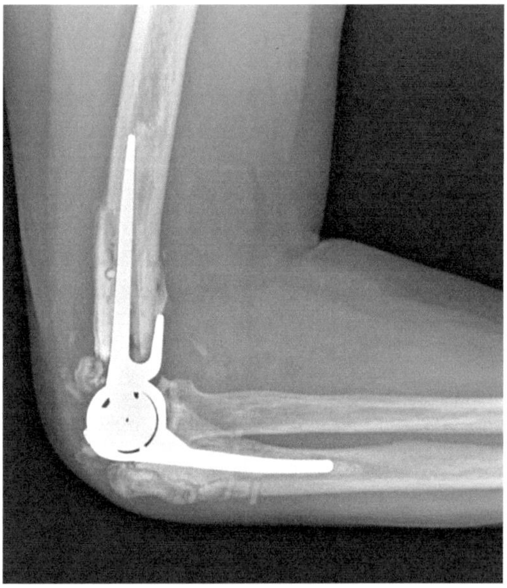

2011/1 elbow prosthesis (septic loosening and humeral periprosthetic fracture)

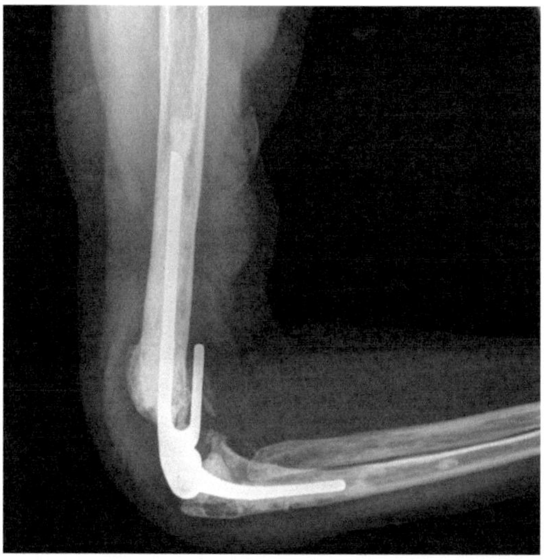

2012/2 Coonrad morrey total elbow prosthesis

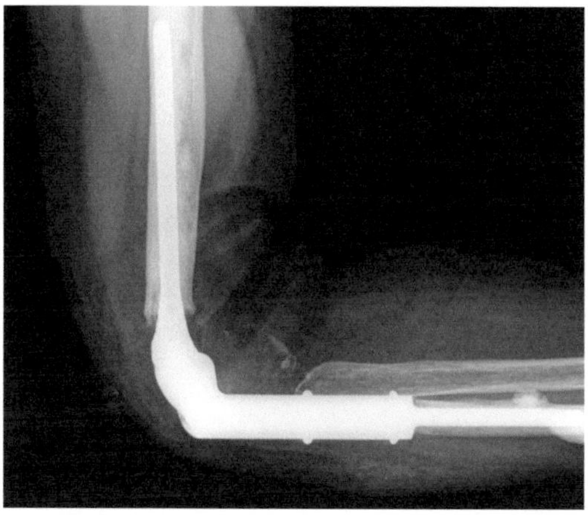

2014/9 proximal Ulna

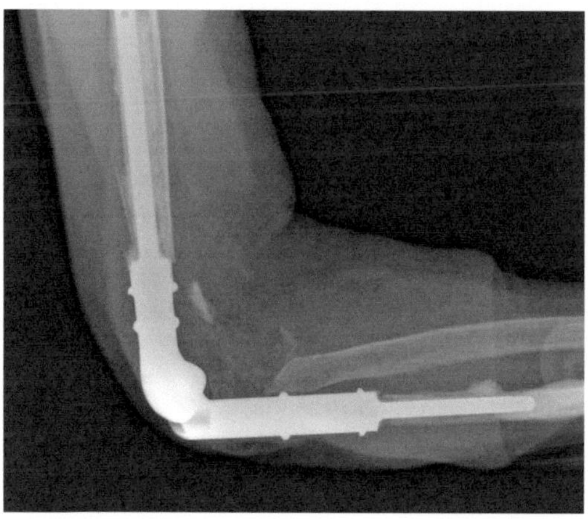

2021/11 total elbow prosthesis

## References


1. Ahmadi S, Lawrence TM, Morrey BF, Sanchez-Sotelo J. The value of intraoperative histology in predicting infection in patients undergoing revision elbow arthroplasty. J Bone Joint Surg Am. 2013;95(21):1976.
2. Ahsan ZS, Somerson JS, Matsen FA 3rd. Characterizing the Propionibacterium load in revision shoulder arthroplasty: a study of 137 culture-positive cases. J Bone Joint Surg Am. 2017;99(2):150.
3. Anakwenze O, Fokin A, Chocas M, Dillon MT, Navarro RA, Yian EH, Singh A. Complications in total shoulder and reverse total shoulder arthroplasty by body mass index. J Shoulder Elb Surg. 2017;26(7):1230.
4. Bohsali KIBA, Wirth MA. Complications of shoulder arthroplasty. J Bone Joint Surg Am. 2017;99(3):256.
5. Bonnevialle N, Dauzères F, Toulemonde J, Elia F, Laffosse JM, Mansat P. Periprosthetic shoulder infection: an overview. EFORT Open Rev. 2017;2(4):104.
6. Contreras ES, Frantz TL, Bishop JY, Cvetanovich GL. Periprosthetic infection after reverse shoulder arthroplasty: a review. Curr Rev Musculoskelet Med. 2020;13(6):757.
7. Cooper ME, Trivedi NN, Sivasundaram L, Karns MR, Voos JE, Gillespie RJ. Diagnosis and Management of Periprosthetic Joint Infection after Shoulder Arthroplasty. JBJS Rev. 2019;7(7):e3.
8. Day JS, Lau E, Ong KL, Williams GR, Ramsey ML, Kurtz SM. Prevalence and projections of total shoulder and elbow arthroplasty in the United States to 2015. J Shoulder Elb Surg. 2010;19(8):1115.
9. Deore VTGE, Monga P. Shoulder arthroplasty—past, present and future. J Arthrosc Joint Surg. 2018;5(1):3–8.
10. Dodson CC, Craig EV, Cordasco FA, Dines DM, Dines JS, Dicarlo E, Brause BD, Warren RF. Propionibacterium acnes infection after shoulder arthroplasty: a diagnostic challenge. J Shoulder Elb Surg. 2010;19(2):303.
11. Egglestone A, Ingoe H, Rees J, Thomas M, Jeavons R, Rangan A. Scoping review: diagnosis and management of periprosthetic joint infection in shoulder arthroplasty. Shoulder Elb. 2019;11(3):167.
12. Everhart JSBJ, Barlow JD. Medical comorbidities and perioperative allogeneic red blood cell transfusion are risk factors for surgical site infection after shoulder arthroplasty. J Shoulder Elb Surg. 2017;26(11):1922.
13. Faria G, Flood C, Muhammed AR, Narang A, Masood Q, Bakti N, Singh B. Prosthetic joint infections of the shoulder: a review of the recent literature. J Orthop. 2022;36:106–13.
14. Fehringer EV, Mikuls TR, Michaud KD, Henderson WG, O'Dell JR. Shoulder arthroplasties have fewer complications than hip or knee arthroplasties in US veterans. Clin Orthop Relat Res. 2010;468(3):717.
15. Flurin L, Greenwood-Quaintance KE, Esper RN, Sanchez-Sotelo J, Patel R. Sonication improves microbiologic diagnosis of periprosthetic elbow infection. J Shoulder Elb Surg. 2021;30(8):1741.

16. Frangiamore SJ, Saleh A, Grosso MJ, Alolabi B, Bauer TW, Iannotti JP, Ricchetti ET. Early versus late culture growth of Propionibacterium acnes in revision shoulder arthroplasty. J Bone Joint Surg Am. 2015;97(14):1149.
17. Garrigues GE, Zmistowski B, Cooper AM, Green A. Proceedings from the 2018 international consensus meeting on orthopedic infections: rationale and methods of the shoulder subgroup. J Shoulder Elb Surg. 2019;28(6S):S4.
18. Garrigues GE, Zmistowski B, Cooper AM, Green A, ICM Shoulder Group. Proceedings from the 2018 international consensus meeting on orthopedic infections: evaluation of periprosthetic shoulder infection. J Shoulder Elb Surg. 2019;28(6S):S4.
19. Garrigues GE, Zmistowski B, Cooper AM, Green A, ICM Shoulder Group. Proceedings from the 2018 international consensus meeting on orthopedic infections: management of periprosthetic shoulder infection. J Shoulder Elb Surg. 2019;28(6S):S4.
20. Garrigues GE, Zmistowski B, Cooper AM, Green A, ICM Shoulder Group. Proceedings from the 2018 international consensus meeting on orthopedic infections: prevention of periprosthetic shoulder infection. J Shoulder Elb Surg. 2019;28(6S):S4.
21. Garrigues GE, Zmistowski B, Cooper AM, Green A, ICM Shoulder Group. Proceedings from the 2018 international consensus meeting on orthopedic infections: the definition of periprosthetic shoulder infection. J Shoulder Elb Surg. 2019;28(6, Supplement):S8–S12.
22. George DA, Volpin A, Scarponi S, Haddad FS, Romanò CL. Does exchange arthroplasty of an infected shoulder prosthesis provide better eradication rate and better functional outcome, compared to a permanent spacer or resection arthroplasty? A systematic review. BMC Musculoskelet Disord. 2016;17:52.
23. Griffin JW, Werner BC, Gwathmey FW, Chhabra AB. Obesity is associated with increased postoperative complications after total elbow arthroplasty. J Shoulder Elb Surg. 2015;24(10):1594.
24. Grosso MJ, Frangiamore SJ, Yakubek G, Bauer TW, Iannotti JP, Ricchetti ET. Performance of implant sonication culture for the diagnosis of periprosthetic shoulder infection. J Shoulder Elb Surg. 2018;27(2):211.
25. Gyftopoulos S, Rosenberg ZS, Roberts CC, Bencardino JT, Appel M, Baccei SJ, Cassidy RC, Chang EY, Fox MG, Greenspan BS, Hochman MG, Jacobson JA, Mintz DN, Newman JS, Shah NA, Small KM, Weissman BN. ACR appropriateness criteria imaging after shoulder arthroplasty. J Am Coll Radiol: JACR. 2016;13(11):1324.
26. Hatta T, Werthel JD, Wagner ER, Itoi E, Steinmann SP, Cofield RH, Sperling JW. Effect of smoking on complications following primary shoulder arthroplasty. J Shoulder Elb Surg. 2017;26(1):1.
27. Hsu JE, Somerson JS, Vo KV, Matsen FA 3rd. What is a "periprosthetic shoulder infection"? A systematic review of two decades of publications. Int Orthop. 2017;41(4):813.
28. Jeon IH, Morrey BF, Anakwenze OA, Tran NV. Incidence and implications of early postoperative wound complications after total elbow arthroplasty. J Shoulder Elb Surg. 2011;20(6):857.
29. Kelly JD 2nd, HE. Positive culture rate in revision shoulder arthroplasty. Clin Orthop Relat Res. 2009;467(9):2343.
30. Kim JYRY, Rhee SM. Clinical outcomes after reverse Total shoulder arthroplasty according to primary diagnosis. Clin Orthop Surg. 2020;12(4):521.
31. Koh CK, Marsh JP, Drinković D, Walker CG, Poon PC. Propionibacterium acnes in primary shoulder arthroplasty: rates of colonization, patient risk factors, and efficacy of perioperative prophylaxis. J Shoulder Elb Surg. 2016;25(5):846.
32. Kunutsor SK, Barrett MC, Whitehouse MR, Craig RS, Lenguerrand E, Beswick AD, Blom AW. Incidence, temporal trends and potential risk factors for prosthetic joint infection after primary total shoulder and elbow replacement: systematic review and meta-analysis. J Infect. 2020;80(4):426.
33. Lenguerrand E, Whitehouse MR, Beswick AD, Kunutsor SK, Foguet P, Porter M, Blom AW, National Joint Registry for England, Wales, Northern Ireland and the Isle of Man. Risk factors associated with revision for prosthetic joint infection following knee replacement: an observational cohort study from England and Wales. Lancet Infect Dis. 2019;19(6):589–600.
34. Martinez-Catalan N, Nguyen NTV, Morrey ME, O'Driscoll SW, Sanchez-Sotelo J. Two-stage reimplantation for deep infection after total elbow arthroplasty. Shoulder Elb. 2022;14(6):668.
35. McFarland EG, Rojas J, Smalley J, Borade AU, Joseph J. Complications of antibiotic cement spacers used for shoulder infections. J Shoulder Elb Surg. 2018;27(11):1996.
36. McGoldrick E, McElvany MD, Butler-Wu S, Pottinger PS, Matsen FA 3rd. Substantial cultures of Propionibacterium can be found in apparently aseptic shoulders revised three years or more after the index arthroplasty. J Shoulder Elb Surg. 2015;24(1):31.
37. Mercurio M, Castioni D, Cosentino O, Familiari F, Iannò B, Gasparini G, Galasso O. Revision surgery for periprosthetic elbow infection: eradication rate, complications, and functional outcomes-a systematic review. Arch Orthop Trauma Surg. 2023;143(2):1117.
38. Moeini S, Rasmussen JV, Salomonsson B, Domeij-Arverud E, Fenstad AM, Hole R, Jensen SL, Brorson S. Reverse shoulder arthroplasty has a higher risk of revision due to infection than anatomical shoulder arthroplasty: 17 730 primary shoulder arthroplasties from the Nordic arthroplasty register association. Bone Joint J. 2019;101-B(6):702.
39. Mook WRGG. Diagnosis and Management of Periprosthetic Shoulder Infections. J Bone Joint Surg Am. 2014;96(11):956.

40. Morris BJ, O'Connor DP, Torres D, Elkousy HA, Gartsman GM, Edwards TB. Risk factors for periprosthetic infection after reverse shoulder arthroplasty. J Shoulder Elb Surg. 2015;24(2):161.
41. Nelson GNDD, Namdari S. Outcomes in the treatment of periprosthetic joint infection after shoulder arthroplasty: a systematic review. J Shoulder Elb Surg. 2016;25(8):1337.
42. National Joint Registry. 14th Annual report: national joint registry for England, Wales, Northern Ireland and the Isle of Man (1 April 2016–31 March 2017). 2017. http://www.njrreports.org.uk/Portals/0/PDFdownload/NJR%2014th%20Annual%20Report%202017.pdf.
43. O'Neill OR, Morrey BF, Tanaka S, An KN. Compensatory motion in the upper extremity after elbow arthrodesis. Clin Orthop Relat Res. 1992;281:89–96.
44. Ortmaier R, Resch H, Hitzl W, Mayer M, Stundner O, Tauber M. Treatment strategies for infection after reverse shoulder arthroplasty. Eur J Orthop Surg Traumatol. 2014;24(5):723–31.
45. Otto RJ, Mulieri PJ, Cottrell BJ, Mighell MA. Arthrodesis for failed total elbow arthroplasty with deep infection. J Shoulder Elb Surg. 2014;23(3):302.
46. Padegimas EM, Maltenfort M, Ramsey ML, Williams GR, Parvizi J, Namdari S. Periprosthetic shoulder infection in the United States: incidence and economic burden. J Shoulder Elb Surg. 2015;24(5):741.
47. Pangaud COM, Argenson JN. Outcome of single-stage versus two-stage exchange for revision knee arthroplasty for chronic periprosthetic infection. EFORT Open Rev. 2019;4(8):495.
48. Park SE, Kim JY, Cho SW, Rhee SK, Kwon SY. Complications and revision rate compared by type of total elbow arthroplasty. J Shoulder Elb Surg. 2013;22(8):1121.
49. Parvizi J, Tan TL, Goswami K, Higuera C, Della Valle C, Chen AF, et al. The 2018 definition of Periprosthetic hip and knee infection: An evidence-based and validated criteria. J Arthroplast. 2018;33(5):1309–1314.e2.
50. Parvizi J, Zmistowski B, Berbari EF, Bauer TW, Springer BD, Della Valle CJ, et al. New definition for Periprosthetic joint infection: from the workgroup of the musculoskeletal infection society. Clin Orthop Relat Res. 2011;469(11):2992.
51. Piper KE, Fernandez-Sampedro M, Steckelberg KE, Mandrekar JN, Karau MJ, Steckelberg JM, Berbari EF, Osmon DR, Hanssen AD, Lewallen DG, Cofield RH, Sperling JW, Sanchez-Sotelo J, Huddleston PM, Dekutoski MB, Yaszemski M, Currier B, Patel R. C-reactive protein, erythrocyte sedimentation rate and orthopedic implant infection. PLoS One. 2010;5(2):e9358.
52. Pope D, Scaife SL, Tzeng TH, Vasdev S, Saleh KJ. Impact of diabetes on early postoperative outcomes after total elbow arthroplasty. J Shoulder Elb Surg. 2015;24(3):348.
53. Pottinger P, Butler-Wu S, Neradilek MB, Merritt A, Bertelsen A, Jette JL, Warme WJ, Matsen FA 3rd. Prognostic factors for bacterial cultures positive for Propionibacterium acnes and other organisms in a large series of revision shoulder arthroplasties performed for stiffness, pain, or loosening. J Bone Joint Surg Am. 2012;94(22):2075.
54. Prkic A, Welsink C, The B, van den Bekerom MPJ, Eygendaal D. Why does total elbow arthroplasty fail today? A systematic review of recent literature. Arch Orthop Trauma Surg. 2017;137(6):761.
55. Rhee YG, Cho NS, Park JG, Song JH. Resection arthroplasty for periprosthetic infection after total elbow arthroplasty. J Shoulder Elb Surg. 2016;25(1):105.
56. Richards J, Inacio MC, Beckett M, Navarro RA, Singh A, Dillon MT, Sodl JF, Yian EH. Patient and procedure-specific risk factors for deep infection after primary shoulder arthroplasty. Clin Orthop Relat Res. 2014;472(9):2809.
57. Rispoli DM, Sperling JW, Athwal GS, Schleck CD, Cofield RH. Pain relief and functional results after resection arthroplasty of the shoulder. J Bone Joint Surg Br. 2007;89(9):1184.
58. Romanò CL, Borens O, Monti L, Meani E, Stuyck J. What treatment for periprosthetic shoulder infection? Results from a multicentre retrospective series. Int Orthop. 2012;36(5):1011.
59. Saltzman MD, Marecek GS, Edwards SL, Kalainov DM. Infection after shoulder surgery. J Am Acad Orthop Surg. 2011;19(4):208.
60. Schairer WW, Nwachukwu BU, Lyman S, Craig EV, Gulotta LV. National utilization of reverse total shoulder arthroplasty in the United States. J Shoulder Elb Surg. 2015;24(1):91.
61. Shah SS, Roche AM, Sullivan SW, Gaal BT, Dalton S, Sharma A, King JJ, Grawe BM, Namdari S, Lawler M, Helmkamp J, Garrigues GE, Wright TW, Schoch BS, Flik K, Otto RJ, Jones R, Jawa A, McCann P, Abboud J, Horneff G, Ross G, Friedman R, Ricchetti ET, Boardman D, Tashjian RZ, Gulotta LV. The modern reverse shoulder arthroplasty and an updated systematic review for each complication: part I. JSES Int. 2020;4(4):929.
62. Singh JA, Sperling JW, Schleck C, Harmsen W, Cofield RH. Periprosthetic infections after shoulder hemiarthroplasty. J Shoulder Elb Surg. 2012;21(10):1304.
63. Singh JA, Sperling JW, Schleck C, Harmsen WS, Cofield RH. Periprosthetic infections after total shoulder arthroplasty: a 33-year perspective. J Shoulder Elb Surg. 2012;21(11):1534.
64. Smucny M, Menendez ME, Ring D, Feeley BT, Zhang AL. Inpatient surgical site infection after shoulder arthroplasty. J Shoulder Elb Surg. 2015;24(5):747.
65. Somerson JS, Boylan MR, Hug KT, Naziri Q, Paulino CB, Huang JI. Risk factors associated with periprosthetic joint infection after total elbow arthroplasty. Shoulder Elb. 2019;11(2):116.
66. Somerson JS, Morrey ME, Sanchez-Sotelo J, Morrey BF. Diagnosis and Management of

Periprosthetic Elbow Infection. J Bone Joint Surg Am. 2015;97(23):1962.
67. Sperling JW, Kozak TK, Hanssen AD, Cofield RH. Infection after shoulder arthroplasty. Clin Orthop Relat Res. 2001;382:206.
68. Svensson K, Rolfson O, Kärrholm J, Mohaddes M. Similar risk of re-revision in patients after one- or two-stage surgical revision of infected Total hip arthroplasty: an analysis of revisions in the Swedish hip arthroplasty register 1979–2015. J Clin Med. 2019;8(4):485.
69. Tai DBG, Hanson S, Brennan P, Suh GA, Esper RN, Sanchez-Sotelo J. Outcomes and risk factors for failure after débridement, antibiotics, and implant retention for elbow periprosthetic joint infection. J Shoulder Elb Surg. 2023;32(3):475.
70. Topolski MS, Chin PY, Sperling JW, Cofield RH. Revision shoulder arthroplasty with positive intraoperative cultures: the value of preoperative studies and intraoperative histology. J Shoulder Elb Surg. 2006;15(4):402.
71. Trappey GJ 4th, O'Connor DP, Edwards TB. What are the instability and infection rates after reverse shoulder arthroplasty? Clin Orthop Relat Res. 2011;469(9):2505.
72. Vergidis P, Greenwood-Quaintance KE, Sanchez-Sotelo J, Morrey BF, Steinmann SP, Karau MJ, Osmon DR, Mandrekar JN, Steckelberg JM, Patel R. Implant sonication for the diagnosis of prosthetic elbow infection. J Shoulder Elb Surg. 2011;20(8):1275.
73. Wainwright TW, Gill M, McDonald DA, Middleton RG, Reed M, Sahota O, et al. Consensus statement for perioperative care in total hip replacement and total knee replacement surgery: enhanced recovery after surgery (ERAS(®)) society recommendations. Acta Orthop. 2020;91(1):3–19.
74. Watts AC, Duckworth AD, Trail IA, Rees J, Thomas M, Rangan A. Scoping review: diagnosis and management of periprosthetic joint infection in elbow arthroplasty. Shoulder Elb. 2019;11(4):282.
75. Welsink CL, Lambers KTA, van Deurzen DFP, Eygendaal D, van den Bekerom MPJ. Total elbow arthroplasty: a systematic review. JBJS Rev. 2017;5(7):e4.
76. Werner BC, Cancienne JM, Burrus MT, Griffin JW, Gwathmey FW, Brockmeier SF. The timing of elective shoulder surgery after shoulder injection affects postoperative infection risk in Medicare patients. J Shoulder Elb Surg. 2016;25(3):390.
77. Werthel JD, Hatta T, Schoch B, Cofield R, Sperling JW, Elhassan BT. Is previous nonarthroplasty surgery a risk factor for periprosthetic infection in primary shoulder arthroplasty? J Shoulder Elb Surg. 2017;26(4):635.
78. Wolfe SW, Figgie MP, Inglis AE, Bohn WW, Ranawat CS. Management of infection about total elbow prostheses. J Bone Joint Surg Am. 1990;72(2):198–212.
79. Zarkadas PC, Cass B, Throckmorton T, Adams R, Sanchez-Sotelo J, Morrey BF. Long-term outcome of resection arthroplasty for the failed total elbow arthroplasty. J Bone Joint Surg Am. 2010;92(15):2576.
80. Zhou H, Orvets ND, Merlin G, Shaw J, Dines JS, Price MD, Eichinger JK, Li X. Total elbow arthroplasty in the United States: evaluation of cost, patient demographics, and complication rates. Orthop Rev. 2016;8(1):6113.
81. Zmistowski B, Della Valle C, Bauer TW, Malizos KN, Alavi A, Bedair H, Booth RE, Choong P, Deirmengian C, Ehrlich GD, Gambir A, Huang R, Kissin Y, Kobayashi H, Kobayashi N, Krenn V, Lorenzo D, Marston SB, Meermans G, Perez J, Ploegmakers JJ, Rosenberg A, Simpfendorfer C, Thomas P, Tohtz S, Villafuerte JA, Wahl P, Wagenaar FC, Witzo E. Diagnosis of periprosthetic joint infection. J Arthroplast. 2014;29(2 Suppl):77–83.
82. Zumstein MA, Pinedo M, Old J, Boileau P. Problems, complications, reoperations, and revisions in reverse total shoulder arthroplasty: a systematic review. J Shoulder Elb Surg. 2011;20(1):146.

# Periprosthetic Joint Infection in Megaprostheses

# 23

Andrea Angelini, Elisa Pala, Giulia Trovarelli, Mariachiara Cerchiaro, Elisa Pagliarini, Alessia Fiumini, and Pietro Ruggieri

## 23.1 Introduction

Treatment of malignant bone tumors has always represented a significant challenge for orthopedic surgeons, which is why the exploration of innovative approaches has been necessary. In the past, amputation was the primary method employed to eradicate cancerous tissue, although with considerable physical and psychological repercussions for patients [1]. The complete removal of the affected limb not only impacted mobility and functionality but also had far-reaching consequences on overall quality of life [2]. With the evolution of medical practices, amputation has gradually taken a backseat, and limb-sparing surgeries have made a gain in both acceptance and use. This paradigm shift can be attributed to several factors, including advancements in imaging studies, the upgrade in adjuvant therapies, a more comprehensive understanding of tumor biology, and the intricacies of tumor–host interactions [3]. Improvements in surgical techniques and prosthetic technologies have also contributed to the growing popularity of limb-sparing surgeries. Surgeons now have access to a wide range of innovative implants and prostheses that not only restore functionality but also enable patients to maintain their mobility and engage in regular activities with minimal restrictions [2–4]. Megaprosthetic reconstruction has become a viable option in approximately 80–85% of cases [1–2]. This surgical technique offers numerous benefits, including early skeletal stability, accelerated rehabilitation, and improved functional outcomes [2].

Nevertheless, it is important to acknowledge that the reported complication rate following the implantation of tumor prostheses is significantly higher compared to conventional total joint arthroplasties, with a range of 5–10 times higher [1]. These complications can be categorized as either biological failures, such as infections, aseptic loosening, and wound/soft tissue breakdowns, or mechanical failures, such as implant breakages and instability [4–5]. Unfortunately, most of these complications necessitate additional procedures, and in many cases, revision of the implants becomes necessary. Therefore, while limb salvage surgery with megaprosthesis or allograft reconstruction has shown promising results in terms of improved survival rates and patient satisfaction, it is crucial to address and manage the associated complications effectively to ensure optimal outcomes [5]. Infection is one of the most frequently observed complications that arise after the initial procedure in the

A. Angelini · E. Pala · G. Trovarelli · M. Cerchiaro · E. Pagliarini · A. Fiumini · P. Ruggieri (✉)
Department of Orthopedics and Orthopedic Oncology, University of Padova, Padova, Italy
e-mail: andrea.angelini@unipd.it; elisa.pala@unipd.it; giulia.trovarelli@unipd.it; mariachiara.cerchiaro@unipd.it; elisa.pagliarini@aopd.veneto.it; pietro.ruggieri@unipd.it



P. Ruggieri et al. (eds.), *Bone and Joint Infections*, https://doi.org/10.1007/978-3-031-96383-4_23

implantation of tumor prostheses, accounting for 8% to 15% [1, 6]. However, the risk of infection escalates significantly following revision surgeries, with rates soaring up to 60% [6–7].

Interestingly, the infection rate remains fairly consistent across various limb-salvage reconstruction techniques, and this suggests that the risk of infection is not influenced by the specific method employed for reconstructing the affected limb [8]. However, it is disconcerting to note that infection of tumor prostheses can lead to the necessity of subsequent amputation, with a risk that spans a wide range, varying from 23.5% to a staggering 87% [6–8]. This highlights the severe consequences that can arise from an infection in the implantation of tumor prostheses and underscores the importance of preventing and managing infections effectively in this procedure. In this chapter, all the aspects related to periprosthetic joint infection (PJI) in megaprostheses will be discussed.

## 23.2 Epidemiology

The infection rate following megaprosthetic reconstruction can vary widely. On average, the overall rate of PJIs after the initial surgery is approximately 10%, but this rate significantly increases to 43–60% after revision surgeries [1, 9–11]. Tumor prostheses are associated with a higher risk of infection in comparison to conventional arthroplasties due to various factors. First, the reconstructive procedures for tumor prostheses are more complex, involving extensive tissue dissection which results in larger bone and soft tissue defects [12]. These larger defects provide a greater opportunity for bacterial colonization and subsequent infection. When analyzing infection rates in relation to specific diagnoses, it has been found that sarcomas exhibit the highest infection rate, reaching 21.7% [11]. This rate surpasses those observed in cases of metastatic or non-metastatic diseases [11]. Interestingly, the highest infection rates are often observed after the resection of chondrosarcomas in comparison to other pelvic tumors [11, 13–15]. This could be attributed to factors such as the large tumor volume and frequent involvement of the acetabulum, which subsequently leads to increased operating time during resection.

The challenges associated with prosthetic reconstruction following the resection of a bone tumor in the proximal tibia are worth noting. The issue of infection after prosthetic replacement following tumor resection is directly related to the difficulties encountered in achieving sufficient soft-tissue coverage [5, 11, 16]. Specifically, patients who undergo proximal tibia replacements are at a significantly higher risk of experiencing PJIs, with reported infection rates of 31% prior to the implementation of the gastrocnemius flap procedure, which decreased the rate to 19.7% [5, 16]. In contrast, proximal femur replacements demonstrate infection rates of only 8% [5]. Larger sizes of tumor implants also contribute because of the larger surface area that provides a wider area for bacterial adhesion and the formation of biofilms, which can further enhance the likelihood of infection [12]. Moreover, the complexity of tumor prosthesis surgery often leads to longer durations and exposure times of surgery.

Patients undergoing megaprostethic implants also tend to have a higher number of previous surgeries. Multiple surgeries can create scar tissue and compromise tissue integrity, making it more difficult for the body to defend against infections. Furthermore, poor nutritional status and immunosuppression commonly found in patients undergoing tumor prosthesis surgery can compromise the immune system's ability to fight off infections [11].

## 23.3 Pathophysiology

The primary cause of PJIs is direct inoculation during surgery or through the spread of infection from a distant source through the bloodstream. All prosthetic implants are susceptible to hematogenous seeding, especially during the initial years following surgery when the surrounding periprosthetic tissues have a high vascularity, which increases the risk of infection. Infections associated with prosthetic joints are typically caused by microbes that grow in biofilms [12,

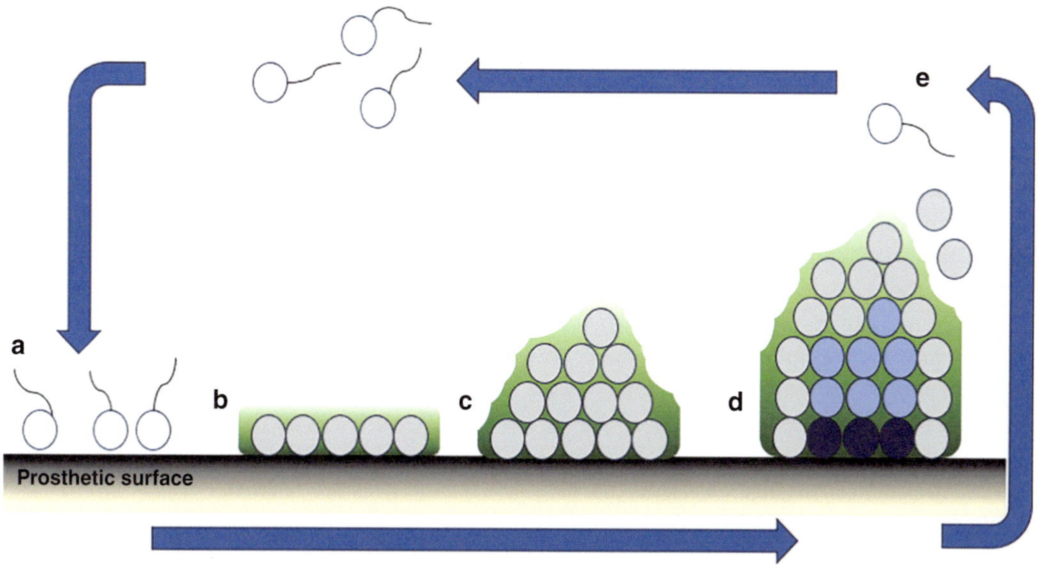


**Fig. 23.1** Schematic drawing about microbial surface colonization shows the main stages in surface attachment and biofilm formation. (**a**) Adsorption, (**b**) irreversible attachment and biofilm formation, (**c**) growth and division, (**d**) mature macrocolony, and (**e**) Dispersion White circles: bacteria in planktonic phase; Grey circles: bacteria producing polymeric matrix; Light blue circles: sessile resistant core; Dark blue circles: persistent cells.

17]. Biofilms are complex communities of microorganisms enclosed in a polymeric matrix, resembling multicellular organisms, in which microorganisms exhibit structural and functional heterogeneity [17–18]. A fully formed biofilm is composed of three layers (Fig. 23.1). The first layer, known as the linking film, consists of glycoproteins and exopolysaccharides secreted by bacteria [18]. This adhesive layer binds the entire biofilm to the surface of tissues or biomaterials. The second layer, called the base film, is a compact assembly of microorganisms responsible for secreting and maintaining the linking film [18]. Finally, the third layer, known as the surface film, exists on the outer side of the biofilm, providing a platform for the emergence and spread of free-floating organisms [17–18].

The importance of biofilms in promoting bacterial infections has been attributed to several factors. High microbial density triggers the release of cell-to-cell signaling molecules (autoinducers, AIs) in sufficient volume to promote the alteration in genetic expression linked to changes in the cell envelope and various proteins [17, 19]. This mechanism known as *quorum sensing* renders bacteria more resilient to current antibiotics [20–21]. Furthermore, the growth rates of bacteria within biofilms often slow down and this contributes to their increased resistance to antimicrobial agents [19]. The slower growth of bacteria also results in a deeper localization within the biofilm, making it challenging for antibiotics to reach and eliminate them effectively. Consequently, bacteria residing within biofilms can withstand concentrations of antimicrobials that are 1000–15,000 times higher than those required to eradicate planktonic bacteria of the same species [19–20].

## 23.4 Etiology

Infections in tumor prostheses are associated with different species of bacteria. Among these, Aerobic gram-positive bacteria, especially Staphylococcus aureus, are responsible for around 82% of cases, making them the most prevalent culprits [1, 19, 22]. This bacteria reigns as the top pathogen linked to tutor prosthesis infections and it typically colonizes implants through hematogenous spread, originating from distant skin or soft tissue infections. Other pathogens like Streptococcus pneumoniae, Enterobacteriaceae species (including Salmonella, Bacteroides, and *S. Gallolyticus*), *Escherichia coli*, *Klebsiella species*, and Viridans Streptococci can also colonize implants through hematogenous spread [1]. These infections may stem from respiratory tract infections, gastrointestinal tract infections, urinary tract infections, or dental procedures, respectively.

Among the coagulase-negative *Staphylococcus* (CoNS) species, *S. Epidermidis* is the most common pathogen causing PJIs and with *Staphylococcus lugdunensis* are part of the normal skin flora in the perineum and hip regions [1, 21–22]. *Staphylococcus lugdunensis* has the ability to mutate under stressful conditions, leading to the formation of genetically modified small-colony variants (SCVs) [21]. The pathogenicity of *S. lugdunensis* is similar to that of *S. aureus*, making it a significant pathogen in periprosthetic infections. Additionally, Group-D Streptococcus species, Enterobacteriaceae species, Enterococcus species, *Pseudomonas aeruginosa*, and various anaerobic species are frequently implicated in these infections [1, 22]. In approximately 25% of cases, multi-pathogen infections are observed in tumor prosthesis infections. The most common pair of pathogens in these cases are CoNS and Enterococcus species [19–23].

The management and treatment of tumor prosthesis infections typically involve a combination of surgical intervention, such as implant removal or debridement, and antibiotic therapy. The choice of antibiotics is usually based on the suspected pathogens and their antibiotic susceptibility patterns [22]. However, the overall success of treatment is influenced by various factors, including the extent of infection, the patient's immune response, and the ability to effectively eradicate the biofilm-associated bacteria. It is also important to note that there is no specific correlation between the presence of certain pathogens and favorable treatment outcomes.

## 23.5 Classifications

The most common approach to classify PJIs in megaprostheses is based on the time of onset of symptoms after implantation. This classification system categorizes infections into three main groups: early, delayed, and late-onset infections.

- Early-onset infections: these infections typically occur within 4 weeks after implantation. They are often related to perioperative contamination during surgery or hematogenous spread of bacteria. Early-onset infections are commonly caused by more virulent organisms, such as *Staphylococcus aureus*, and often have an abrupt onset of clinical symptoms. If left untreated, early infections can progress to chronic infections characterized by the presence of sinuses, bacteremia, and sepsis [9, 24].
- Delayed onset infections: these infections occur between 1and 24 months after implantation. They are usually associated with low-grade infections, often caused by organisms with lower virulence, such as Coagulase-negative Staphylococci [9]. Delayed onset infections can result from a variety of factors, including persistent contamination, biofilm formation, or hematogenous spread. These infections may present with more subtle signs, such as persistent chronic inflammation and postoperative discomfort.
- Late-onset infections: these infections develop more than 24 months after implantation and are often associated with hematogenous spread from a distant site or contiguous spread from a nearby infected focus. Late-onset infections are commonly caused by low-virulence organisms as well as by the reactivation of dormant bacteria [10].

This classification provides a practical approach to understanding the timeline and potential causes of PJIs. It helps guide clinical management decisions, such as the choice and duration of antibiotic therapy and the need for surgical intervention. It is important to note that this classification system is not comprehensive and may not capture all possible variations and complexities of PJIs. Therefore, it is often used in combination with other classification systems, such as the PJI-TNM classification, to provide a more holistic understanding of the infection [25]. This system is inspired by the conventional TNM oncologic score for malignant tumors, considering that there are certain similarities between tumors and PJIs such as the need for wide removal of affected tissue. Just as tumors require the removal of malignant cells to prevent further spread, PJIs necessitate the removal of infected tissue to eradicate the infection and promote healing [25]. In 2020 Alt and coworkers proposed a standardized framework for evaluating and classifying PIJs, the PJI-TNM classification (Table 23.1) [25] This system builds upon the principles of the TNM system in oncology and incorporates crucial parameters specific to periprosthetic joint infections such as the type of implant, surrounding soft tissue conditions, the causative microorganism, and the host [25–26]. This categorization system utilizes three significant letters: T, N, and M. 'T' represents the local situation of the tissue and the indwelling implant. This includes factors such as the extent of tissue involvement and the severity of implant-related complications. 'N' stands for the causative non-human bacterial and/or fungal organisms, indicating the type and virulence of the infecting microorganism. Lastly, 'M' represents the morbidity of the patient, taking into consideration factors such as the patient's overall health status and the presence of comorbidities that may impact the management and outcome of the infection [25–26]. Each item is further specified by numbers indicating the severity or extent. The PJI-TNM classification system includes the name of the affected joint in front of the TNM letters to clearly indicate the body region involved. In

**Table 23.1** The PJI-TNM classification system

| T | Tissue and implant conditions | | |
|---|---|---|---|
| **T** | T0 | a | Stable standard implant without important soft tissue defect |
| | | b | Stable revision implant without important soft tissue defect |
| | T1 | a | Loosened standard implant without important soft tissue defect |
| | | b | Loosened revision implant without important soft tissue defect |
| | T2 | a | Severe soft tissue defect with standard implant |
| | | b | Severe soft tissue defect with revision implant |
| N | Non-human cells (bacteria and fungi) | | |
| **N** | N0 | a | No mature biofilm formation, directly postoperatively |
| | | b | No mature biofilm formation, late haematogeneous |
| | N1 | a | Mature biofilm formation without "difficult to treat bacteria" |
| | | b | Mature biofilm formation, with culture negative infection |
| | N2 | a | Mature biofilm formation with "difficult to treat bacteria" |
| | | b | Mature biofilm formation, with polymicrobial infection |
| | | c | Mature biofilm formation with fungi |
| M | Morbidity of the patient | | |
| **M** | M0 | | Not or only mildly compromised (CCI: 0–1)[a] |
| | M1 | | Moderately compromised patient (CCI: 2–3) |
| | M2 | | Severely compromised patient (CCI: 4–5) |
| | M3 | a | Patient refuses surgical treatment |
| | | b | Patient does not benefit from surgical treatment |
| | | c | Patient does not survive surgical treatment |
| r | Reinfection | | |
| | If the infection involves a previously infected implant, the situation is considered as "reinfection" and an "r" is put in front of the classification | | |

[a]CCI: Charlson Comorbidity Index

cases of recurrent infections, the letter 'r' is added to emphasize reinfection.

However, there are limitations to this classification system. One limitation is the use of biofilm formation maturity in the 'N' section. While it is a step forward in classifying PJIs, accurately determining the exact time differentiation between immature and mature biofilm formation is challenging with current diagnostic methods. Additionally, the complexity of the use of three letters and further sub-specification can make it more difficult to use in daily clinical practice compared to the simple differentiation between early, delayed, and late classifications [25–26].

## 23.6 Diagnosis

Early diagnosis is extremely important for the successful treatment of PJIs, especially in megaprostheses. However, the diagnosis of these infections can be quite difficult due to the wide range of symptoms that can occur and the absence of specific laboratory tests and procedures. To address these challenges, a comprehensive and multidisciplinary approach is often required. This approach typically involves the collaboration of orthopedic surgeons, infectious disease specialists, and microbiologists. By working together, these professionals can utilize a combination of different methods to establish an accurate diagnosis.

The symptoms of PJIs can vary widely and may overlap with other postoperative complications. In fact, pain, swelling, redness, warmth, and limited range of motion can also be present in aseptic loosening or other non-infectious complications [9, 12]. This overlap makes it challenging to differentiate between infectious and non-infectious causes. To confirm the diagnosis of a PJI the presence of pus, sinus discharge, or positive cultures from the affected area is required [9–10].

### 23.6.1 Lab Test

Laboratory tests play a crucial role in the diagnostic process. While there may not be specific tests for periprosthetic infections, various blood tests can help indicate the presence of inflammation or infection in the body. These tests may include a complete blood count (especially white blood cell count WBC), erythrocyte sedimentation rate (ESR), and C-reactive protein (CRP) levels [10, 12].

Considering the lack of specificity, it is crucial to interpret these results in conjunction with clinical findings. For example, during the early postoperative period (within the first 2 weeks), these markers can be elevated as part of the normal inflammatory response to surgery, whereas after the initial 2-week period, consistently high levels of CRP and WBC count become more indicative of an ongoing infection [12]. Furthermore, the conventional laboratory procedures used to detect and identify bacteria are mainly designed to detect planktonic bacteria (which are freely floating in a liquid medium), but they may not effectively identify bacteria that are present within biofilms [12, 20–21]. This limitation poses a significant challenge in identifying and diagnosing biofilm-related infections, further complicating the problem.

### 23.6.2 Imaging

Imaging studies are also commonly used to aid in the diagnosis. X-rays, magnetic resonance imaging (MRI), computed tomography (CT), ultrasonography (US), and bone scintigraphy scans can provide valuable information about the condition of the prosthesis, surrounding tissues, and potential signs of infection such as fluid collections or bone destruction [24, 27]. While simple radiographs can be useful in ruling out other causes of periprosthetic pain, they have limitations when it comes to early infection detection [27]. A series of plain radiographs taken over a period of time after implantation can demonstrate loosening of the implant and periprosthetic osteolysis, but it can also occur without an infection development [27–28]. Computed tomography (CT) offers a comprehensive evaluation of bone structures, including a detailed analysis of cortical and trabecular anatomy. The administration of intravenous contrast during a CT scan further enhances the contrast between various soft tissues, facilitating the identification and highlighting of pathological changes. Dual-energy CT is an advanced technique that can detect bone marrow edema, making it particularly valuable in the context of infection [28]. Ultrasound (US) is an invaluable diagnostic tool that offers a wealth of detailed information about the soft tissues surrounding a prosthetic joint [29]. Unlike other imaging techniques that may be hindered by metallic artifacts, the US offers clear visualization of these tissues allowing for a comprehensive examination of the painful site [27–29]. While it may not be the ideal method for evaluating the prosthesis and periprosthetic bone due to the limitations of sound beams in penetrating metal or bone, US excels in detecting joint effusion and identifying extra-articular fluid collections. In cases where it is feasible to perform aspiration or biopsy on the affected joints, it is highly recommended to do so.

MRI is widely considered the most effective imaging technique for diagnosing musculoskeletal infections [30], but while it is highly effective in diagnosing infections on native bone, its use in cases of PJIs has traditionally been limited due to susceptibility artefacts produced by metallic implants [28]. To overcome this challenge, modified and advanced MRI pulse sequences have been developed to minimize the metal artefacts between the implant components and the neighboring tissues. These pulse sequences are specifically designed to enhance the performance of the 1.5 Tesla MRI system, allowing for a substantial reduction in artefacts around metallic implants [28]. MRI with intravenous gadolinium-based contrast agents provides more anatomical detail, spatial resolution, and soft tissue contrast, allowing for accurate and precise imaging. One of the key strengths of MRI is its ability to detect pathological processes by imaging edema, which often leads to an increase in water content. This is especially valuable in identifying infectious pathologies, which can be best visualized using fluid-sensitive, fat-suppressed sequences. For more specific situations, additional sequences like diffusion-weighted imaging (DWI) and gradient echo (GRE) sequences can be employed to investigate fluid collections, and tumors and identify blood products respectively [27–29]. Despite its many advantages, MRI does have some drawbacks. Limited availability, long scanning times, and high costs can make it less accessible for some patients. Bone scintigraphy, in combination with 111In-labeled leukocytes and radiotracers such as 99mTechnetium-sulfur colloid or Gallium citrate 67 can be used to aid in the diagnosis of PJIs [31–33].

### 23.6.3 Cultures

Microbiological analysis is an essential component of the diagnostic process. This involves obtaining samples from the affected area and sending them to the laboratory for culture and sensitivity testing. This allows the healthcare team to identify the specific bacteria or other microorganisms causing the infection, as well as determine the most effective treatment options. In order to identify the specific pathogens causing PJIs, tissue cultures from multiple sites have long been regarded as the most dependable method [12, 24, 34]. However, these cultures have been found to have a sensitivity ranging from 70% to 90% and a specificity ranging from 67% to 91% [35]. Additionally, it typically takes 7–9 days to receive results from these cultures.

Joint aspiration is highly recommended for the evaluation of PJIs, as it allows for thorough histological and microbiological testing of the synovial fluid [34]. However, there are certain factors that can affect the accuracy of these tests: (1) it is important to discontinue the use of antimicrobial agents at least 14 days before surgery [34–35]; (2) it is important to understand that a negative result from joint aspiration does not necessarily rule out the presence of infection (in up to 50% of PJI cases, the infecting organism is not isolated in cultures) [35]; (3) it is also important to avoid relying solely on sinus tract cultures for diagnosis, as they have a high risk of contamination by normal skin flora, which can lead to false positive results [35].

Cultures and diagnostic tests are valuable tools in the evaluation of periprosthetic infections, but they are not foolproof. False positive results can occur due to the detection of contaminants or secondary microorganisms, as well as indirect signs of infection that may not accurately guide treatment decisions [34].

### 23.6.4 Polymerase Chain Reaction (PCR) and Next-Generation Sequencing (NGS)

There has been a growing interest in exploring faster and more accurate molecular techniques to improve the sensitivity of diagnosing PJIs. PCR is a non-culture-based method that utilizes specific oligodeoxynucleotide primers to enzymatically amplify bacterial DNA, allowing for its detection [36–38]. It requires a small volume of synovial fluid, tissue samples, or fluid from sonicated implants, and can deliver results within 5–24 h of collection. It has been found to have higher diagnostic accuracy in terms of sensitivity and specificity compared to tissue cultures [34, 38, 39]. In addition to traditional quantitative PCR, another alternative method for detecting bacterial pathogens is broad-range PCR, which targets the 16S ribosomal DNA (rDNA) [40, 41].

Metagenomic next-generation sequencing (mNGS) technology is a powerful tool that can directly detect pathogens and other functional genes in clinical samples without the need for pre-amplification of target sequences [42]. It utilizes DNA sequencing to identify a wide range of pathogens, including bacteria and fungi but reports a higher rate of false positive results [43]. Whenever possible, the best way to obtain a diagnostic material is the sonication of implants after removal and the culture of the sonication fluid [44–47].

## 23.7 Risk Factors

Identifying and understanding the key risk factors associated with infections in megaprostheses is crucial for healthcare professionals to develop effective strategies for prevention and management. By considering patient-related, disease-related, and procedure-related risk factors, healthcare professionals can optimize patient outcomes and reduce the incidence of infections in patients undergoing reconstructive surgery for tumors.

***Patient-Related Risk Factors*** Malnutrition, male gender, advanced age, diabetes mellitus, obesity, smoking, alcohol abuse, previous native joint infection, skin diseases, peripheral vascular disease, and, pre-existing joint disease (particularly rheumatoid arthritis) have been identified as significant risk factors for infections in tumor prostheses [12, 48–50]. About lab exams, lower preoperative hemoglobin and albumin levels, neutropenia [51–55], elevated C-reactive protein (CRP) levels and a decreased white blood cell count have been associated with an increased risk of infection following reconstructive surgery [1, 51, 56].

***Disease-Related Risk Factors*** Tumor site is an important predictor, with the proximal tibia, proximal femur, and pelvis being associated with a higher risk of infection [13, 16, 50, 57]. Conversely, the distal femur and proximal humerus are linked to a lower infection rate [50, 58–59]. Interestingly, periprosthetic joint infections in the knee have been found to have a worse prognosis compared to infections in other locations [1, 50, 60–62]. The connection between the tumor's metastatic spread and its histological features, along with the occurrence of infections, remains ambiguous. Several studies suggest a continuing discussion on whether primary tumors or metastatic sites are more prone to infection development. [59, 63]. Tissue damage caused by radiation therapy [20, 64–65], as well as chemotherapy-induced leukocytopenia and neutropenia [59, 66–68] are believed to increase the risk of postoperative deep infection. Patients who receive radiation therapy have an infection rate of 9.8%, compared to 20.7% in those who receive preoperative radiation therapy, and 35.3% in those who receive postoperative radiation therapy [64]. The available evidence on the link between infection rates and the time lapse between neoadjuvant therapy and prosthetic reconstructions in tumor patients is scarce. [69–72]. Currently, the decision on the timing of surgery after neoadjuvant treatment is typically based on individual hospital protocols and physician preferences. However, it is generally recommended to avoid surgery immediately after radiotherapy, and a waiting period of 4–6 weeks is often necessary to allow for the restoration of normal tissue properties [69–72].

***Procedure-Related Risk Factors*** Surgical procedures and surgical techniques performed can also affect the risk of infections in megaprostheses [73–74]. For example, an inadequate debridement of infected tissues, improper wound closure, and poor surgical technique can increase the risk of infection. Surgeons must ensure meticulous surgical technique and adhere to strict aseptic protocols to minimize the risk of any kind of complications. The association between the duration of surgery and infection risk is controversial and may vary depending on various factors, such as patient population, surgical technique, and infection prevention measures [75–79]. Moreover, the amount of blood loss during the procedure and the resulting need for blood transfusion, preoperative hospitalization for more than 48 h, or postoperative access to intensive care have been identified as potential risk factors [1]. The use of surgical drains in musculoskeletal tumor surgery is a common practice even though there is limited evidence supporting its beneficial effect and/or its link to an increased risk of infection [80–87]. Certain characteristics of the implant itself can contribute to the risk of infection. For example, prostheses with rough surfaces or those made of materials that promote bacterial adhesion can increase the risk of infection [50] whereas silver-coated prostheses have been found to have antibacterial properties that disrupt DNA synthesis and cellular membranes [88–90]. Several studies on silver-coated prostheses have shown promising results, with a significant decrease in infection rates (7,9% silver-coated prosthesis vs 11,6% uncoated ones) and a higher success rate of two-stage revision surgery for infected silver-coated prostheses compared to infected uncoated implants [87–90]. The association between infection rates and the type of fixation (cemented vs. cementless) in musculoskeletal tumor surgeries has been investigated in several studies, but the results are highly variable [48, 91–95].

***Antibiotic Prophylaxis*** The standard guidelines for antibiotic prophylaxis in total joint arthroplasty suggest a single preoperative dose of antibiotics to be administered 60 min prior to the procedure and should be discontinued within 24 h after the completion of the surgery [96–98]. In musculoskeletal oncology, it is generally recommended to administer additional doses of antibiotics during the procedure if it exceeds the half-life of the prophylactic antimicrobial agent or lasts longer than 3–4 h [97]. The selection of an antibiotic for prophylaxis during surgery is primarily determined by its spectrum of action [99]. Numerous studies have indicated that the most suitable antibiotic for perioperative prophylaxis is a first- or second-generation cephalosporin, such as cefazolin or cefuroxime, administered intravenously in a dose adjusted according to the patient's weight [100–101]. Due to their effectiveness against gram-positive bacteria that are resistant to other antibiotics, glycopeptide antibiotics like vancomycin and teicoplanin have been recommended as alternative prophylactic agents [102–103]. While methicillin-sensitive Staphylococcus aureus (MRSA) remains largely susceptible to cephalosporin antibiotics, the prevalence of MRSA infections is on the rise [104–106]. Bone cement is commonly used to secure implants. To prevent infection, antimicrobial agents are often added to the bone cement (i.e. vancomycin, gentamycin, clindamycin) [107–109].

## 23.8 Surgical Treatment

The aim of treating PJIs associated with megaprostheses is to eliminate the infection while preserving the functionality of the affected limb

[110]. Currently, there are various treatment options available, including non-operative methods such as long-term antibiotic suppression, debridement, and implant retention (DAIR), as well as surgical interventions like one- or two-stage revision arthroplasty [111]. It is still uncertain which approach is superior between the two-stage replacement, one-stage exchange, or debridement with retention since these different options have not been tested in a randomized fashion in a homogenous patient population. The choice of surgical approach relies on the surgeon's personal experience, postoperative lag, infection classification, condition of the implant and surrounding soft tissues, as well as the patient's comorbidity.

### 23.8.1 Debridement, Antibiotics, and Implant Retention (DAIR)

The approach known as DAIR is a treatment option for infected prostheses that involves several key principles. To begin with, antibiotics are withheld prior to surgery, and the joint is aspirated to identify the specific organism causing the infection [112]. The surgical procedure itself consists of surgical irrigation, debridement, antibiotic therapy, and the decision to either retain the existing implant with or without exchanging the polyethylene component [12, 112]. During debridement, various elements are removed, including hematoma, fibrous membranes, sinus tracts, as well as any devitalized bone and soft tissue [12, 110]. The DAIR treatment approach offers several advantages compared to more invasive options: (1) it is less technically demanding, resulting in lower morbidity for the patient; (2) it also allows for shorter hospital stays and better preservation of bone stock; (3) the economic burden associated with this approach is lower. However, it is important to note that DAIR is suitable only if the infection occurs within 14–28 days after the initial surgery, if it is confirmed through histopathology and microbiology, if the implants remain stable, and if the isolated pathogen is susceptible to an effective oral antibiotic [113]. When all these criteria are met, the reported rate of infection eradication following this procedure is 42.8% [113]. Intravenous antibiotics are typically administered for a period of at least 2–6 weeks following the DAIR procedure [110]. Several studies have evaluated the effectiveness of this protocol in cases of infected megaprostheses, with success rates ranging from 39% to 70% [11, 62, 113–116]. These studies have reported eradication rates of 42% with irrigation and debridement without implant exchange, 70% after a single-stage debridement with the exchange of modular components, and 62% after a two-stage revision surgery [117].

In cases where the DAIR procedure fails to eradicate the infection, alternative surgical options become necessary. The two-stage revision surgery has long been considered the "gold standard" in these cases. However, for patients with relatively healthy bone and soft tissue, no prior revision surgeries, or treatment involving effective antibiotics against biofilm-active microorganisms, a one-stage exchange would be the treatment of choice [110, 118–120].

### 23.8.2 One-Stage Revision Surgery

There is a shortage of high-quality studies examining the outcomes of single-stage revision surgery PJIs [14, 19, 61–62]. Single-stage revision treatment entails comprehensive debridement and revision of all implants simultaneously, with the aim of improving infection eradication rates. The success of resolving these infections is closely linked to the extent of soft tissue debridement and subsequent reduction in bioburden [14]. Nevertheless, the question remains as to whether it is necessary to remove and revise all implants during a one-stage revision surgery, or if some implants can be retained. In cases where complete removal of all implants is not feasible, it is recommended to thoroughly irrigate the retained implants using solutions such as povidone-iodine or chlorhexidin [121]. One of the potential advantages of one-stage reimplantation is the reduction in the waiting period for delayed reimplantation, leading to improved joint function. Additionally, it eliminates the need for a second complex procedure, which carries inherent risks and complications, including the possibility of developing a new infection. However, there is a higher risk of persistence or recurrence of the original infection if the debridement is inadequate or if the antibiotic treatment is insufficient.

This is why the decision to perform a one-stage revision surgery is typically based on the patient's characteristics and circumstances. Generally, patients with PJIs caused by unknown microbial organisms, difficult-to-treat organisms (such as multi-resistant strains), the presence of a fistula, or the need for bone reconstruction are excluded from undergoing one-stage revision surgery. In these cases, a two-stage revision surgery is preferred [122].

### 23.8.3 Two-Stage Revision Surgery

Two-stage revision surgery is widely considered the most effective treatment approach for infections in megaprostheses, with reported success rates ranging from 63% to 100% [61, 115]. During a two-stage revision surgery, the implants are initially removed and replaced with antibiotic-loaded bone cement spacers (Fig. 23.2). These

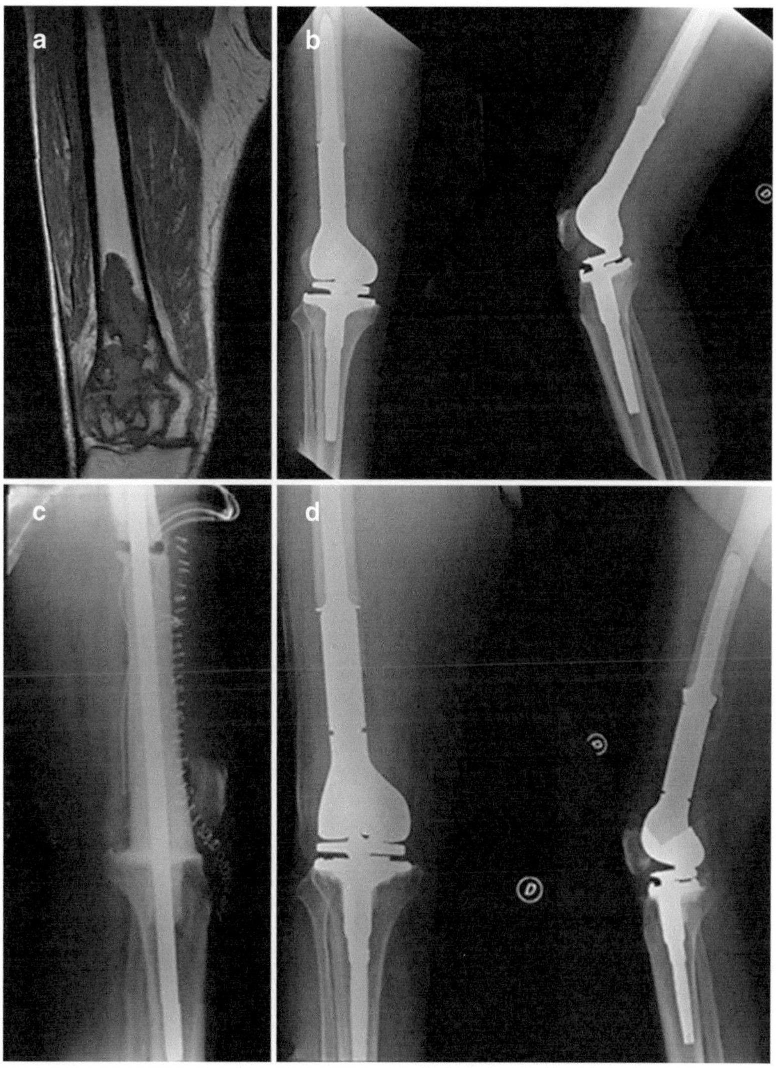

**Fig. 23.2** Chondrosarcoma of the distal femur in a 73-year-old male. (**a**) Coronal MRI shows the intramedullary extension of the disease. (**b**) Postoperative radiographs after distal femur resection and reconstruction with megaprosthesis. (**c**) Removal of the prosthesis and implantation of an antibiotic cement spacer for an early infection. (**d**) 5-year follow-up after reimplantation of similar megaprosthesis 4 months after the first revision stage

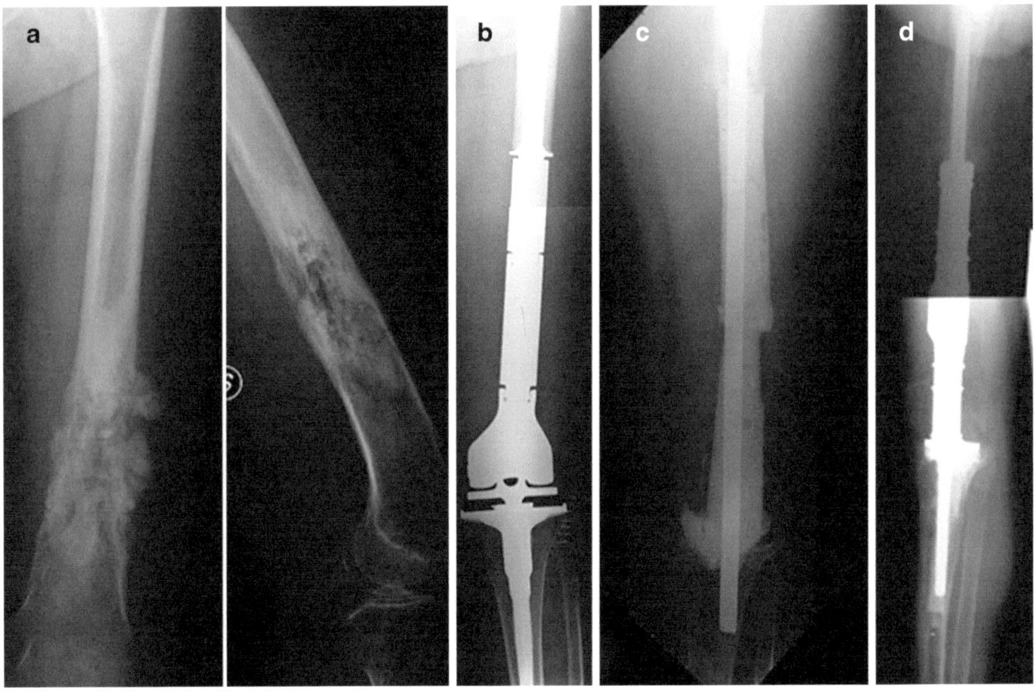


**Fig. 23.3** Osteoblastic osteosarcoma of the distal femur in a 57-year-old male. (**a**) AP and lateral radiographs show the extensive involvement of bone and soft tissue. (**b**) Postoperative radiographs after wide resection and megaprosthetic reconstruction combined with chemotherapy. (**c**) Removal of the prosthesis and implant of a vancomycin and tobramycin cement spacer after 4 months follow-up due to S. Epidermidis infection. (**d**) Modular arthrodesis with silver implant (MUTARS system, Implantcast Ltd., Buxtehude, Germany) 6 months later

spacers remain in place for a period of 2–3 months, during which systemic antibiotics are administered [123]. The choice and duration of antibiotics may vary depending on the results of microbial cultures. In the second stage, the spacers are removed and replaced with the final implants after a minimum of 2 weeks without antibiotics [61, 123]. Re-implantation is typically recommended at least 2–6 weeks after the infected prosthesis has been explanted [61], but is not always possible to preserve the joint function (Fig. 23.3). Patients who are recommended to undergo a two-stage revision surgery include those with persistent or high-grade infections, infections caused by antibiotic-resistant pathogens, or individuals who have previously undergone unsuccessful one-stage revision surgery [61, 124]. In cases where cementless modular megaprostheses are securely fixed, infected implants can be revised in two stages while retaining the anchorage stem [124]. However, the use of the two-stage revision surgery technique remains controversial due to several factors. These include the extended duration of hospital stay, increased bone loss and risk of osteoporosis resulting from lack of use, and the potential for limb shortening [125–126].

## 23.9 Conclusions

The prevention of postoperative infections in prosthetic reconstruction is crucial, particularly in tumor patients. A comprehensive and multidisciplinary approach involving orthopedic surgeons and specialists from various disciplines is essential to recognize risk factors, make a proper diagnosis, and plan the best therapeutic approach. The treatment goals include resolving the infection and preserving the functionality of the affected limb. Various treatment strategies have been employed for managing megaprosthetic infections, such as DAIR, one-stage and two-stage revision surgery. Unfortunately, in some cases, amputation becomes the final option when other treatment strategies fail. Two-stage revision surgery has exhibited superior functional outcomes and elevated success rates, making it the current gold standard for addressing chronic infections in tumor prostheses. Nonetheless, for patients harboring isolated pathogens highly susceptible to antibiotics, one-stage revision surgery could serve as a feasible alternative. This approach involves removing the infected implant and replacing it with a new prosthesis in a single surgical procedure. In some cases, implant exchange may not be necessary, depending on the severity of the infection and the effectiveness of the antibiotic treatment.

## 23.10 Declarations

**Author Contributions** Conceptualization, project administration: AA, PR; data curation and formal analysis: AA, AF; supervision: AA, PR; writing-original draft: AA, MCC, GT, EP, AF; writing-review and editing: AA, EP, PR; drawings: AA; All authors have read and agreed to the published version of the manuscript.

**Institutional Review Board Statement** Not applicable.

**Informed Consent Statement** Written informed consent was obtained from patients at the time of admission to our Institute. However, all pictures have been reported anonymized.

**Consent for Publication (Include Appropriate Statements)** We confirm that this paper, including related data, figures, and tables, has not been published previously, it is not under consideration for publication elsewhere, and, if accepted, it will not be published elsewhere in the same form, in English or in any other language, without the written consent of the publisher.

**Conflicts of Interest/Competing Interests (Include Appropriate Disclosures)** Ruggieri P is a consultant for Stryker and Exactech (not relevant to the present manuscript). The other authors declare that there are no relationships/conditions/circumstances that present a potential conflict of interest with the present manuscript.

**Availability of Data and Material (Data Transparency)** Manuscript data are embedded in the text and fully available on specific request.

**Funding** There was no external funding source in support of this study.

## References

1. Tsantes AG, Altsitzioglou P, Papadopoulos DV, Lorenzo D, Romanò CL, Benzakour T, et al. Infections of tumor prostheses: an updated review on risk factors, microbiology, diagnosis, and treatment strategies. Biology (Basel). 2023;12(2):314.
2. DiCaprio MR, Friedlaender GE. Malignant bone tumors: limb sparing versus amputation. J Am Acad Orthop Surg. 2003;11(1):25–37.
3. Haijie L, Dasen L, Tao J, Yi Y, Xiaodong T, Wei G. Implant survival and complication profiles of Endoprostheses for treating tumor around the knee in adults: a systematic review of the literature over the past 30 years. J Arthroplast. 2018;33(4):1275–1287.e3.
4. Ahlmann ER, Menendez LR, Kermani C, Gotha H. Survivorship and clinical outcome of modular endoprosthetic reconstruction for neoplastic disease of the lower limb. J Bone Joint Surg Br. 2006;88(6):790–5.
5. Henderson ER, Groundland JS, Pala E, Dennis JA, Wooten R, Cheong D, Windhager R, Kotz RI, Mercuri M, Funovics PT, Hornicek FJ, Temple HT, Ruggieri P, Letson GD. Failure mode classification for tumor endoprostheses: retrospective review of five institutions and a literature review. J Bone Joint Surg Am. 2011;93(5):418–29. https://doi.org/10.2106/JBJS.J.00834.
6. Shehadeh A, Noveau J, Malawer M, Henshaw R. Late complications and survival of endoprosthetic reconstruction after resection of bone tumors. Clin Orthop Relat Res. 2010;468(11):2885–95.
7. Gundavda MK, Katariya A, Reddy R, Agarwal MG. Fighting megaprosthetic infections: what are the chances of winning? Indian J Orthop. 2020;54(4):469–76.
8. Grimer RJ, Belthur M, Chandrasekar C, Carter SR, Tillman RM. Two-stage revision for infected endo-

prostheses used in tumor surgery. Clin Orthop Relat Res. 2002;395:193–203.
9. Morii T, Yabe H, Morioka H, Beppu Y, Chuman H, Kawai A, et al. Postoperative deep infection in tumor endoprosthesis reconstruction around the knee. J Orthop Sci. 2010;15(3):331–9.
10. Nobile M, Navone P, Domeniconi G, Della Valle A, Daolio PA, Buccino NA, et al. Surgical site infections in oncologic orthopaedic prosthetics surgery. Ann Ig. 2015;27(5):711–7.
11. Kapoor SK, Thiyam R. Management of infection following reconstruction in bone tumors. J Clin Orthop Trauma. 2015;6(4):244–51.
12. Zimmerli W, Trampuz A, Ochsner PE. Prosthetic-joint infections. N Engl J Med. 2004;351(16):1645–54.
13. Angelini A, Drago G, Trovarelli G, Calabrò T, Ruggieri P. Infection after surgical resection for pelvic bone tumors: an analysis of 270 patients from one institution. Clin Orthop Relat Res. 2014;472(1):349–59. https://doi.org/10.1007/s11999-013-3250-x.
14. Biau D, Faure F, Katsahian S, Jeanrot C, Tomeno B, Anract P. Survival of total knee replacement with a megaprosthesis after bone tumor resection. J Bone Joint Surg Am. 2006;88(6):1285–93.
15. Mavrogenis AF, Angelini A, Drago G, Merlino B, Ruggieri P. Survival analysis of patients with chondrosarcomas of the pelvis. J Surg Oncol. 2013;108(1):19–27. https://doi.org/10.1002/jso.23351.
16. Mavrogenis AF, Pala E, Angelini A, Ferraro A, Ruggieri P. Proximal tibial resections and reconstructions: clinical outcome of 225 patients. J Surg Oncol. 2013;107(4):335–42. https://doi.org/10.1002/jso.23216.
17. Chandki R, Banthia P, Banthia R. Biofilms: a microbial home. J Indian Soc Periodontol. 2011;15(2):111–4.
18. Silverstein A, Donatucci CF. Bacterial biofilms and implantable prosthetic devices. Int J Impot Res. 2003;15(S5):S150–4.
19. Jeys LM, Grimer RJ, Carter SR, Tillman RM. Periprosthetic infection in patients treated for an orthopaedic oncological condition. J Bone Joint Surg Am. 2005;87(4):842–9.
20. Rutherford ST, Bassler BL. Bacterial quorum sensing: its role in virulence and possibilities for its control. Cold Spring Harb Perspect Med. 2012;2(11):a012427.
21. Jeys LM, Grimer RJ, Carter SR, Tillman RM, Abudu A. Post operative infection and increased survival in osteosarcoma patients: are they associated? Ann Surg Oncol. 2007;14(10):2887–95.
22. Patel R. Periprosthetic joint infection. N Engl J Med. 2023;388(3):251–62.
23. Hardes J, von Eiff C, Streitbuerger A, Balke M, Budny T, Henrichs MP, et al. Reduction of periprosthetic infection with silver-coated megaprostheses in patients with bone sarcoma. J Surg Oncol. 2010;101(5):389–95.
24. Moran E, Byren I, Atkins BL. The diagnosis and management of prosthetic joint infections. J Antimicrob Chemother. 2010;65(Suppl 3):iii45–54.
25. Alt V, Rupp M, Langer M, Baumann F, Trampuz A. Can the oncology classification system be used for prosthetic joint infection?: the PJI-TNM system. Bone Joint Res. 2020;9(2):79–81.
26. Alt V, Rupp M, Langer M, Baumann F, Trampuz A. Infographic: can the oncology classification system be used for prosthetic joint infection?: the PJI-TNM system. Bone Joint Res. 2020;9(2):77–8.
27. Chin TY, Peh WC. Imaging update on musculoskeletal infections. J Clin Orthop Trauma. 2021;22:101600.
28. Verberne SJ, Raijmakers PG, Temmerman OPP. The accuracy of imaging techniques in the assessment of Periprosthetic hip Infection: a systematic review and meta-analysis. J Bone Joint Surg Am. 2016;98(19):1638–45.
29. Douis H, Dunlop DJ, Pearson AM, O'Hara JN, James SLJ. The role of ultrasound in the assessment of post-operative complications following hip arthroplasty. Skeletal Radiol. 2012;41(9):1035–46.
30. Shufen C, Jinmin L, Xiaohui Z, Bin G. Diagnostic value of magnetic resonance imaging for patients with periprosthetic joint infection: a systematic review. BMC Musculoskelet Disord. 2023;24(1):801.
31. Palestro CJ, Torres MA. Radionuclide imaging in orthopedic infections. Semin Nucl Med. 1997;27(4):334–45.
32. Mulamba L, Ferrant A, Leners N, de Nayer P, Rombouts JJ, Vincent A. Indium-111 leucocyte scanning in the evaluation of painful hip arthroplasty. Acta Orthop Scand. 1983;54(5):695–7.
33. Palestro CJ, Love C, Tronco GG, Tomas MB, Rini JN. Combined labeled leukocyte and technetium 99m sulfur colloid bone marrow imaging for diagnosing musculoskeletal infection. Radiographics. 2006;26(3):859–70.
34. Higgins E, Suh GA, Tande AJ. Enhancing diagnostics in orthopedic infections. J Clin Microbiol. 2022;60(6):e0219621.
35. Achermann Y, Vogt M, Leunig M, Wüst J, Trampuz A. Improved diagnosis of periprosthetic joint infection by multiplex PCR of sonication fluid from removed implants. J Clin Microbiol. 2010;48(4):1208–14.
36. Marín M, Garcia-Lechuz JM, Alonso P, Villanueva M, Alcalá L, Gimeno M, et al. Role of universal 16S rRNA gene PCR and sequencing in diagnosis of prosthetic joint infection. J Clin Microbiol. 2012;50(3):583–9.
37. Bergin PF, Doppelt JD, Hamilton WG, Mirick GE, Jones AE, Sritulanondha S, et al. Detection of periprosthetic infections with use of ribosomal RNA-based polymerase chain reaction. J Bone Joint Surg Am. 2010;92(3):654–63.
38. Morgenstern C, Cabric S, Perka C, Trampuz A, Renz N. Synovial fluid multiplex PCR is superior to culture for detection of low-virulent pathogens caus-

ing periprosthetic joint infection. Diagn Microbiol Infect Dis. 2018;90(2):115–9.
39. Esteban J, Gómez-Barrena E. An update about molecular biology techniques to detect orthopaedic implant-related infections. EFORT Open Rev. 2021;6(2):93–100.
40. Bourbour S, Emaneini M, Jabalameli M, Mortazavi SMJ, Tahmasebi MN, Taghizadeh A, et al. Efficacy of 16S rRNA variable regions high-resolution melt analysis for bacterial pathogens identification in periprosthetic joint infections. BMC Microbiol. 2021;21(1):112.
41. Wang CX, Huang Z, Fang X, Li W, Yang B, Zhang W. Comparison of broad-range polymerase chain reaction and metagenomic next-generation sequencing for the diagnosis of prosthetic joint infection. Int J Infect Dis. 2020;95:8–12.
42. Wang C, Huang Z, Li W, Fang X, Zhang W. Can metagenomic next-generation sequencing identify the pathogens responsible for culture-negative prosthetic joint infection? BMC Infect Dis. 2020;20(1):253.
43. Torchia MT, Austin DC, Kunkel ST, Dwyer KW, Moschetti WE. Next-generation sequencing vs culture-based methods for diagnosing Periprosthetic joint Infection after Total knee arthroplasty: a cost-effectiveness analysis. J Arthroplast. 2019;34(7):1333–41.
44. Portillo ME, Salvadó M, Alier A, Martínez S, Sorli L, Horcajada JP, et al. Advantages of sonication fluid culture for the diagnosis of prosthetic joint infection. J Infect. 2014;69(1):35–41.
45. Puig-Verdié L, Alentorn-Geli E, González-Cuevas A, Sorlí L, Salvadó M, Alier A, et al. Implant sonication increases the diagnostic accuracy of infection in patients with delayed, but not early, orthopaedic implant failure. Bone Joint J. 2013;95-B(2):244–9.
46. Trampuz A, Piper KE, Jacobson MJ, Hanssen AD, Unni KK, Osmon DR, et al. Sonication of removed hip and knee prostheses for diagnosis of infection. N Engl J Med. 2007;357(7):654–63.
47. Rothenberg AC, Wilson AE, Hayes JP, O'Malley MJ, Klatt BA. Sonication of arthroplasty implants improves accuracy of Periprosthetic joint Infection cultures. Clin Orthop Relat Res. 2017;475(7):1827–36.
48. Capanna R, Morris HG, Campanacci D, Del Ben M, Campanacci M. Modular uncemented prosthetic reconstruction after resection of tumours of the distal femur. J Bone Joint Surg Br. 1994;76(2):178–86.
49. Gaur AH, Liu T, Knapp KM, Daw NC, Rao BN, Neel MD, et al. Infections in children and young adults with bone malignancies undergoing limb-sparing surgery. Cancer. 2005;104(3):602–10.
50. Miwa S, Shirai T, Yamamoto N, Hayashi K, Takeuchi A, Tada K, et al. Risk factors for postoperative deep infection in bone tumors. PLoS One. 2017;12(11):e0187438.
51. Gafter-Gvili A, Paul M, Fraser A, Leibovici L. Effect of quinolone prophylaxis in afebrile neutropenic patients on microbial resistance: systematic review and meta-analysis. J Antimicrob Chemother. 2007;59(1):5–22.
52. Bodey GP, Buckley M, Sathe YS, Freireich EJ. Quantitative relationships between circulating leukocytes and infection in patients with acute leukemia. Ann Intern Med. 1966;64(2):328–40.
53. Lima SSS, França MS, Godoi CCG, Martinho GH, de Jesus LA, de Romanelli RMC, et al. Neutropenic patients and their infectious complications at a university hospital. Rev Bras Hematol Hemoter. 2013;35(1):18–22.
54. Gulack BC, Englum BR, Lo DD, Nussbaum DP, Keenan JE, Scarborough JE, et al. Leukopenia is associated with worse but not prohibitive outcomes following emergent abdominal surgery. J Trauma Acute Care Surg. 2015;79(3):437–43.
55. Ghert M, Deheshi B, Holt G, Randall RL, Ferguson P, Wunder J, et al. Prophylactic antibiotic regimens in tumour surgery (PARITY): protocol for a multicentre randomised controlled study. BMJ Open. 2012;2(6):e002197.
56. Cruciani M, Rampazzo R, Malena M, Lazzarini L, Todeschini G, Messori A, et al. Prophylaxis with fluoroquinolones for bacterial infections in neutropenic patients: a meta-analysis. Clin Infect Dis. 1996;23(4):795–805.
57. Trovarelli G, Cappellari A, Angelini A, Pala E, Ruggieri P. What is the survival and function of modular reverse Total shoulder prostheses in patients undergoing tumor resections in whom an innervated deltoid muscle can be preserved? Clin Orthop Relat Res. 2019;477(11):2495–507. https://doi.org/10.1097/CORR.0000000000000899.
58. Pala E, Trovarelli G, Angelini A, Ruggieri P. Distal femur reconstruction with modular tumour prostheses: a single institution analysis of implant survival comparing fixed versus rotating hinge knee prostheses. Int Orthop. 2016;40(10):2171–80. https://doi.org/10.1007/s00264-016-3232-1.
59. Pugh LR, Clarkson PW, Phillips AE, Biau DJ, Masri BA. Tumor endoprosthesis revision rates increase with peri-operative chemotherapy but are reduced with the use of cemented implant fixation. J Arthroplast. 2014;29(7):1418–22.
60. Brigman BE, Hornicek FJ, Gebhardt MC, Mankin HJ. Allografts about the knee in young patients with high-grade sarcoma. Clin Orthop Relat Res. 2004;421:232–9.
61. Hardes J, Gebert C, Schwappach A, Ahrens H, Streitburger A, Winkelmann W, et al. Characteristics and outcome of infections associated with tumor endoprostheses. Arch Orthop Trauma Surg. 2006;126(5):289–96.
62. Funovics PT, Hipfl C, Hofstaetter JG, Puchner S, Kotz RI, Dominkus M. Management of septic complications following modular endoprosthetic reconstruction of the proximal femur. Int Orthop. 2011;35(10):1437–44.

63. Mayilvahanan N, Paraskumar M, Sivaseelam A, Natarajan S. Custom mega-prosthetic replacement for proximal humeral tumours. Int Orthop. 2006;30(3):158–62.
64. Davis AM, O'Sullivan B, Turcotte R, Bell R, Catton C, Chabot P, et al. Late radiation morbidity following randomization to preoperative versus postoperative radiotherapy in extremity soft tissue sarcoma. Radiother Oncol. 2005;75(1):48–53.
65. Jeys LM, Luscombe JS, Grimer RJ, Abudu A, Tillman RM, Carter SR. The risks and benefits of radiotherapy with massive endoprosthetic replacement. J Bone Joint Surg Br. 2007;89(10):1352–5.
66. McDonald DJ, Capanna R, Gherlinzoni F, Bacci G, Ferruzzi A, Casadei R, et al. Influence of chemotherapy on perioperative complications in limb salvage surgery for bone tumors. Cancer. 1990;65(7):1509–16.
67. Montassier E, Gastinne T, Vangay P, Al-Ghalith GA, Bruley des Varannes S, Massart S, et al. Chemotherapy-driven dysbiosis in the intestinal microbiome. Aliment Pharmacol Ther. 2015;42(5):515–28.
68. Galloway-Peña JR, Smith DP, Sahasrabhojane P, Ajami NJ, Wadsworth WD, Daver NG, et al. The role of the gastrointestinal microbiome in infectious complications during induction chemotherapy for acute myeloid leukemia. Cancer. 2016;122(14):2186–96.
69. Denham JW, Hauer-Jensen M. The radiotherapeutic injury–a complex "wound". Radiother Oncol. 2002;63(2):129–45.
70. Griffin AM, Dickie CI, Catton CN, Chung PWM, Ferguson PC, Wunder JS, et al. The influence of time interval between preoperative radiation and surgical resection on the development of wound healing complications in extremity soft tissue sarcoma. Ann Surg Oncol. 2015;22(9):2824–30.
71. Keam J, Bilsky MH, Laufer I, Shi W, Zhang Z, Tam M, et al. No association between excessive wound complications and preoperative high-dose, hypofractionated, image-guided radiation therapy for spine metastasis. J Neurosurg Spine. 2014;20(4):411–20.
72. Sugita S, Hozumi T, Yamakawa K, Goto T, Kondo T. Risk factors for surgical site infection after posterior fixation surgery and intraoperative radiotherapy for spinal metastases. Eur Spine J. 2016;25(4):1034–8.
73. Namba RS, Inacio MCS, Paxton EW. Risk factors associated with deep surgical site infections after primary total knee arthroplasty: an analysis of 56,216 knees. J Bone Joint Surg Am. 2013;95(9):775–82.
74. Bozic KJ, Ward DT, Lau EC, Chan V, Wetters NG, Naziri Q, et al. Risk factors for periprosthetic joint infection following primary total hip arthroplasty: a case control study. J Arthroplast. 2014;29(1):154–6.
75. Cheng H, Chen BPH, Soleas IM, Ferko NC, Cameron CG, Hinoul P. Prolonged operative duration increases risk of surgical site infections: a systematic review. Surg Infect. 2017;18(6):722–35.
76. Pulido L, Ghanem E, Joshi A, Purtill JJ, Parvizi J. Periprosthetic joint infection: the incidence, timing, and predisposing factors. Clin Orthop Relat Res. 2008;466(7):1710–5.
77. de Boer AS, Geubbels EL, Wille J, Mintjes-de Groot AJ. Risk assessment for surgical site infections following total hip and total knee prostheses. J Chemother. 2001;13(1):42–7.
78. Wymenga AB, van Horn JR, Theeuwes A, Muytjens HL, Slooff TJ. Perioperative factors associated with septic arthritis after arthroplasty. Prospective multicenter study of 362 knee and 2,651 hip operations. Acta Orthop Scand. 1992;63(6):665–71.
79. Suzuki G, Saito S, Ishii T, Motojima S, Tokuhashi Y, Ryu J. Previous fracture surgery is a major risk factor of infection after total knee arthroplasty. Knee Surg Sports Traumatol Arthrosc. 2011;19(12):2040–4.
80. Kurtz SM, Ong KL, Lau E, Bozic KJ, Berry D, Parvizi J. Prosthetic joint infection risk after TKA in the Medicare population. Clin Orthop Relat Res. 2010;468(1):52–6.
81. Morii T, Mochizuki K, Tajima T, Ichimura S, Satomi K. Surgical site infection in malignant soft tissue tumors. J Orthop Sci. 2012;17(1):51–7.
82. Lerman DM, Blank AT, Billig JI, Karia R, Rapp TB. Identification of risk factors for acute surgical site infections in musculoskeletal tumor patients using CDC/NHSN criteria. Bull Hosp Jt Dis (2013). 2015;73(4):233–8.
83. Patel VP, Walsh M, Sehgal B, Preston C, DeWal H, Di Cesare PE. Factors associated with prolonged wound drainage after primary Total hip and knee arthroplasty. J Bone Joint Surg. 2007;89(1):33–8.
84. Dogar SA, Khan MAM. Implantable port devices in paediatric oncology patients: a clinical experience from a tertiary care hospital. J Pak Med Assoc. 2013;63(10):1248–51.
85. Bratzler DW, Houck PM, Richards C, Steele L, Dellinger EP, Fry DE, et al. Use of antimicrobial prophylaxis for major surgery: baseline results from the National Surgical Infection Prevention Project. Arch Surg. 2005;140(2):174–82.
86. Jeys LM, Grimer RJ, Carter SR, Tillman RM. Risk of amputation following limb salvage surgery with endoprosthetic replacement, in a consecutive series of 1261 patients. Int Orthop. 2003;27(3):160–3.
87. Zeegen EN, Aponte-Tinao LA, Hornicek FJ, Gebhardt MC, Mankin HJ. Survivorship analysis of 141 modular metallic endoprostheses at early followup. Clin Orthop Relat Res. 2004;420:239–50.
88. Trovarelli G, Angelini A, Pala E, Cappellari A, Breda A, Ruggieri P. Infection in orthopaedic oncology: crucial problem in modern reconstructive techniques. Eur Rev Med Pharmacol Sci. 2019;23(2 Suppl):271–8. https://doi.org/10.26355/eurrev_201904_17501.
89. Wafa H, Grimer RJ, Reddy K, Jeys L, Abudu A, Carter SR, et al. Retrospective evaluation of the incidence of early periprosthetic infection with silver-treated

endoprostheses in high-risk patients: case-control study. Bone Joint J. 2015;97-B(2):252–7.
90. Zajonz D, Zieme A, Prietzel T, Moche M, Tiepoldt S, Roth A, et al. Periprosthetic joint infections in modular endoprostheses of the lower extremities: a retrospective observational study in 101 patients. Patient Saf Surg. 2016;10:6.
91. Sharma S, Turcotte RE, Isler MH, Wong C. Experience with cemented large segment endoprostheses for tumors. Clin Orthop Relat Res. 2007;459:54–9.
92. Mittermayer F, Krepler P, Dominkus M, Schwameis E, Sluga M, Heinzl H, et al. Long-term followup of uncemented tumor endoprostheses for the lower extremity. Clin Orthop Relat Res. 2001;388:167–77.
93. Griffin AM, Parsons JA, Davis AM, Bell RS, Wunder JS. Uncemented tumor endoprostheses at the knee: root causes of failure. Clin Orthop Relat Res. 2005;438:71–9.
94. Unwin PS, Cannon SR, Grimer RJ, Kemp HB, Sneath RS, Walker PS. Aseptic loosening in cemented custom-made prosthetic replacements for bone tumours of the lower limb. J Bone Joint Surg Br. 1996;78(1):5–13.
95. Pala E, Mavrogenis AF, Angelini A, Henderson ER, Douglas Letson G, Ruggieri P. Cemented versus cementless endoprostheses for lower limb salvage surgery. J BUON. 2013;18(2):496–503.
96. Prokuski L. Prophylactic antibiotics in orthopaedic surgery. J Am Acad Orthop Surg. 2008;16(5):283–93.
97. Francesco R, Arthur M, Francesco C, Daniel C. What is the Most appropriate perioperative prophylactic antibiotic (Agent, route and number of doses) for patients undergoing primary Total joint arthroplasty (TJA) to reduce the risk of subsequent surgical site infections/Periprosthetic joint infections (SSIs/PJIs)? [Internet]. ICM Philly. 2019;
98. Schneider P, Heels-Ansdell D, Thabane L, Ghert M, PARITY Investigators. Prophylactic antibiotic regimens in tumor surgery (PARITY): a multi-center randomized controlled study comparing alternative antibiotic regimens in patients undergoing tumor resections with endoprosthetic replacements-a statistical analysis plan. Trials. 2021;22(1):223.
99. Meehan J, Jamali AA, Nguyen H. Prophylactic antibiotics in hip and knee arthroplasty. J Bone Joint Surg Am. 2009;91(10):2480–90.
100. Veltman ES, Lenguerrand E, Moojen DJF, Whitehouse MR, Nelissen RGHH, Blom AW, et al. Similar risk of complete revision for infection with single-dose versus multiple-dose antibiotic prophylaxis in primary arthroplasty of the hip and knee: results of an observational cohort study in the Dutch arthroplasty register in 242,179 patients. Acta Orthop. 2020;91(6):794–800.
101. Neu HC. Cephalosporin antibiotics as applied in surgery of bones and joints. Clin Orthop Relat Res. 1984;190:50–64.
102. Tornero E, García-Ramiro S, Martínez-Pastor JC, Bori G, Bosch J, Morata L, et al. Prophylaxis with teicoplanin and cefuroxime reduces the rate of prosthetic joint infection after primary arthroplasty. Antimicrob Agents Chemother. 2015;59(2):831–7.
103. Bolon MK, Morlote M, Weber SG, Koplan B, Carmeli Y, Wright SB. Glycopeptides are no more effective than beta-lactam agents for prevention of surgical site infection after cardiac surgery: a meta-analysis. Clin Infect Dis. 2004;38(10):1357–63.
104. Gafter-Gvili A, Fraser A, Paul M, van de Wetering M, Kremer L, Leibovici L. Antibiotic prophylaxis for bacterial infections in afebrile neutropenic patients following chemotherapy. Cochrane Database Syst Rev. 2005;1(4):CD004386.
105. Zhanel GG, Adam HJ, Low DE, Blondeau J, Decorby M, Karlowsky JA, et al. Antimicrobial susceptibility of 15,644 pathogens from Canadian hospitals: results of the CANWARD 2007-2009 study. Diagn Microbiol Infect Dis. 2011;69(3):291–306.
106. Costelloe C, Metcalfe C, Lovering A, Mant D, Hay AD. Effect of antibiotic prescribing in primary care on antimicrobial resistance in individual patients: systematic review and meta-analysis. BMJ. 2010;18(340):c2096.
107. Hashimoto K, Nishimura S, Shinyashiki Y, Ito T, Kakinoki R, Akagi M. Novel reconstruction method by mega-prosthesis wrapped with vancomycin-containing cement after resection of malignancies. Medicine. 2022;101(48):e31547.
108. Lee SH, Tai CL, Chen SY, Chang CH, Chang YH, Hsieh PH. Elution and mechanical strength of vancomycin-loaded bone cement: in vitro study of the influence of brand combination. PLoS One. 2016;11(11):e0166545.
109. Bishop AR, Kim S, Squire MW, Rose WE, Ploeg HL. Vancomycin elution, activity and impact on mechanical properties when added to orthopedic bone cement. J Mech Behav Biomed Mater. 2018;87:80–6.
110. Longo UG, De Salvatore S, Bandini B, Lalli A, Barillà B, Budhiparama NC, et al. Debridement, antibiotics, and implant retention (DAIR) for the early prosthetic joint infection of total knee and hip arthroplasties: a systematic review. J ISAKOS. 2023;9:62.
111. Giulieri SG, Graber P, Ochsner PE, Zimmerli W. Management of infection associated with total hip arthroplasty according to a treatment algorithm. Infection. 2004;32(4):222–8.
112. Qasim SN, Swann A, Ashford R. The DAIR (debridement, antibiotics and implant retention) procedure for infected total knee replacement – a literature review. SICOT J. 2017;3:2.
113. Dhanoa A, Ajit Singh V, Elbahri H. Deep infections after Endoprosthetic replacement operations in orthopedic oncology patients. Surg Infect. 2015;16(3):323–32.
114. Li X, Moretti VM, Ashana AO, Lackman RD. Perioperative infection rate in patients with osteosarcomas treated with resection and pros-

thetic reconstruction. Clin Orthop Relat Res. 2011;469(10):2889–94.
115. Mavrogenis AF, Pala E, Angelini A, Calabro T, Romagnoli C, Romantini M, et al. Infected prostheses after lower-extremity bone tumor resection: clinical outcomes of 100 patients. Surg Infect. 2015;16(3):267–75.
116. Mavrogenis AF, Papagelopoulos PJ, Coll-Mesa L, Pala E, Guerra G, Ruggieri P. Infected tumor prostheses. Orthopedics. 2011;34(12):991–8. quiz 999–1000
117. Allison MDMFD, Huang ME, Ahlmann ME, Carney MS, Wang PCL, Menendez MFL. Peri-prosthetic Infection in the orthopedic tumor patient. Reconstr Rev. 2014;4(3):13–7.
118. Sherrell JC, Fehring TK, Odum S, Hansen E, Zmistowski B, Dennos A, et al. The Chitranjan Ranawat award: fate of two-stage reimplantation after failed irrigation and débridement for periprosthetic knee infection. Clin Orthop Relat Res. 2011;469(1):18–25.
119. Choi HR, von Knoch F, Zurakowski D, Nelson SB, Malchau H. Can implant retention be recommended for treatment of infected TKA? Clin Orthop Relat Res. 2011;469(4):961–9.
120. Gardner J, Gioe TJ, Tatman P. Can this prosthesis be saved?: implant salvage attempts in infected primary TKA. Clin Orthop Relat Res. 2011;469(4):970–6.
121. Stockley I, Mockford BJ, Hoad-Reddick A, Norman P. The use of two-stage exchange arthroplasty with depot antibiotics in the absence of long-term antibiotic therapy in infected total hip replacement. J Bone Joint Surg Br. 2008;90(2):145–8.
122. El Amiri L, Clavert P, Gaudias J, Klein S, Rondé Oustau C, Antoni M. High infection control rate after systematic one-stage procedure for shoulder arthroplasty chronic infection. Int Orthop. 2023;47(11):2809–26.
123. Bejon P, Berendt A, Atkins BL, Green N, Parry H, Masters S, et al. Two-stage revision for prosthetic joint infection: predictors of outcome and the role of reimplantation microbiology. J Antimicrob Chemother. 2010;65(3):569–75.
124. Flint MN, Griffin AM, Bell RS, Wunder JS, Ferguson PC. Two-stage revision of infected uncemented lower extremity tumor endoprostheses. J Arthroplast. 2007;22(6):859–65.
125. Younger AS, Duncan CP, Masri BA. Treatment of infection associated with segmental bone loss in the proximal part of the femur in two stages with use of an antibiotic-loaded interval prosthesis. J Bone Joint Surg Am. 1998;80(1):60–9.
126. Ure KJ, Amstutz HC, Nasser S, Schmalzried TP. Direct-exchange arthroplasty for the treatment of infection after total hip replacement. An average ten-year follow-up. J Bone Joint Surg Am. 1998;80(7):961–8.

# Antibiotic Spacers Used for Prosthetic Joint Infections

# 24

Claire Park, Yazan Kadkoy, Luis Vallejo, Ashley Castan, Joseph A. Ippolito, and Joseph Benevenia

## 24.1 Introduction

Following treatment of prosthetic joint infection (PJI), antibiotic-eluting spacers are frequently utilized to fill bone defects left behind after debridement and removal of prior reconstructive components. This chapter will span a variety of anatomic locations and spacer types. This may include static spacers, articulating spacers, and hybrid spacers which may be considered for long-term use. Given the diversity of patients who suffer from PJI and in consideration of an oncologic and revision arthroplasty populations with large bone defects, possible immunocompromised status, and wide varieties of microorganisms, decisions on spacer type are best left to a careful discussion between the surgeon and patient. While other chapters will discuss the very important considerations for adequate debridement, laboratory studies, and antibiotic stewardship, the objective of this chapter is to provide surgeons with a review of the literature and a framework of ideas that empower surgeons to utilize their technical skills, creativity, and understanding of patient goals to achieve optimal results in the aim of limb salvage.

## 24.2 Knee

### 24.2.1 Overview

Infection at the knee is the most common site of PJI following arthroplasty. In addition to being among the most common anatomic locations for total joint replacement, the distal femur and proximal tibia remain among the most operated sites for tumor resection and reconstruction. Furthermore, given the demands upon the knee, antibiotic spacers in this region must be of durability and elute of antibiotics.

### 24.2.2 Spacers After Primary Adult Reconstruction

Following the explant of components and debridement, if the collateral ligamentous structures can be preserved at the knee, either static or articulating spacer components can be considered to help clear infection [1–5]. Static spacers have been used historically and can be fashioned from a sim-

C. Park
Department of Surgery, Rutgers NJMS,
Newark, NJ, USA
e-mail: cp906@njms.rutgers.edu

Y. Kadkoy · A. Castan · J. A. Ippolito · J. Benevenia (✉)
Department of Orthopaedics, Rutgers NJMS,
Newark, NJ, USA
e-mail: yk399@njms.rutgers.edu;
aqc3@njms.rutgers.edu; ippolija@njms.rutgers.edu;
benevejo@njms.rutgers.edu

L. Vallejo
University Hospital, Newark, NJ, USA
e-mail: vallejl2@uhnj.org



P. Ruggieri et al. (eds.), *Bone and Joint Infections*, https://doi.org/10.1007/978-3-031-96383-4_24

ple block of antibiotic cement with or without intramedullary stabilization [2]. Potential advantages of articulating spacers include more effective maintenance of the joint space, reduction in bone loss, and maintenance of range of motion [3, 4]. Traditionally, these spacers have been comprised of an articulating femoral and tibial component which can be either cement-on-cement, cement-on-polyethylene, or metal-on-polyethylene [5].

For cement-only molds, several options exist for surgeons, including pre-fabricated antibiotic molds with multiple sizes and molds that can be modified intraoperatively [3]. While numerous options in industry exist, the main difference between prefabricated molds and intraoperative molds is the ability to add additional or different antibiotic/antifungal powder to the mold.

Utilization of a with an all-polyethylene tibial component has grown increasingly popular over the past several years, particularly in patients with acute or low virulence organisms [4]. In these patients, the new components are implanted in a fashion that allows ease of ease component removal for a second-stage surgery [6]. However, several studies have highlighted the ability of patients to retain their metallic femur and all-poly tibia antibiotic spacer for longer durations with satisfactory functional outcomes [5–12]. This may be particularly useful in patients with medical comorbidities or wound issues that undermine their ability to tolerate a second-stage procedure [13–16].

## Articulating Antibiotic Spacers Following Primary TKA

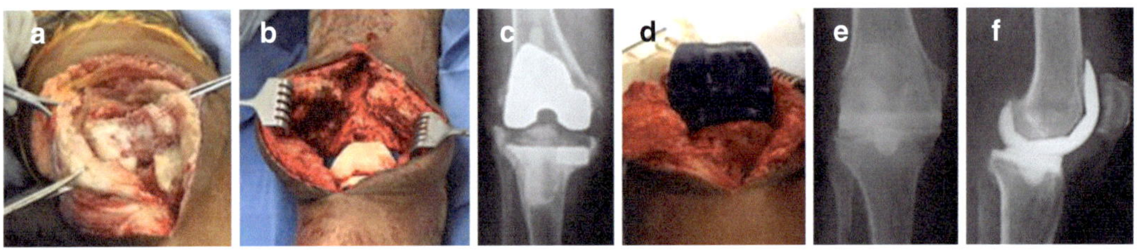


*Articulating primary total knee arthroplasty spacer*: A. post-explant bone loss B. intraoperative view of all cement mold spacer C. Metallic femur with all poly tibia with augment D. Intraoperative view of metal-backed cement mold E, F. AP & lateral xrays

1. Prior to explant, we recommend placement of two drill bits above and below the anticipated hardware explant (one in the femur, one in the tibia) and measuring the gap between these for later restoration of limb lengths and soft tissue tension.
2. Following radical debridement of infected tissue and explant of prior implants, assess the proper sizing of articulating spacer construct.
3. Once sizing is complete, prepare the appropriate amount of required additional antibiotic-impregnated cement, ideally tailored to pre-operative cultures and microbiology sensitivities. We recommend utilizing a high-viscosity cement to enable a more workable material that stays intact.
4. We recommend preparing the side with less bone loss first, then working from there to restore length on the higher bone loss side by "floating" the cemented articulating spacer device with the leg at restored pre-surgical length.
5. Usually, this framework leads to the tibia being prepared first. Ideally, this cement is allowed to cure into a "sticky" form before

implantation to avoid cement dropping down the canal and molding around the tibia polyethylene. Once the tibial component is implanted in a satisfactory alignment and rotation and all loose cement is removed from the knee, the femoral component can be addressed.

6. For the preparation of the second construct (usually the femur), an assistant pulls traction on the leg and the extension gap distance is re-checked to anticipate the ideal position of the cemented component. Similarly, cement is placed on the femur and the femoral component individually, with an emphasis on preventing cement from being pushed far up into the femur to facilitate removal for future revisions.

### 24.2.3 Static Spacers

Depending on the extent of debridement required, patients with severe bone loss, collateral ligament insufficiency, periarticular fracture, and an insufficient functional extensor mechanism may be good candidates for static spacers [17–19]. In these settings, we prefer the utilization of either an antibiotic cement dowel or a metallic rod coated in cement to provide temporary arthrodesis and improved stability around an antibiotic-eluting cement block. After removal of infected components, polymethylmethacrylate (PMMA) cement can be mixed with numerous heat-stable antibiotic or antifungal medications, including tobramycin, vancomycin, and amphotericin B on the back table. A small amount of cement can be retrieved to create a cement dowel by rolling cement out on the mayo stand and frequently irrigating it. This can then be inserted into the intramedullary canals of the tibia and femur. Next, the remaining amount of cement is placed in the manually held gap between the distal femur and proximal tibia and gently pressed together to form an arthrodesis. The coated metallic rod technique will be discussed in the later section on larger segmental defect spacers.

### 24.2.4 Static Versus Articulating Spacers

Several studies have examined the outcomes of static and articulating spacers. To preface a brief discussion of these findings, there are numerous confounding variables, including the type of infective organism and the retention or not of various anatomical structures that can influence the choice of static or articulating antibiotic spacer. In a systematic review of 47 articles, articulating spacers had lower rates of infection, greater range of motion, less bone loss, and favorable conditions for reimplantation [19]. In a review of 34 articles examining types of articulating spacers among pre-fabricated, handmade, custom molds, and new knee components implanted with antibiotic cement, there were no differences in rates of reinfection or difficulty in reimplantation [20]. However, there were fewer spacer-specific complications with the new metal femoral and all-poly tibial components compared to other spacer types.

### 24.2.5 Distal Femoral or Proximal Tibial Replacement Infection

Following infection of a distal femoral replacement (DFR) or proximal tibial replacement (PTR), considerations in addition to the infecting organism(s) must be held, including the status of the extensor mechanism, surrounding soft tissues, and history of a gastrocnemius flap and possible future need for one [21]. In addition to explant of components, these patients must undergo a radical debridement which includes intramedullary reaming to remove all residual infectious tissue [21].

The author's preference is to perform a multistage procedure that includes a debridement may be repeated with an interim antibiotic eluting spacer construct prior to reimplantation of segmental arthroplasty components. Compared to patients with PJI following primary or revision knee arthroplasty, patients with PJI following

DFR/PTR require more robust stabilization for the interim with articulating or arthrodesis type implants between stages 1 and 2 [21–26]. Additionally, these patients may be more likely to present with polymicrobial infection and require more than one debridement procedure prior to consideration for reimplantation [27, 28].

### 24.2.6 Stage 1 Arthrodesis Spacers

Segmental arthrodesis antibiotic spacers can be constructed in various ways, including the use of a femorotibial fusion nail, the use of a knee fusion metallic spacer surrounded by cement, or the use of two standard intramedullary nails linked together and surrounded by cement [29, 30]. For all these scenarios, pre-operative measurement of the patient's segmental defect and rotational alignment of the limb should be performed to minimize limb length discrepancy and maximize the success of reimplantation [31, 33].

If utilizing two intramedullary nails, securing a configuration that allows for a straight leg can be slightly challenging if utilizing a tibial nail and femoral nail. An alternative to this is using a short femoral nail with a large radius of curvature on the tibial side and articulating this with a femoral nail proximally. The nail can be secured with either cerclage or interlocking screws to fasten the nails together, followed by hand molding antibiotic cement around the structure.

**Massive Bone Loss at Knee Spacers: Intramedullary Nail Construct**

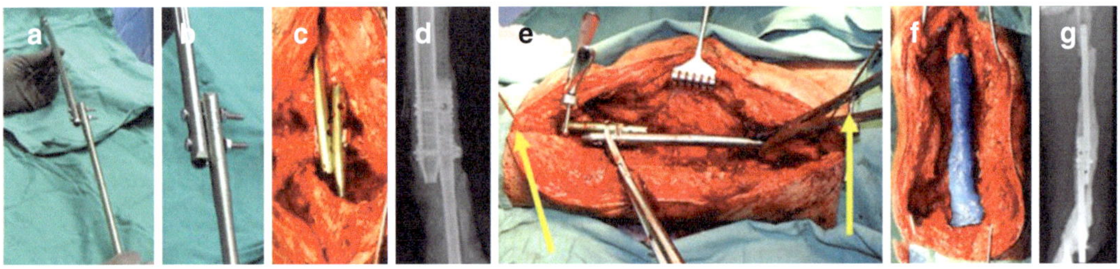


*Static intramedullary nail spacer for massive bone loss at knee*: A. Two intramedullary nails assembled and locked together B. Interlocking screws with nut to link nails C. Tensioned cable to lock nails D. Wiring of nails together in addition to interlocking screws E. Large bone defect stabilized with intramedullary nails and demonstration of two drill bits placed prior to explant to confirm restoration of limb length after nail implantation F. PMMA molded around intramedullary nail G. Two intramedullary nails spanning a 32 cm defect after tumor endoprosthesis explant

1. Prior to explant, we recommend placement of two drill bits above and below the anticipated hardware explant (one in femur, one in tibia, fig. E) and measuring the gap between these for later restoration of limb lengths and soft tissue tension.
2. Once prior implants are removed and debridement is performed, continue debridement of the intramedullary canal, either with standard reamers or with a reamer irrigator aspirator system to ensure the removal of infected components.
3. Nail size selection is typically 1–1.5 cm smaller than the largest reamer used. We recommend templating the ideal length of nails to retain limb length pre-operatively and confirming during surgery.
4. If there is more than minimal bone loss at the tibia, two femoral nails may be optimal for use (one at femur, one at tibia) and allow for easier linking of the two nails by various methods shown above. A femoral and tibial nail can be linked but may require cabling due to the interlocking holes not matching up as well.

5. Once the length has been restored and re-measured with nails in place, antibiotic cement can be molded around the nails. A high-viscosity cement may allow for a more moldable construct around the nails. The surgical team should ensure that copious irrigation is available to prevent thermal injury to adjacent soft tissues during the curing process.

For femorotibial fusion nails, our technique includes inserting the rod through a large chest tube that is situated over the templated region where there is a bone defect between the femur and tibia. The chest tube is then filled with cement, which is allowed to cure. Once the cement is cured, the chest tube can be incised sharply and cut off from around the cement. This allows for a contained spacer with a uniform slim shape to promote soft tissue reapproximation at the conclusion of the procedure. In very large defects, Steinmann pins can be situated throughout the chest tube, with cement filled around the pins, to create a stronger rebar effect.

**Massive Bone Loss at Knee Spacers: Femoral-Tibial Fusion Nail Spacer**

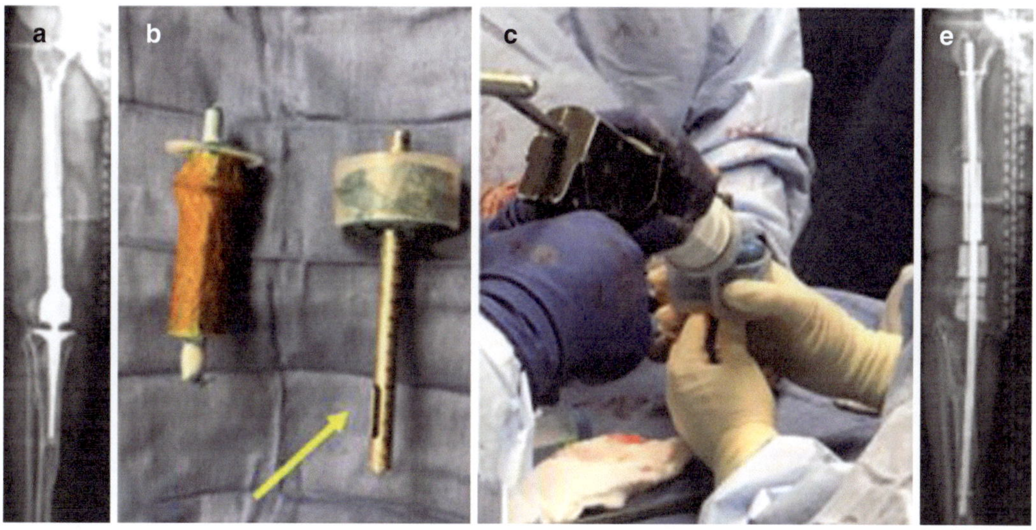


**Femoral-Tibial Fusion Nail Spacer**

A. Patient with PJI after tumor endoprosthesis.
B. To facilitate sufficient antibiotic cement along the length of the long defect, several spacers can be pre-made to slide over the nail. In this instance, a Toomey syringe was cut in half, filled with Steinmann pins for rebar effect, and cement inserted, over a trephine reamer that was well lubricated and larger than the nail diameter. Once the cement begins to harden, the trephine reamer is carefully removed.
C. This technique can be repeated to create several smaller rings of cement using a spacer mold and the trephine reamer (arrow).
D. Final construct demonstrating several spacer molds and fusion nails in place. While multiple molds may contribute to a weaker construct, this technique facilitates easier removal for later revision. An alternative to this would be to form a single long column of cement (demonstrated in another figure in this chapter). This decision is best left to the surgeon based on their individual discussion with the patient.

For arthrodesis spacers, off-the-shelf arthrodesis implants can be utilized. This allows for greater preservation of the native bone above and below the prior implant. Similar to the femorotibial fusion nail, these robust constructs enable the possible retention of an arthrodesis spacer for the remainder of the patient's life if they are unable to undergo a repeat surgical procedure. Technical pearls to these arthrodesis implants include hollowing out sufficient amounts of bone circumferentially to accommodate a large amount of antibiotic cement to help eradicate infection.

**Massive Bone Loss at Knee Spacers: Knee Arthrodesis Nail**

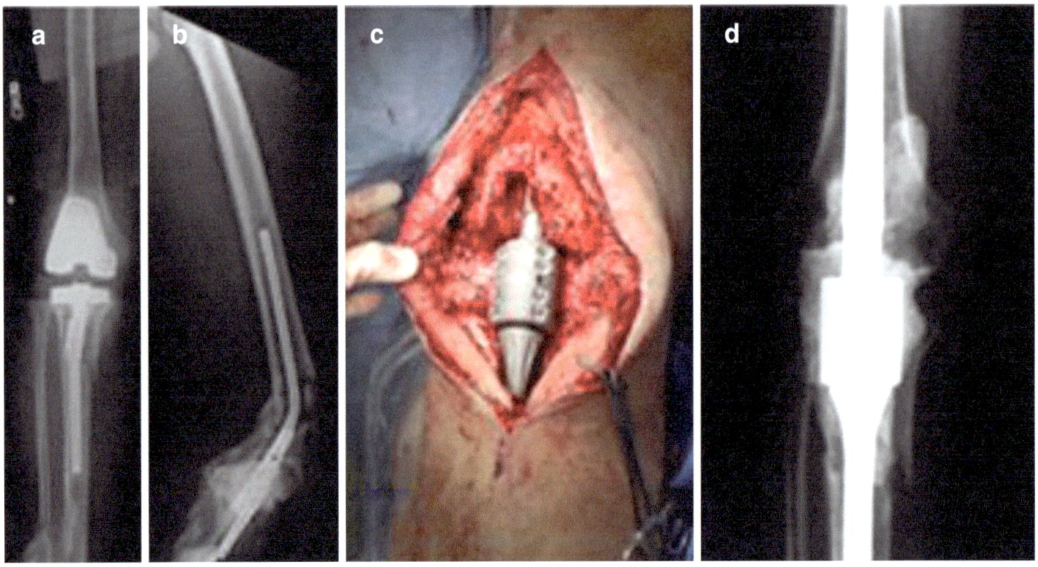


**Femoral-Tibial Fusion Nail Spacer**

A. Patient with PJI and proximal tibia fracture.
B. Following the explant of components, there was severe bone loss and concern with the patient's ability to tolerate limited weight-bearing status. Intramedullary nail constructs have been seen to bend and fail if patients are non-compliant with these restrictions.
C. An arthrodesis nail allows for immediate weight-bearing. These stems can be placed in a cemented or press-fit manner. Our preference is to tightly fit a stem from this system without canal cementation to facilitate future removal with ease if needed.
D. Once the nail is set in place, antibiotic cement can be placed by hand around the arthrodesis nail. It benefits the surgeon to ensure the femur and tibia are appropriately recessed to accommodate antibiotic cement around the nail. Having a burr available for these canals is very helpful for this purpose.

### 24.2.7 Articulating DFR/PTR Spacers

In settings of low virulence organisms or in patients with severely compromised soft tissues or medical status that will likely not be amenable to a later reimplantation procedure, surgeons can consider reimplantation of a large segmental prosthesis after explant of all infected components. If this is planned, it is paramount to have two distinct sterile back table setups to prevent cross-contamination, as well as to have all surgical staff completely change their gown and gloves between the explant and reimplantation components of the procedure. If this method is chosen, consideration of the implant design can be helpful in selecting a reconstruction that balances infection clearance and structural stability.

At the distal femur, selecting a shorter segmental body and a longer stem that sits proudly at the femur may be helpful. This allows for hand molding of cement around the residual stem not inserted inside of the femur. Our preference is to make our limb length and rotation analyses as described above, coat the distal portion of the femoral stem not being inserted inside of the femur, and let this cure before performing a pressurized cementation procedure at the distal femur.

At the proximal tibia, the method described above is typically more challenging to perform [34–37]. However, the selection of a shorter segmental body on the proximal tibial component and using a long stem that sits proudly proximal to the tibia may similarly be considered. If planning on using this technique, using a stem long and large enough to maintain some stability at the distal tibia prior to building up the absent tibial metaphyseal region with cement should be favored.

## Articulating Massive Bone Loss Antibiotic Spacers

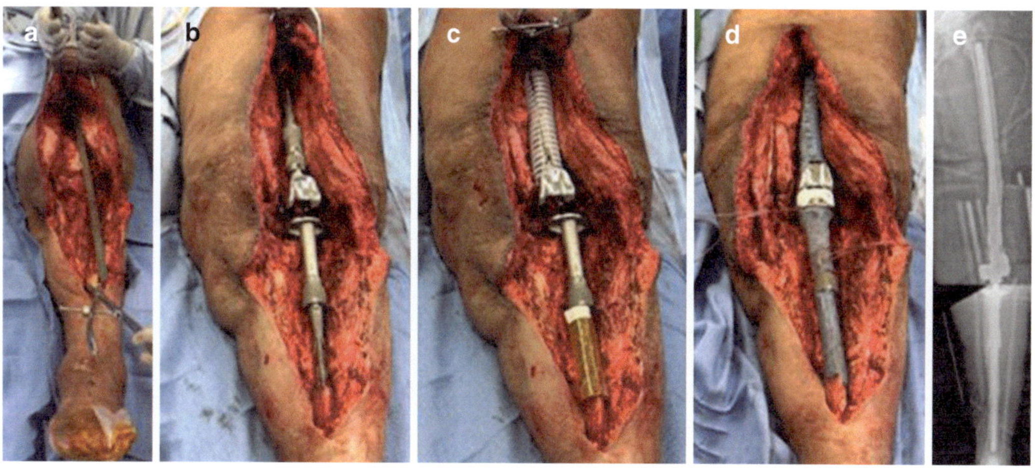


**Articulating Massive Bone Loss Antibiotic Spacers**

A. 50 cm bone defect after explant of prior implants and radical debridement of bone and soft tissues.
B. Segmental hinged distal femoral replacement. In this setting, it is our preference to utilize a grit-blasted stem in a line-to-line manner, reaming either to the size of the anticipated stem. In some cases, it is required to ream 0.5 mm over the size of the stem to facilitate stem implantation. At the conclusion of the implantation, the stems should have a tight fit with provisional axial and rotational stability. It is our preference to utilize the smallest distal femoral component available and minimal segmental bodies, to facilitate for antibiotic eluting cement to be fashioned around the stems. Performing this method of cementation reserves the possibility of later stem removal and bone stock preservation in the setting of the revision procedure.
C. Proximally, a sterile coiled plastic sleeve is cur longitudinally and wrapped around the femoral stem. Distally, a Toomey syringe is cut longitudinally, with loban wrapped around it to link the two half shells together.

Prior to cement placement, these tubes are filled with lube to facilitate easy separation of plastic from cured cement. Next, cement is laid into the plastic shells. The shells are squeezed together by hand initially and can be held together by bone-holding clamps.

D. Cemented coated distal femur and proximal tibia replacement stems with sutures tied to the proximal tibia component and embedded in cement for extensor mechanism reconstruction in addition to gastrocnemius flap.
E. X-ray of construct.

## 24.3 Hip

Infected primary hip replacements are typically managed with two-stage revisions, which have a high rate of survivorship after reimplantation [38]. After the explantation of the infected prosthetic components and the removal of devitalized tissue, it has been demonstrated that the use of antibiotic-impregnated cement spacers can significantly enhance patient outcomes by effectively delivering high local concentrations of antibiotics, thus reducing infection rates, and improving the chances for successful limb salvage [4, 39]. During these staged revisions, there are many considerations that need to be taken including choice of antibiotics, type of spacer, and chemical and mechanical properties of cement, among many other features. Evidence does not indicate an unequivocally superior spacer or method for periprosthetic hip infection management. Rather, the debate continues whether there are differences in rates of infection eradication between articulating and static spacers as well as between spacers made only with cement or real components [40].

### 24.3.1 Static Spacers

In situations where there is extensive bone loss, large acetabular defects, deficient ligamentous structures, or inadequate flap coverage, static spacers can be considered. It is essential that the spacer is molded with antibiotic-loaded cement in such a way that does not promote tissue ingrowth to allow for uncomplicated removals. While hip static spacers cannot prevent all hip motion, they restrict patients from any weight bearing [41]. They are usually constructed with an antibiotic-impregnated cement ball placed into the acetabulum with antibiotic cement beads or cement-covered rod for the femoral canal. While these spacers are adept at eliminating infection with possibly increased surface area for antibiotic exposure, they unfortunately will usually lead to large limb length discrepancy and soft tissue contracture. Furthermore, prior to final reimplantation, patients must be non-weight bearing, leading to decreased patient satisfaction.

**Static Hip Spacer**

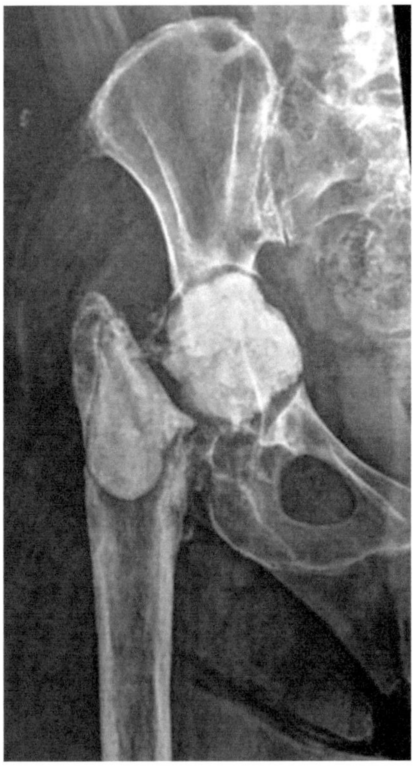

### 24.3.2 Articulating Spacers

Articulating spacers are beneficial in preserving hip mobility and has been shown to be as efficient at eradicating infection. They may allow for an easier surgery when transitioning to the final implant. They are only contraindicated in situations with acetabular insufficiency, pelvic discontinuity, or loss of the abductor mechanism. The different methods of construction range from handmade to 3D-printed custom articulating spacers. The methods of construction generally utilize similar underlying principles-utilizing a metal endoskeleton to allow for greater load endurance, preventing spacer fracture with weight-bearing. The major tradeoffs between these different methods remain preoperative and intraoperative time and cost versus mechanical complication risk [42].

Articulating spacers can be categorized by their mode of reconstruction or their design of cement-on-bone hemiarthroplasty versus a metal or ceramic head articulating with a cemented polyethylene liner. Handmade spacers are constructed in the shape of a hemiarthroplasty- when the size of the femoral head matches, it is useful to utilize the bulb syringe as a mold. This method is low cost but requires knowledge and familiarity with the method by the surgical team. While these are associated with an increased risk of mechanical failure or dislocation, preventative measures can be taken to reduce this risk. To reduce the risk of dislocation with these spacers, the head should be only 2–3 mm smaller than the acetabular socket to ensure optimal seating and geometric congruence to optimize joint mechanics. To ensure sufficient fixation of the femoral spacer stem, a cement collar can be formed, allowing for better control of the spacer height and anteversion, without increasing difficulty during removal. Many different methods of creating spacers have been documented including intraoperative sterilization of the prosthetic components to construct a mold. These molded spacers have been associated with higher procedural cost and mechanical complication rates. Preformed articulating spacers are another option. They decrease cost and intraoperative time, but are less universal, limited by sizes and shapes. Cases with significant proximal femoral bone loss should utilize custom-made spacers, including cemented femoral stems.

A hemiarthroplasty design can be utilized with a cement femoral component articulating with the native acetabulum [41]. This has been associated with greater limitations in hip function and pain with possible bony erosion. The more commonly utilized design consists of a metal or ceramic head on a cemented polyethylene liner. While the additional implants increase surgical costs, patients may experience improved functional movement and less pain. Notably, the polyethylene liner may increase the risk of harboring bacteria due to its propensity for biofilm.

To avoid common complications associated with articulating spacers such as dislocation, careful attention must be brought to maintaining an appropriate neck-head ratio to avoid acetabular impingement as well as preservation of femoral offset to keep appropriate muscle tension. When determining whether the articulating spacer should be made of cement versus a real component, no significant differences were found in outcomes regarding reinfection and reoperation rates, and time to reimplantation. The only consideration pertains to patient comfort and healthcare cost with significant differences in leg length in the all-cement groups after the second stage and with patients in the real-component group having a higher probability of being discharged after the first and second-stage surgeries.

## Articulating Antibiotic Spacers Following Primary THA

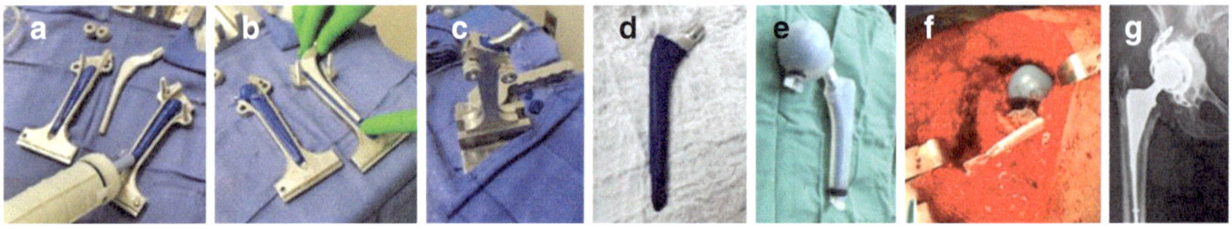


*Articulating primary total hip arthroplasty spacer*: A. Metal-backed cement spacer with open clam shell being filled with high viscosity cement B. Metallic prosthesis is laid into mold C. Clamp applied to compress cement around the metallic implant. Take care to clear off cement from the superior aspect and prevent cement from extending to trunnion D. Completed pre-molded metal-backed antibiotic cement device E. Hemiarthroplasty mold F. Intra-operative view of hemiarthroplasty mold G. AP X-Ray of total hip spacer comprised of metal-backed cement femoral stem and flanged acetabular component for patient with severe acetabular bone loss at time of explant

1. Prior to explant, we recommend a pre-operative CT to evaluate for extent of bone loss and the likelihood of requiring certain instrumentation or osteotomy techniques for implant removal.
2. Several antibiotic cement total hip spacer molds exist on the market. Once all prior components are removed and debridement is completed, most systems allow for a broaching system to be used and estimate the appropriate stem size for final implantation.
3. In instances of severe bone loss or considerable soft tissue loss from infection and debridement, the option of cementing a constrained liner might be of value to the surgeon. We recommend familiarizing yourself with the taper of the antibiotic cement total hip arthroplasty stems.
4. The total hip stem is created on the back table, with a mold and metallic compression system to facilitate proper shaping. Usually, we prefer a high-viscosity cement.
5. Depending on the surgical situation, a cemented all poly acetabular liner, with or without constraint, can be implanted for an infected total hip. Alternatively, for infected hemiarthroplasties, a large cement head can be facilitated from a mold similar to the femoral stem.

**Massive Bone Loss at Hip Spacers: Intramedullary Nail Constructs**

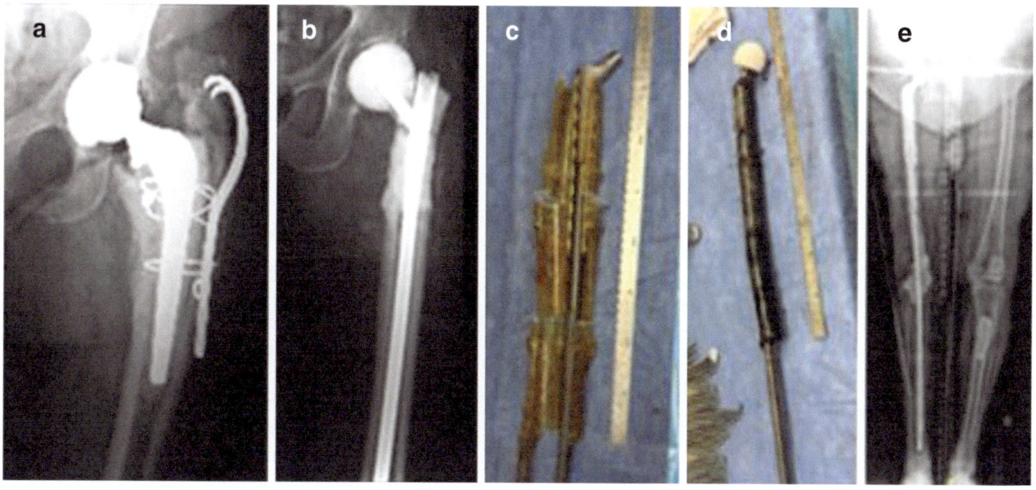


**Massive Bone Loss at Hip Spacers: Intramedullary Nail Constructs**

A. Patient with PJI after revision of total hip for periprosthetic fracture.
B. Intramedullary nail with cement ball fashioned from bulb syringe. A modern alternative to this is to utilize pre-made hemiarthroplasty molds as shown in another figure in this chapter and cement this to the cephallomedullary screw of the nail construct.
C. Arthroplasty stem impacted into the top of a femoral-tibial fusion nail and secured with two stainless steel plates, with screws and nuts placed through proximal interlocking holes of the nail.
D. Proximal construct coated in antibiotic cement on the back table. With a bipolar hemiarthroplasty head impacted on top of device.
E. Mechanical axis series of total femur articulating hip and static knee spacer. The patient was able to ambulate post-operatively on this device.

### 24.3.3 Static Versus Articulating Spacers

Several studies have retrospectively analyzed outcomes between static and articulating spacers and consistently found relatively comparable results in their ability to eradicate infection and complication rates. A large retrospective study demonstrated articulating spacers had significantly lower operative time with final implantation as well as slightly higher rates of treatment success. The financial burden must be taken into consideration with longer hospital stays associated with patients receiving static spacers rather than articulating spacers.

Importantly, evidence may be influenced by the selection of statics spacers in more challenging cases including those with more extensive bone loss and poor soft tissue coverage. A randomized control trial determined that static and articulating spacers have comparable operative times during second-stage reimplantation, functional outcome scores, and postoperative complications. The main significant difference identified between them was a longer hospital admission, implying a potential economic burden. Given these tradeoffs, articulating spacers should be the default spacer utilized in hip prosthetic infections unless otherwise contraindicated.

## References


1. Flint MN, et al. Two-stage revision of infected uncemented lower extremity tumor endoprostheses. J Arthroplast. 2007;22(6):859–65.
2. Grimer RJ, et al. Two-stage revision for infected endoprostheses used in tumor surgery. Clin Orthop Relat Res. 2002;395:193–203.
3. Nickinson RS, et al. Two stage revision knee arthroplasty for infection with massive bone loss. A technique to achieve spacer stability. Knee. 2012;19(1):24–7.
4. Bickels J, et al. Distal femur resection with endoprosthetic reconstruction: a long-term followup study. Clin Orthop Relat Res. 2002;400:225–35.
5. Jeys LM, et al. Periprosthetic infection in patients treated for an orthopaedic oncological condition. J Bone Joint Surg Am. 2005;87(4):842–9.
6. Alvand A, et al. Clinical outcome of massive Endoprostheses used for managing Periprosthetic joint infections of the hip and knee. J Arthroplast. 2018;33(3):829–34.
7. Graci C, et al. Infection following bone tumor resection and reconstruction with tumoral prostheses: a literature review. Int J Immunopathol Pharmacol. 2010;23(4):1005–13.
8. Hanssen AD, Rand JA. Evaluation and treatment of infection at the site of a total hip or knee arthroplasty. Instr Course Lect. 1999;48:111–22.
9. Eckardt JJ, et al. The UCLA experience in limb salvage surgery for malignant tumors. Orthopedics. 1985;8(5):612–21.
10. Holzer G, Windhager R, Kotz R. One-stage revision surgery for infected megaprostheses. J Bone Joint Surg Br. 1997;79(1):31–5.
11. Teeny SM, et al. Treatment of infected total knee arthroplasty. Irrigation and debridement versus two-stage reimplantation. J Arthroplast. 1990;5(1):35–9.
12. Insall JN, Thompson FM, Brause BD. Two-stage reimplantation for the salvage of infected total knee arthroplasty. J Bone Joint Surg Am. 1983;65(8):1087–98.
13. Bejon P, et al. Two-stage revision for prosthetic joint infection: predictors of outcome and the role of reimplantation microbiology. J Antimicrob Chemother. 2010;65(3):569–75.
14. Gathen M, et al. Comparison of two-stage revision arthroplasty and intramedullary arthrodesis in patients with failed infected knee arthroplasty. Arch Orthop Trauma Surg. 2018;138:1443.
15. Pignatti G, et al. Two stage hip revision in periprosthetic infection: results of 41 cases. Open Orthop J. 2010;4:193–200.
16. Bian T, et al. Tests for predicting reimplantation success of two-stage revision for periprosthetic joint infection: a systematic review and meta-analysis. Orthop Traumatol Surg Res. 2018;104:1115.
17. Calton TF, Fehring TK, Griffin WL. Bone loss associated with the use of spacer blocks in infected total knee arthroplasty. Clin Orthop Relat Res. 1997;345:148–54.
18. Fehring TK, et al. Articulating versus static spacers in revision total knee arthroplasty for sepsis. The Ranawat Award. Clin Orthop Relat Res. 2000;380:9–16.
19. Lichstein P, et al. Treatment of Periprosthetic knee infection with a two-stage protocol using static spacers. Clin Orthop Relat Res. 2016;474(1):120–5.
20. Guild GN, Wu B, Scuderi GR. Articulating vs. static antibiotic impregnated spacers in revision total knee arthroplasty for sepsis. A systematic review. J Arthroplast. 2014;29(3):558–63.
21. Parvizi J, Gehrke T, Chen AF. Proceedings of the international consensus on periprosthetic joint infection. Bone Joint J. 2013;95-B(11):1450–2.
22. Parvizi J, et al. The 2018 definition of Periprosthetic hip and knee infection: an evidence-based and validated criteria. J Arthroplast. 2018;33(5):1309–1314.e2.
23. Parvizi J, et al. New definition for periprosthetic joint infection: from the workgroup of the musculoskeletal infection society. Clin Orthop Relat Res. 2011;469(11):2992–4.
24. Zimmerli W, Trampuz A, Ochsner PE. Prosthetic-joint infections. N Engl J Med. 2004;351(16):1645–54.
25. Restrepo C, et al. Antibiotic treatment and timing of reimplantation. J Orthop Res. 2014;32(Suppl 1):S136–40.
26. Tan TL, et al. Surgical treatment of chronic Periprosthetic joint infection: fate of spacer exchanges. J Arthroplast. 2019;34(9):2085–2090.e1.
27. Manoso MW, et al. Limb salvage of infected knee reconstructions for cancer with staged revision and free tissue transfer. Ann Plast Surg. 2006;56(5):532–5. discussion 535
28. Hannigan GD, et al. Current concepts and ongoing research in the prevention and treatment of open fracture infections. Adv Wound Care (New Rochelle). 2015;4(1):59–74.
29. Glueck DA, Charoglu CP, Lawton JN. Factors associated with infection following open distal radius fractures. Hand (N Y). 2009;4(3):330–4.
30. Warth LC, Hadley CJ, Grossman EL. Two-stage treatment for total knee arthroplasty infection utilizing an articulating prefabricated antibiotic spacer. J Arthroplast. 2020;35(3S):S57–62.
31. Kini SG, et al. Two-stage revision for Periprosthetic hip and knee joint infections. Open Orthop J. 2016;10:579–88.

32. Koschnick M, Bruener S, Germann G. Free tissue transfer: an advanced strategy for postinfection soft-tissue defects in the upper extremity. Ann Plast Surg. 2003;51(2):147–54.
33. Zalavras CG, et al. Infected fractures of the distal tibial metaphysis and plafond: achievement of limb salvage with free muscle flaps, bone grafting, and ankle fusion. Clin Orthop Relat Res. 2004;427:57–62.
34. Pu LL, et al. Free tissue transfer to a difficult wound of the lower extremity. Ann Plast Surg. 2004;53(3):222–8.
35. Isenberg JS, et al. Salvage and reconstruction of complex post-extirpative knee wounds: a successful surgical protocol. J Reconstr Microsurg. 1999;15(2):115–8.
36. Funovics PT, et al. Management of septic complications following modular endoprosthetic reconstruction of the proximal femur. Int Orthop. 2011;35(10):1437–44.
37. Hardes J, et al. Characteristics and outcome of infections associated with tumor endoprostheses. Arch Orthop Trauma Surg. 2006;126(5):289–96.
38. Chen WS, Fu TH, Wang JW. Two-stage reimplantation of infected hip arthroplasties. Chang Gung Med J. 2009;32(2):188–97.
39. Marson BA, et al. Two-stage revision surgery for infected total knee replacements: reasonable function and high success rate with the use of primary knee replacement implants as temporary spacers. Eur J Orthop Surg Traumatol. 2018;28(1):109–15.
40. Biau D, et al. Survival of total knee replacement with a megaprosthesis after bone tumor resection. J Bone Joint Surg Am. 2006;88(6):1285–93.
41. Kugelman D, Roof M, Egol A, Guanche I, Chen AF, Scwarzkopf R, Aggarwal VK. Comparing articulating spacers for Periprosthetic joint infection after primary Total hip arthroplasty: all-cement versus real-component articulating spacers. J Arthroplast. 2022;37(7):S657–63.
42. Nahhas CR, Chalmers PN, Parvizi J, Sporer SM, Deirmengian GK, Chen AF, Culvern CN, Moric M, Della Valle CJ. Randomized trial of static and articulating spacers for treatment of the infected Total hip arthroplasty. J Arthroplast. 2021;36(6):2171–7.

# 25 Native Hip Joint Infection

Agustin Albani-Forneris, Martin A. Buttaro, and Pablo A. Slullitel

## 25.1 Introduction

Infection of the native hip joint, either in isolation or associated with previous hardware, is both a limb- and life-threatening problem, being considered as a medical emergency when presented in an acute fashion [1]. Most research about perioperative hip joint infection has been developed in the setting of a previous hip replacement [2]. However, literature about native hip joint infection and peri-implant hip joint infection in adult patients is not so abundant. Within this chapter, the authors will review the epidemiology, etiology, diagnosis and treatment of the most common non-prosthetic hip joint infection scenarios: (i) septic arthritis of the native hip joint, (ii) infection following hip preservation surgery, and (iii) following plating or nailing of a previous hip fracture.

A. Albani-Forneris · M. A. Buttaro · P. A. Slullitel (✉)
Hip Surgery Unit, Institute of Orthopaedics 'Carlos E. Ottolenghi', Hospital Italiano Buenos Aires, Buenos Aires, Argentina
e-mail: agustin.albani@hiba.org.ar; martin.buttaro@hiba.org.ar; pablo.slullitel@hiba.org.ar

## 25.2 Native Hip Arthritis in the Adult Patient

### 25.2.1 Epidemiology

Septic arthritis (SA) is a rare disease that affects 2 persons per 100,000 inhabitants each year [3], being the hip the second most affected joint in 20–25% of all joints after the knee. The main risk factors for SA of the hip joint are age over 80 years (due to age-related changes in the immune system), diabetes, inflammatory joint diseases such as rheumatoid arthritis, recent joint surgery, skin infection [4], intravenous drug use, and patients undergoing hemodialysis (e.g., renal failure) [5]. The most frequent means of infection is hematogenous dissemination, being unusual direct inoculation by either trauma, surgical procedure, or an animal bite. Nonetheless, joint injections with corticosteroids are a rare cause of infection, affecting about 4 patients per 10,000 injections [6].

The highly vascularized synovium that lacks a protective membrane is fertile soil for bacterial infiltration [7]. Once microorganisms proliferate inside the joint, an inflammatory reaction is triggered, which in combination with bacterial toxins and enzymes is responsible for joint damage [8]. The cartilage's nutrition is mainly dependent on oxygen diffusion. However, with the increase in joint pressure due to purulent exudate and


P. Ruggieri et al. (eds.), *Bone and Joint Infections*, https://doi.org/10.1007/978-3-031-96383-4_25

inflammatory reaction, the blood flow decreases causing anoxia of the cartilage [9].

### 25.2.2 Etiology

In adults the most common causes of SA of the hip joint are gram-positive organisms, being *Staphylococcus aureus* responsible for about 37–56% of cases, especially in those patients suffering from uncontrolled diabetes or rheumatoid arthritis (prevalence of up to 80% of infections). In the latter group, polyarticular infections caused by this bacterium are more prevalent. The increase in cases of methicillin-resistant *Staphylococcus aureus* (MRSA) strains, whose sensitivity to antibiotics varies according to the communities and in-hospital infections, is currently a cause for concern [3, 9]. *Streptococcus pyogenes* (group A—Beta-haemolytic) is second in frequency (8–16% of cases). In patients with immunodeficiency, and gastrointestinal or urinary tract infections, it is important to consider group B, C, and G *streptococci* as potential offending organisms. Gram-negative bacilli should also be suspected in immunocompromised patients, as well as in the elderly population and intravenous drug users [10]. Following inclusion in the immunization schedule, the incidence of *Haemophilus influenzae*-joint infections has decreased considerably in the neonatal and pediatric population [11], as has in the adult population as well.

*Mycobacterium tuberculosis*-joint infections are rare (2%), with chronic and silent presentations being the most common types, exhibiting progressive, late symptoms similar to those of primary osteoarthritis. Only about 50% of these patients are found to have thoracic radiographs with signs of tuberculosis infection. Therefore, its diagnosis is late and advanced joint damage is commonly seen [12].

Gonococcal septic arthritis was the main cause of septic arthritis in young adults in the 80's; today its prevalence has fallen to 1% or less. Some believe, however, that its incidence may increase due to antibiotic resistance and current sexual behaviors [13]. Women are mainly affected, usually presenting with migratory polyarthritis. The isolation of gonococcus in cultures is approximately 50%. Fortunately, treatment is usually effective, and joint sequelae are rare [14].

### 25.2.3 Clinical Presentation

The clinical presentation of septic hip arthritis can vary depending on age, the underlying cause of the infection, the patient's general health, and immune status. However, some common signs and symptoms of septic hip arthritis are: (i) pain in the groin area, which is usually the most prominent symptom, is often severe, constant and worsens with movement; (ii) fever, although chills and high fever are unusual; (iii) limited range of motion and stiffness; and (iiii) swelling and local redness, with the adjacent skin being warm. Weight-bearing is usually difficult with the affected leg, with patients usually limping or needing walking assistance. In some cases, patients with septic hip arthritis are also likely to experience systemic symptoms such as fatigue, malaise, and loss of appetite. Due to joint effusion, the hip is usually flexed, abducted, and externally rotated, a position in which the joint capsule has greater volume [10, 13].

### 25.2.4 Diagnosis

The gold standard for the diagnosis of native hip arthritis is the confirmation of an offending organism in the synovial fluid by culture, for which it is of paramount importance to perform an arthrocentesis (i.e., hip joint aspiration) prior to antibiotic treatment. The synovial fluid (SF) white blood-cell count (WBC) is usually >50,000 cells/mm$^3$ but its reported sensitivity ranges from 53 to 100% with a specificity of 66%-97%. The polymorphonuclear leukocyte ratio >90% has shown a sensitivity of 42–82% and specificity of 67–89% [15]. Gram stain usually provides rapid results but its low sensitivity of 45% limits its utility [16].

Elevated inflammatory markers such as C-reactive protein (CRP), erythrosedimentation rate (ESD) in addition to serum WBC >10,000 cells/mm$^3$ are non-specific for the diagnosis of septic arthritis, however, they are very sensitive, and when correlated with the patient's clinical picture and a synovial fluid WBC value of >50,000 cells/mm$^3$ the specificity increases and the combined sensitivity reaches almost 100% [17]. Measurement of CRP in synovial fluid is as useful as serum measurement, although it increases the specificity. Serum CRP >20 mg/l is a strong independent risk factor for septic arthritis (odds ratio 81.9, $p < 0.001$) [18]. On the other hand, the synovial CRP threshold seems to be around 10 mg/l [19], similar to what has been described for cases with periprosthetic joint infection [20]. Recent studies have shown that the synovial fluid and serum neutrophil-to-lymphocyte ratio (SF- and SR-NLR), with a cut-off value of 25, had 78% sensitivity and 81% specificity in the diagnosis of native hip arthritis. It seems to be a very useful tool for diagnosis at no additional cost [21]. However, these results should be validated in prospective studies.

Diagnostic imaging studies focus on identifying inflammation, adjacent tissue involvement, and joint damage. Sometimes, they are not able to accurately differentiate whether it is an infectious or non-infectious cause. Ultrasonography can evidence an increase in joint fluid with very low specificity but is very helpful in performing a guided and safe arthrocentesis, which is almost always needed. Radiographic images are useful when compared with previous radiographs if they are available, initially a widening of the joint space and fat pad displacement can be visualized, but in cases of late diagnosis, joint erosion and space narrowing can be seen.

In cases where adjacent bone involvement is suspected, magnetic resonance imaging (MRI) is useful for diagnosis and for assessing the extent of infection in adjacent tissue (Fig. 25.1). The area of the edema and inflammation may help the surgeon guide the extent of the debridement [22].

### 25.2.5 Differential Diagnoses

When diagnosing SA it is important to consider other differential diagnoses of pathologies with acute mono- or oligo-articular involvement, such as crystalloid arthritis, reactive arthritis, rheumatoid arthritis, and Lyme disease. Intra-articular accumulation of monosodium urate crystals (gout) or calcium pyrophosphate (pseudogout) can produce symptoms similar to SA, thus being the main diagnosis to be excluded. The diagnosis is confirmed by direct visualization of crystals by polarized light microscopy in synovial fluid. In patients with gout, high serum urate levels, the presence of tophi as well as first metatarsophalangeal joint involvement are useful to clinically assess the diagnosis. However, the intra-articular presence of crystals or the absence of positive cultures does not definitively exclude the diagnosis of SA [23, 24].

Reactive arthritis occurs in patients with a history of gastrointestinal or genitourinary infections, usually after 2–4 weeks. Joint symptoms are caused by bacteria that share the characteristic of being intracellular organisms, such as *Chlamydia trachomatis* (which has genitourinary transmission). In these situations, treatment should be symptomatic and the use of broad-spectrum antibiotics is not recommended [25]. When symptoms are symmetrical and polyarticular, with three or more joints involved, often affecting the joints of the hands and is associated with morning stiffness, the diagnosis of rheumatoid arthritis should be considered [26]. However, these patients are at increased risk for SA and therefore should be suspected in cases that present with acute monoarticular symptoms.

Patients presenting with joint swelling and pain who are inhabitants of or recent travelers to areas where Lyme disease is endemic should be suspected of *B. burgdorferi* infection. The history of a slowly expanding skin lesion (*erythema migrans*) at the site of a tick bite orients the diagnosis which can be confirmed by serology [27].

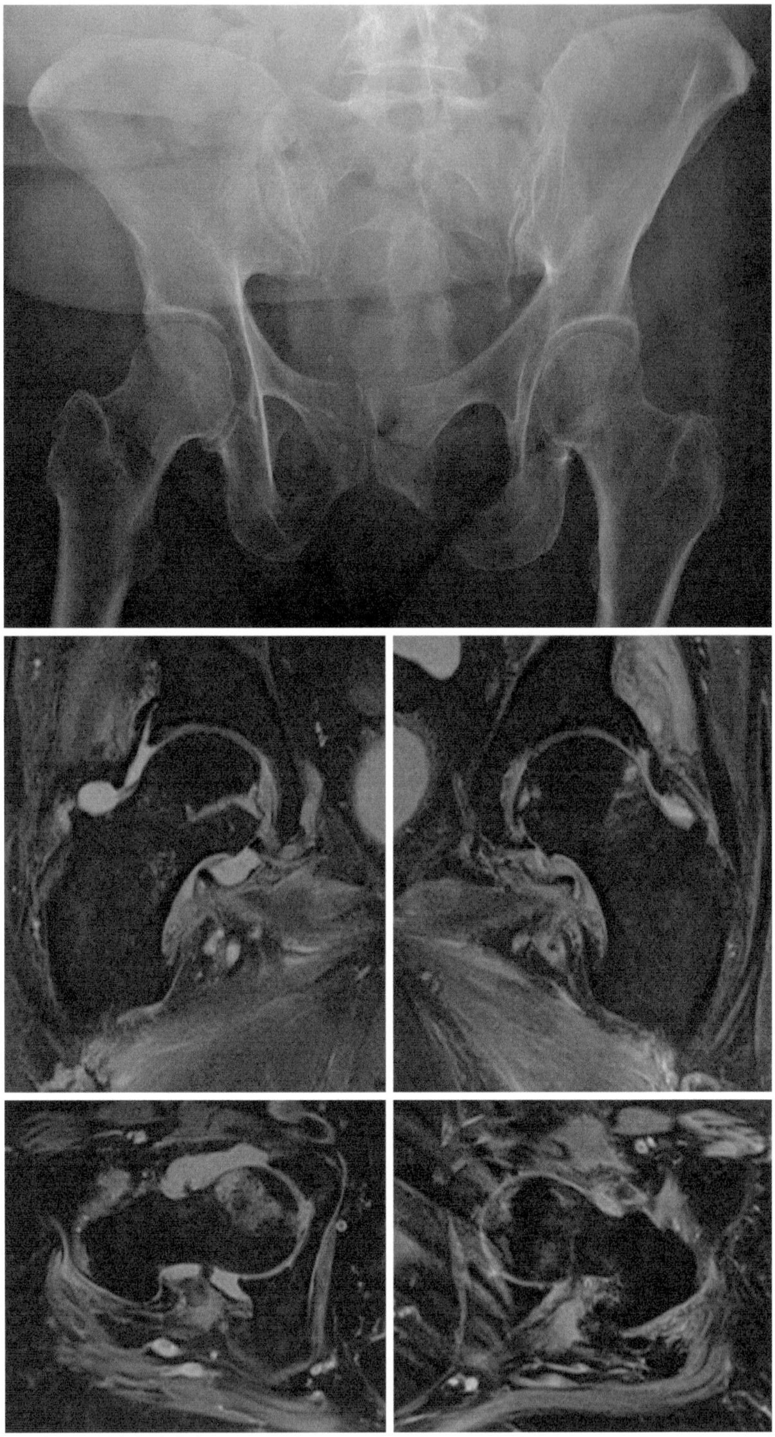

**Fig. 25.1** Radiographic and magnetic resonance imaging (MRI) of a 57-year-old female, with a history of acute myeloid leukemia under prolonged treatment with immunosuppressive drugs. The patient presented with fever and severe pain in both hips that increased with weight bearing (she was unable to walk). Radiographs did not show any acute pathology. MRI revealed abundant effusion, cartilage erosion and signs of atypical insufficiency fractures of both hips. Positive cultures for *Klebsiella pneumoniae* after bilateral hip joint aspiration

### 25.2.6 Treatment

Septic arthritis is an orthopedic emergency, and should not be delayed since its aggressive behavior leads to irreversible osteoarticular damage in the short-term. Antibiotic treatment must always be accompanied by surgical debridement of the joint. Empirical antibiotic treatment must start immediately without waiting for culture results. Only after the offending germ has been identified, the antibiotic therapy should be targeted to the specific germ. Surgical debridement can be performed either open or arthroscopically. Hip arthroscopy has proven to be a safe treatment option for patients with acute native infection [28]. However, this requires specific equipment to be available at the orthopedic theater, as well as specific surgical training and skills. For this reason, the authors of this chapter recommend performing the surgical debridement in an open fashion, through a minimally invasive direct anterior (Hueter) approach, which provides straightforward access to the joint.

Given the high prevalence of methicillin-resistant *Staphylococcus aureus* (MRSA) in the community, an antibiotic effective against MRSA, such as vancomycin, should always be included [29]. Only in areas where methicillin-sensitive strains are prevalent, cefazolin can be used empirically. Patients with risk factors for gram-negative bacteria such as those immunosuppressed, intravenous drug users, elderly, or critically ill patients would benefit from the empirical use of antibiotics effective against these germs. Under suspicion of disseminated gonococcal disease, ceftriaxone should be used. The duration of the antibiotic treatment is determined by the causal germ in case it is identified.

If SA is diagnosed in a late scenario or chronically, then the benefit of debridement and antibiotherapy remains unclear. Therefore, when the hip joint presents with space narrowing at index diagnosis or it has advanced cartilage damage upon complementary imaging, one- or two-stage total hip arthroplasty should be considered. Patients with a history of native joint infections are at higher risk of periprosthetic joint infection (PJI), especially smokers. Sultan et al. showed that in patients with a history of treated same-joint native septic arthritis, the proportion of PJI was five of 62 patients (8%). The Kaplan-Meier analysis demonstrated overall survivorship free from PJI of 92% at 14.5 ± 1.14 years (95% confidence interval [CI] = 12.3–16.8 years) [30]. Surprisingly, failures were reported in the knee joint only, whereas no cases of hips with previous native hip arthritis had to be reoperated. However, it has also been shown that less than a 1-year quiescent period after septic arthritis has been associated with 38-times increased risk and 22-times risk for post-THA PJI, at 0 and 6 months and 6 and 12 months, respectively [31]. Despite patients undergoing THA 6 months after their septic arthritis treatment having a decreased risk (compared to those between 0 and 6 months), the risks of further infection thereafter are still high. Therefore, the authors of this chapter suggest doing a two-stage arthroplasty with an articulating spacer in between to perform the most aggressive debridement possible. Often, delayed septic arthritis is diagnosed in patients with a systemic infection that will have prolonged hospitalization times. Functional spacers (Kiwi-type spacers) are especially useful in critically ill patients in which the time to the second stage remains unknown [32] (Fig. 25.2).

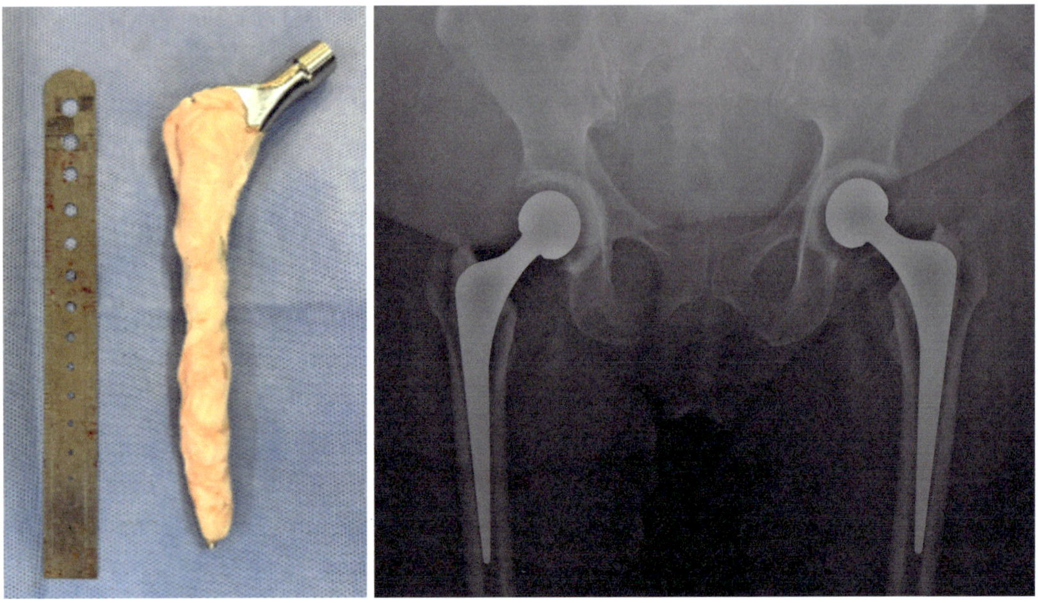

**Fig. 25.2** Image of functional femoral spacer assembled to a polished stem, coated with antibiotic-loaded cement; and postoperative radiographs of implanted bilateral functional spacers

## 25.3 Infection Following Hip Preservation Surgery

### 25.3.1 Hip Arthroscopy

#### 25.3.1.1 Epidemiology

The overall estimated incidence of septic arthritis after hip arthroscopy is less than 1% [33], ranging from 0% to 1.2% [34, 35]. Although the frequency of this complication is higher in the knee and the shoulder, the native hip is not an exception. In very rare cases, abdominal or scrotal infection may develop after fluid effusion into those compartments in case increased articular pressure is needed to perform the arthroscopy [36].

The history of intra-articular anesthetic, cortisone injection, or contrast agents for enhanced computed tomography or magnetic resonance imaging, increases the risk of joint infection. After analyzing a large administrative database, Wang et al. defined the risk of post-hip arthroscopy infection by separating the population into three groups based on the interval between preoperative injection and ipsilateral hip arthroscopy: <3 months, 3–6 months, 6–12 months [35]. In this study, preoperative hip injection within 3 months of hip arthroscopy was associated with a higher risk of postoperative infection as compared to both privately insured and medicare controls (2.16%, odds ratio [OR] 6.1, $P < .001$; and 2.80%, OR 1.99, $P = .037$, respectively). This 2- to 6-fold risk was not associated with any other demographic risk factor.

Nonetheless, some other factors such as obesity, inflammatory arthritis, chronic kidney disease, coronary artery disease, and depression have been associated with post-hip arthroscopy acute infection [37–40]. These factors, however, had been associated with overall complications and 30-day readmissions and not specifically with postoperative infection.

Surprisingly, the addition of hip arthroscopy as an adjuvant procedure to other hip preservation surgeries such as periacetabular osteotomy has not increased the complication rate of both procedures when performed in isolation [41]. In a prospective series of 248 hips analyzed by Sabbag et al. [41] the authors described 3 cases with postoperative infection and 1 additional case which required haematoma exploration, being such incidence below or in line with previously described prevalence percentages of post-hip arthroscopy infection.

Despite hip arthroscopy being increasingly indicated and performed in the last 20 years, evidence of antibiotic prophylaxis for this procedure has been under-reported [42]. In a recent systematic review including 9 studies, which comprised 592 patients, only 390 received routine antibiotic prophylaxis, while 160 patients did not and 42 received prophylaxis only if an additional implant was used [42]. This calls for the development of Delphi-based guidelines on antibiotic prophylaxis in hip arthroscopy specifically. Despite being based on an arthroplasty-driven study [43], the authors of this chapter believe that prophylaxis should always be done intravenously during anesthetic induction with cefazolin, whenever possible. We believe that one prophylactic dose of antibiotics is as effective as multiple doses [44, 45].

#### 25.3.1.2 Diagnosis

Diagnosis of an acute infection following hip arthroscopy is usually straightforward. Although fever and chills may be absent, pain (when loading or rotating the hip) and persistent wound drainage with elevated C-reactive protein and erythrosedimentation rate are usually present. If in doubt, hip joint aspiration should be performed to obtain appropriate samples for culture, cytologic analysis (including percentage of polymorphonuclears and synovial C-reactive protein), and physicochemical analysis. Whether doubt persists following this algorithm, an open debridement to obtain further samples should be performed.

If diagnosis is performed after 4–6 weeks, the infection can be considered as chronic, with an increased risk of failure of an eventual irrigation and debridement procedure. In this scenario, the senior author strongly recommends performing a magnetic resonance imaging (STIR volume) [46] to discard osteomyelitis and further plan a one- or two-stage primary total hip replacement. This helps determine the exact extension of the intraosseous edema, being useful for preoperative planning so that all regions affected by the infection can be resected.

#### 25.3.1.3 Differential Diagnoses

Several situations may mimic an acute hip infection, although none of them usually presents with excruciating pain and wound drainage. The following diagnoses should be strongly considered:

- Nerve damage, especially to the femoro-cutaneous or pudendal nerves
- Fluid extravasation, which may be associated with massive wound drainage [47]
- Complex regional pain syndrome, previously described after hip surgery [48]
- Ganglion cyst arising from the hip joint [49]
- Femoral neck fracture (prevalence, 0.08% to 0.12%) [50]

#### 25.3.1.4 Treatment

In case of an acute infection, the authors of this chapter suggest performing an open instead of arthroscopic debridement through an extensile anterior (Hueter) approach. This enables the surgeon to remove all fibrotic and necrotic, infected tissue while preserving the vascularity of the femoral head provided by the deep rami of the medial femoral circumflex artery. A 'bikini'-type incision can be performed connecting the anterolateral and mid-anterior portals in the most superficial plane, while the deeper dissection must be done following the Hueter interval to reach the hip joint.

There is, however, room for the indication of arthroscopic treatment following an infected hip arthroscopy [28, 51]. Lee et al. reported 9 patients with native septic arthritis treated with arthroscopic debridement without major complications and with only one of them with infection relapse at a mean follow-up of 19.4 months [52]. From the senior author's point of view, arthroscopy can be especially better for treating infected hip arthroscopy in the pediatric population, for being less invasive and having good-to-excellent functional and infection-free results at a minimum 2-year follow-up [53].

If a chronic infection is diagnosed, a primary total hip arthroplasty is advocated, either in one or two stages. In this scenario, there is no room for an arthroscopic approach. Preferably, two stages are recommended in order to perform a wide debridement in the first stage, with the removal of all infected tissue including capsule, synovium, subcutaneous tissue, and bone. If a posterior or a lateral approach is chosen, the authors of this chapter strongly recommend performing an anterior debridement at least through the arthroscopic portals, since the infection is supposed to be anteriorly 'grounded'. Otherwise, an anterior approach is preferred to excise the previous scars and remove a sinus tract, if any. A case example is shown in Figs. 25.3, 25.4 and 25.5.

### 25.3.2 Periacetabular Osteotomy

#### 25.3.2.1 Epidemiology

The first description of the surgical technique and outcomes of periacetabular osteotomy (PAO) was performed by Ganz in 1988 [54]. Since that

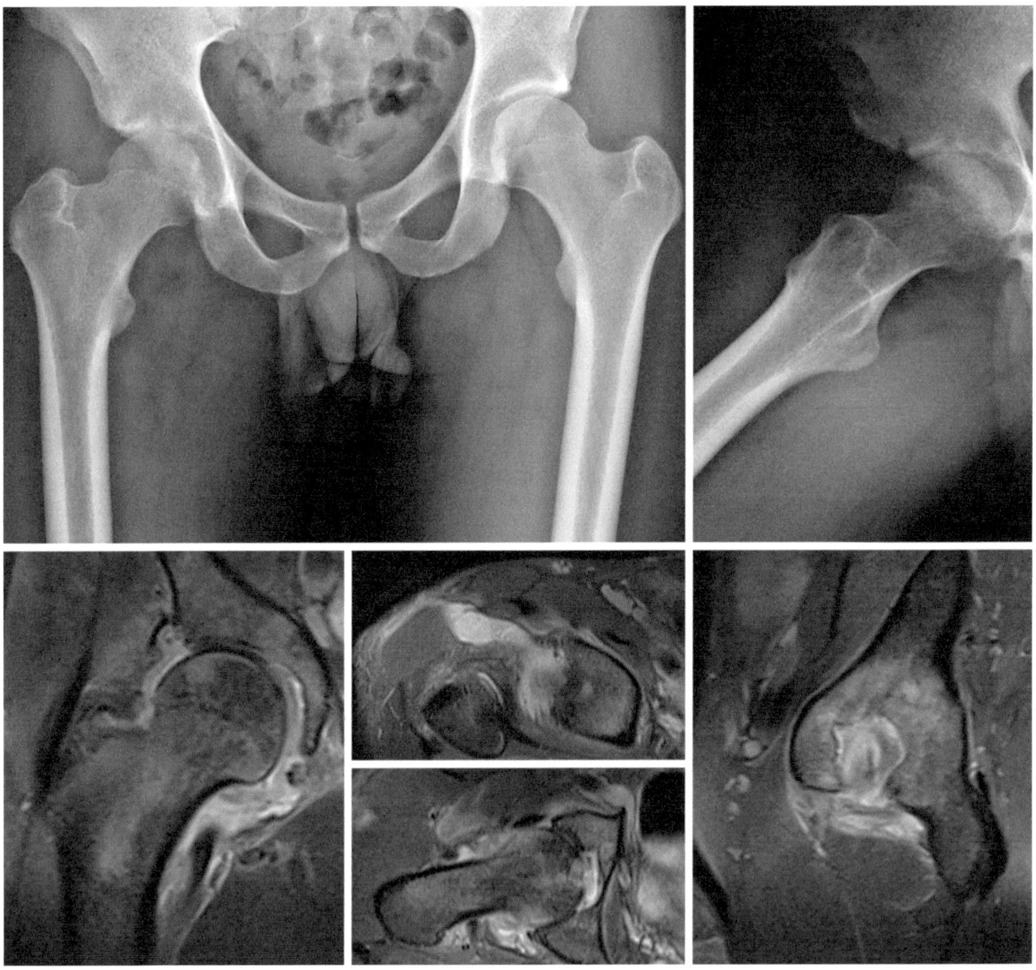

**Fig. 25.3** Radiographic and magnetic resonance imaging (MRI) of a 26-year-old male who underwent right hip arthroscopy due to femoroacetabular impingement at another institution 1 month before referral to our institution. The patient presented with excruciating pain, inability to walk independently, and persistent wound drainage. Radiographs evidenced chondral collapse with joint space narrowing, while revealing massive effusion associated with an anterior collection as well as bony acetabular and femoral head edema

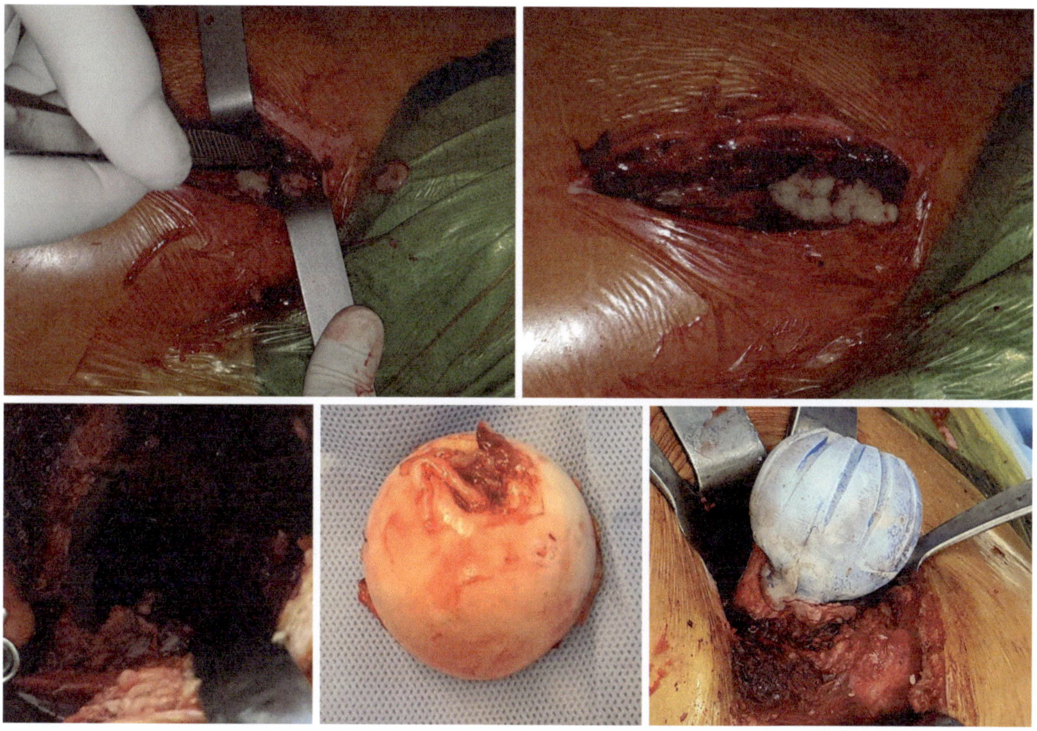

**Fig. 25.4** Intraoperative images show massive drainage of pus after performing an anterior approach joining both arthroscopic portals, followed by resection of a compromised femoral head with chondral delamination and implantation of an antibiotic-loaded spacer

report, the development of this technique has been globalized and the indication has substantially increased in the past 20 years, as has the development of fellowship training in hip preservation surgery. It has been further shown that the more this procedure is performed, the fewer complications are seen, especially after the first 40 PAOs [55]. In this concise report performed by Novais et al. that analyzed the surgeon's learning curve, the three infections detected (out of 81 cases, 3.7%) were associated with extended surgical procedure time since the median operative time was 320 minutes.

In a series of 238 PAOs operated between 1994 and 2008, only 3 cases (1.26%) developed a deep infection that required open debridement [56]. In a prospective multicenter study of 205 consecutive unilateral periacetabular osteotomies performed at seven institutions by ten surgeons, Zaltz et al. reported 2 patients (0.97%) that required incision and drainage of a deep infection, one of which required a primary hip replacement years after the PAO [57]. Likewise, in a systematic review performed by Ali and Malviya [58], the incidence of superficial infection was 1.03%, whereas deep infections represented 0.69%. While minimally invasive procedures had not been associated with neither infection nor wound complications, abductor-sparing modified Smith-Petersen and two-incision approaches were the most associated with this complication.

#### 25.3.2.2 Diagnosis

Even though there is no specific research study focusing on how to make an accurate diagnosis of deep infection following hip preservation surgery, any wound with erythema and persistent drainage should be inspected and eventually explored. In the 'Hip Arthroscopy' section, the authors suggest ordering blood work and performing aspiration of any suspicious collection if there is any doubt.

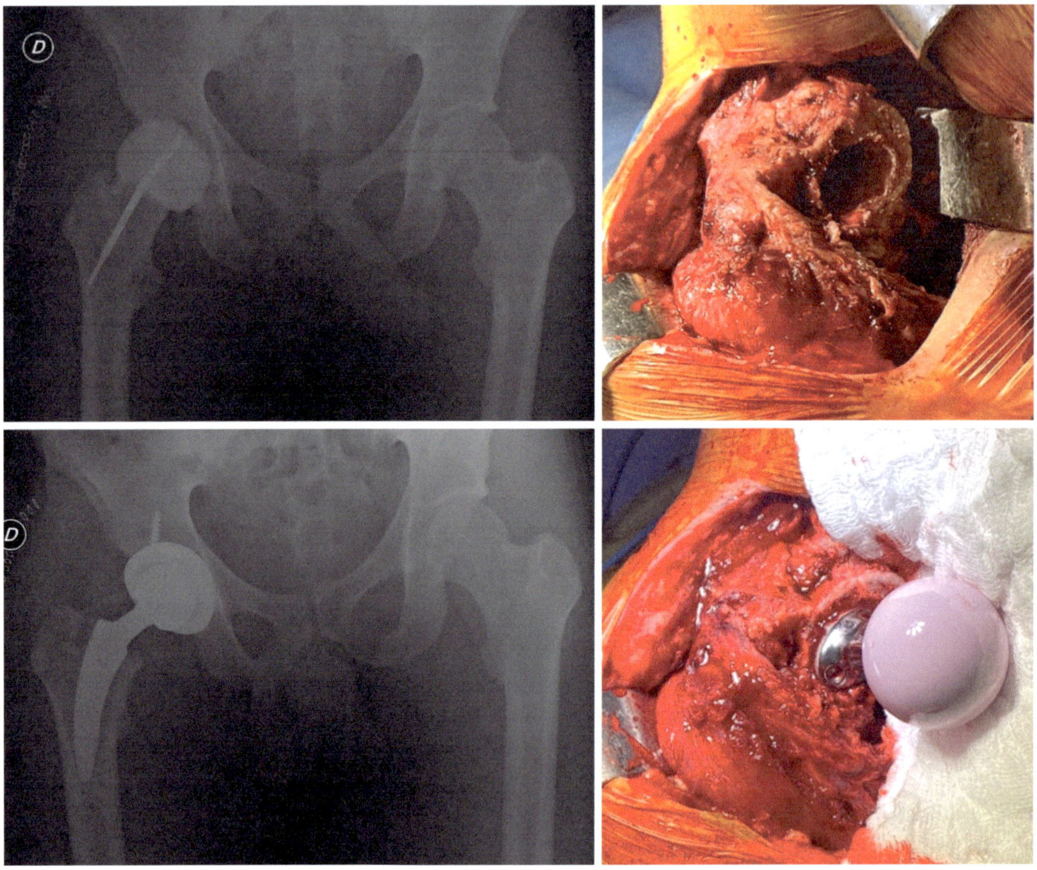

**Fig. 25.5** After 5 weeks of the first stage and following normalization of the serum biomarkers, the patient underwent implantation of a short femoral neck-preserving cementless stem and a cementless acetabular component with a ceramic-on-polyethylene bearing surface. The figure depicts both radiographic and intraoperative images (right hip)

#### 25.3.2.3 Classification

In 2012, Sink et al. published a modified Dindo-Clavien classification adapted for hip preservation surgery to better classify complications following surgery, with good-to-excellent intra- and inter-observer reliability [59]. This has been further validated for the pediatric population undergoing hip preservation surgery [60].

In this classification, a superficial infection is classified as grade 1, 'without clinical relevance'. On the other hand, a deep wound infection can be classified as grade 2 if it only requires medical treatment, or grade 3 if it needs 'surgical therapy or unplanned hospitalization'. The following table (Table 25.1) depicts the Dindo-Clavien classification adjusted for PAO and other hip-preserving surgeries [59, 61].

#### 25.3.2.4 Treatment

A superficial wound infection following PAO can be safely treated with oral antibiotics and observation. On the other hand, surgical debridement is the gold standard for the treatment of a deep infection. Sometimes, a new osteotomy of the anterior-superior iliac spine is needed to evacuate fluid collection lying medially to the inner table. Oral antibiotherapy is usually indicated unless a multi-drug resistant bacteria is isolated, in which case intravenous administration of antibiotics may be needed.

**Table 25.1** Dindo-Clavien classification adjusted for PAO and other hip-preserving surgeries

| Grade | Complication |
|---|---|
| 1. Complication without clinical relevance | Urinary tract infection |
| | Superficial wound infection |
| | Heterotopic ossifications grades 1–2 (Brooker) |
| | Postoperative fever |
| 2. Complications treated with conservative or medical therapy (outpatient) | Paraesthesia of femoro-cutaneous nerve |
| | Transient neuropraxia of the femoral or sciatic nerves |
| | Blood loss (>5 blood conserves administered) |
| | Avulsion of the anterior-superior iliac spine |
| | Trochanteric delayed union |
| | Stress fracture of the ischium |
| 3. Complication treated with surgery, intervention, or requiring unplanned readmission | Deep wound infection |
| | Haematoma requiring evacuation |
| | Migration of the acetabular fragment |
| | Revision surgery for non-union |
| | Heterotopic ossification grades 3–4 (Brooker) |
| | Intra-articular osteotomy (fracture) |
| | Trochanteric non-union |
| | Deep vein thrombosis |
| 4. Life-threatening complication, requirement of intensive care unit, or requirement of salvage procedure (total hip replacement), or complication not treatable with potential for permanent disability | Conversion to total hip replacement (necrosis of the acetabular fragment or femoral head) |
| | Permanent nerve injury |
| | Pulmonary embolism |
| | Organ dysfunction |
| 5. Death | – |

### 25.3.3 Surgical Hip Dislocation

#### 25.3.3.1 Epidemiology

Infection following surgical hip dislocation (SHD) is also a rare complication. In the first series described with this technique, no infections were reported in 213 hips [62]. In a retrospective multicenter study of complications following SHD on 334 hips carried out before the publication of Sink et al.'s classification of complications, only one (0.3%) deep infection was found (treated with surgical debridement), whereas two superficial wound infections (0.6%) were diagnosed (and treated with observation only) [63]. In other series, surgical site infections were reported to be as high as 3.8% [64]. In the setting of complex hip deformities, such complications are reported to be more prevalent, given the extended surgical time required for appropriate correction [65]: superficial infection, 4.34%; and deep infection, 2.17%.

When performing SHD for the treatment of femoral head fractures, infection may arise and be as high as 3.2%, being the most common complication following surgical treatment [66]. However, the modernization of this technique has led to almost zero infections in cases where this technique was performed by fellowship-trained surgeons [67].

#### 25.3.3.2 Classification, Diagnosis and Treatment

The authors of the chapter suggest reading the previous section ('Periacetabular osteotomy'), since classification, diagnosis, and treatment are the same.

## 25.4 Infection Following Plating or Nailing of a Previous Hip Fracture

### 25.4.1 Epidemiology

Infection following failed fixation after hip fracture is not uncommon despite many of them being treated with minimally invasive approaches, especially because such fractures occur in a very fragile population. In a randomized controlled trial comparing 203 cases treated with intramedullary nailing versus 197 patients treated with sliding hip screw, signs of superficial infection were found in 6 (2.9%) patients in the former group, compared with 4 (2.0%) in the latter group [68]. Additionally, deep wound infection was detected in 3 (1.4%) nail patients and 2 (1%) sliding hip screw patients [68]. In a recent meta-analysis, no difference was found between the two types of fixation with regard to infection when treating unstable A3 intertrochanteric fractures (1.8% vs. 2.57%, $p = 0.1$) [69]. Similar findings (without differences between treatment options) were found in another meta-analysis by Wessels et al., in which infection was a secondary outcome of the study [70]. Although there seems to be a lower reoperation rate for intramedullary nails than for sliding hip screws due to failure of fixation in unstable fractures, there is no apparent benefit of one treatment choice over the other in terms of infection prevention [71]. Likewise, Madariaga et al. studied 55 cases who underwent hip arthroplasty with concomitant hardware removal (cannulated screws, intramedullary nail, or dynamic hip screw) from 2005 to 2018, finding that 9% required reoperation for early postoperative infection [72]. Surprisingly, although 16% of cases had at least one positive intraoperative culture (out of 46 cases analyzed), none of them developed a postoperative infection.

### 25.4.2 Diagnosis

Diagnosis of an implant-related infection can sometimes be challenging, especially in the chronic setting. Early postoperative infection (<4 weeks) is usually characterized by erythema, local hyperthermia, delayed wound/bone healing, and an unhealed wound with drainage. Late/chronic infections may be more difficult to diagnose. A fracture-related infection (FRI) diagnosis can be done with either confirmatory or suggestive criteria [73, 74]. If a confirmatory criterion is present, surgical exploration should be done; whereas if a suggestive one is detected, observation can be performed. However, if one such isolated suggestive criterion is persistent drainage, this should enhance deep sampling for culture [73]. Confirmatory criteria include the following:

(a) sinus tract or wound breakdown (with communication to the bone or the implant);
(b) purulent drainage from the wound or presence of pus during surgery;
(c) phenotypically indistinguishable pathogens identified by culture from at least two separate deep tissue/implant (including sonication-fluid) specimens taken during an operative intervention; and
(d) presence of microorganisms in deep tissue taken during an operative intervention, as confirmed by histopathological examination using specific staining techniques for bacteria or fungi, or the presence of >5 polymorphonuclear neutrophils (PMNs)/high power field (HPF) in chronic/late-onset cases [73, 74].

On the other hand, suggestive criteria include the following:

(a) clinical signs such as unbearable pain, local redness or swelling, and fever
(b) radiological signs such as peri-implant or peri-fracture bony lysis, implant loosening, sequestrations (suggesting chronicity), non-union, and/or periosteal reaction. Magnetic resonance imaging can be useful to identify extension of osteomyelitis [75].
(c) identification by culture analysis from a single deep tissue specimen
(d) elevated serum C-reactive protein and erythrosedimentation rate (the value of white blood cell count is limited)
(e) new onset of joint effusion or persistent drainage: when drainage is still not evident but a collection of fluid is suspected, a contrast-CT scan can be useful [75].

In case of using tissue samples, multiple specimens (≥3) should be taken, using always clean and unused instruments (superficial and sinus tract swabs should be avoided). For this matter, a cold knife is preferred rather than diathermy. In cases of joint effusion arising in a joint contiguous to a fractured bone, fluid samples obtained by aspiration should be performed.

In 2017, Gittings et al. reported that erythrosedimentation rate >30 mm/h (odds ratio 28.8, 95% confidence interval 2.6–315.4, $P$ = .001) and C-reactive protein >1.0 mg/dL (odds ratio 11.5, 95% confidence interval 1.6–85.2, $P$ = .01) values were strongly associated with the development of infection after conversion to total hip arthroplasty [76]. In line with these findings, Cichos et al. reported that since patients undergoing conversion total hip arthroplasty from internal fixation of hip/acetabular fractures are at high risk for suffering periprosthetic joint infection, all should have a preoperative screening with inflammatory markers (C-reactive protein and erythrosedimentation rate) as part of the preoperative diagnostic work-up, especially C-reactive protein, which had an optimal cutoff value of 12 mg/L (area under the curve = 0.77, 95% confidence interval 0.58–0.97; 75% sensitivity, 84% specificity, 43% positive predictive value, and 95% negative predictive value) [77]. Xu et al. additionally demonstrated that combining C-reactive protein with neutrophil-to-lymphocyte ratio (cut-off value, 2.38) increases the sensitivity of diagnosing fracture-related infection to 89.5% and specificity to 91.5% before total hip arthroplasty [78]. All these serum biomarkers are cheap and available worldwide, so the authors of this chapter suggest ordering them since they are part of the suggestive criteria for fracture-related infection [73, 74].

### 25.4.3 Treatment

There is no doubt that in the acute setting, an FRI of the hip should be treated with irrigation, debridement, and implant retention (DAIR) as long as there is no complication related to the implant fixation. Whether to remove the hardware or not depends on both the chronicity of the infection and the stability of the construct [79]. It is pointless to retain unstable hardware even if the fracture was treated weeks ago [74]. In case of chronic infection with a sinus tract, not only the hardware has to be removed, but also peri-implant bone, the surrounding necrotic/infected tissue, and the sinus tract must be detached.

Usually, chronic hardware infections around the hip are associated with implant failure, including cut-out, cut-through, non-union, secondary avascular necrosis of the femoral head, etc. All these complications are characterized by the inability to walk independently, unremitting pain, and limb shortening. In this scenario, conversion to total hip arthroplasty is usually the treatment of choice. This procedure (i.e., complex primary total hip replacement) has been associated with great complications when compared to regular total hip arthroplasty, namely infection (6.2% vs. 2.6%), dislocation (8.1% vs. 4.5%), all-cause revision (8.4% vs. 4.3%), revision for infection (1.1% vs. 0.37%), and revision for dislocation (2.2% vs. 0.6%) [80].

It has been shown that a complex primary total hip arthroplasty is not just a 'more difficult' primary replacement. When comparing preoperative characteristics, intraoperative factors, and 30-day postoperative complications among primary, conversion and revision total hip arthroplasties, the first two differed in as much as 23 variables, whereas conversion hip arthroplasties and revisions differed in only one variable, being therefore quite similar procedures in terms of baseline characteristics and complications [81]. The disproportionate number of different variables between conversion and primary hip arthroplasties may be even more pronounced if the hardware to be removed in the conversion arthroplasty is already infected. These findings suggest that patients undergoing conversion hip arthroplasties mostly resemble patients undergoing revisions rather than primary surgeries [82].

In the case of a chronic FRI around the hip, conversion to total hip arthroplasty can be performed either in one or two stages, like in the treatment of chronic periprosthetic joint infection [83, 84]. This depends on the presence of a sinus tract, the clinical status of the patient, and the preoperative isolation of the infecting organism [85]. The authors of this chapter also believe that bone stock is also a variable to be considered when choosing between both approaches, since deficient bone stock (especially in the femur), can be associated with failure of a one-stage procedure [84]. Usually, patients with a failed fixation following a hip fracture are extremely frail and comorbid [86], which leads to resolving such cases in one stage. The following figure (Fig. 25.6) depicts a case with infected hardware following treatment of a previous hip fracture, treated by the senior author in a one-stage approach. Although some believe doing this surgery in one stage may carry a higher risk (5.8%) of an eventual new early infection around the prosthesis [52], a comprehensive approach should be performed in a case-based fashion. In a retrospective study of 41 cases with infected failed fixation following treatment of hip fracture, 12% of cases required an irrigation and debridement procedure [87]. Nonetheless, following Madariaga et al.'s study [72], which found no association between the positivity of intraop-

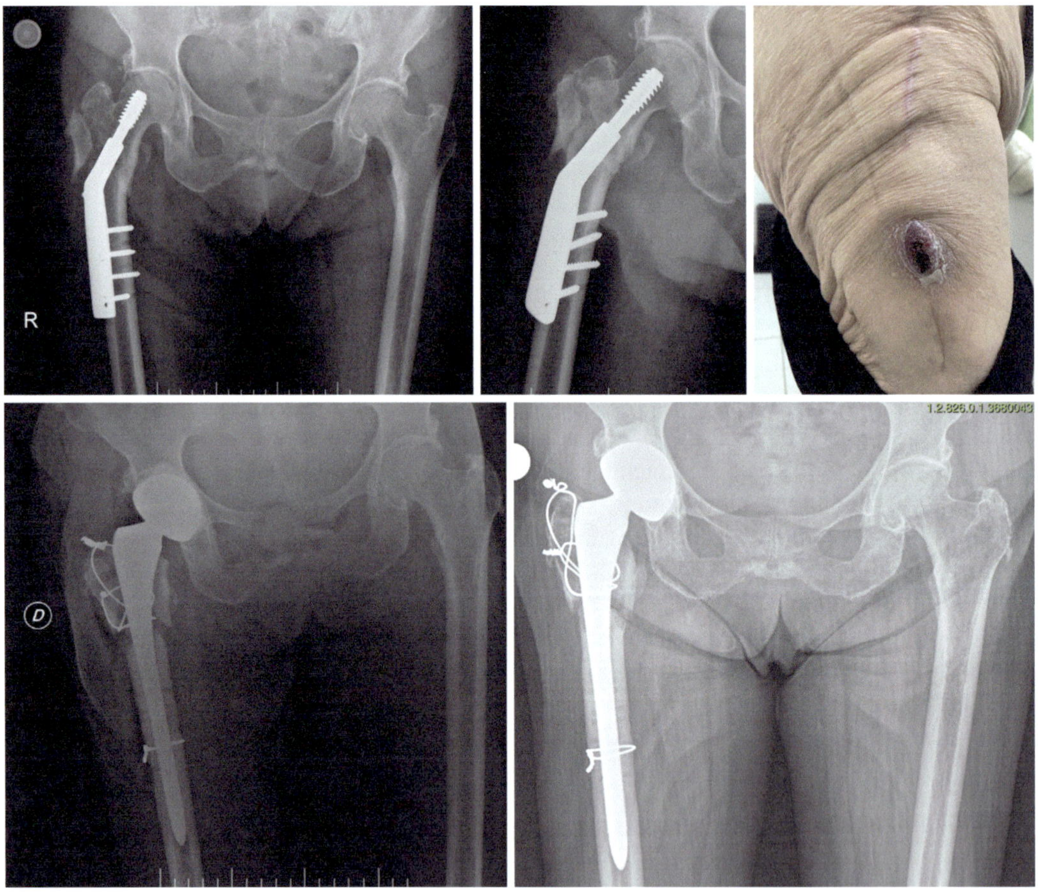

**Fig. 25.6** The first two images in the upper side are preoperative radiographs of an 84-year-old female who underwent treatment for a right intertrochanteric fracture. She evolved with unremitting pain, and inability to ambulate, and, one year after the index surgery, she presented with drainage and a sinus tract at the distal end of the wound (upper right image). Previous aspiration and bony samples evidenced a positive culture of methicillin-resistant Staphylococcus aureus. The patient was treated with a one-stage conversion to a cementless non-modular fit-and-fill stem and a cemented dual mobility acetabular component (lower left radiograph). The evolution was very good and at a 2-year follow-up, she is walking again with a cane (lower right radiograph), with the previous fracture site healed around the new implant

erative cultures and further development of infection, it seems adequate to perform a conversion total hip arthroplasty in a one-stage manner as long as other criteria are fulfilled.

When choosing a one-stage procedure, it is always preferred to use cement for fixation of both femoral and acetabular components, in order to load antibiotics for the preoperatively isolated organism (or broad-spectrum antibiotics in case the cultures are negative). Whether the bone loss is massive on the femoral side (>Paprosky 3A), an extensively porous-coated stem is preferred to enhance a better fixation [88, 89]. With regard to the acetabular side, the authors of this chapter prefer to use a dual mobility component (either cemented or cementless) since trochanteric non-union is frequent both before and after conversion to arthroplasty [90]. In the case of choosing a two-stage approach, the authors recommend using articulating spacers with the 'Kiwi' technique so that the patient can at least partially bear weight and ambulate [91]. One should take into account that many of these patients may not be fit enough to undergo the second stage for medical reasons [92, 93]; thus, using functional spacers could be of value in this population.

Following surgical treatment, patients should receive intravenous antibiotics while in-hospital waiting for cultures to be finalized, under close monitoring of an infectious diseases specialist. After discharge, oral antibiotics can be safely indicated whether the infecting organism is sensitive to them [94]. Irrespective of the route of administration, antibiotics should be prescribed for at least 12 weeks [95, 96].

## References


1. Kim B, Boukebous B, White D, Baker JF. Septic arthritis of the native hip joint: a multi-pattern, multi-outcome disease. Eur J Orthop Surg Traumatol. 2023;33:2587–94.
2. Ennis H, Chen CJ-L, Bondar K, McCormick J, Zieminski C, Hernandez VH. Influential literatures in periprosthetic infection following joint arthroplasty: a bibliometric review. J Orthopaed Trauma Rehabil. 2021;28:22104917211009777.
3. Mathews CJ, Weston VC, Jones A, Field M, Coakley G. Bacterial septic arthritis in adults. Lancet. 2010;375:846–55.
4. Kaandorp CJ, Van Schaardenburg D, Krijnen P, Habbema JD, van de Laar MA. Risk factors for septic arthritis in patients with joint disease. A prospective study. Arthritis Rheum. 1995;38:1819–25.
5. Al-Nammari SS, Gulati V, Patel R, Bejjanki N, Wright M. Septic arthritis in haemodialysis patients: a seven-year multi-centre review. J Orthop Surg. 2008;16:54–7.
6. Geirsson AJ, Statkevicius S, Víkingsson A. Septic arthritis in Iceland 1990–2002: increasing incidence due to iatrogenic infections. Ann Rheum Dis. 2008;67:638–43.
7. Goldenberg DL, Reed JI. Bacterial arthritis. N Engl J Med. 1985;312:764–71.
8. Shirtliff ME, Mader JT. Acute septic arthritis. Clin Microbiol Rev. 2002;15:527–44.
9. Stevens CR, Williams RB, Farrell AJ, Blake DR. Hypoxia and inflammatory synovitis: observations and speculation. Ann Rheum Dis. 1991;50:124–32.
10. Goldenberg DL. Septic arthritis. Lancet. 1998;351:197–202.
11. Iliadis AD, Ramachandran M. Paediatric bone and joint infection. EFORT Open Rev. 2017;2:7–12.
12. Gardam M, Lim S. Mycobacterial osteomyelitis and arthritis. Infect Dis Clin N Am. 2005;19:819–30.
13. Ross JJ. Septic arthritis of native joints. Infect Dis Clin N Am. 2017;31:203–18.
14. Goldenberg DL, Brandt KD, Cathcart ES, Cohen AS. Acute arthritis caused by gram-negative bacilli: a clinical characterization. Medicine. 1974;53:197–208.
15. Walinga AB, Stornebrink T, Langerhuizen DWG, Struijs PAA, Kerkhoffs GMMJ, Janssen SJ. What are the best diagnostic tests for diagnosing bacterial arthritis of a native joint?: a systematic review of 27 studies. Bone Joint J. 2021;103-B:1745–53.
16. Faraj AA, Omonbude OD, Godwin P. Gram staining in the diagnosis of acute septic arthritis. Acta Orthop Belg. 2002;68:388–91.
17. Li SF, Cassidy C, Chang C, Gharib S, Torres J. Diagnostic utility of laboratory tests in septic arthritis. Emerg Med J. 2007;24:75–7.
18. Singhal R, Perry DC, Khan FN, Cohen D, Stevenson HL, James LA, Sampath JS, Bruce CE. The use of CRP within a clinical prediction algorithm for the differentiation of septic arthritis and transient synovitis in children. J Bone Joint Surg Br. 2011;93:1556–61.
19. Dey M, Al-Attar M, Peruffo L, Coope A, Zhao SS, Duffield S, Goodson N. Assessment and diagnosis of the acute hot joint: a systematic review and meta-analysis. Rheumatology. 2023;62:1740–56.
20. Buttaro MA, Martorell G, Quinteros M, Comba F, Zanotti G, Piccaluga F. Intraoperative synovial C-reactive protein is as useful as frozen section to detect periprosthetic hip infection. Clin Orthop Relat Res. 2015;473:3876–81.

21. Varady NH, Schwab P-E, Kheir MM, Dilley JE, Bedair H, Chen AF. Synovial fluid and serum neutrophil-to-lymphocyte ratio: novel biomarkers for the diagnosis and prognosis of native septic arthritis in adults. J Bone Joint Surg Am. 2022;104:1516–22.
22. Coakley G, Mathews C, Field M, et al. BSR & BHPR, BOA, RCGP and BSAC guidelines for management of the hot swollen joint in adults. Rheumatology. 2006;45:1039–41.
23. Dalbeth N, Merriman TR, Stamp LK. Gout. Lancet. 2016;388:2039–52.
24. Hassan AS, Rao A, Manadan AM, Block JA. Peripheral bacterial septic arthritis: review of diagnosis and management. J Clin Rheumatol. 2017;23:435–42.
25. García-Kutzbach A, Chacón-Súchite J, García-Ferrer H, Iraheta I. Reactive arthritis: update 2018. Clin Rheumatol. 2018;37:869–74.
26. Scott DL, Wolfe F, Huizinga TWJ. Rheumatoid arthritis. Lancet. 2010;376:1094–108.
27. Steere AC. Lyme disease. N Engl J Med. 2001;345:115–25.
28. Fukushima K, Uekusa Y, Koyama T, Ohashi Y, Uchiyama K, Takahira N, Takaso M. Efficacy and safety of arthroscopic treatment for native acute septic arthritis of the hip joint in adult patients. BMC Musculoskelet Disord. 2021;22:318.
29. Hassoun A, Linden PK, Friedman B. Incidence, prevalence, and management of MRSA bacteremia across patient populations – a review of recent developments in MRSA management and treatment. Crit Care. 2017;21:211.
30. Sultan AA, Mahmood B, Samuel LT, George J, Faour M, Pelt CE, Anderson MB, Klika AK, Higuera CA. Patients with a history of treated septic arthritis are at high risk of periprosthetic joint infection after total joint arthroplasty. Clin Orthop Relat Res. 2019;477:1605–12.
31. Dubin JA, Chen Z, Bains SS, Hameed D, Mont MA, Delanois RE, Nace J. Less than 1-year quiescent period after septic arthritis of the hip is associated with high risk of periprosthetic joint infection following total hip arthroplasty. J Arthroplasty. 2023;38:930–934.e1.
32. Tsung JD, Rohrsheim JAL, Whitehouse SL, Wilson MJ, Howell JR. Management of periprosthetic joint infection after total hip arthroplasty using a custom made articulating spacer (CUMARS); the Exeter experience. J Arthroplasty. 2014;29:1813–8.
33. Bauer T, Boisrenoult P, Jenny JY. Post-arthroscopy septic arthritis: current data and practical recommendations. Orthop Traumatol Surg Res. 2015;101:S347–50.
34. Malviya A, Raza A, Jameson S, James P, Reed MR, Partington PF. Complications and survival analyses of hip arthroscopies performed in the national health service in England: a review of 6,395 cases. Arthroscopy. 2015;31:836–42.
35. Wang D, Camp CL, Ranawat AS, Coleman SH, Kelly BT, Werner BC. The timing of hip arthroscopy after intra-articular hip injection affects postoperative infection risk. Arthroscopy. 2017;33:1988–1994.e1.
36. Griffin DR, Dickenson EJ, Wall PDH, et al. Hip arthroscopy versus best conservative care for the treatment of femoroacetabular impingement syndrome (UK FASHIoN): a multicentre randomised controlled trial. Lancet. 2018;391:2225–35.
37. Clarke MT, Arora A, Villar RN. Hip arthroscopy: complications in 1054 cases. Clin Orthop Relat Res. 2003:84–8.
38. Cvetanovich GL, Chalmers PN, Levy DM, Mather RC 3rd, Harris JD, Bush-Joseph CA, Nho SJ. Hip arthroscopy surgical volume trends and 30-day postoperative complications. Arthroscopy. 2016;32:1286–92.
39. Du JY, Knapik DM, Trivedi NN, Sivasundaram L, Mather RC 3rd, Nho SJ, Salata MJ. Unplanned admissions following hip arthroscopy: incidence and risk factors. Arthroscopy. 2019;35:3271–7.
40. Truntzer JN, Hoppe DJ, Shapiro LM, Abrams GD, Safran M. Complication rates for hip arthroscopy are underestimated: a population-based study. Arthroscopy. 2017;33:1194–201.
41. Sabbag CM, Nepple JJ, Pascual-Garrido C, Lalchandani GR, Clohisy JC, Sierra RJ. The addition of hip arthroscopy to periacetabular osteotomy does not increase complication rates: a prospective case series. Am J Sports Med. 2019;47:543–51.
42. Ekhtiari S, Haldane CE, de SA D, Simunovic N, Wong IH, Farrokhyar F, Ayeni OR. The use of antibiotic prophylaxis in hip arthroscopy is under-reported and lacks evidence-based guidelines: a systematic review and survey. J ISAKOS. 2018;3:105–9.
43. Wyles CC, Hevesi M, Osmon DR, Park MA, Habermann EB, Lewallen DG, Berry DJ, Sierra RJ. 2019 John Charnley Award: Increased risk of prosthetic joint infection following primary total knee and hip arthroplasty with the use of alternative antibiotics to cefazolin: the value of allergy testing for antibiotic prophylaxis. Bone Joint J. 2019;101-B:9–15.
44. Ryan SP, Kildow BJ, Tan TL, Parvizi J, Bolognesi MP, Seyler TM, American Association of Hip and Knee Surgeons Research Committee. Is there a difference in infection risk between single and multiple doses of prophylactic antibiotics? A Meta-analysis. Clin Orthop Relat Res. 2019;477:1577–90.
45. Veltman ES, Lenguerrand E, Moojen DJF, Whitehouse MR, Nelissen RGHH, Blom AW, Poolman RW. Similar risk of complete revision for infection with single-dose versus multiple-dose antibiotic prophylaxis in primary arthroplasty of the hip and knee: results of an observational cohort study in the Dutch Arthroplasty Register in 242,179 patients. Acta Orthop. 2020;91:794–800.
46. Zalavras CG, Rigopoulos N, Lee J, Learch T, Patzakis MJ. Magnetic resonance imaging findings in hematogenous osteomyelitis of the hip in adults. Clin Orthop Relat Res. 2009;467:1688–92.
47. Ekhtiari S, Haldane CE, de Sa D, Simunovic N, Ayeni OR. Fluid extravasation in hip arthroscopy: a systematic review. Arthroscopy. 2017;33:873–80.

48. Zanotti G, Slullitel PA, Comba FM, Buttaro MA, Piccaluga F. Three cases of type-1 complex regional pain syndrome after elective total hip replacement. SICOT J. 2017;3:52.
49. Burnett RA, Westermann R, Bedard N, Liu S, Callaghan JJ. Ganglion cyst as a rare complication of hip arthroscopy resolved with THA: a case report. Iowa Orthop J. 2018;38:87–91.
50. Zimmerer A, Sobau C, Ries C, Miehlke W. Femoral neck fracture is a rare complication after arthroscopic femoroplasty for femoroacetabular impingement with no known prognostic factors and few reported risk factors: a systematic review. J ISAKOS. 2017;2:147–51.
51. de SA D, Cargnelli S, Catapano M, Peterson D, Simunovic N, Larson CM, Ayeni OR. Efficacy of hip arthroscopy for the management of septic arthritis: a systematic review. Arthroscopy. 2015;31:1358–70.
52. Lee Y-K, Park K-S, Ha Y-C, Koo K-H. Arthroscopic treatment for acute septic arthritis of the hip joint in adults. Knee Surg Sports Traumatol Arthrosc. 2014;22:942–5.
53. Duman S, Camurcu Y, Ucpunar H, Çöbden A, Karahan N, Sofu H. Arthroscopic treatment of acute septic arthritis of the hip joint in pediatric patients aged 10 years or younger. Arthroscopy. 2020;36:464–72.
54. Ganz R, Klaue K, Vinh TS, Mast JW. A new periacetabular osteotomy for the treatment of hip dysplasias: technique and preliminary results. 1988. Clin Orthop Relat Res. 2004:3–8.
55. Novais EN, Carry PM, Kestel LA, Ketterman B, Brusalis CM, Sankar WN. Does surgeon experience impact the risk of complications after bernese periacetabular osteotomy? Clin Orthop Relat Res. 2017;475:1110–7.
56. Wells J, Schoenecker P, Petrie J, Thomason K, Goss CW, Clohisy JC. Are complications after the bernese periacetabular osteotomy associated with subsequent outcomes scores? Clin Orthop Relat Res. 2019;477:1157–63.
57. Zaltz I, Baca G, Kim Y-J, et al. Complications associated with the periacetabular osteotomy: a prospective multicenter study. J Bone Joint Surg Am. 2014;96:1967–74.
58. Ali M, Malviya A. Complications and outcome after periacetabular osteotomy – influence of surgical approach. Hip Int. 2020;30:4–15.
59. Sink EL, Leunig M, Zaltz I, Gilbert JC, Clohisy J, Academic Network for Conservational Hip Outcomes Research Group. Reliability of a complication classification system for orthopaedic surgery. Clin Orthop Relat Res. 2012;470:2220–6.
60. Dodwell ER, Pathy R, Widmann RF, Green DW, Scher DM, Blanco JS, Doyle SM, Daluiski A, Sink EL. Reliability of the modified clavien-dindo-sink complication classification system in pediatric orthopaedic surgery. JB JS Open Access. 2018;3:e0020.
61. Hanke MS, Lerch TD, Schmaranzer F, Meier MK, Steppacher SD, Siebenrock KA. Complications of hip preserving surgery. EFORT Open Rev. 2021;6:472–86.
62. Ganz R, Gill TJ, Gautier E, Ganz K, Krügel N, Berlemann U. Surgical dislocation of the adult hip a technique with full access to the femoral head and acetabulum without the risk of avascular necrosis. J Bone Joint Surg Br. 2001;83:1119–24.
63. Sink EL, Beaulé PE, Sucato D, et al. Multicenter study of complications following surgical dislocation of the hip. J Bone Joint Surg Am. 2011;93:1132–6.
64. Kargin D, Albayrak A, Atici Y, Yapici F, İlvan G, Balioğlu MB. The complications after open hip dislocation in hip surgery. Acta Orthop Belg. 2017;83:74–80.
65. Edelstein AI, Duncan ST, Akers S, Pashos G, Schoenecker PL, Clohisy JC. Complications associated with combined surgical hip dislocation and periacetabular osteotomy for complex hip deformities. J Hip Preserv Surg. 2019;6:117–23.
66. Giannoudis PV, Kontakis G, Christoforakis Z, Akula M, Tosounidis T, Koutras C. Management, complications and clinical results of femoral head fractures. Injury. 2009;40:1245–51.
67. Massè A, Aprato A, Alluto C, Favuto M, Ganz R. Surgical hip dislocation is a reliable approach for treatment of femoral head fractures. Clin Orthop Relat Res. 2015;473:3744–51.
68. Adams CI, Robinson CM, Court-Brown CM, McQueen MM. Prospective randomized controlled trial of an intramedullary nail versus dynamic screw and plate for intertrochanteric fractures of the femur. J Orthop Trauma. 2001;15:394–400.
69. Yu F, Tang Y-W, Wang J, Lin Z-C, Liu Y-B. Does intramedullary nail have advantages over dynamic hip screw for the treatment of AO/OTA31A1-A3? A meta-analysis. BMC Musculoskelet Disord. 2023;24:588.
70. Wessels JO, Bjarnesen MP, Erichsen JL, Palm H, Gundtoft PH, Viberg B. Sliding hip screw vs intramedullary nail for AO/OTA31A1-A3: a systematic review and meta-analysis. Injury. 2022;53:1149–59.
71. Grønhaug KML, Dybvik E, Matre K, Östman B, Gjertsen J-E. Intramedullary nail versus sliding hip screw for stable and unstable trochanteric and subtrochanteric fractures: 17,341 patients from the Norwegian Hip Fracture Register. Bone Joint J. 2022;104-B:274–82.
72. Madariaga S, Vargas-Reverón C, Tornero E, Alías A, Capurro B, Combalia A, Fernández-Valencia JÁ, Muñoz-Mahamud E. Outcomes of hip arthroplasty with concomitant hardware removal: influence of the type of implant retrieved and impact of positive intraoperative cultures. Arch Orthop Trauma Surg. 2021;141:333–9.
73. Metsemakers WJ, Morgenstern M, McNally MA, et al. Fracture-related infection: a consensus on definition from an international expert group. Injury. 2018;49:505–10.
74. Obremskey WT, Metsemakers W-J, Schlatterer DR, Tetsworth K, Egol K, Kates S, McNally M, ICM Orthopaedic Trauma Work Group, ICM Orthopaedic Trauma Work Group. Musculoskeletal infection in orthopaedic trauma: assessment of the 2018 interna-

tional consensus meeting on musculoskeletal infection. J Bone Joint Surg Am. 2020;102:e44.
75. McNally M, Govaert G, Dudareva M, Morgenstern M, Metsemakers W-J. Definition and diagnosis of fracture-related infection. EFORT Open Rev. 2020;5:614–9.
76. Gittings DJ, Courtney PM, Ashley BS, Hesketh PJ, Donegan DJ, Sheth NP. Diagnosing infection in patients undergoing conversion of prior internal fixation to total hip arthroplasty. J Arthroplasty. 2017;32:241–5.
77. Cichos KH, Christie MC, Heatherly AR, McGwin G Jr, Quade JH, Ghanem ES. The value of serological screening prior to conversion total hip arthroplasty. J Arthroplasty. 2020;35:S319–24.
78. Xu H, Xie J-W, Liu L, Wang D, Huang Z-Y, Zhou Z-K. Combination of CRP with NLR is a sensitive tool for screening fixation-related infection in patients undergoing conversion total hip arthroplasty after failed internal fixation for femoral neck fracture. Bone Joint J. 2021;103-B:1534–40.
79. Berkes M, Obremskey WT, Scannell B, Ellington JK, Hymes RA, Bosse M, Southeast Fracture Consortium. Maintenance of hardware after early postoperative infection following fracture internal fixation. J Bone Joint Surg Am. 2010;92:823–8.
80. Smith A, Denehy K, Ong KL, Lau E, Hagan D, Malkani A. Total hip arthroplasty following failed intertrochanteric hip fracture fixation treated with a cephalomedullary nail. Bone Joint J. 2019;101-B:91–6.
81. Baghoolizadeh M, Schwarzkopf R. The Lawrence D. Dorr Surgical Techniques & Technologies Award: conversion total hip arthroplasty: is it a primary or revision hip arthroplasty. J Arthroplasty. 2016;31:16–21.
82. Raiford ME, Barra MF, Myers TG. A conversion total hip arthroplasty is not a primary total hip arthroplasty. Oper Tech Orthop. 2019;29:100725.
83. Slullitel PA, Oñativia JI, Cima I, Zanotti G, Comba F, Piccaluga F, Buttaro MA. Patients with no recurrence of infection five years after two-stage revision hip arthroplasty may be classified as periprosthetic infection "in remission". Bone Joint J. 2021;103-B:79–86.
84. Slullitel PA, Oñativia JI, Zanotti G, Comba F, Piccaluga F, Buttaro MA. One-stage exchange should be avoided in periprosthetic joint infection cases with massive femoral bone loss or with history of any failed revision to treat periprosthetic joint infection. Bone Joint J. 2021;103-B:1247–53.
85. Citak M, Friedenstab J, Abdelaziz H, Suero EM, Zahar A, Salber J, Gehrke T. Risk factors for failure after 1-stage exchange total knee arthroplasty in the management of periprosthetic joint infection. J Bone Joint Surg Am. 2019;101:1061–9.
86. Slullitel PA, Lucero CM, Soruco ML, et al. Prolonged social lockdown during COVID-19 pandemic and hip fracture epidemiology. Int Orthop. 2020;44:1887–95.
87. George R, Hariharan TD, Arunshankar A, Elangovan D, Lal B, Chandy VJ, Oommen AT, Poonnoose PM. Is it safe to do a single-stage implant exit and primary hip replacement? Clinical and microbiological profiling. Indian J Med Microbiol. 2019;37:531–5.
88. Mathur HH, Shah HS, Vishwanathan K. Functional outcome of conversion total hip arthroplasty (CTHA) using uncemented distally loading femoral stem for failed fixation of proximal femoral nail – a case series. J Orthop. 2022;34:14–20.
89. Godoy-Monzon D, Diaz Dilernia F, Piccaluga F, Cid Casteulani A, Turus L, Buttaro M. Conversion total hip arthroplasty with a proximally modular, distal fixation reconstruction prosthesis following cephalomedullar nail failure. Hip Int. 2020;30:26–33.
90. Shi T, Fang X, Huang C, Li W, You R, Wang X, Xia C, Zhang W. Conversion hip arthroplasty using standard and long stems after failed internal fixation of intertrochanteric fractures. Orthop Surg. 2023;15:124–32.
91. Craig A, King SW, van Duren BH, Veysi VT, Jain S, Palan J. Articular spacers in two-stage revision arthroplasty for prosthetic joint infection of the hip and the knee. EFORT Open Rev. 2022;7:137–52.
92. Choi H-R, Freiberg AA, Malchau H, Rubash HE, Kwon Y-M. The fate of unplanned retention of prosthetic articulating spacers for infected total hip and total knee arthroplasty. J Arthroplasty. 2014;29:690–3.
93. Petis SM, Perry KI, Pagnano MW, Berry DJ, Hanssen AD, Abdel MP. Retained antibiotic spacers after total hip and knee arthroplasty resections: high complication rates. J Arthroplasty. 2017;32:3510–8.
94. Li H-K, Rombach I, Zambellas R, et al. Oral versus intravenous antibiotics for bone and joint infection. N Engl J Med. 2019;380:425–36.
95. Bernard L, Arvieux C, Brunschweiler B, et al. Antibiotic therapy for 6 or 12 weeks for prosthetic joint infection. N Engl J Med. 2021;384:1991–2001.
96. Yang J, Parvizi J, Hansen EN, Culvern CN, Segreti JC, Tan T, Hartman CW, Sporer SM, Della Valle CJ, Knee Society Research Group. 2020 Mark Coventry Award: microorganism-directed oral antibiotics reduce the rate of failure due to further infection after two-stage revision hip or knee arthroplasty for chronic infection: a multicentre randomized controlled trial at a minimum of two years. Bone Joint J. 2020;102-B:3–9.

# 26 Infective Complications After Trauma Surgeries

Khaled M. Emara, Ahmed K. Emara, and Mohamed O. Eissa

## 26.1 Introduction

Infection after orthopedic trauma surgeries remains a catastrophic disease for both clinicians and patients despite great efforts in its various fields. Although these infections share similarities with prosthetic joint infection (PJI) they have unique features. One of the typical characteristics is its high heterogeneity. Although diagnosis is established based on different tools, presentations of clinical symptoms, and imaging tests, serum levels of inflammatory biomarkers, microorganism culture results, and even treatment strategies differ among different patients with infection.

## 26.2 Definition

There have been numerous words used to characterize the start of infection after fracture. The usage of terms such as osteomyelitis, osteitis, and deep surgical site infection can be confusing and does not provide a clear indication of the association between the condition and a fracture. In 2018, the FRI Consensus Group issued the initial definition criteria and adopted the term fracture-related infection (FRI) to encompass all infections that occur in the setting of a fracture. This includes early infection surrounding fracture implants, infected non-unions, hematogenous infections following fracture healing, and infections in fractures without internal fixation. [1]

## 26.3 Epidemiology

The typical incidence of FRI ranges from 1% (closed fractures) to over 30% (open fractures), with a maximum incidence rate of 55%. [1] The incidence of FRI varies amongst fracture locations. The FRI incidence of distal femoral joint fracture fixation was found to be 1.5 [2], tibial plateau fractures 7% [3], ankle fractures 6% [4], and calcaneal fractures 3% [5]. Infection rates following intramedullary nail (IMN) insertion for femoral and tibial diaphyseal fractures were 8.59 percent at 3 months and 11.8 percent at 12 months [6].

## 26.4 Risk Factors

In addition to the location and severity of the injury, the chance of developing an FRI is influenced by the amount of concurrent injuries and preexisting comorbidities. Polytraumatized patients are at high risk because severe trauma is usually accompanied by complex musculoskeletal injuries and an impaired host immune

K. M. Emara · A. K. Emara · M. O. Eissa (✉)
Department of Orthopedic Surgery, Ain Shams University, Cairo, Egypt



P. Ruggieri et al. (eds.), *Bone and Joint Infections*, https://doi.org/10.1007/978-3-031-96383-4_26

response. Risk factors can be classified as external factors and internal factors. [7]

External factors (environmental factors)

1. injury type and degree
2. injury site
3. pathogen virulence
4. prophylaxis and treatment methods
5. geographical location and seasonal factor

Internal factors (host factors)

1. immune status
2. lifestyle
3. comorbidity of the patients

## 26.5 Pathogenesis

FRI arises exogenously as a result of the initial trauma (in the event of an open fracture), fracture fixation, or disrupted wound healing, or late soft-tissue coverage. In FRIs, hematogenous transmission of bacteria to the implant is a rare source of infection. [8]

The most common microorganisms involved in FRI include *Staphylococcus aureus* (30–42%), coagulase-negative staphylococci (20–39%), enterobacterial (14–27%), anaerobes (16%), and streptococci (11%). Polymicrobial infections (20–35%) occur typically in patients with open fractures [1, 9].

Biofilm formation on the surface of foreign material is crucial in the pathogenesis of FRI. Biofilm-dwelling microorganisms are able to withstand significantly higher antibiotic concentrations than planktonic microorganisms; hence, most systematically administered antibiotics fail to achieve the required therapeutic doses. For this reason, successful management of FRI requires a combination of surgical and antimicrobial treatment. [10]

Time is an important aspect in the pathogenesis of FRI for the following reasons. First, the maturation of biofilms over weeks impacts the efficiency of antimicrobial therapy. [11] Second, fracture healing leading to bone consolidation is essential for infection cure and takes weeks to months to occur. Third, the degree of bone involvement must be considered while formulating a treatment plan. Despite the presence of microorganisms on the implant, two weeks after fracture fixation, the bone does not exhibit symptoms of osteomyelitis or osteolysis, according to preclinical models. [1] Over the course of the following weeks, histological signs become present.

## 26.6 Classification

According to the duration from fracture or fracture intervention to the onset of infection FRI can be classified as:

1. *Early (shorter than 2 weeks)*, Bacteria may have already established a biofilm, however, this biofilm may still be in an "immature" phase; despite the presence of bacteria, the bone does not exhibit signs of osteomyelitis or osteolysis; bone healing is in the "inflammatory or soft callus stage"
   Clinical features
   (a) persistent pain after initial bone fixation.
   (b) The wound is characterized by erythema, hyperthermia, swelling, or wound discharge of turbid fluid or even pus.
   (c) In addition to being risk factors for FRI, prolonged secretion, wound edge necrosis, and hematoma may also indicate an already-established infection. Therefore, these clinical symptoms should prompt a rapid surgical evaluation for diagnostic and therapeutic objectives, thereby increasing the likelihood of implant retention until fracture consolidation.

In the early phase after fracture fixation, the diagnosis 'superficial wound infection' should be avoided, as it may delay the investigation and treatment of a deep implant infection.

2. *Delayed (2–10 weeks)*, biofilm is mature and more resistant to antibiotic therapy. Although normal bone healing can take up to 10 weeks (the "hard callus stage" is between 3 and 16 weeks), the presence of bacteria impairs callus formation. In this phase, bacterial bone

invasion and inflammation (osteomyelitis) frequently occur.

Clinical features: pain and wound healing disturbances, but occasionally patients report low-grade fever.

This type of infection is generally acquired during the perioperative period but is diagnosed with a delay because:

(a) low virulence of the infecting agent
(b) previous empiric antimicrobial therapy without diagnostic workup
(c) misinterpretation of nonspecific symptoms such as wound healing disturbances.

3. *Late (over 10 weeks) infections*, it's either acquired during the perioperative period or via hematogenous seeding. Primarily caused by micro-organisms of low virulence like *S. Epidermidis* [12]

Clinical features: uneventful postoperative course and a sudden onset of symptoms, mostly pain and swelling.

The Cierny–Mader (C-M) classification [13] for OM is often selected, especially for those in the chronic stage. In 2017, Hotchen et al. [14] recommended that the following four aspects should be emphasized when classifying OM: (1) bone involvement, (2) antimicrobial resistance patterns of the causative pathogens, (3) coverage of soft tissue, and (4) host status. Based on this theory, the authors proposed the B.A.C.H classification and assessed this system, and they concluded that such a system can be applied accurately by users with different clinical backgrounds [14].

## 26.7 Diagnosis of FRI

Diagnosis of FRI is established based on comprehensive considerations of the medical history, clinical signs and symptoms, imaging tests, and laboratory tests. The diagnostic criteria of FRI were proposed by an international consensus in 2018 [15] and updated later [16], including confirmatory criteria and suggestive criteria.

### 26.7.1 Confirmatory Criteria for FRI

1. Fistula, sinus, or wound breakdown (with communication to the bone or the implant).
2. Purulent drainage from the wound or presence of pus during surgery.
3. Phenotypically indistinguishable pathogens identified by culture from at least two separate deep tissue/implant (including sonication-fluid) specimens taken during an operative intervention. In the case of tissue, multiple specimens ($\geq$ 3) should be taken, each with clean instruments (not superficial or sinus tract swabs). In cases of joint effusion, arising in a joint adjacent to a fractured bone, fluid samples obtained by sterile puncture may be included as a single sample.
4. Presence of microorganisms in deep tissue taken during an operative intervention, as confirmed by histopathological examination using specific staining techniques for bacteria or fungi.
5. Presence of more than five PMNs/HPF, was confirmed by histopathological examination.

### 26.7.2 Suggestive Criteria for FRI

1. Clinical signs: any one of
    - pain (without weight bearing, increasing over time, new-onset)
    - local redness
    - local swelling
    - increased local temperature
    - fever (single oral temperature measurement of $\geq$38.3 °C (101 °F))
    - persistent, increasing or new-onset wound drainage, beyond the first few days postoperatively, without solid alternative explanation
    - new-onset of joint effusion in fracture patients. Surgeons should be aware that FRI can present as an adjacent septic arthritis in the following cases: Implant material which penetrates the joint capsule (e.g. femoral nailing) or intra-articular fractures

2. Radiological signs: any one of
   - bone lysis (at the fracture site, around the implant)
   - implant loosening
   - sequestration (occurring over time)
   - failure of progression of bone healing (i.e. non-union)
   - presence of periosteal bone formation (e.g. at localizations other than the fracture site or in case of a consolidated fracture)
3. A pathogenic organism identified by culture from a single deep tissue/implant (including sonication fluid) specimen taken during an operative intervention.
4. Elevated serum inflammatory markers:
   - erythrocyte sedimentation rate (ESR)
   - white blood cell count (WBC)
   - C-reactive protein (CRP)

## 26.8 Treatment

The general treatment principles for FRI include:

1. radical debridement
2. implant handling
3. systemic and local antibiotics
4. defects reconstruction of bone and soft tissues
5. functional recovery

Multidisciplinary teams, including surgeons, infectious diseases specialists, pharmacists, and microbiologists, are recommended to improve the treatment efficacy [17]. Selection of the specific treatment methods should consider many factors, such as infection site and duration, pathogen type and virulence, host immunity and requirements, and expectations of the patients.

### 26.8.1 Radical Debridement

Radical debridement is one of the most efficient methods for reducing the bacterial burden of affected tissues, which is the key to reducing the risk of infection recurrence. Excision of bone or tissue, excision of poorly perfused tissue, and removal of all non-essential foreign bodies (e.g., broken screws, sutures) are typical components of debridement [18]. Although 'oncologic resection' of infected bone has been proposed, a more prudent strategy with bone excision until uniform punctate bleeding is detected is indicated [19]. This is predicated on the concept that viable infected bone can recover with antibiotic treatment (i.e. systemic and local).

The purpose of irrigation is to reduce bacterial load and remove loose debris. To prevent bacterial seeding in soft tissue and bone, it should be conducted using normal saline at low pressure [20]. Currently, the use of chemicals is not recommended since they may increase cell toxicity [21]. In order to fully clean the surgical field and reduce the bacterial burden after debridement, a significant amount (depending on the anatomic location) of irrigation fluid should be employed.

### 26.8.2 Implant Handling

The existence of a fracture is one of the key characteristics that distinguish FRI from PJI. Fracture stability is crucial not only for fracture union but also for infection prevention and treatment [22]. As fracture fixation devices primarily target fracture consolidation, they can be removed after the fracture has healed (in contrast to PJI), eliminating the biofilm with a high likelihood of eradicating the infection and preventing chronic infection. This indicates that total eradication of an infection may not always be the primary objective. In select circumstances, antibiotic suppression therapy has been established as an alternative [1].

Based on this, two main surgical concepts should be considered. The first concept consists of debridement, antimicrobial therapy, and implant retention (DAIR). The second consists of debridement, antimicrobial therapy, and implant removal if the fracture is healed or implant exchange (in one or multiple stages) if the fracture is not healed.

In every case, special attention should be paid to the stability of the fracture in order to obtain union and treat the infection [23].

Several criteria determine whether the implant should be removed or not. Implants should be removed or exchanged when the implant and fracture are unstable, reduction is not acceptable, or the host physiology is substantially impaired. In uncommon circumstances when healing cannot occur due to a compromised host or a severe infection, amputation, or a nonsurgical method with or without (lifelong) antibiotic suppression may be the only therapy option (e.g., in elderly patients with compromised host physiology) [1].

### 26.8.3 Systemic and Local Antibiotics

As soon as culture results and corresponding antibiotic susceptibility patterns from the intraoperatively obtained samples are available, empiric antibiotics are changed to targeted therapy. Initial empiric therapy should be broad-spectrum and include a lipo/ glycopeptide and a gram-negative bacillus-targeting drug.

The current recommendation is that IV therapy be switched to oral antibiotics after 1–2 weeks, when the soft tissues are stable, and the wounds are dry [9]. In case of implant retention or exchange, a total treatment duration of 12 weeks is recommended. If the internal device is removed, antibiotics are given for in total of 6 weeks [9].

Biofilm-active antibiotics include rifampicin for staphylococcal infections and fluoroquinolones for Gram-negative bacteria, assuming susceptibility testing. They should be administered only after thorough debridement to reduce bacterial burden and when wounds are dry to prevent superinfection with resistant germs [24]. Because of the rapid emergence of resistant microorganisms, rifampicin must be given with a companion antibiotic [25].

The presence of an infection that is difficult to treat determines whether the antibiotic regimen is curative or suppressive. In the latter scenario, antimicrobial therapy controls the infection until the fracture heals and the implant may be removed.

All FRI patients should have a baseline blood analysis available, especially patients who will receive IV antimicrobial therapy, including baseline inflammatory markers, full blood count, electrolytes, and liver- and renal function tests. They should be repeated at least twice weekly, as common side effects of high-dose IV antibiotics include bone marrow suppression, hepatitis, and nephrotoxicity.

## 26.9 Local Antimicrobial Therapy

The benefit of achieving a very high local concentration of antimicrobials with limited systemic exposure is persuasive, especially in light of decreased blood flow to the site of infection and necrotic bone tissue [1, 26]. Furthermore, after an extensive debridement they can be an important treatment option for dead space management.

The drug release has its peak within the first 7 days and rapidly decreases thereafter [26]. Standard antibacterial agents in spacers and beads are aminoglycosides (e.g., gentamicin, tobramycin), either alone or in combination with vancomycin. Antibiotics have traditionally been incorporated into PMMA cement [27]. PMMA carriers must be removed in a second procedure three to four weeks after insertion. A bioabsorbable substance as a vehicle for local antibiotic delivery, on the other hand, does not necessitate a second surgical procedure and may permit bone regrowth [28]. Studies on bioabsorbable bone substitutes (BBS) impregnated with antibiotics for the management of FRI reported reinfection rates ranging from 0% to 14.3% [28]. Calcium sulfate with hydroxyapatite, when used as an antibiotic carrier, has been proposed to enhance bone growth [29].

### 26.9.1 Defects Reconstruction of Bone and Soft Tissue

Autogenous bone graft remains the gold standard for the treatment of bone defects shorter than 2.5 cm [30]. As for large segmental bone defects, the selection of reconstruction procedures depends on numerous aspects, such as the surgeons' experience, the location and extent of the bone defect, comorbidities, and compliance of the patient. The Ilizarov technique, the Masquelet approach, and the free vascularized fibular grafting technique are the most common procedures for reconstructing segmental bone defects.

#### 26.9.1.1 Ilizarov Technique

If the defect is small (<2 cm), the limb can be shortened to give good bone contact and allow skin closure. If the defect is up to 4 cm in the tibia and 6 cm in the femur, the limb can be acutely shortened to give bone contact, but this will produce a significant limb length discrepancy that must be addressed. Within the Ilizarov fixator, it is possible to relengthen the bone through a separate corticotomy, away from the site of infection. In larger defects, gradual defect filling by Ilizarov bone transport has been shown to be a safe and effective method of securing union and eradicating infection.

Several recent studies have demonstrated the advantages of double-level bone transport over single-level bone transport, including shorter time with external fixation, faster bone healing time, fewer problems, and greater function recovery [31].

#### 26.9.1.2 The Masquelet Technique

Also known as the induced membrane technique, is another effective way to repair large bone defects. A membrane is produced around the cement block. After some weeks, the cement can be removed, and bone graft packed into the defect inside the carefully preserved membrane. If the bone remains stable, this graft may consolidate and remodel over many months [32].

#### 26.9.1.3 Free Vascularized Fibular Grafting

Vascularized fibula graft is a successful method for reconstructing a bone defect; however, a well-trained multidisciplinary team is essential to eliminate the high risk of potential consequences, such as stress fractures [33].

#### 26.9.1.4 3D Printing

Recently, with the advent of three-dimensional (3D) printing technology, individualized and accurate reconstruction and repair are no longer inaccessible. Liu et al. [34] reported employing 3D-printed porous Ti6Al4V scaffolds to repair severe diaphyseal defects of the lower limbs and achieving satisfactory postoperative functionality and minimal complication rates in prospective research.

## 26.10 Repair of Soft Tissue Defects

In the absence of an adequate soft-tissue envelope ideal definitive soft-tissue coverage within an orthoplastic technique should be conducted as soon as possible.

Free faps, skin grafts, and rotational faps were the most often selected methods for reconstructing soft tissues. Multiple criteria, including the microsurgical experience of the surgeons, the patient's age, smoking status, the presence of comorbidities, and the location and size of the soft tissue defect, must be taken into account when determining the precise techniques to repair soft tissue defects.

Negative pressure wound therapy (NPWT) can provide significant convenience in the treatment of both open fractures and FRI. Regarding the use of NPWT in FRI therapy, there was insufficient evidence to support its usage as a definitive FRI treatment [35]. Negative pressure wound therapy (NPWT) should be utilized just as a bridge to definitive soft tissue covering. It cannot serve as a substitute for definitive soft tissue reconstruction in FRI and should not be utilized for longer than approximately one week. Extended NPWT may result in the colonization of resistant organisms and an increase in infection rates [36].

## 26.11 Rehabilitation and Follow-Up

Early customized functional rehabilitation is essential for all orthopedic trauma patients, especially when infection develops. As FRI frequently involves a lengthy course of treatment, psychological support should also be made accessible.

It is recommended to follow up the patient in regular intervals for a minimum of 12 months after cessation of therapy in a specialized inter-disciplinary outpatient clinic [37]. Follow-up outpatient visits generally consist of a wound inspection, radiological evaluation of the fracture, and monitoring for complications or recurrence of infection.

## 26.12 Prevention of FRI

Several preventive measures are currently considered as very effective with a high level of evidence (grade IA) according to guidelines [38]. These include:

### 26.12.1 Pre-operative Measures

#### 26.12.1.1 Skin Preparation Solutions

Chlorhexidine, iodine, and alcohol are the most common solutions used for skin preparation in orthopedic surgery. Due to its limited duration of action, alcohol is typically utilized in conjunction with other antiseptics. There is no consensus on the recommended solution.

#### 26.12.1.2 Skin Hair Management

There may be little difference in SSI risk between using clippers or hair removal lotion versus not removing hair (evidence of low certainty) [39]. However, there are likely fewer SSIs when hair is not removed when compared to razor shaving (moderate-certainty evidence). There may be a little reduction in SSIs when hair is removed on the day of surgery as opposed to the day prior.

### 26.12.2 Peri-operative Management

#### 26.12.2.1 Drapes

Adhesive drapes, especially those with antimicrobial characteristics, have been demonstrated to reduce the incidence of wound contamination. However, if drape adherence is impaired and wound edge peeling occurs, this advantage may be lost and the danger of wound infection may increase [40].

#### 26.12.2.2 Double Gloving

Double gloving reduces perforations, yet there is no data of high quality addressing the relationship between gloving techniques and FRI rates [41].

#### 26.12.2.3 Antibiotics Coated Implants

According to numerous preclinical research, antibacterial coatings have been proposed to reduce bacterial adherence and biofilm development [42].

## References

1. Metsemakers WJ, Kuehl R, Moriarty TF, Richards RG, Verhofstad MHJ, Borens O, et al. Infection after fracture fixation: current surgical and microbiological concepts. Injury. 2018;49:511–22.
2. Lu K, Zhang J, Cheng J, Liu H, Yang C, Yin L, et al. Incidence and risk factors for surgical site infection after open reduction and internal fixation of intra-articular fractures of distal femur: a multicentre study. Int Wound J. 2019;16:473–8.
3. Zhu Y, Liu S, Zhang X, Chen W, Zhang Y. Incidence and risks for surgical site infection after adult tibial plateau fractures treated by ORIF: a prospective multicentre study. Int Wound J. 2017;14:982–8.
4. Olsen LL, Møller AM, Brorson S, Hasselager RB, Sort R. The impact of lifestyle risk factors on the rate of infection after surgery for a fracture of the ankle. Bone Joint J. 2017;99-B:225–30.
5. Wang H, Pei H, Chen M, Wang H. Incidence and predictors of surgical site infection after ORIF in calcaneus fractures, a retrospective cohort study. J Orthop Surg Res. 2018;13:293.
6. Oliveira PR, Leonhardt MC, Carvalho VC, Kojima KE, Silva JS, Rossi F, et al. Incidence and risk factors associated with infection after intramedullary nailing of femoral and tibial diaphyseal fractures: prospective study. Injury [Internet] 2018 [cited 2023 Jul 13];49:1905–11. Available from: http://www.injuryjournal.com/article/S002013831830408X/fulltext
7. Sagi HC, Donohue D, Cooper S, Barei DP, Siebler J, Archdeacon MT, et al. Institutional and seasonal variations in the incidence and causative organisms for posttraumatic infection following open fractures. J Orthop Trauma. 2017;31:78–84.
8. Murdoch DR, Roberts SA, Fowler VGJ, Shah MA, Taylor SL, Morris AJ, et al. Infection of orthopedic

prostheses after Staphylococcus aureus bacteremia. Clin Infect Dis. 2001;32:647–9.
9. Depypere M, Morgenstern M, Kuehl R, Senneville E, Moriarty TF, Obremskey WT, et al. Pathogenesis and management of fracture-related infection. Clin Microbiol Infect. 2020;26:572–8.
10. Zimmerli W, Sendi P. Orthopaedic biofilm infections. APMIS [Internet]. 2017;125:353–64. Available from: https://onlinelibrary.wiley.com/doi/abs/10.1111/apm.12687
11. Barberán J, Aguilar L, Carroquino G, Giménez M-J, Sánchez B, Martínez D, et al. Conservative treatment of staphylococcal prosthetic joint infections in elderly patients. Am J Med [Internet]. 2006;119(993):e7–10. Available from: https://doi.org/10.1016/j.amjmed.2006.03.036
12. Lalani T, Chu VH, Grussemeyer CA, Reed SD, Bolognesi MP, Friedman JY, et al. Clinical outcomes and costs among patients with Staphylococcus aureus bacteremia and orthopedic device infections. Scand J Infect Dis. 2008;40:973–7.
13. Cierny G 3rd, Mader JT, Penninck JJ. A clinical staging system for adult osteomyelitis. Clin Orthop Relat Res 2003;7–24.
14. Hotchen AJ, Mcnally MA, Sendi P. The classification of long bone osteomyelitis: a systemic review of the literature. J Bone Jt Infect [Internet]. 2017 [cited 2023 Jul 6];2:167–74. Available from: https://pubmed.ncbi.nlm.nih.gov/29119075/
15. Metsemakers WJ, Morgenstern M, McNally MA, Moriarty TF, McFadyen I, Scarborough M, et al. Fracture-related infection: a consensus on definition from an international expert group. Injury [Internet]. 2018 [cited 2023 Sep 26];49:505–10. Available from: http://www.injuryjournal.com/article/S0020138317305636/fulltext
16. McNally M, Govaert G, Dudareva M, Morgenstern M, Metsemakers W-J. Definition and diagnosis of fracture-related infection. EFORT Open Rev. 2020;5:614–9.
17. Walter N, Rupp M, Baertl S, Alt V. The role of multidisciplinary teams in musculoskeletal infection. Bone Joint Res England. 2022:6–7.
18. Metsemakers WJ, Kortram K, Morgenstern M, Moriarty TF, Meex I, Kuehl R, et al. Definition of infection after fracture fixation: a systematic review of randomized controlled trials to evaluate current practice. Injury. 2018;49:497–504.
19. Kavolus JJ, Schwarzkopf R, Rajaee SS, Chen AF. Irrigation fluids used for the prevention and treatment of Orthopaedic infections. J Bone Joint Surg Am. 2020;102:76–84.
20. Draeger RW, Dahners LE. Traumatic wound debridement: a comparison of irrigation methods. J Orthop Trauma. 2006;20:83–8.
21. Yun HC, Murray CK, Nelson KJ, Bosse MJ. Infection after Orthopaedic trauma: prevention and treatment. J Orthop Trauma [Internet]. 2016:30. Available from: https://journals.lww.com/jorthotrauma/fulltext/2016/10001/infection_after_orthopaedic_trauma__prevention_and.6.aspx
22. Schmidt AH, Swiontkowski MF. Pathophysiology of infections after internal fixation of fractures. J Am Acad Orthop Surg. 2000;8:285–91.
23. Hak DJ, Fitzpatrick D, Bishop JA, Marsh JL, Tilp S, Schnettler R, et al. Delayed union and nonunions: epidemiology, clinical issues, and financial aspects. Injury. 2014;45(Suppl 2):S3–7.
24. Gonzalez Moreno M, Trampuz A, Di Luca M. Synergistic antibiotic activity against planktonic and biofilm-embedded Streptococcus agalactiae, Streptococcus pyogenes and Streptococcus oralis. J Antimicrob Chemother. 2017;72:3085–92.
25. Werner Z, Parham S. Role of rifampin against staphylococcal biofilm infections in vitro, in animal models, and in orthopedic-device-related infections. Antimicrob Agents Chemother [Internet]. 2019;63. Available from: https://doi.org/10.1128/aac.01746-18
26. Metsemakers W-J, Fragomen AT, Moriarty TF, Morgenstern M, Egol KA, Zalavras C, et al. Evidence-based recommendations for local antimicrobial strategies and dead space Management in Fracture-Related Infection. J Orthop Trauma. 2020;34:18–29.
27. Kanellakopoulou K, Giamarellos-Bourboulis EJ. Carrier systems for the local delivery of antibiotics in bone infections. Drugs. 2000;59:1223–32.
28. Ferguson J, Athanasou N, Diefenbeck M, McNally M. Radiographic and histological analysis of a synthetic bone graft substitute eluting gentamicin in the treatment of chronic osteomyelitis. J Bone Jt Infect. 2019;4:76–84.
29. Pesch S, Hanschen M, Greve F, Zyskowski M, Seidl F, Kirchhoff C, et al. Treatment of fracture-related infection of the lower extremity with antibiotic-eluting ceramic bone substitutes: case series of 35 patients and literature review. Infection. 2020;48:333–44.
30. Nauth A, Schemitsch E, Norris B, Nollin Z, Watson JT. Critical-size bone defects: is there a consensus for diagnosis and treatment? J Orthop Trauma [Internet]. 2018:32. Available from: https://journals.lww.com/jorthotrauma/fulltext/2018/03003/critical_size_bone_defects__is_there_a_consensus.2.aspx
31. Yushan M, Ren P, Abula A, Alike Y, Abulaiti A, Ma C, et al. Bifocal or trifocal (double-level) bone transport using unilateral rail system in the treatment of large Tibial defects caused by infection: a retrospective study. Orthop Surg. 2020;12
32. Masquelet AC, Begue T. The concept of induced membrane for reconstruction of long bone defects. Orthop Clin North Am. 2010;41:27–37. table of contents
33. Antonini A, Rossello C, Salomone C, Iacoviello P, Chiarlone F, Burastero G. Bone defect management with vascularized fibular grafts in the treatment of grade III-IV osteomyelitis. Handchirurgie, Mikrochirurgie, plastische Chirurgie: Organ der Deutschsprachigen Arbeitsgemeinschaft fur Handchirurgie: Organ der Deutschsprachigen Arbeitsgemeinschaft fur

Mikrochirurgie der Peripheren Nerven und Gefasse: Organ der V. 2019;51:444–452.
34. Liu B, Hou G, Yang Z, Li X, Zheng Y, Wen P, et al. Repair of critical diaphyseal defects of lower limbs by 3D printed porous Ti6Al4V scaffolds without additional bone grafting: a prospective clinical study. J Mater Sci Mater Med. 2022;33:64.
35. Haidari S, Ijpma FFA, Metsemakers WJ, Maarse W, Vogely HC, Ramsden AJ, et al. The role of negative-pressure wound therapy in patients with fracture-related infection: a systematic review and critical appraisal: Biomed Res Int 2021;2021.
36. Oosthuysen W, Venter R, Tanwar Y, Ferreira N. Bioactive glass as dead space management following debridement of type 3 chronic osteomyelitis. Int Orthop. 2020;44:421–8.
37. Metsemakers W-J, Morgenstern M, Senneville E, Borens O, Govaert GAM, Onsea J, et al. General treatment principles for fracture-related infection: recommendations from an international expert group. Arch Orthop Trauma Surg. 2020;140:1013–27.
38. Berriós-Torres SI, Umscheid CA, Bratzler DW, Leas B, Stone EC, Kelz RR, et al. Centers for disease control and prevention guideline for the prevention of surgical site infection, 2017. JAMA Surg [Internet]. 2017 [cited 2023 Sep 26];152:784–91. Available from: https://jamanetwork.com/journals/jamasurgery/fullarticle/2623725
39. Tanner J, Melen K. Preoperative hair removal to reduce surgical site infection. Cochrane Database Syst Rev. 2021;8:CD004122.
40. Mundi R, Nucci N, Ekhtiari S, Wolfstadt J, Ravi B, Chaudhry H. Do adhesive drapes have an effect on infection rates in Orthopaedic surgery? A systematic review and Meta-analysis. Clin Orthop Relat Res. 2022;480:551–9.
41. Tanner J, Parkinson H. Double gloving to reduce surgical cross-infection. Cochrane Database Syst Rev. 2002:CD003087.
42. Shirai T, Shimizu T, Ohtani K, Zen Y, Takaya M, Tsuchiya H. Antibacterial iodine-supported titanium implants. Acta Biomater. 2011;7:1928–33.

# 27 Infective Complications After Open Fractures

Khaled M. Emara, Ramy A. Diab,
and Mohamed O. Eissa

## 27.1 Introduction

Open fractures are serious injuries with a reported incidence of 30.7 per 100,000 persons each year [1]. Infection remains one of the most significant complications in the treatment of open fractures, despite the fact that outcomes have improved over the past century. The underlying bone is susceptible to direct contact with contaminating agents if the tissue barrier between the fracture zone and the environment is compromised.

An open fracture is an injury where the fractured bone and/or fracture hematoma are exposed to the external environment via a traumatic violation of the soft tissue and skin. The skin wound may lie at a site distant from the fracture and not directly over it. Therefore, any fracture that has a concomitant wound should be considered open until proven otherwise [2].

Classification of open fractures is of the utmost importance, as the severity and extent of soft tissue damage determine a complex treatment concept involving surgical and non-surgical measures. In 1976, Gustilo and colleagues established their classification system [3], which allowed them to draw therapeutic conclusions for an individual fracture which was then modified in 1984 [4].

Other classification systems like the classification system of Tscherne and Oestern [5] and the AO Müller Classification [6] provide more refined descriptions of the local situation, as lesions of bone, soft tissues, and neurovascular structures are evaluated separately, along with the level of contamination. On the other hand, their detailed classification of various parameters in an open fracture results in a descriptive complexity that makes daily communication more challenging than Gustillo's classification. After the initial debridement, the classification of an open fracture must be reassessed [5].

## 27.2 Epidemiology

The risk of fracture-related infection (FRI) in high-impact open fractures is up to 30% [7]. Weiz-Marschall [8] reported in a survey of the literature the risk of acute infection in open fractures and it was 0% infection rate in Gustilo type I, up to 12% in type II, and up to 50% in type III fractures.

## 27.3 Pathophysiology

### 27.3.1 Contamination and Virulence

Rates of primary colonization have been reported to be between 70 and 80 percent, depending on the nature of the accident. Smears reveal Gram-

K. M. Emara · R. A. Diab · M. O. Eissa (✉)
Department of Orthopedic Surgery, Ain Shams University, Cairo, Egypt



P. Ruggieri et al. (eds.), *Bone and Joint Infections*, https://doi.org/10.1007/978-3-031-96383-4_27

positive *Staph. aureus* and epidermidis and Gram-negative Bacilli, Pseudomonas, Acinetobacter, or Enterobacteria the majority of the time [7, 9, 10].

Most infections in open fractures are of nosocomial origin as the causative micro-organisms of infection differ from those found in initial smears [11].

Following an open fracture, polymicrobial infections are associated with increased antibiotic requirements and an increase in amputations. A higher fracture grade (III), working in agriculture, the need for a blood transfusion, or the need for additional surgical debridement are all associated with the development of a polymicrobial infection following an open fracture [12].

## 27.4 Risk Factors

A variety of factors determine the clinical results following an open fracture. Polytraumatized patients are at high risk because severe trauma is commonly accompanied by complex musculoskeletal injuries and a compromised host immune response [13]. Risk factors can be divided into:

External factors (environmental factors) [14]:

1. Injury type and degree.
2. Injury site.
3. Pathogen virulence.
4. Prophylaxis and treatment methods.

Internal factors (host factors)

1. Immune status.
2. Lifestyle.
3. Comorbidity of the patients.

## 27.5 Clinical Presentation and Investigations

The clinical presentation depends on; duration of infection, type of microorganism, anatomic localization, mechanism of the trauma leading to fracture, and type of surgery that has been performed.

### 27.5.1 Laboratory Examination

Due to multiple influencing factors and differences in half-life times of serum inflammatory makers, their diagnostic values on FRI differ.

- WBC usually rises to the highest level from day 1 to day 3 after surgery and is back to normal within 4 to 6 days [15].
- ESR usually increases to the highest level from day 7 to day 11 after surgery and decreases to normal after 6 weeks gradually [16].
- CRP usually goes up to the highest level on the second day following surgery and returns to normal after 2 weeks [17]. If serum CRP level continuously increases from fourth to seventh day after surgery, a high probability of FRI should be considered after the exclusion of infection in other systems or persistent systemic inflammatory stress status of the patient [18].
- Aside from surgery, bacterial type and virulence can also affect the levels of the inflammatory markers, meaning that high-virulence and drug-resistant bacteria are often associated with higher levels [19].

New markers:

(a) Serum D-dimer may be a useful indicator for the evaluation of infected nonunion, with sensitivity and specificity at 75% and 91.2% [20, 21].
(b) Interleukin-6 (IL-6) had a similar diagnostic value for FRI, in comparison to ESR and CRP [22].
(c) Platelet count to mean platelet volume ratio [23].
(d) Wound alpha defensin [24].
(e) Cluster of differentiation (CD) 64 [25].

### 27.5.2 Imaging Procedures

The indications to request diagnostic imaging:

1. Assessment of fracture healing, fracture reduction, and stability of the osteosynthesis construct.

2. Acquire more certainty regarding the presence or absence of FRI.
3. Visualization of the anatomic details of the infection such as its extension, the presence of sequestra, sinus tracts, and subcortical abscess [26].

## 27.6 Nuclear Imaging

Applying radioisotopes to detect and track physiological and pathophysiological changes, such as fracture healing, bone remodeling, and the inflammatory response to an infection. Recently, the use of hybrid camera systems that combine nuclear imaging with CT (single photon emission computed tomography (SPECT)) (SPECT/CT, PET/CT, or PET/MRI) has resulted in improved accuracy and more anatomical details [27]. The consensus definition classifies nuclear imaging as suggestive despite its excellent diagnostic accuracy in establishing the diagnosis of FRI [26].

## 27.7 Microbiology

Surgical exploration and microbiological sampling are the pillars of diagnosis and, more critically, the key determinants for antimicrobial treatment. Intraoperative sample collection is crucial to the diagnostic process since it permits the interpretation of histological and microbiological tests. It is essential to identify the causative pathogen(s) for antimicrobial therapy to be effective [28].

Recommendations during sample collection:

1. Collect preferably five, representative deep tissue samples from the site of perceived infection and adjacent to implants [9, 26].
2. Unused surgical instruments should be used for each sample obtained to avoid cross-contamination [29].
3. The samples should be numbered and labelled with the anatomical localization and sent for microbiological and histopathological investigation.
4. Superficial swabs and surface biopsies from open wounds should be avoided as there is a high chance of culturing bacteria belonging to the skin microbiome colonizing the wound [9].
5. Whenever possible (except in septic patients), systemic antibiotics should be avoided 2 weeks prior to sampling to avoid false-negative culture results [9].
6. Different culture media should be considered to cover both aerobic and anaerobic pathogens. It is advised that the culture time is generally for 7 day.s but can be extended to 14 days in suspicion of slow-growing strains, such as Cutibacterium acnes [9, 26].

If a highly virulent pathogen (such as *Staphylococcus aureus*) is found in a single sample of deep tissue, a strong suspicion of infection should be raised [30].

Several institutes include the sonication of extracted implants in their diagnostic procedures. Sonication is a valuable supplement to conventional tissue culture in implant-associated infections, particularly in patients who have been pre-treated with antibiotics. However, its diagnostic value in FRIs still needs to be established, and tissue cultures remain the gold standard [26, 31, 32].

## 27.8 Molecular Technologies

1. Polymerase Chain Reaction.

Scientific data on molecular techniques, such as PCR, in the field of FRI are scarce [31]. These tests are fast diagnostic procedures that can distinguish between viable and nonviable bacteria. However, the high sensitivity of PCR carries the risk of producing false positive results due to contamination [33].

2. Next-generation sequencing (NGS).

Capable of sequencing all DNA contained in a given sample, providing a full image of the microbial genomes present; proven effective in culture-negative settings for the detection of pathogens [34, 35].

## 27.9 Histopathology

The presence of visible microorganisms in deep tissue, as confirmed by histological investigation using particular staining procedures for bacteria (e.g., Gram stain, Ziehl-Neelsen stain for tuberculosis, or Grocott methenamine silver stain for fungi), is considered confirmation of FRI. [30] In late FRIs, an infection can be reliably confirmed if the histological investigation reveals the presence of more than five polymorphonuclear neutrophils (PMNs) per high-power field. Aseptic nonunion can be identified by the absence of neutrophils in any high-power field [36].

## 27.10 Management of Open Fractures

The goals of treating an open fracture are well-known and include preventing infection, achieving bony union, and restoring function. In order to accomplish the other goals, the prevention of infection is the most important measure. Post-traumatic bone infection (fracture-related infection) is a devastating complication that frequently impedes the patient's rehabilitation and treatment. This infection increases treatment costs and duration, causes physical and social losses, and diminishes patients' quality of life and functional independence.

### 27.10.1 Principles of Surgical Care for Open Fractures

#### 27.10.1.1 Initial Assessment and Stabilization

A trauma patient must be evaluated according to Advanced Trauma Life Support (ATLS) and institutional protocols. Then, open fracture wounds can be dressed with sterile, moist gauze, and clinical realignment of the limb can be achieved using a temporary splint or traction.

**Irrigation**

Washing the wound with large volumes of fluid will eliminate macro-level contamination and clots that may obscure the view of deeper levels of contamination or damaged tissue. Once the macro contamination has been eradicated, irrigation serves to reduce the bacterial contamination of the remaining healthy tissue.

#### 27.10.1.2 Appropriate Intravenous Antibiotics

**Type of Antibiotic**

Administration of antibiotics is best considered therapeutic, rather than prophylactic, because of the high risk of infection in the absence of antibiotics [37].

Although debate still surrounds some aspects of antibiotic administration for open fractures, [38] the following generalizations can be made:

- Type I injuries should receive cefazolin 1–2 grams/8 hours or equivalent gram-positive coverage.
- Type II or type III injuries likely benefit from the addition of adequate gram-negative coverage, typically with an aminoglycoside (gentamycin 80 mg/8–12 hours) or a fourth-generation cephalosporin. Ampicillin-sulbactam may be an acceptable alternative for type IIIa fractures [39].
- Injuries at risk for anaerobic infections (eg, farm injuries, severe tissue necrosis) probably benefit from the addition of penicillin (five million-ten million units/24 hours) or clindamycin and consider metronidazole.
- *Tetanus immunization and Prophylaxis.*

A tetanus toxoid booster should be administered to any patient with an open fracture who has not completed the tetanus toxoid immunization or has not received a booster within the past 5 years. If the wound is susceptible to Clostridium tetani contamination, tetanus toxoid should be combined with 250.500 IU of human tetanus immune globulin (HTIG). In addition, if it has been more than 10 years since the patient's last tetanus booster or if the patient's immune system is compromised, both tetanus toxoid and HTIG should be administered [40]. The HTIG will offer most patients 3 weeks of protection.

#### Duration of Antibiotic Administration

The ideal duration of antibiotic administration has been controversial. A 2017 systematic review by Messner et al. could not support the administration of antibiotics for longer than 72 hours following an open long-bone fracture [41]. A 2019 study discovered a correlation between extended antibiotic prophylaxis (>72 hours after definitive wound closure) and an increase in surgical-site infections (SSIs) in mildly contaminated wounds, but a significant reduction in SSIs in severely contaminated wounds [42]. A 2020 review article also could not support antibiotic administration beyond 24 hours after either debridement with sterile dressings or definitive coverage [43].

#### Timing

Early antibiotic prophylaxis has been identified as the single most important factor in preventing infection and further complications [44]. Earlier studies recommended administration within 3 hours of facility presentation; however, more recent studies suggest a stricter guideline of administration within 1 hour [45].

#### Local Antibiotics

Local antibiotics may be beneficial for the treatment of certain open fractures. Antibiotics placed in the zone of injury can achieve high local drug concentrations, typically without systemic side effects [46].

### 27.10.1.3 Meticulous Injury Zone Excision (Debridement)

In general, the purpose is to eliminate damaged tissue that could serve as a bacterial breeding ground without causing extensive additional surgical trauma through unnecessary periosteal stripping or undermining of skin flaps.

Debridement of an open fracture must be performed cautiously so as to avoid leaving behind devitalized tissue or contamination.

(a) Traumatic wounds must be extended, and muscle compartments opened and explored.
(b) The skin edges should be trimmed to a healthy bleeding edge.
(c) Loose subcutaneous fat should also be removed, along with any severely contused or noncontractile muscle.
(d) Bone should also be removed if it is free of soft-tissue attachment. Major articular fragments may be an exception to this rule; whenever possible, they should be retained so that attempts can be made to restore joint stability and motion.

#### Timing of Debridement

The timing of surgical irrigation and debridement remains a controversial topic. Traditionally, 6 hours was regarded as a traditional for reduce the risk of infection following an open fracture. Multiple studies indicate that early surgical irrigation and debridement should be emphasized to reduce the risk of infection. Surgical treatment should be administered no later than 24 hours post-injury for open fractures of grades I and II, and within 12 hours for open fractures of grade III, although earlier treatment may be preferred [47, 48].

#### Irrigation

Irrigation combined with debridement assists in removing contamination from open fractures and reducing the risk of infection. The fluid lavage of open wounds (FLOW) study compared and contrasted various lavage fluids and irrigation pressures. They discovered that, regardless of irrigation pressure, normal saline solution appeared to reduce the reoperation rate [49]. Other studies suggest that low-pressure irrigation with saline offers an effective, low-cost option for the irrigation of open fractures [50].

It has been demonstrated that the addition of antiseptics, surfactants, or antibiotics to the fluid is inferior to normal saline in preventing infection and limiting the rate of reoperation [50]. The ideal volume of irrigant has not been determined [50]. An example of a common regimen calls for 3, 6, and 9 L of irrigant for grade I, II, and III fractures respectively [51].

#### 27.10.1.4 Fracture Stabilization

The injured patient receives numerous benefits from the prompt stabilization of open fractures. It protects the soft tissues surrounding the injury site from further damage caused by mobile fracture fragments. Additionally, length, alignment, and rotation are restored. This restoration of length also aids in the reduction of soft tissue dead spaces which has been demonstrated in studies to reduce infection rates in open fractures [52]. Lastly, early fixation allows improved access to soft tissues surrounding the injury and facilitates the patient's early return to normal function [53].

When selecting fixation constructs, the surgeon has numerous options, including skeletal traction, external fixation, and intramedullary nails and plates. The choice of fixation depends on the fractured bone and its location (intraarticular, metaphyseal, diaphyseal), the degree of soft-tissue injury and contamination, and the patient's physiologic status [54].

It appears that grades I and II open fractures can be treated similarly to grades I and II closed fractures, with appropriate antibiotic prophylaxis, wound debridement, and closure [55], and in the case of tibial fractures, the use of reamed intramedullary nails seems reasonable [56].

In the management of grade III open fractures, there are more controversies. In grade IIIA fractures with minimal bone defect, the use of non-reamed intramedullary nails appears to be a good and safe option (superior) compared to temporary external fixation, with minimal complications and good union rates [57]. In grade IIIB open tibial fractures, recent research indicates that reamed nailing is functionally equivalent to unreamed nailing [58]. If we are in the presence of a bone defect, the use of a protocoled treatment with temporary external fixation may be useful for definitive treatment. Conversion from external fixation to an intramedullary nail is safe given two parameters: conversion in less than 2 weeks and absence of pin site infections. Conversion after pin site infections may require additional time and antibiotic treatment after removing the external fixator and placement of the intramedullary nail [59].

#### 27.10.1.5 Second Look

Forty-eight hours after the original debridement, it is generally advisable to reinspect the injury zone under anesthesia. This affords the opportunity to:

- Assess the viability of the soft tissues.
- Conduct any necessary further tissue excision.
- Wash out any accumulated blood clot, tissue fluid coagulum, or remaining foreign material.

#### 27.10.1.6 Soft Tissue Closure

Options for wound closure in the treatment of open fractures include primary closure of the skin, split-thickness skin-grafting, and the use of either free or local muscle flaps.

##### Timing of Primary Closure

(a) *Immediate* (at the time of the initial surgical intervention) certain criteria should be met [60]:
   - Debridement performed within 12 h.
   - No excess skin loss primarily or secondarily during debridement.
   - Skin approximation is possible without tension.
   - No gross soil or other similar contamination.
   - No vascular insufficiency.

(b) *Early* (within the 24–72 h window).

(c) *Delayed* (closure extends beyond 3 days).

##### Contraindications of Primary Closure

- Gross contamination, stagnant water contamination, and farm injuries or freshwater boating injuries.
- Delay of 12 hours after injury for delivery of antibiotics.
- Confounding comorbidities.
- Doubt about the adequacy of the initial debridement [8].

Closure with local, or free flaps is appropriate for larger and more complicated wounds and for open joints, as soon as staged wound excision is complete. It is important to close a complex wound, especially involving a joint, as soon as the wound appears healthy (preferably at 5–7 days), rather than to leave it open and risk hospital infection.

### 27.10.2 Negative Pressure Wound Therapy (NPWT)

Used in dealing with open fracture wounds and may decrease the need for free tissue transfer or rotational flap coverage in high-energy open fractures [61]. Negative wound therapy is an option for the temporary closure of wounds in patients whose conditions preclude reconstruction (e.g. polytrauma patients who are not suitable for surgery).

#### 27.10.2.1 Advantages

1. Reduce the risk of infection and accelerate wound healing in open fractures [62].
2. Decreased the incidence of deep infection and flap failure as compared with conventional dressings after open fractures that were not amenable to early closure [63].

In many cases, abundant granulation tissue forms after NPWT, and residual soft-tissue defects can be covered effectively with basic skin grafts.

### 27.10.3 Primary Amputation in Open Fractures

Primary amputation must be considered in most severe soft tissue damage, to avoid prolonged disability and a limb without function after many reconstruction attempts. Discrimination between salvageable or non-salvageable extremities may be supported by the Mangled extremity severity score [64].

It represents a relatively easily assessable scoring system, where values of >7 are absolute predictable for amputation.

### 27.10.4 Management of Established Infection

The most effective method to prevent infection in open fractures is optimal primary treatment. In the case of an established infection, surgical treatment must concentrate on eradicating the inflamed area completely. Management of acutely infected wounds is primarily surgical, relying on removal of remaining foreign bodies and debris, debridement of necrotic and devascularized tissue, and drainage of fluid collections. Orthopaedic hardware is frequently affected, which would ideally be removed or replaced given biofilm involvement.

Typically, empiric antimicrobial treatment is a broad spectrum, but therapy should be as narrow as possible based on culture data.

The duration of antibiotic therapy is determined by the depth and extent of the infection; superficial wound infections may require nothing except debridement, deep-wound infections frequently require 1–2 weeks of systemic antibiotics, and osteomyelitis typically requires 4–6 weeks of therapy, which is frequently prolonged when orthopedic hardware is involved [65].

## References

1. Sop JL, Sop A. Open fracture management. Treasure Island (FL); 2023.
2. Morris R, Jones NC, Pallister I. The use of personalised patient information leaflets to improve patients' perceived understanding following open fractures. Eur J Orthop Surg Traumatol. 2019;29:537–43.
3. Gustilo RB, Anderson JT. Prevention of infection in the treatment of one thousand and twenty-five open fractures of long bones: retrospective and prospective analyses. J Bone Joint Surg Am. 1976;58:453–8.
4. Gustilo RB, Mendoza RM, Williams DN. Problems in the management of type III (severe) open fractures: a

new classification of type III open fractures. J Trauma. 1984;24:742–6.
5. Tscherne H, Oestern HJ. A new classification of soft-tissue damage in open and closed fractures (author's transl). Unfallheilkunde. 1982;85:111–5.
6. Marsh JL, Slongo TF, Agel J, Broderick JS, Creevey W, DeCoster TA, et al. Fracture and dislocation classification compendium – 2007: orthopaedic trauma association classification, database and outcomes committee. J Orthop Trauma. 2007;21:S1–133.
7. Metsemakers WJ, Kuehl R, Moriarty TF, Richards RG, Verhofstad MHJ, Borens O, et al. Infection after fracture fixation: current surgical and microbiological concepts. Injury. 2018;49:511–22.
8. Weitz-Marshall AD, Bosse MJ. Timing of closure of open fractures. J Am Acad Orthop Surg. 2002;10:379–84.
9. Depypere M, Morgenstern M, Kuehl R, Senneville E, Moriarty TF, Obremskey WT, et al. Pathogenesis and management of fracture-related infection. Clin Microbiol Infect. 2020;26:572–8.
10. Kuehl R, Tschudin-Sutter S, Morgenstern M, Dangel M, Egli A, Nowakowski A, et al. Time-dependent differences in management and microbiology of orthopaedic internal fixation-associated infections: an observational prospective study with 229 patients. Clin Microbiol Infect. 2019;25:76–81.
11. Merritt K. Factors increasing the risk of infection in patients with open fractures. J Trauma. 1988;28:823–7.
12. Jorge LS, Fucuta PS, Oliveira MGL, Nakazone MA, de Matos JA, Chueire AG, et al. Outcomes and risk factors for Polymicrobial posttraumatic osteomyelitis. J Bone Jt Infect. 2018;3:20–6.
13. Stylianaki A, Stanic B, Morgenstern M, Richards GR, Moriarty FT, Thompson K. Humoral factors from musculoskeletal Polytrauma patients impair antibacterial responses of neutrophils in vitro. J Bone Jt Infect. 2019;4:280–4.
14. Sagi HC, Donohue D, Cooper S, Barei DP, Siebler J, Archdeacon MT, et al. Institutional and seasonal variations in the incidence and causative organisms for posttraumatic infection following open fractures. J Orthop Trauma. 2017;31:78–84.
15. Kraft CN, Krüger T, Westhoff J, Lüring C, Weber O, Wirtz DC, et al. CRP and leukocyte-count after lumbar spine surgery: fusion vs. nucleotomy. Acta Orthop. 2011;82:489–93.
16. Kunakornsawat S, Tungsiripat R, Putthiwara D, Piyakulkaew C, Pluemvitayaporn T, Pruttikul P, et al. Postoperative kinetics of C-reactive protein and erythrocyte sediment rate in one-, two-, and multilevel posterior spinal decompressions and instrumentations. Global Spine J [Internet]. 2017;7:448–51. Available from: https://doi.org/10.1177/2192568217699389
17. Schutz R, Boukebous B, Boutroux P, Guillon P. C-reactive protein levels for early detection of early postoperative complications after proximal femoral fracture surgery. European Journal of Orthopaedic Surgery and Traumatology [Internet]. 2018 [cited 2023 Jul 6];28:907–13. Available from: https://link.springer.com/article/10.1007/s00590-017-2080-z
18. Jiang N, Wang B-W, Chai Y-M, Wu X-B, Tang P-F, Zhang Y-Z, et al. Chinese expert consensus on diagnosis and treatment of infection after fracture fixation. Injury. 2019;50:1952–8.
19. Kheir MM, Tan TL, Shohat N, Foltz C, Parvizi J. Routine diagnostic tests for Periprosthetic joint infection demonstrate a high false-negative rate and are influenced by the infecting organism. J Bone Joint Surg Am. 2018;100:2057–65.
20. Shahi A, Kheir MM, Tarabichi M, Hosseinzadeh HRS, Tan TL, Parvizi J. Serum D-dimer test is promising for the diagnosis of Periprosthetic joint infection and timing of Reimplantation. J Bone Joint Surg Am. 2017;99:1419–27.
21. Wang Z, Zheng C, Wen S, Wang J, Zhang Z, Qiu X, et al. Usefulness of serum D-dimer for preoperative diagnosis of infected nonunion after open reduction and internal fixation. Infect Drug Resist. 2019;12:1827–31.
22. Zhao X-Q, Wan H-Y, Qin H-J, Jiang N, Yu B. Interleukin-6 versus common inflammatory biomarkers for diagnosing fracture-related infection: utility and potential influencing factors. J Immunol Res. 2021;2021:1461638.
23. Strony J, Paziuk T, Fram B, Plusch K, Chang G, Krieg J. An adjunct indicator for the diagnosis of fracture-related infections: platelet count to mean platelet volume ratio. J Bone Jt Infect. 2020;5:54–9.
24. Kumar P, Mittal A, Bansal P, Aggarwal S, Rajnish RK, Dadra A, et al. Wound alpha defensin levels are significantly higher in patients with fracture related infection: a pilot, prospective cohort study. Injury. 2023;54:416–21.
25. Raikwar A, Singh A, Verma V, Mehdi AA, Kushwaha NS, Kushwaha R. Analysis of risk factors and Association of Cluster of differentiation (CD) markers with conventional markers in delayed fracture related infection for closed fracture. Cureus. 2021;13:e20124.
26. Govaert GAM, Kuehl R, Atkins BL, Trampuz A, Morgenstern M, Obremskey WT, et al. Diagnosing fracture-related infection: current concepts and recommendations. J Orthop Trauma. 2020;34:8–17.
27. Glaudemans AWJM, Bosch P, Slart RHJA, IJpma FFA, Govaert GAM. Diagnosing fracture-related infections: can we optimize our nuclear imaging techniques? Eur J Nucl Med Mol Imaging Germany. 2019;46:1583–7.
28. Morgenstern M, Kühl R, Eckardt H, Acklin Y, Stanic B, Garcia M, et al. Diagnostic challenges and future perspectives in fracture-related infection. Injury. 2018;49(Suppl 1):S83–90.
29. Hellebrekers P, Rentenaar RJ, McNally MA, Hietbrink F, Houwert RM, Leenen LPH, et al. Getting it right first time: the importance of a structured tissue sampling protocol for diagnosing fracture-related infections. Injury. 2019;50:1649–55.
30. Metsemakers WJ, Morgenstern M, McNally MA, Moriarty TF, McFadyen I, Scarborough M, et al.

Fracture-related infection: a consensus on definition from an international expert group. Injury. 2018;49:505–10.
31. Onsea J, Depypere M, Govaert G, Kuehl R, Vandendriessche T, Morgenstern M, et al. Accuracy of tissue and sonication fluid sampling for the diagnosis of fracture-related infection: a systematic review and critical appraisal. J Bone Jt Infect. 2018;3:173–81.
32. Dudareva M, Barrett L, Figtree M, Scarborough M, Watanabe M, Newnham R, et al. Sonication versus tissue sampling for diagnosis of prosthetic joint and other orthopedic device-related infections. J Clin Microbiol. 2018;56
33. Panousis K, Grigoris P, Butcher I, Rana B, Reilly JH, Hamblen DL. Poor predictive value of broad-range PCR for the detection of arthroplasty infection in 92 cases. Acta Orthop. 2005;76:341–6.
34. Tarabichi M, Shohat N, Goswami K, Alvand A, Silibovsky R, Belden K, et al. Diagnosis of Periprosthetic joint infection: the potential of next-generation sequencing. J Bone Joint Surg Am. 2018;100:147–54.
35. Street TL, Sanderson ND, Atkins BL, Brent AJ, Kevin C, Dona F, et al. Molecular diagnosis of orthopedic-device-related infection directly from sonication fluid by metagenomic sequencing. J Clin Microbiol [Internet]. 2017;55:2334–47. Available from: https://doi.org/10.1128/jcm.00462-17
36. Morgenstern M, Athanasou NA, Ferguson JY, Metsemakers W, Atkins BL, McNally MA. The value of quantitative histology in the diagnosis of fracture-related infection. Orthopaedic Proc. 2018;100-B:2–2:966.
37. Zalavras CG, Patzakis MJ. Open fractures: evaluation and management. J Am Acad Orthop Surg. 2003;11:212–9.
38. Samai K, Vilella A. Update in therapeutics: prophylactic antibiotics in open fractures. J Trauma Nurs. 2018;25:83–6.
39. Takahara S, Tokura T, Nishida R, Uefuji A, Ichimura K, Nishihara H, et al. Ampicillin/sulbactam versus cefazolin plus aminoglycosides for antimicrobial prophylaxis in management of Gustilo type IIIA open fractures: a retrospective cohort study. Injury. 2022;53:1517–22.
40. Rhee P, Nunley MK, Demetriades D, Velmahos G, Doucet JJ. Tetanus and trauma: a review and recommendations. J Trauma. 2005;58:1082–8.
41. Messner J, Papakostidis C, Giannoudis PV, Kanakaris NK. Duration of Administration of Antibiotic Agents for open fractures: meta-analysis of the existing evidence. Surg Infect. 2017;18:854–67.
42. Stennett CA, O'Hara NN, Sprague S, Petrisor B, Jeray KJ, Leekha S, et al. Effect of extended prophylactic antibiotic duration in the treatment of open fracture wounds differs by level of contamination. J Orthop Trauma. 2020;34:113–20.
43. Garner MR, Sethuraman SA, Schade MA, Boateng H. Antibiotic prophylaxis in open fractures: evidence, evolving issues, and recommendations. J Am Acad Orthop Surg. 2020;28:309–15.
44. Lack WD, Karunakar MA, Angerame MR, Seymour RB, Sims S, Kellam JF, et al. Type III open tibia fractures: immediate antibiotic prophylaxis minimizes infection. J Orthop Trauma. 2015;29:1–6.
45. Chang Y, Bhandari M, Zhu KL, Mirza RD, Ren M, Kennedy SA, et al. Antibiotic prophylaxis in the Management of Open Fractures: a systematic survey of current practice and recommendations. JBJS Rev. 2019;7:e1.
46. Zalavras CG, Patzakis MJ, Holtom P. Local Antibiotic Therapy in the Treatment of Open Fractures and Osteomyelitis. Clin Orthop Relat Res [Internet]. 2004 [cited 2023 Jul 14];427:86–93. Available from: https://journals.lww.com/clinorthop/Fulltext/2004/10000/Local_Antibiotic_Therapy_in_the_Treatment_of_Open.16.aspx
47. Foote CJ, Tornetta P 3rd, Reito A, Al-Hourani K, Schenker M, Bosse M, et al. A reevaluation of the risk of infection based on time to debridement in open fractures: results of the GOLIATH meta-analysis of observational studies and limited trial data. J Bone Joint Surg Am. 2021;103:265–73.
48. Srour M, Inaba K, Okoye O, Chan C, Skiada D, Schnüriger B, et al. Prospective evaluation of treatment of open fractures: effect of time to irrigation and debridement. JAMA Surg. 2015;150:332–6.
49. Petrisor B, Sun X, Bhandari M, Guyatt G, Jeray KJ, Sprague S, et al. Fluid lavage of open wounds (FLOW): a multicenter, blinded, factorial pilot trial comparing alternative irrigating solutions and pressures in patients with open fractures. J Trauma. 2011;71:596–606.
50. Heckmann N, Simcox T, Kelley D, Marecek GS. Wound irrigation for open fractures. JBJS Rev. 2020;8:e0061.
51. Cross WW 3rd, Swiontkowski MF. Treatment principles in the management of open fractures. Indian J Orthop. 2008;42:377–86.
52. Worlock P, Slack R, Harvey L, Mawhinney R. The prevention of infection in open fractures: an experimental study of the effect of fracture stability. Injury. 1994;25:31–8.
53. Gustilo RB, Merkow RL, Templeman D. The management of open fractures. J Bone Joint Surg Am. 1990;72:299–304.
54. Zalavras CG, Marcus RE, Levin LS, Patzakis MJ. Management of open fractures and subsequent complications. J Bone Joint Surg Am United States. 2007;89:884–95.
55. Godfrey J, Pace JL. Type I open fractures benefit from immediate antibiotic administration but not necessarily immediate surgery. J Pediatr Orthop. 2016;36(Suppl 1):S6–10.
56. Duyos OA, Beaton-Comulada D, Davila-Parrilla A, Perez-Lopez JC, Ortiz K, Foy-Parrilla C, et al. Management of Open Tibial Shaft Fractures: does the timing of surgery affect outcomes? J Am Acad Orthop Surg. 2017;25:230–8.

57. Foote CJ, Guyatt GH, Vignesh KN, Mundi R, Chaudhry H, Heels-Ansdell D, et al. Which surgical treatment for open Tibial shaft fractures results in the fewest reoperations? A network meta-analysis. Clin Orthop Relat Res. 2015;473:2179–92.
58. Shao Y, Zou H, Chen S, Shan J. Meta-analysis of reamed versus unreamed intramedullary nailing for open tibial fractures. J Orthop Surg Res [Internet]. 2014;9:74. Available from: https://doi.org/10.1186/s13018-014-0074-7
59. Nowotarski PJ, Turen CH, Brumback RJ, Scarboro JM. Conversion of external fixation to intramedullary nailing for fractures of the shaft of the femur in multiply injured patients*. J Bone Joint Surg. 2000;82:781–8.
60. Rajasekaran S. Early versus delayed closure of open fractures. Injury. 2007;38:890–5.
61. Dedmond BT, Kortesis B, Punger K, Simpson J, Argenta J, Kulp B, et al. The use of negative-pressure wound therapy (NPWT) in the temporary treatment of soft-tissue injuries associated with high-energy open tibial shaft fractures. J Orthop Trauma. 2007;21:11–7.
62. Liu X, Zhang H, Cen S, Huang F. Negative pressure wound therapy versus conventional wound dressings in treatment of open fractures: a systematic review and meta-analysis. Int J Surg. 2018;53:72–9.
63. Grant-Freemantle MC, Ryan ÉJ, Flynn SO, Moloney DP, Kelly MA, Coveney EI, et al. The effectiveness of negative pressure wound therapy versus conventional dressing in the treatment of open fractures: a systematic review and meta-analysis. J Orthop Trauma. 2020;34:223–30.
64. Helfet DL, Howey T, Sanders R, Johansen K. Limb salvage versus amputation. Preliminary results of the mangled extremity severity score. Clin Orthop Relat Res. 1990:80–6.
65. Morgenstern M, Kuehl R, Zalavras CG, McNally M, Zimmerli W, Burch MA, et al. The influence of duration of infection on outcome of debridement and implant retention in fracture-related infection. Bone Joint J. 2021;103-B:213–21.

# Infections in Orthopedic Oncology

# 28

Alberto Crimì, Elisa Pala, Giulia Trovarelli, Andrea Angelini, and Pietro Ruggieri

## 28.1 Introduction

This chapter focuses on Infections in Orthopedic Oncology in those cases when there is no reconstruction after tumor resection, after curettage surgeries, and when the reconstruction after resection is not a prosthetic reconstruction. The wider topic of infections in Megaprosthesis is discussed in another chapter of this book.

The rate of Surgical Site Infections (SSI) in Orthopaedics ranges between 0.2% and 4.2%, it is lower in arthroplasties (around 0.2%) [1] and higher in spine surgery (reaching 4.2%) [2, 3]. In Orthopaedic Oncology the infection rate is higher [4–19] than in Traumatology and standard Orthopaedics, due to the different typology of patients, the associated therapies (chemotherapy and radiation therapy), and the often more invasive surgery (Fig. 28.1).

While the rate of infection in megaprosthesis is well studied and ranges between 9.3% and 20.4% [4, 5], depending on the site of the prosthetic reconstruction [20], the infections in other types of Orthopaedic Oncology surgeries have been described in the scientific literature, but with a less homogeneous approach compared to the megaprosthesis, and usually presented not as a standing alone topic but together with outcomes and other complications.

The analysis of infection risk in Orthopaedic Oncology shows a higher patient-specific risk of SSI in case of malignancy, smoking history, and a higher American Society of Anesthesiologists (ASA) score. While procedure-specific risk factors for SSI are considered surgical time, blood loss, blood transfusion volume, neoadjuvant chemotherapy, neoadjuvant radiation therapy, inpatient type of surgery, and number of previous surgeries on the same site [21]. These last two factors are highlighted to be independent predictors of SSI. Another study shows the same risk factors, adding to the list of risk factors also age, preexisting implants, concomitant infection at another site, and body mass index (BMI) [22].

As presented in the previous paragraph both Radiation Therapy (XRT) and Chemotherapy (CHT) are considered a risk factor for SSI in Orthopaedic Oncology.

XRT is considered a risk factor for SSI because of subsequent tissue damage, it has been studied in the scientific literature but its real influence on post-operative infections is still debated and only few papers focused specifically on this topic [5, 22–24]. Some studies [23, 24] do not demonstrate a statistically significant increased risk of infection after XRT, while in another study XRT is found to be asso-

A. Crimì · E. Pala · G. Trovarelli · A. Angelini · P. Ruggieri (✉)
Department of Orthopedic and Orthopedic Oncology, University of Padova, Padova, Italy
e-mail: alberto.crimi@aopd.veneto.it; elisa.pala@unipd.it; giulia.trovarelli@unipd.it; andrea.angelini@unipd.it; pietro.ruggieri@unipd.it



P. Ruggieri et al. (eds.), *Bone and Joint Infections*, https://doi.org/10.1007/978-3-031-96383-4_28

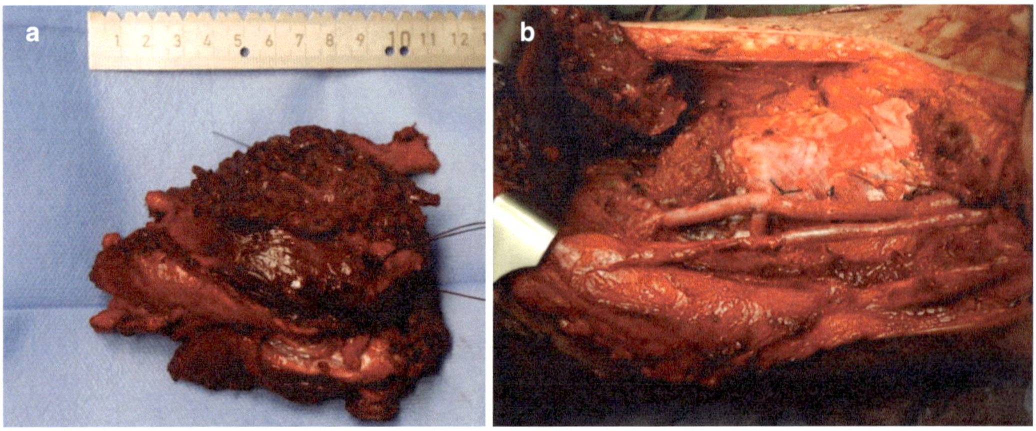


**Fig. 28.1** Wide surgical exposure is required for resection of a (**a**) large Synovial Sarcoma of the popliteal fossa with (**b**) neurovascular structures identification and protection

ciated with a higher risk of SSI in spine metastatic tumors [5], a significantly higher risk of SSI is also highlighted in a series of 1034 patients who had preoperative XRT and in patients with a remote history of XRT [22].

CHT is considered a s risk factor for SSI because it can induce leukocytopenia and neutropenia, also in this case the real influence of CHT on SSI is debated. Neoadjuvant CHT is considered a risk factor for SSI in all types of cancer surgeries [25]. In Orthopaedic Oncology there are some works reporting CHT as a risk factor for SSI [21, 22, 24, 26], but there are some works that do not report a statistically significant higher risk of SSI in patients who had CHT [23, 27, 28], in these last studies more than CHT itself a lower number of White Blood Cells (WBC) is correlated with a higher risk of SSI. In the studies supporting the correlation between CHT and SSI, in a first study on 1521 patients [22], a post-operative CHT in the first month after surgery was associated with a higher risk of SSI, in another study [21] there an SSI rate of 34% was found in patients who had neoadjuvant-CHT while the rate in patients who did not have neoadjuvant-CHT was 13%, with a statistically significant difference. A CHT-associated preoperative lower count of WBC was found to be a predictor for SSI in patients with allograft reconstruction after resection of the proximal tibia [26].

SSIs have terrible consequences, bringing the burden of longer hospital admission times, worse function, higher costs for the health system (long times of expensive antibiotics administration, multiple surgeries, difficult reconstructions), and increased mortality (also considering the possible effect of delaying pivotal treatment as chemotherapy and radiation therapy [29].

## 28.2 Infections in Resection without Reconstruction

### 28.2.1 Infections in Soft Tissue Sarcomas Resection

Surgical Site Infection (SSI) in soft tissue sarcoma resection is more common in junctional areas, like the groin and the axilla [30], and when the reconstruction is with a cutaneous-fascial flap. It is pivotal for optimal reconstruction after STS resection multidisciplinary teamwork with Plastic Surgery [31] in the so-called Ortho-plastic approach [32].

SSI in soft tissue sarcoma resection is not a rare complication, the rate of SSI ranges between 8.3% [33] and 43.3% [34]; the highest rate was found in resection of STS of the pelvis [35]. It was found a trend of higher rates of SSI in immediate reconstruction and in patients who underwent neoadjuvant radiation, without being statistically significant in some series [34]. A wider series showed that a higher incidence of SSI was significantly correlated with tumor dimensions >5 cm and preoperative XRT [36].

SSI was shown to be an independent risk factor for the length of hospitalization [33]. Furthermore, patients with SSI after STS resection had higher local recurrence rates, lower survival, and worse oncological outcomes [33]. Because SSI can delay or prevent other crucial therapies for local and systemic control, in 13% of patients an SSI delayed post-operative XRT and CHT while 8% of patients did not receive any XRT due to SSI [36].

Among the consequences of SSI, there were repeated fluid collections aspirations and prolonged need of dressing of the wound [37], and in the same series, 18% of patients required a surgical revision for SSI [37]. In a recent series, wound dehiscence and SSI were the most frequent complications after STS surgery (as high as 34%) [38]. In short-term follow-up of STS resection, acute wound complications were the first complication, while the long-term complications were chronic radiation-related limb complications, part of them SSI. It is interesting to note that XRT complications in STS resection show a higher rate for tumors located in the groin area and are related to acute wound complications [36], (Fig. 28.2).

Smoke was significantly associated with major complications after STS resection, while obesity and bone exposure after resection showed a trend of association with SSI, that was not statistically significant [37]. Multiple other risk factors for SSI were investigated without highlighting strong statistical significance [33].

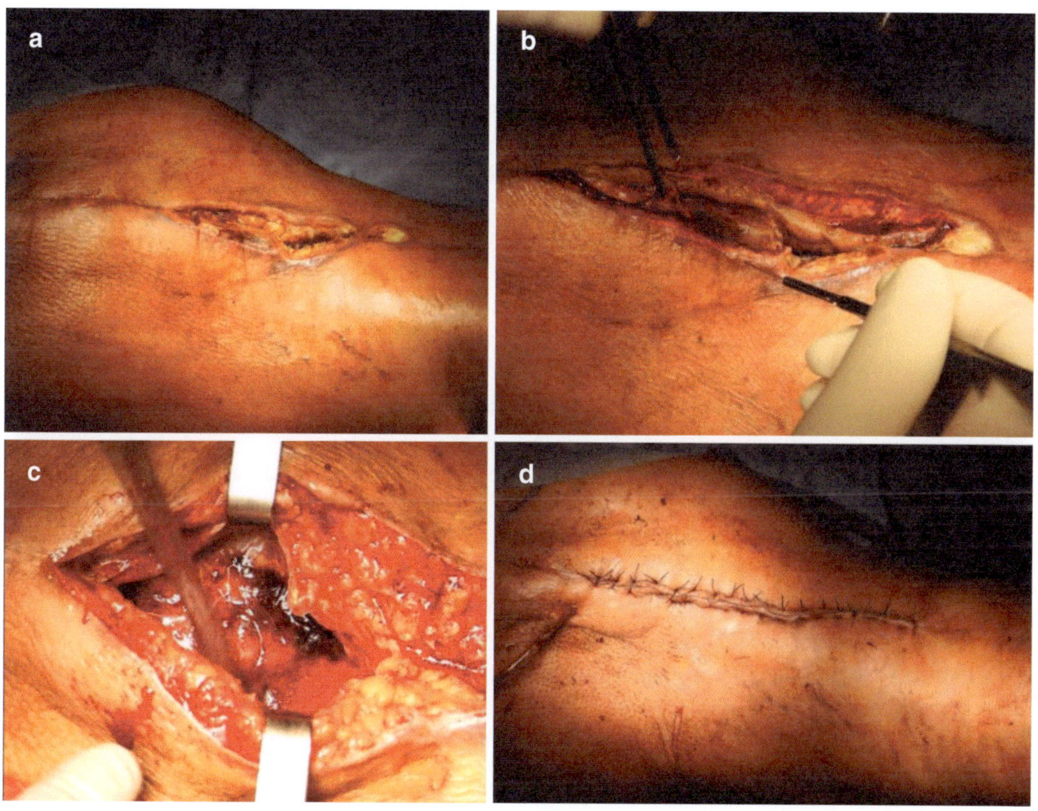


**Fig. 28.2** (**a**) Surgical Site Infection in a 64 years old female patient after pre-operative XRT and resection of a thigh high-grade liposarcoma, (**b**, **c**) debridement of necrotic tissues and irrigation, (**d**) wound closure

### 28.2.2 Infections in Resection of 'Expendable' Bones Without Reconstruction

Surgical site infection (SSI) after resection of expendable bones is a difficult topic, few bones are considered really expendables and not worth reconstruction, but the scapula and fibula are among the sites where is still debated the possibility of reconstruction and what there are data on SSI rate.

SSI in scapular resections can occur when there are large soft tissue defects, and an adequate reconstruction is not possible. In scapular resection, the SSI reported rate varies between 3% [39] and 9% [40]. The cases are deep SSI post-scapulectomy in a patient with radiation-induced osteosarcoma and superficial SSI post-scapulectomies, wound complications successfully treated with a course of antibiotics [39, 40]. This rate of SSI is comparable to the SSI rate in other resections around the shoulder joint, between 0% and 5.4% [41–43].

Prosthetic reconstruction of the scapula shows a better function but a higher SSI rate, due to the more difficult soft tissue coverage and the presence of hardware [44]. As shown by a series of prosthetic reconstructions of the humeral-scapular joint, with partial resection of the scapula, where the rate of patients that required hardware removal for SSI was 25% [45].

A possible option of reconstruction without endoprosthesis is a humeral suspension (using remaining rotator cuff tendons), in this case of soft tissue-only reconstruction the SSI rate was 4% to 9% [46], patients treated successfully with antibiotic therapy, 1 patient of a series required reoperation with debridement and subsequent targeted antibiotic therapy [44].

In the fibula resection for bone tumors, the SSI rate widely varies between 9% and 17.5% [47, 48]. Due to the limited number of patients in the series, the different entities of the resection, and the different sites of the resection (proximal, intercalary, and distal) have to be carefully taken into consideration, together with the definition of SSI. When considering SSI as a deep infection the distal fibula resection seems to have a higher risk of SSI, while considering the wound healing problems as SSI, the proximal fibula resection bears the highest rate of wound complications [47, 48].

Neoadjuvant and adjuvant chemo/radiation therapy can lead to a higher rate of SSI, the rate of SSI is higher also with the use of grafts for the reconstruction of the resected fibula [49, 50]. Autografts are less affected by SSI compared to allografts [51]. Good soft tissue coverage is pivotal to reducing the dead space around the reconstruction (or the cavity left by the resection), reducing the SSI rate in fibula resection [52].

## 28.3 Infections in Resection with Reconstruction

This paragraph discusses the Surgical Site Infection (SSI) in resections for bone tumors followed by reconstruction without an endoprosthesis, meaning SSI after allograft reconstruction.

SSI in allograft reconstruction varies between 11.9% and 13.5% [53] in the extremities, reaching 50% in pelvic allograft reconstruction, the last topic is treated in another paragraph of this chapter. The overall free survival from infection for allograft reconstruction at 5 years is 92% [53]. In the extremities, the proximal tibia has a higher risk of SSI after an allograft reconstruction, with up to 15% of deep infection and 48% of soft tissue complications [54].

The high incidence of SSI in allograft reconstruction was associated with the characteristics of the allograft itself, being non-vital bone (acellular and avascular) and with high porosity, being a very favorable environment for bacterial infection [55]. Bacteria, once seeded on an allograft, easily form a glycocalyx matrix (biofilm) preventing immune response ed. effectiveness of antibiotics [56].

Multiple risk factors analyzed show a statistically significant influence on the rate of SSI in allograft reconstruction. Tibia allografts, male sex, and longer post-operative antibiotic prophylaxis are associated with a higher SSI rate [53]. There is a reported higher rate of SSI in patients with allograft reconstruction who received high doses of corticosteroids and chemo/radiation therapy [57, 58].

The onset of SSI in allograft reconstructions is usually within 4 months, a careful follow-up can lead to an early detection and treatment of SSI with better outcomes for patients [59].

Treatment for SSI in allograft reconstruction is first, surgical debridement followed by targeted antibiotic therapy (effective in 18% of cases), usually effective in low-grade single microbial infections [60].

Usually, antibiotic treatment is administered intravenously for 2 weeks and then prolonged orally for 16 weeks [61, 62]. Other than the normal preoperative antibiotic prophylaxis, careful antisepsis in the OR, and reduction of operative times, other attempted preventive treatments for SSI are the use of antibiotic-impregnated bone allografts [55, 62] and the use of antibiotic-loaded bone cement [63].

If debridement and antibiotic administration fails, the SSI treatment is allograft removal, temporary antibiotic-loaded cement spacer, and targeted antibiotic therapy for 3 months (a 2-stages treatment), followed by reconstruction with another allograft or prosthesis [59].

After the second reconstruction, the SSI rate rises to 34%. Similarly, Mankin [64] describes a higher risk of SSI after a second (revision) allograft surgery, rising from 7.9% to 12.8%. The failure of the 2-stage treatment can lead in severe cases to amputation [53].

## 28.4 Infections in Curettage Surgeries

Surgical Site Infection (SSI) rate after curettage surgery in orthopedic oncology can widely vary, based on what is considered SSI, it can range between 4.1% [65] and 10.7% [66], when considered as SSI also wound infections and superficial infections.

Overall complications rate in curettage surgery is reported to be around 9.6% [66] of these complications up to 10.7% are infections (Fig. 28.3). Anyway, it is important to remember that the most common post-operative complication after a curettage surgery is a post-operative fracture, representing almost 26% of all complications [66], but SSI can lead to a higher rate of graft failure and subsequent post-curettage fracture [67].

Risk factors analysis for SSI in curettage shows that smoking history, a distal tumor location (like distal femur), and low serum albumin are associated with a higher rate of SSI [65]. In some sites of curettage, complications and SSI rates are more frequently reported, like in the radius and distal radius [68].

Cavity filling after curettage with antibiotic-loaded polymethylmethacrylate (PMMA) bone cement has a reduced risk of infection [65], while the use of allografts to fill the cavity after benign bone tumor curettage has a higher rate of infection, with an associated low, but possible, risk of disease transmission and immune rejection [67].

As in other cases of SSI in Orthopaedic Oncology, a careful follow-up can bring to early detection and prompt treatment of SSI after curettage surgery, leading to better outcomes [29].

Treatment is usually debridement, possibly cavity-filling removal and substitution with antibiotic-loaded PMMA, targeted antibiotic therapy, and adequate soft tissue coverage [65].

## 28.5 Infections in Resection in Pelvis with and Without Reconstruction

Surgical Site Infection (SSI) in pelvis surgery is a rather common and at the same time dangerous complication. The necessity to obtain adequate exposure to identify and protect the neurovascular structures and to obtain wide margins of resection in tumor surgery, associated with larger soft tissue damage and longer surgical times brings to a high infection rate. Reconstruction with prosthesis and allograft after pelvis bone tumor resection is often required to have a good function in case of internal hemipelvectomy or to give back integrity to the pelvic ring, while in some minor soft tissue or bone resections, without compromising the integrity of the pelvic ring,

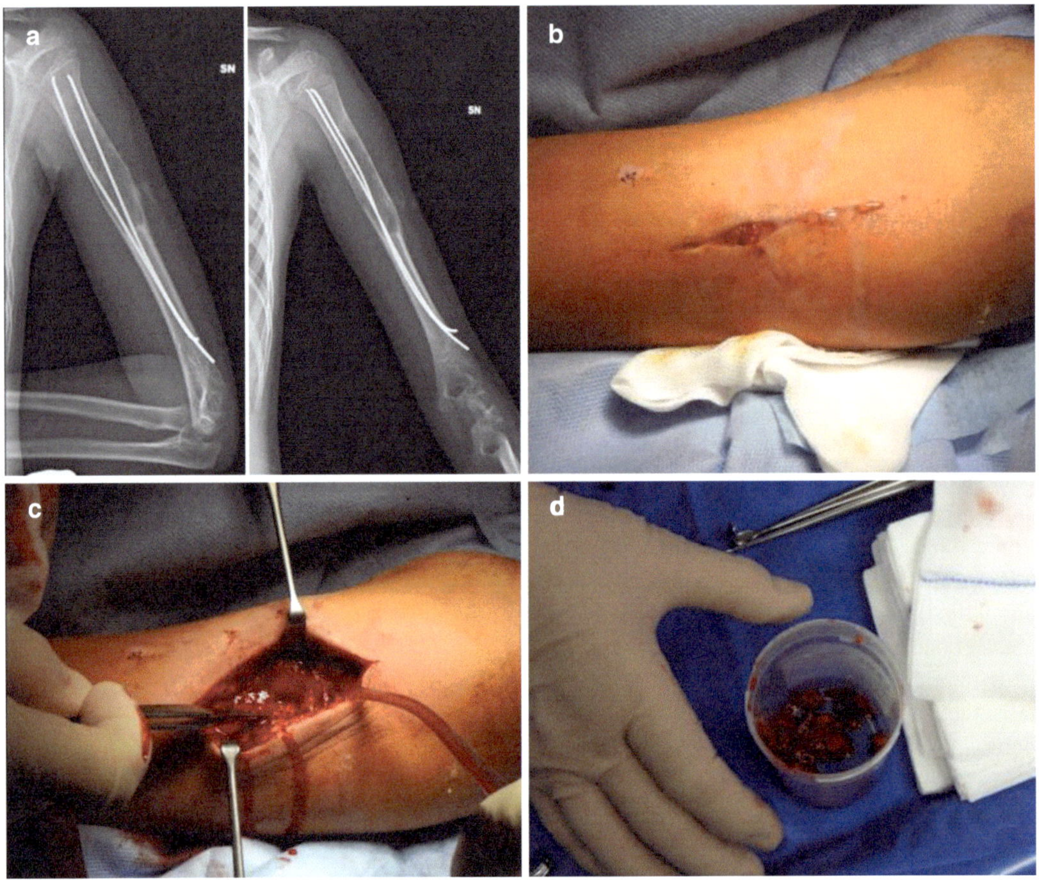


**Fig. 28.3** (**a**) X-rays after curettage, Titanium Elastic Nails fixation, and allograft filling of a Unicameral Bone Cyst in an 8 years old female patient, (**b**) surgical site infection, 40 days after surgery, (**c**, **d**) surgical debridement, irrigation, and microbiology samples for cultures and susceptibilities

no prosthetic or allograft reconstruction is needed [69, 70].

Pelvis orthopedic oncology surgery shows a rate of infection between 10% and 47% of patients [10–15, 70–87]. SSI has a lower rate in resections without reconstruction, between 10% and 15%, while there is a higher SSI rate in allograft reconstructions, reaching the highest rate of SSI, 47% [17]. It is known that infection is the most dreadful complication after allograft reconstruction in pelvic tumor surgery [10, 75, 88].

A study shows a higher SSI rate in allograft reconstruction compared to prosthetic reconstruction [89], while another study highlights a similar 38% SSI rate between allograft and prosthetic reconstruction [79]. A large series [17] of pelvis resection and reconstruction surgeries showed that prosthetic reconstruction has a 30% SSI rate, allograft reconstruction has a 28% SSI rate, composite allograft, and prosthetic reconstruction has a 20% SSI rate, surgeries without reconstruction have a 15% SSI rate [17].

Risk factors analyzed as a type of surgical resection, oncological stage, and chemo/radiation therapy do not show a significantly higher risk of SSI, the only predictor of complications is an age >50 years [76]. Radiation and chemotherapy are significantly correlated to a higher risk of SSI in univariate analysis, this significance is no longer present in multivariate analysis, with pelvic reconstruction being the only independent prognostic factor for SSI [17].

SSI onset is at a mean of 6–8 months after surgery, but it is still possible up to 2 years post-

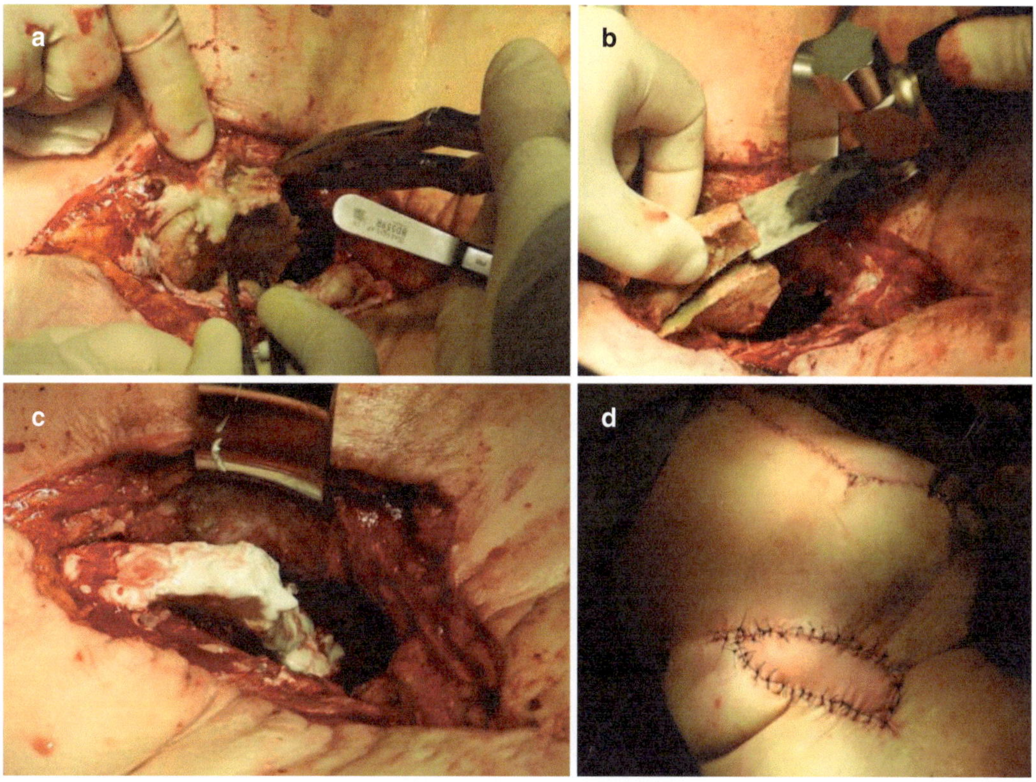

**Fig. 28.4** (**a**) Surgical site infection after soft tissue sarcoma resection and partial iliac wing resection, without reconstruction, (**b**) debridement, irrigation, and resection of necrotic/infected bone, (**c**) antibiotic-loaded bone cement, (**d**) soft tissue reconstruction with a vertical rectus abdominis musculocutaneous flap

operatively. A careful follow-up can determine early detection and prompt treatment, with better outcomes [10, 73].

Treatment of SSI in pelvis cases is accurate debridement (multiple times when required), antibiotic treatment (targeted on the bacteria and susceptibilities obtained from microbiology samples), and adequate soft tissue reconstruction after resection [10–14, 70–83, 86, 87]. The multidisciplinary approach with the Plastic Surgeon to obtain good soft tissue coverage is crucial at the time of the first surgery and in the treatment of the possible infective complications [90, 91], (Fig. 28.4).

In wound complications, superficial SSI, and deep SSI in pelvis cases without reconstruction, the success rate of this treatment can possibly be 80%. The worst case is represented by a deep SSI in pelvis reconstruction cases, it leads to an implant/allograft removal in almost 46% of cases, with loss of function and worse outcomes. External hemipelvectomy as the endpoint of SSI treatment is a last-step option rarely needed [17].

SSI in pelvis oncology cases has the burden of longer hospital admissions, delayed adjuvant therapies, higher costs of treatments, higher morbidity, and higher mortality [17].

## 28.6 Infections in Resection in Spine and Sacrum with/Without Reconstruction

Surgical site infection (SSI) in sacrectomy without reconstruction is a common complication, with a range between 32% [91] and 56% [92] in surgeries for chordomas, while in sacrectomies for giant cell tumor of the bone (27 cases from a single institution) a series shows no cases of deep infections [93]. Surgical treatment for Chordomas is known to have a high risk of infective complications [94].

SSI onset is most frequent in between 2 [92] and 4 weeks [93] post-operatively, in almost 70% of cases and in all cases within 6 months from surgery, usually the infection is multi-microbial (up to 74% of cases) with Enterococcus, *Escherichia coli*, and *Pseudomonas aeruginosa* being the most frequent pathogens [92, 93].

Multiple risk factors are investigated to understand a possible influence on SSI rate. There is not statistically significant higher risk of SSI correlated to previous treatments, level of resections, presence of colostomy, operating time, bowel incontinence, age, and tumor volume [93]. There is a trend of higher risk of SSI with neoadjuvant radiation therapy [92]. In another study, radiation therapy is associated with a higher rate of wound complications and a higher risk of infection in other studies [95, 96].

Deep surgical site infection and wound complications are the most common reasons for re-operation [97]. Up to 31% of SSI cases require another surgery [91]. Treatment of deep surgical site infections in chordoma consists of multiple debridement surgeries associated with microbiological cultures and tailored antibiotic treatment based on susceptibilities [93]. The use of rectus abdomini flaps, for soft tissue defect reconstruction, showed a statistically significant lower risk of wound dehiscence and SSI [98], (Fig. 28.5).

SSI in a debilitated patient after a demolitive chordoma surgery can be a dreadful complication, leading to sepsis and, in the worst cases, death of the patient, in a series sepsis was shown to be the cause of death for 5% of patients [98].

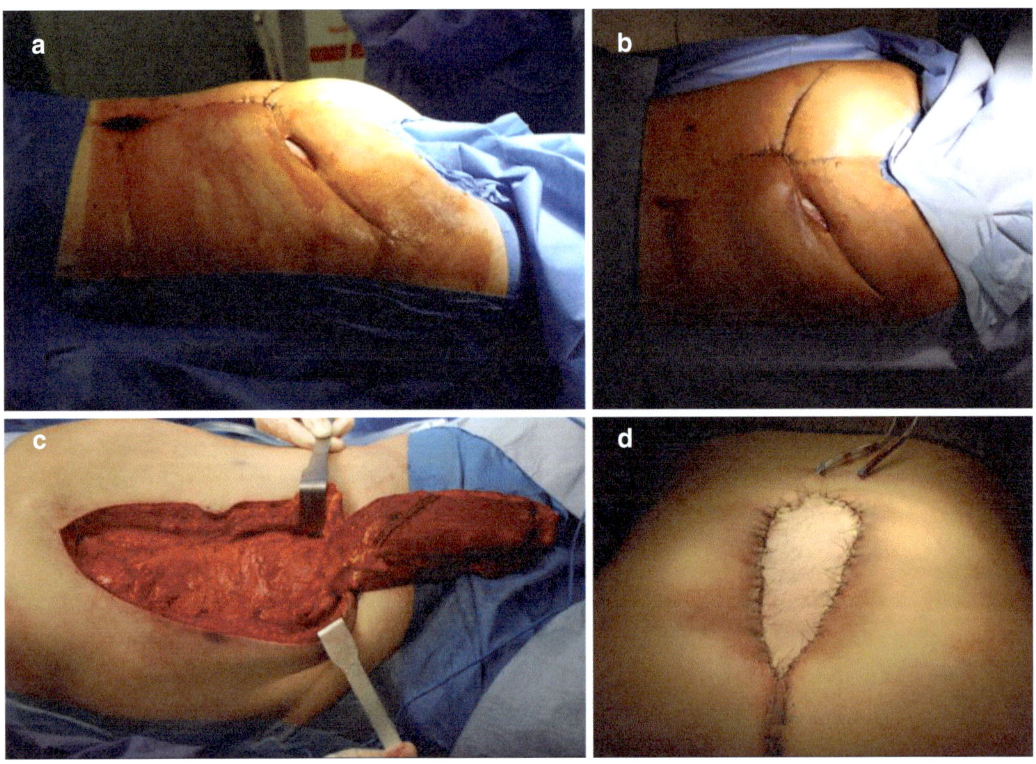


**Fig. 28.5** (**a**, **b**) Deep surgical site infection and superficial wound complications after chordoma surgery are quite common, (**c**, **d**) reconstruction of the soft tissue defects can be performed successfully with a vertical rectus abdominis musculocutaneous flap

## References


1. Bourget-Murray J, Bansal R, Soroceanu A, Piroozfar S, Railton P, Johnston K, Johnson A, Powell J. Assessment of risk factors for early-onset deep surgical site infection following primary total hip arthroplasty for osteoarthritis. J Bone Jt Infect. 2021;6:443–50.
2. Pei H, Wang H, Chen M, Ma L, Liu G, Ding W. Surgical site infection after posterior lumbar interbody fusion and instrumentation in patients with lumbar degenerative disease. Int Wound J. 2021;18:608–15.
3. Matsumoto H, Larson EL, Warren SI, Hammoor BT, Bonsignore-Opp L, Troy MJ, Barrett KK, Striano BM, Li G, Terry MB, et al. A clinical risk model for surgical site infection following pediatric spine deformity surgery. J Bone Jt Surg Am. 2022;104:364–75.
4. Staals EL, Sambri A, Campanacci DA, Muratori F, Leithner A, Gilg MM, Gortzak Y, Van De Sande M, Dierselhuis E, Mascard E, et al. Expandable distal femur megaprosthesis: a European musculoskeletal oncology society study on 299 cases. J Surg Oncol. 2020;122:760–5.
5. Pala E, Trovarelli G, Calabro T, Angelini A, Abati CN, Ruggieri P. Survival of modern knee tumor megaprostheses: failures, functional results, and a comparative statistical analysis. Clin Orthop Relat Res. 2015;473:891–9.
6. Lee SY, Jeon DG, Cho WH, Song WS, Kim BS. Are pasteurized autografts durable for reconstructions after bone tumor resections? Clin Orthop Relat Res. 2018;476:1728–37.
7. Araki Y, Yamamoto N, Hayashi K, Takeuchi A, Miwa S, Igarashi K, Higuchi T, Abe K, Taniguchi Y, Yonezawa H, et al. Clinical outcomes of frozen autograft reconstruction for the treatment of primary bone sarcoma in adolescents and young adults. Sci Rep. 2021;11:17291.
8. Severyns M, Briand S, Waast D, Touchais S, Hamel A, Gouin F. Postoperative infections after limb-sparing surgery for primary bone tumors of the pelvis: incidence, characterization and functional impact. Surg Oncol. 2017;26:171–7.
9. Abudu A, Grimer RJ, Cannon SR, Carter SR, Sneath RS. Reconstruction of the hemipelvis after the excision of malignant tumours. Complications and functional outcome of prostheses. J Bone Jt Surg Br. 1997;79:773–9.
10. Jaiswal, P.K.; Aston,W.J.; Grimer, R.J.; Abudu, A.; Carter, S.; Blunn, G.; Briggs, T.W.; Cannon, S. Periacetabular resection and endoprosthetic reconstruction for tumours of the acetabulum. J Bone Jt Surg Br 2008, 90, 1222–1227.
11. Aljassir F, Beadel GP, Turcotte RE, Griffin AM, Bell RS, Wunder JS, Isler MH. Outcome after pelvic sarcoma resection reconstructed with saddle prosthesis. Clin Orthop Relat Res. 2005;438:36–41.
12. Cottias P, Jeanrot C, Vinh TS, Tomeno B, Anract P. Complications and functional evaluation of 17 saddle prostheses for resection of periacetabular tumors. J Surg Oncol. 2001;78:90–100.
13. Ozaki T, Hillmann A, Bettin D, Wuisman P, Winkelmann W. High complication rates with pelvic allografts. Experience of 22 sarcoma resections. Acta Orthop Scand. 1996;67:333–8.
14. Guo,W.; Li, D.; Tang, X.; Ji, T. Surgical treatment of pelvic chondrosarcoma involving periacetabulum. J Surg Oncol 2010, 101, 160–165.
15. Ham SJ, Schraffordt Koops H, Veth RPH, van Horn JR, Eisma WH, Hoekstra HJ. External and internal hemipelvectomy for sarcomas of the pelvic girdle: consequences of limb-salvage treatment. Eur J Surg Oncol (EJSO). 1997;23:540–6.
16. Miwa S, Shirai T, Yamamoto N, Hayashi K, Takeuchi A, Tada K, Kajino Y, Higuchi T, Abe K, Aiba H, et al. Risk factors for surgical site infection after malignant bone tumor resection and reconstruction. BMC Cancer. 2019;19:33.
17. Angelini A, Drago G, Trovarelli G, Calabro T, Ruggieri P. Infection after surgical resection for pelvic bone tumors: an analysis of 270 patients from one institution. Clin Orthop Relat Res. 2014;472:349–59.
18. Fujiwara T, Ogura K, Christ A, Bartelstein M, Kenan S, Fabbri N, Healey J. Periacetabular reconstruction following limb-salvage surgery for pelvic sarcomas. J Bone Oncol. 2021;31:100396.
19. Wu, J.; Xie, K.; Luo, D.;Wang, L.;Wu,W.; Yan, M.; Ai, S.; Dai, K.; Hao, Y. Three-dimensional printing-based personalized limb salvage and reconstruction treatment of pelvic tumors. J Surg Oncol 2021, 124, 420–430.
20. Trovarelli G, Angelini A, Pala E, Cappellari A, Breda A, Ruggieri P. Infection in orthopaedic oncology: crucial problem in modern reconstructive techniques. Eur Rev Med Pharmacol Sci. 2019;23(2 Suppl):271–8.
21. Anatone AJ, Danford NC, Jang ES, Smartt A, Konigsberg M, Tyler WK. Risk factors for surgical site infection in orthopaedic oncology. J Am Acad Orthop Surg. 2020;28(20):e923–8.
22. Gradl G, de Witte PB, Evans BT, Hornicek F, Raskin K, Ring D. Surgical site infection in orthopaedic oncology. JBJS. 2014;96(3):223–30.
23. Miwa S, Shirai T, Yamamoto N, Hayashi K, Takeuchi A, Tada K, Kajino Y, Inatani H, Higuchi T, Abe K, et al. Risk factors for postoperative deep infection in bone tumors. PLoS One. 2017;12:e0187438.
24. Morris CD, Sepkowitz K, Fonshell C, Margetson N, Eagan J, Miransky J, Boland PJ, Healey J. Prospective identification of risk factors for wound infection after lower extremity oncologic surgery. Ann Surg Oncol. 2003;10:778–82.
25. Anaya DA, Cormier JN, Xing Y, Koller P, Gaido L, Hadfield D, Chemaly RF, Feig BW. Development and validation of a novel stratification tool for identifying cancer patients at increased risk of surgical site infection. Ann Surg. 2012;255:134–9.

26. Lozano-Calderon SA, Swaim SO, Federico A, Anderson ME, Gebhardt MC. Predictors of soft-tissue complications and deep infection in allograft reconstruction of the proximal tibia. J Surg Oncol. 2016;113:811–7.
27. Langit MB, Miwa S, Yamamoto N, Hayashi K, Takeuchi A, Igarashi K, Tada K, Higuchi T, Yonezawa H, Morinaga S, et al. Risk factors for postoperative deep infection after malignant bone tumor surgery of the extremities. Anticancer Res. 2020;40:3551–7.
28. Fujiwara T, Ebihara T, Kitade K, Setsu N, Endo M, Iida K, Matsumoto Y, Matsunobu T, Oda Y, Iwamoto Y, et al. Risk factors of Periprosthetic infection in patients with tumor prostheses following resection for musculoskeletal tumor of the lower limb. J Clin Med. 2020;9:3133.
29. Miwa S, Yamamoto N, Hayashi K, Takeuchi A, Igarashi K, Tsuchiya H. Surgical site infection after bone tumor surgery: risk factors and new preventive techniques. Cancer. 2022;14(18):4527.
30. Farhan-Alanie OM, Ha TT, Doonan J, Mahendra A, Gupta S. Inflammatory prognostic scoring systems are risk factors for surgical site infection following wide local excision of soft tissue sarcoma. Eur J Orthop Surg Traumatol. 2021;32:1–9.
31. Miyamoto S, Fujiki M, Nakatani F, Kobayashi E, Sakisaka M, Sakuraba M. Reconstruction of complex groin defects after sarcoma resection. Ann Plast Surg. 2017;78(4):443–7.
32. Angelini A, Tiengo C, Cerchiaro MC, Soto F, Biz C, Messana F, et al. Ortho-oncoplastic surgery in foot and ankle: a narrative overview on reconstruction of soft-tissue defects after oncologic resections. Microsurgery. 2024;44(4):e31168.
33. Morii T, Mochizuki K, Tajima T, Ichimura S, Satomi K. Surgical site infection in malignant soft tissue tumors. J Orthop Sci. 2012;17:51–7.
34. Perrault DP, Lee GK, Roy PY, Carre AL, Chattha A, Johnson MB, et al. Risk factors for wound complications after soft tissue sarcoma resection. Ann Plast Surg. 2021;86(3S):S336–41.
35. Bensaid S, Contejean A, Morand P, Enser M, Eyrolle L, Charlier C, et al. Surgical site infection after pelvic bone and soft tissue sarcoma resection: risk factors, microbiology, and impact of extended postoperative antibiotic prophylaxis. J Surg Oncol. 2023;128(2):344–9.
36. Cannon CP, Ballo MT, Zagars GK, Mirza AN, Lin PP, Lewis VO, et al. Complications of combined modality treatment of primary lower extremity soft-tissue sarcomas. Cancer. 2006;107(10):2455–61.
37. Bisson-Patoué A, Bourdais-Sallot A, Janoray G, Rosset P, Samargandi R, Le Nail LR. Factors associated with complications after resection of soft tissue sarcomas of the groin. Orthop Traumatol Surg Res. 2022;108(4):103158.
38. Pagnoni C, Zoccali G, di Uccio AS, Sperati F, Favale L, Valeri S, et al. Soft tissue sarcomas of the proximal adductor area of the thigh: indications, results and complications at medium follow-up in a series of 43 surgically treated patients. J Orthop. 2024;58:16.
39. Tsuda Y, Fujiwara T, Evans S, Kaneuchi Y, Abudu A. Extra-articular resection of shoulder joint for bone sarcomas: oncologic and limb-salvage outcomes of 32 cases compared with shoulder disarticulation and forequarter amputation. J Surg Oncol. 2020;121(4):612–9.
40. Mayil Vahanan N, Mohanlal P, Bose JC, Gangadharan R, Karthisundar V. The functional and oncological results after scapulectomy for scapular tumours: 2–16-year results. Int Orthop. 2007;31:831–6.
41. Voggenreiter G, Assenmacher S, Schmit-Neuerburg KP. Tikhoff- Linberg procedure for bone and soft tissue tumors of the shoulder girdle. Arch Surg. 1999;134:252–7.
42. Angelini A, Mavrogenis AF, Trovarelli G, et al. Extra-articular shoulder resections: outcomes of 54 patients. J Shoulder Elb Surg. 2017;26:e337–45.
43. Xie L, Tang XD, Yang RL, Guo W. Interscapulothoracic resection of tumours of shoulder with a note on reconstruction. Bone Joint J. 2014;96-B(5):684–90.
44. Pritsch T, Bickels J, Wu CC, Squires MH, Malawer MM. Is scapular endoprosthesis functionally superior to humeral suspension? Clin Orthop Relat Res. 2007;1976-2007(456):188–95.
45. Capanna R, van Horn JR, Biagini R, et al. The Tikhoff-Linberg procedure for bone tumors of the proximal humerus: the classical "extensive" technique versus a modified "transglenoid" resection. Arch Orthop Trauma Surg. 1990;109:63–7.
46. Yu XJ, Liu QK, Wang YG, Wang SX, Lu R, Xu HR, et al. Oncologic and functional outcomes of different reconstruction modalities after resection of chondrosarcoma of the scapula: a medium-to long-term follow-up study. BMC Musculoskelet Disord. 2022;23(1):758.
47. Dieckmann R, Gebert C, Streitbürger A, Henrichs MP, Dirksen U, Rödl R, et al. Proximal fibula resection in the treatment of bone tumours. Int Orthop. 2011;35:1689–94.
48. Dieckmann R, Ahrens H, Streitbürger A, Budny TB, Henrichs MP, Vieth V, et al. Reconstruction after wide resection of the entire distal fibula in malignant bone tumours. Int Orthop. 2011;35:87–92.
49. Capanna R, van Horn JR, Biagini R, Ruggieri P, Bettelli G, Campanacci M. Reconstruction after resection of the distal fibula for bone tumor. Acta Orthop Scand. 1986;57:290–4. https://doi.org/10.3109/17453678608994394.
50. Wang J, Du Z, Yang R, Tang X, Guo W. Lateral malleolus en bloc resection for the distal fibula osteosarcoma based on a new classification and proposed reconstruction choice: analysis of 6 cases prognosis and literature review. Foot Ankle Surg. 2020;26:855–63. https://doi.org/10.1016/j.fas.2019.11.003.
51. Kiyokawa K, Tanaka S, Kiduka Y, Inoue Y, Yamauchi T, Tai Y. Reconstruction of the form and function of lateral malleolus and ankle joint.

J Reconstr Microsurg. 2005;21:371–6. https://doi.org/10.1055/s-2005-915204.
52. Angelini A, Bohacek I, Plecko M, Biz C, Trovarelli G, Cerchiaro M, et al. Reconstructive surgery after distal fibular resection due to bone tumors: a technical report on surgical strategies and results from the PROSPERO international register of systematic reviews. EFORT Open Rev. 2024;9(6):503–16.
53. Aponte-Tinao LA, Ayerza MA, Muscolo LD, Farfalli GL. What are the risk factors and management options for infection after reconstruction with massive bone allografts? Clin Orthop Relat Res. 2016;474(3):669–73.
54. Lozano-Calderón SA, Swaim SO, Federico A, Anderson ME, Gebhardt MC. Predictors of soft-tissue complications and deep infection in allograft reconstruction of the proximal tibia. J Surg Oncol. 2016;113(7):811–7.
55. Witso E, Persen L, Benum P, Bergh K. Cortical allograft as a vehicle for antibiotic delivery. Acta Orthop. 2005;76:481–6.
56. Ketonis C, et al. Bacterial colonization of bone allograft. Establishment and effect of antibiotics. Clin Orthop Relat Res. 2010;468(8):2113–21.
57. Mankin H, Doppelt S, Tomford W. Clinical experience with allograft implantation. The first ten years. Clin Orthop. 1983;174:69–86.
58. Fricdlaender GE, Toss RE, Doganis AC, Kirkwood JM, Barron R. Effects of cheinothcrapculic agents on bone. J Bone Joint Surg Am. 1984;66(4):602–7.
59. Lord CF, Gebhardt MC, Tomford WW, Mankin HJ. Infection in bone allografts. Incidence, nature, and treatment. J Bone Joint Surg Am. 1988;70:369–76.
60. Kapoor SK, Thiyam R. Management of infection following reconstruction in bone tumors. J Clin Orthopaed Trauma. 2015;6(4):244–51.
61. Dick HM, Strauch RJ. Infection of massive bone allografts. Clin Orthop Relat Res. 1994;306(September):46–53.
62. Degroot H, Donati D, Di Liddo M, Gozzi E, Mercuri M. The use of cement in osteoarticular allografts for proximal humerus bone tumors. Clin Orthop Relat Res. 2004;427:190–7.
63. Ortiz-Cruz E, Gebhardt MC, Jennings LC, Springfield DS, Mankin HJ. The results of transplantation of intercalary allografts after resection of tumors. Long term follow up study. J Bone Joint Surg Am. 1997;79-A:97–106.
64. Mankin HJ, Hornicek FJ, Raskin KA. Infection in massive bone allografts. Clin Orthop Relat Res (1976–2007). 2005;(432):210–6.
65. Sukpanichyingyong S, Poosiripinyo T, Salang K, Simsin S. Impact of antibiotic-loaded bone cement prophylaxis on infection rates after curettage and cementation for bone tumor. J Orthopaed Rep. 2024;3(4):100331.
66. Smolle MA, Roessl V, Leithner A. Effect of local adjuvants following curettage of benign and intermediate tumours of bone: a systematic review of the literature. Cancer. 2023;15(17):4258.
67. Gava NF, Engel EE. Treatment alternatives and clinical outcomes of bone filling after benign tumour curettage. A systematic review. Orthop Traumatol Surg Res. 2022;108(4):102966.
68. Seth I, Bulloch G, Lim B, Xie Y, Seth N, Rozen WM, Ng SKH. Evaluating extended curettage and adjuvant therapy against wide resection and reconstruction in the management of distal radius giant cell tumors: a systematic review and meta-analysis. Hand. 2024;15589447241245736
69. Enneking WF. Pelvis. In: Enneking WF, editor. Musculoskeletal tumor surgery. New York: Churchill-Livingstone; 1983. p. 483–90.
70. Satcher RL Jr, O'Donnell RJ, Johnston JO. Reconstruction of the pelvis after resection of tumors about the acetabulum. Clin Orthop Relat Res. 2003;409:209–17.
71. Aboulafia AJ, Buch R, Mathews J, Li W, Malawer MM. Reconstruction using the saddle prosthesis following excision of primary and metastatic periacetabular tumors. Clin Orthop Relat Res. 1995;314:203–13.
72. Abudu A, Grimer RJ, Cannon SR, Carter SR, Sneath RS. Reconstruction of the hemipelvis after the excision of malignant tumours: complications and functional outcome of prostheses. J Bone Joint Surg Br. 1997;79:773–9.
73. Biau D, The'venin F, Dumaine V, Babinet A, Tomeno B, Anract P. Ipsilateral femoral autograft reconstruction after resection of a pelvic tumor. J Bone Joint Surg Am. 2009;91:142–51.
74. Capanna R, van Horn JR, Guernelli N, Briccoli A, Ruggieri P, Biagini R, Bettelli G, Campanacci M. Complications of pelvic resections. Arch Orthop Trauma Surg. 1987;106:71–7.
75. Delloye C, Banse X, Brichard B, Docquier PL, Cornu O. Pelvic reconstruction with a structural pelvic allograft after resection of a malignant bone tumor. J Bone Joint Surg Am. 2007;89:579–87.
76. Gebert C, Wessling M, Hoffmann C, Roedl R, Winkelmann W, Gosheger G, Hardes J. Hip transposition as a limb salvage procedure following the resection of periacetabular tumors. J Surg Oncol. 2011;103:269–75.
77. Guo W, Li D, Tang X, Yang Y, Ji T. Reconstruction with modular hemipelvic prostheses for periacetabular tumor. Clin Orthop Relat Res. 2007;461:180–8.
78. Harrington KD. The use of hemipelvic allografts or autoclaved grafts for reconstruction after wide resections of malignant tumors of the pelvis. J Bone Joint Surg Am. 1992;74:331–41.
79. Hillmann A, Hoffmann C, Gosheger G, Rodl R, Winkelmann W, Ozaki T. Tumors of the pelvis: complications after reconstruction. Arch Orthop Trauma Surg. 2003;123:340–4.
80. Laffosse JM, Pourcel A, Reina N, Tricoire JL, Bonnevialle P, Chiron P, Puget J. Primary tumor of the periacetabular region: resection and reconstruction using a segmental ipsilateral femur autograft. Orthop Traumatol Surg Res. 2012;98:309–18.

81. Langlais F, Lambotte JC, Thomazeau H. Long-term results of hemipelvis reconstruction with allografts. Clin Orthop Relat Res. 2001;388:178–86.
82. Ozaki T, Hoffmann C, Hillmann A, Gosheger G, Lindner N, Winkelmann W. Implantation of hemipelvic prosthesis after resection of sarcoma. Clin Orthop Relat Res. 2002;396:197–205.
83. Puri A, Gulia A, Jambhekar NA, Laskar S. Results of surgical resection in pelvic Ewing's sarcoma. J Surg Oncol. 2012;106:417–22.
84. Rodl RW, Hoffmann C, Gosheger G, Leidinger B, Jurgens H, Winkelmann W. Ewing's sarcoma of the pelvis: combined surgery and radiotherapy treatment. J Surg Oncol. 2003;83:154–60.
85. Schwameis E, Dominkus M, Krepler P, Dorotka R, Lang S, Windhager R, Kotz R. Reconstruction of the pelvis after tumor resection in children and adolescents. Clin Orthop Relat Res. 2002;402:220–35.
86. Windhager R, Karner J, Kutschera HP, Polterauer P, Salzer-Kuntschik M, Kotz R. Limb salvage in periacetabular sarcomas: review of 21 consecutive cases. Clin Orthop Relat Res. 1996;331:265–76.
87. Wirbel RJ, Schulte M, Maier B, Mutschler WE. Megaprosthetic replacement of the pelvis: function in 17 cases. Acta Orthop Scand. 1999;70:348–52.
88. Yoshida Y, Osaka S, Mankin HJ. Hemipelvic allograft reconstruction after periacetabular bone tumor resection. J Orthop Sci 2000;5:198–204.sgs.
89. Zeifang F, Buchner M, Zahlten-Hinguranage A, Bernd L, Sabo D. Complications following operative treatment of primary malignant bone tumours in the pelvis. Eur J Surg Oncol. 2004;30:893–9.
90. Tiengo C, Monticelli A, Sonda R, Angelini A, Ruggieri P, Bassetto F. Role of plastic surgery in the treatment of pelvic tumors. In: Surgery of pelvic bone tumors. Springer; 2021. p. 225–32.
91. Zuckerman SL, Lee SH, Chang GJ, Walsh GL, Mehran RJ, Gokaslan ZL, et al. Outcomes of surgery for sacral chordoma and impact of complications: a report of 50 consecutive patients with long-term follow-up. Global Spine J. 2021;11(5):740–50.
92. Marmouset D, Haseny B, Dukan R, Saint-Etienne A, Missenard G, Court C, Bouthors C. Characteristics, survivals and risk factors of surgical site infections after En Bloc sacrectomy for primary malignant sacral tumors at a single center. Orthop Traumatol Surg Res. 2022;108(4):103197.
93. Ruggieri P, Angelini A, Pala E, Mercuri M. Infections in surgery of primary tumors of the sacrum. Spine. 2012;37(5):420–8.
94. Varga PP, Szoverfi Z, Fisher CG, et al. Surgical treatment of sacral chordoma: prognostic variables for local recurrence and overall survival. Eur Spine J. 2015;24(5):1092–101.
95. Houdek MT, Rose PS, Hevesi M, Schwab JH, Griffin AM, Healey JH, et al. Low dose radiotherapy is associated with local complications but not disease control in sacral chordoma. J Surg Oncol. 2019;119(7):856–63.
96. Ji T, Guo W, Yang R, Tang X, Wang Y, Huang L. What are the conditional survival and functional outcomes after surgical treatment of 115 patients with sacral chordoma? Clin Orthop Relat Res. 2017;475(3):620–30.
97. Kolz JM, Wellings EP, Houdek MT, Clarke MJ, Yaszemski MJ, Rose PS. Surgical treatment of primary mobile spine chordoma. J Surg Oncol. 2021;123(5):1284–91.
98. Schwab J, Healey J, Rose P, Casas-Ganem J, Boland PJ. The surgical Management of Sacral Chordomas. Spine. 2009;34(24):2700–4.

# Infective Complications After Spinal Instrumentation

# 29

Andrea Angelini, Giovanni Baldin, Ron Batash, and Pietro Ruggieri

## 29.1 Introduction

Surgical site infection (SSI) is an uncommon complication of spine surgery, but when it happens, it represents a huge challenge both for the surgeon and the patient, with potentially catastrophic consequences if not treated quickly [1–3]. In fact, patients with post-operative spine infection require longer hospital lengths of stay, have higher re-operation rates, and are put at high risk of chronic pain, neurological complications, pseudarthrosis that can lead to implant failure, and even death if they involve the spinal cord. Progress was made in reducing the risk of infection by adopting a standardized protocol in the management of the patient both pre-, intra-, and post-operative, and by better understanding of risk factors. Early diagnosis and treatment are mandatory to treat those kinds of complications.

## 29.2 Incidence and Risk Factors

The reported incidence of SSI ranges between 1 and 18% [4–7]. This wide range is due to the different variety present in spine surgery depending on the surgical complexity and patient risk factors, both concerning the type of operation and the surgical approach. Conventionally the elements accountable for SSI are divided into two main categories, the unchangeable (patient-related) and changeable (procedure-related) [8–11]. Patient's related risk factors are age (>65 years old), American Society of Anesthesiologist (ASA) score, diabetes mellitus, cardiovascular disease, obesity, smoking, steroid use, nutritional status, and immunologic competence. Smoking and substance abuse negatively impact wound healing and immune function, and malnourished patients are 15 times more likely to present SSI [12–16]. Procedure-related risk factors are linked to the duration of surgery, blood loss, presence of instrumentation, and prolonged preoperative hospital stay. Anterior approaches have shown the least amount of postoperative infection, meanwhile, the posterior lumbar approach is the one with the greatest risk of infections. This is due to the proximity of the surgical site with the anus and the genitourinary tract, with a high risk of involuntary contamination after the surgery [1, 17–19]. Also, it appears that simpler operations without implants present a lower incidence of SSI when compared with major operations with instrumented fusion. Those findings are linked to the fact that major surgery also means more blood loss, longer surgical time, and longer hospitalization of the patient. The presence of instrumentation can provide bacteria (such as Staphylococcus species) with a

A. Angelini · G. Baldin · R. Batash · P. Ruggieri (✉)
Department of Orthopedics and Orthopedic Oncology, University of Padova, Padova, Italy
e-mail: andrea.angelini@unipd.it; pietro.ruggieri@unipd.it



P. Ruggieri et al. (eds.), *Bone and Joint Infections*, https://doi.org/10.1007/978-3-031-96383-4_29

suitable foreign surface for a polysaccharide biofilm called "glycocalyx," a barrier against antibiotics and the host immune system [20]. This biofilm makes infections difficult to eradicate.

## 29.3 Types of SSI

The SSI's type can be mainly divided into superficial SSI and deep SSI. Superficial SSI is limited to the skin or the subcutaneous layers, meanwhile, deep SSI involves the muscular fascia or even the paraspinal musculature; it can present huge potential dangers when in proximity to the spine cord and the neural elements. Thalgott et al. [21] have described a classification based not on the depth but on the severity of the infection and the patient's immune system response. The severity of infection was divided into three groups: (1) superficial/deep infection caused by a single germ; (2) deep infection caused by multiple germs; (3) deep infection with muscular necrosis caused by multiple or drug-resistant germs. The immune system response was categorized too into three subgroups: (1) normal general immune defenses, without vascular defects or metabolic diseases; (2) general diffused infection or tumors; (3) malnourished or immunodeficient patient.

Moreover, these infections are typically classified based on their timing: early (within 3 months post-surgery), delayed (3 to 12 months), and late (more than 12 months). Early infections are often caused by more virulent organisms like Staphylococcus aureus, including methicillin-resistant *Staphylococcus aureus* (MRSA). Delayed and late infections are frequently associated with less virulent organisms, such as coagulase-negative staphylococci [20, 22].

## 29.4 Diagnosis

Diagnosis usually made both by clinical and radiological findings considering that superficial and deep SSI can have different characteristics. While superficial SSI can be clinically evident from the early stage, deep SSI can hide for a long time showing just few general symptoms before rapid worsening. Especially in those cases, early diagnosis is crucial [10–11, 23]. The surgeon should always use all the weapons at his disposal to investigate the presence of SSI when suspected. Surgical site infection can be a difficult task even for experienced surgeons, starting from the diagnosis; an early diagnosis can significantly improve the outcome and simplify the management of the patient. The clinician should always suspect an infection in a patient complaining of excessive back pain after surgery and a pain-free interval, especially if are also present other general signs like fever. There can also be more evident symptoms that can lead the examiner to the suspicion of SSI, like wound dehiscence or necrosis and the presence of purulent material on the surgical site [24].

Usually, superficial SSI shows early local redness, swollen skin, and pain, with local secretion, meanwhile deep SSI can be more difficult to diagnose due to low to no local symptoms. When they become clear they show local pain and can have general symptoms like fever [25–26]. First of all, draw multiple blood cultures during fever and take additional laboratory tests. In SSI those present elevated white blood cell (WBC), increased C-reactive protein (CRP), and erythrocytes sedimentation rate (ESR). Polymorphonuclear cells increase is an important indication of infection, and should always be monitored for some days after surgery. ESR tends to increase right after surgery (with peak in about 4–5 days), but should go back to normal value by 14 days; a tendency to a high value of ESR is suggestive of SSI. The CRP value usually peaks in few days after surgery and decreases more rapidly than ESR. Progression of the CRP value or persistently elevated value is a valid indicator or SSI [27–30]. After the first line of blood exams, radiological imaging has a pivotal role in the diagnosis. Plain radiographs do not provide relevant information, especially in early infections because bacteria had no time to alter the bone or implant. Meanwhile, in case of late infection, an X-ray can show bone lysis or lytic areas around the instrumentation [31]. Ultrasound can be used to investigate the presence of hematoma in early infection and even guide a puncture of it. Computed tomography (CT) and magnetic resonance imaging (MRI) provide the best data for diagnosis and should be acquired with the use of an intravenous contrast medium if possible [32–35]. CT scans can show changes in the vertebrae, bone lysis, and even fluid collection. Also, CT can be used to guide biopsy. MRI is essential, in particular, if a discitis or epidural abscess are suspected. Discitis diagnosis is suggested by a high-intensity signal in the disc and the adjacent vertebral bodies on T2 sequences with close-by fluid collection. Elements suggesting infection of instrumentation at the MRI are enhanced high-intensity T2 signal on soft tissue or ringed enhancement of fluid collection after gadolinium injection.

Instrumentation can complicate the radiographic examination due to the presence of artifacts. Nowadays is possible to obtain sequences with reduced artifacts software. The choice between CT and MRI is made considering the presence or not of instrumentation and the type of infection suspected, and can help to determine the extension of the infection. One of the most critical steps when diagnosing an SSI is to determine the specific regions of the spine involved. It is essential to rule out medullary involvement, such as meningitis. Additionally, if instrumentation is present, assessing the stability of the implant is crucial.

## 29.5 Treatment

After diagnosis, it is essential to begin treatment of the infection promptly, as spinal surgical site infections (SSIs) can be challenging to eradicate. These infections typically require a multidisciplinary approach with long-term antibiotic therapy and multiple meticulous surgical sessions for debridement [36–38]. The causative bacteria must be identified through blood cultures or cultures obtained from biopsy samples or surgical debridement. After the samples are taken a broad-spectrum antibiotic therapy should always be started, to be switched to a more specific one after the pathogenic agent is identified. The infectious disease specialist should always be addressed in those parts of the treatment [39–41]. In extremely superficial SSI, limited just to the suture or skin incision, local treatment associated with antibiotic therapy can be enough. However, those cases are quite rare. In the majority of cases SSI, both superficial or deep, can be quite difficult to eradicate and can make the surgeon face difficult decisions.

For early post-operative infections where spinal instrumentation is present, the hardware is maintained in order to prevent spinal instability; every loose bone graft should be carefully removed, keeping only one integrated. If there are signs of mobility in the implants they should be removed and replaced with new instrumentation [42–46]. For late post-operative infections involving spinal instrumentation where solid bone graft fusion has occurred, hardware removal is highly recommended. This action helps prevent pathogens from forming a glycocalyx, which contributes to antibiotic resistance. Furthermore, removing the hardware allows for more thorough debridement of any infected tissue. Abbey et al. [47] developed a treatment algorithm, where they suggest removing the implantation only when debridement and long period antibiotics have failed. Picada et al. [48] proposed that instrumentation removal is not necessary in acute infections. The wound is closed on an aspiration drain. It is advised to perform a second look 48 to 72 hours after the initial surgery if there is a severe infection [49–51].

The efficacy of treatment is monitored with clinical monitoring and periodic blood exams. There is still no clear consensus on the duration of the antibiotic regimen, but usually, long-term IV antibiotics are followed by oral suppressive antibiotics [4, 6, 46, 52–54].

## 29.6 Prevention of Postoperative Infections

Prevention of SSI should focus on the changeable factors listed previously. The sterile technique in the operating room is of course paramount and should always be as accurate as possible. As described by other authors, to cause an infection, bacteria must be present in significant quantity [20, 55–56]. The surgeon should always investigate and rule out the presence of any kind of infectious disease (urinary tract, pulmonary system) before performing surgery, and treat them as a priority [57]. As stated before, the risk of post-operative infection is highly dependent on the type of surgery performed; therefore, the surgeon should always try to prioritize less invasive methods when possible.

## 29.7 Conclusions

SSI after spine surgery is a challenging problem with a major toll on the patient, the surgeon, and the healthcare national system. Infection is a major complication both in short and long term due to being challenging to diagnose, and even more to treat. It often requires prolonged medical therapy and sometimes more than one surgical debridement. Many factors play a role in determining the risk of SSI, both changeable or unchangeable; the surgeon should look to minimize the risk of postoperative infection by taking action on the changeable elements. A strict follow-up in the post-operative short and long time period is mandatory. SSI should be investigated every time there is an anomalous postoperative course, using blood exams and radiological exams; an early diagnosis is the key to success. Once diagnosed, a treatment strategy can be defined. It is advised to obtain blood cultures and local tissue samplings to identify the pathogenic agent responsible for the infection; broad-spectrum IV antibiotics are mandatory until results are obtained, and it is possible to switch to a more specific antibiotic. Treatment can change based on the patient's clinical history, the site of infection (superficial or deep), the postoperative infection timing (early or late), and the type of surgery (presence or absence of spine implant), but it is usually based on long-term antibiotic and local surgical debridement. Implant removal is usually avoided but can be necessary in difficult cases when neurological symptoms are present.

**Declarations Author Contributions:** Conceptualization, project administration: AA, PR; data curation and formal analysis: AA, RB; supervision: AA, PR; writing-original draft: GB; writing-review and editing: AA, PR; All authors have read and agreed to the published version of the manuscript.

**Funding:** There was no external funding source in support of this study.

**Institutional Review Board Statement:** Not applicable.

**Informed Consent Statement:** Written informed consent was obtained from patients at the time of admission to our Institute. However, all pictures have been reported anonymized.

**Consent for Publication (Include Appropriate Statements)**

We confirm that this paper, including related data, figures, and tables, has not been published previously, it is not under consideration for publication elsewhere, and, if accepted, it will not be published elsewhere in the same form, in English or in any other language, without the written consent of the publisher.

**Conflicts of Interest/Competing Interests (Include Appropriate Disclosures)**

Ruggieri P is a consultant for Stryker and Exactech (not relevant to the present manuscript). The other authors declare that there are no relationships/conditions/circumstances that present a potential conflict of interest with the present manuscript.

**Availability of Data and Material (Data Transparency)**

Manuscript data are embedded in the text and fully available on specific request.

## References

1. Beiner JM, Grauer J, Kwon BK, Vaccaro AR. Postoperative wound infections of the spine. Neurosurg Focus. 2003;15(3) https://pubmed.ncbi.nlm.nih.gov/15347232/
2. Zimmerli W. Clinical practice. Vertebral osteomyelitis. N Engl J Med. 2010;362:1022–9.
3. Pola E, Logroscino C, Gentiempo M, Colangelo D, Mazzotta V, Meco E, et al. Medical and surgical treatment of pyogenic spondylodiscitis. Eur Rev Med Pharmacol Sci. 2012;16(Suppl 2):35–49.
4. Brown EM, Pople IK, De Louvois J, Hedges A, Bayston R, Eisenstein SM, et al. Spine update: prevention of postoperative infection in patients undergoing spinal surgery. Spine (Phila Pa 1976). 2004;29(8):938–45. https://pubmed.ncbi.nlm.nih.gov/15083000/
5. Tsantes AG, Papadopoulos DV, Vrioni G, Sioutis S, Sapkas G, Benzakour A, Benzakour T, Angelini A, Ruggieri P, Mavrogenis AF. World association against infection in orthopedics and trauma W A I O T study group on bone and joint infection definitions. Spinal

Infect Update Microorg. 2020;8(4):476. https://doi.org/10.3390/microorganisms8040476.

6. Glassman SD, Dimar JR, Puno RM, Johnson JR. Salvage of instrumental lumbar fusions complicated by surgical wound infection. Spine (Phila Pa 1976) [Internet]. 1996 Sep 15 [cited 2024 Apr 2];21(18):2163–9. Available from: https://pubmed.ncbi.nlm.nih.gov/8893444/
7. Rechtine GR, Bono PL, Cahill D, Bolesta MJ, Chrin AM. Postoperative wound infection after instrumentation of thoracic and lumbar fractures. J Orthop Trauma [Internet]. 2001 [cited 2024 Apr 2];15(8):566–9. Available from: https://pubmed.ncbi.nlm.nih.gov/11733673/
8. Attenello J, Allen RT. Postoperative spine infections. Semin Spine Surg. 2019;31(4):176–83.
9. Pawar AY, Biswas SK. Postoperative Spine Infections. Asian Spine J [Internet]. 2016 Feb [cited 2024 Apr 2];10(1):176–83. Available from: http://www.ncbi.nlm.nih.gov/pubmed/26949475
10. Pull Ter Gunne AF, Cohen DB. Incidence, prevalence, and analysis of risk factors for surgical site infection following adult spinal surgery. Spine (Phila Pa 1976) [Internet]. 2009 Jun 1 [cited 2024 Apr 2];34(13):1422–8. Available from: https://europepmc.org/article/med/19478664
11. Koutsoumbelis S, Hughes AP, Girardi FP, Cammisa FP, Finerty EA, Nguyen JT, et al. Risk factors for postoperative infection following posterior lumbar instrumented arthrodesis. J Bone Joint Surg Am [Internet]. 2011 Sep 7 [cited 2024 Apr 2];93(17):1627–33. Available from: https://pubmed.ncbi.nlm.nih.gov/21915578/
12. Klein JD, Hey LA, Yu CS, Klein BB, Coufal FJ, Young EP, et al. Perioperative nutrition and postoperative complications in patients undergoing spinal surgery. Spine (Phila Pa 1976) [Internet]. 1996 Nov 15 [cited 2024 Apr 10];21(22):2676–82. Available from: https://pubmed.ncbi.nlm.nih.gov/8961455/
13. Levin R, Bono CM, Garfin SR. Vertebral Discitis and Osteomyelitis. Core Knowl Orthop Spine [Internet]. 2004 Jan 1 [cited 2024 Apr 10];212–25. Available from: https://www.researchgate.net/publication/288813986_Vertebral_Discitis_and_Osteomyelitis
14. Patel N, Bagan B, Vadera S, Maltenfort MG, Deutsch H, Vaccaro AR, et al. Obesity and spine surgery: relation to perioperative complications. J Neurosurg Spine. 2007;6(4):291–7.
15. He Z, Zhou K, Tang K, Quan Z, Liu S, Su B. Perioperative hypoalbuminemia is a risk factor for wound complications following posterior lumbar interbody fusion. J Orthop Surg Res. 2020;15(1):538.
16. Adogwa O, Martin JR, Huang K, Verla T, Fatemi P, Thompson P, et al. Preoperative serum albumin level as a predictor of postoperative complication after spine fusion. Spine (Phila Pa 1976). 2014;39(18):1513–9.
17. Massie JB, Heller JG, Abitbol JJ, McPherson D, Garfin SR. Postoperative posterior spinal wound infections. Clin Orthop Relat Res. 1992;284:99–108.
18. Weinstein MA, McCabe JP, Cammisa J. Postoperative spinal wound infection: a review of 2,391 consecutive index procedures. J Spinal Disord. 2000;13(5):422–6.
19. Willems P. Decision making in surgical treatment of chronic low back pain: the performance of prognostic tests to select patients for lumbar spinal fusion. Acta Orthop. 2013;84(SUPPL.349):1–37.
20. Chaudhary SB, Vives MJ, Basra SK, Reiter MF. Postoperative spinal wound infections and post-procedural diskitis. J Spinal Cord Med [Internet]. 2007 [cited 2024 Apr 2];30(5):441. Available from: /pmc/articles/PMC2141723/
21. Thalgott JS, Cotler HB, Sasso RC, LaRocca H, Gardner V. Postoperative infections in spinal implants. Classification and analysis--a multicenter study. Spine (Phila Pa 1976) [Internet]. 1991 [cited 2024 Apr 10];16(8):981–4. Available from: https://pubmed.ncbi.nlm.nih.gov/1948385/
22. Sasso RC, Garrido BJ. Postoperative spinal wound infections. J Am Acad Orthop Surg [Internet]. 2008 [cited 2024 Apr 2];16(6):330–7. Available from: https://pubmed.ncbi.nlm.nih.gov/18524984/
23. Viola RW, King HA, Adler SM, Wilson CB. Delayed infection after elective spinal instrumentation and fusion. A retrospective analysis of eight cases. Spine (Phila Pa 1976) [Internet]. 1997 Oct 15 [cited 2024 Apr 10];22(20):2444–51. Available from: https://pubmed.ncbi.nlm.nih.gov/9355228/
24. Hadjipavlou AG, Mader JT, Necessary JT, Muffoletto AJ. Hematogenous pyogenic spinal infections and their surgical management. Spine (Phila Pa 1976). 2000;25(13):1668–79.
25. Zippelius T, Bürger J, Schömig F, Putzier M, Matziolis G, Strube P. Clinical presentation and diagnosis of acute postoperative spinal implant infection (Psii). J Spine Surg. 2020;6(4):765–71.
26. Prinz V, Vajkoczy P. Surgical revision strategies for postoperative spinal implant infections (PSII). J spine Surg (Hong Kong) [Internet]. 2020 Dec [cited 2024 Apr 10];6(4):777–84. Available from: http://www.ncbi.nlm.nih.gov/pubmed/33447683
27. Meyer B, Schaller K, Rohde V, Hassler W. The C-reactive protein for detection of early infections after lumbar microdiscectomy. Acta Neurochir (Wien) [Internet]. 1995 Sep [cited 2024 Apr 10];136(3–4):145–50. Available from: https://pubmed.ncbi.nlm.nih.gov/8748845/
28. Wang L, Yang B, Yin B, Zhang Z, Zhang L, Tang L, et al. Clinical significance of PCT, CRP, ESR, WBC count as predictors in postoperative early infectious complications with fever after posterior lumbar internal fixation. Zhongguo Gu Shang. 2015;28(1):66–70.
29. Kalfas F, Severi P, Scudieri C. Infection with spinal instrumentation: a 20-year, single-institution experience with review of pathogenesis, diagnosis, prevention, and management. Asian J Neurosurg [Internet]. 2019 Dec [cited 2024 Apr 10];14(4):1181–9. Available from: http://www.ncbi.nlm.nih.gov/pubmed/31903360

30. Kang BU, Lee SH, Ahn Y, Choi WC, Choi YG. Surgical site infection in spinal surgery: detection and management based on serial C-reactive protein measurements clinical article. J Neurosurg Spine. 2010 Aug;13(2):158–64.
31. Stambough JL, Beringer D. Postoperative wound infections complicating adult spine surgery. J Spinal Disord [Internet]. 1992 [cited 2024 Apr 10];5(3):277–85. Available from: https://pubmed.ncbi.nlm.nih.gov/1520986/
32. Hayashi D, Roemer FW, Mian A, Gharaibeh M, Müller B, Guermazi A. Imaging features of postoperative complications after spinal surgery and instrumentation. AJR Am J Roentgenol. 2012;199(1):123–9.
33. Girão MMV, Miyahara LK, Dwan VSY, Baptista E, Taneja AK, Gotfryd A, et al. Imaging features of the postoperative spine: a guide to basic understanding of spine surgical procedures. Insights Imaging [Internet]. 2023 Dec 1 [cited 2024 Apr 10];14(1):1–10. Available from: https://insightsimaging.springeropen.com/articles/10.1186/s13244-023-01447-0
34. Ortiz AO, de Moura A, Johnson BA. Postsurgical spine: techniques, expected imaging findings, and complications. Semin Ultrasound CT MR. 2018;39(6):630–50.
35. Thakkar RS, Malloy JP, Thakkar SC, Carrino JA, Khanna AJ. Imaging the postoperative spine. Radiol Clin North Am. 2012;50(4):731–47.
36. Horan TC, Culver DH, Gaynes RP, Jarvis WR, Edwards JR, Reid CR. Nosocomial infections in surgical patients in the United States, January 1986-June 1992. National Nosocomial Infections Surveillance (NNIS) System. Infect Control Hosp Epidemiol [Internet]. 1993 Feb [cited 2024 Apr 11];14(2):73–80. Available from: https://pubmed.ncbi.nlm.nih.gov/8440883/
37. Richards MJ, Edwards JR, Culver DH, Gaynes RP. Nosocomial infections in medical intensive care units in the United States. Crit Care Med. 1999;27(5):887–92.
38. Cunningham ME, Girardi F, Papadopoulos EC, Cammisa FP. Spinal infections in patients with compromised immune systems. Clin Orthop Relat Res [Internet]. 2006 [cited 2024 Apr 11];444:73–82. Available from: https://pubmed.ncbi.nlm.nih.gov/16523130/
39. Levi ADO, Dickman CA, Sonntag VKH. Management of postoperative infections after spinal instrumentation. J Neurosurg [Internet]. 1997 [cited 2024 Apr 2];86(6):975–80. Available from: https://pubmed.ncbi.nlm.nih.gov/9171176/
40. Silber JS, Anderson DG, Vaccaro AR, Anderson PA, McCormick P. Management of postprocedural discitis. Spine J [Internet]. 2002 Jul 8 [cited 2024 Apr 2];2(4):279–87. Available from: https://pubmed.ncbi.nlm.nih.gov/14589480/
41. Pull Ter Gunne AF, Mohamed AS, Skolasky RL, Van Laarhoven CJHM, Cohen DB. The presentation, incidence, etiology, and treatment of surgical site infections after spinal surgery. Spine (Phila Pa 1976). 2010 Jun 1;35(13):1323–8.
42. Lall RR, Wong AP, Lall RR, Lawton CD, Smith ZA, Dahdaleh NS. Evidence-based management of deep wound infection after spinal instrumentation. J Clin Neurosci [Internet]. 2015 Feb 1 [cited 2024 Apr 11];22(2):238–42. Available from: https://pubmed.ncbi.nlm.nih.gov/25308619/
43. Yin D, Liu B, Chang Y, Gu H, Zheng X. Management of late-onset deep surgical site infection after instrumented spinal surgery. BMC Surg. 2018;18(1):121.
44. Núñez-Pereira S, Pellisé F, Rodríguez-Pardo D, Pigrau C, Bagó J, Villanueva C, et al. Implant survival after deep infection of an instrumented spinal fusion. Bone Joint J [Internet] 2013 [cited 2024 Apr 11];95-B(8):1121–6. Available from: https://pubmed.ncbi.nlm.nih.gov/23908430/
45. Chen SH, Lee CH, Huang KC, Hsieh PH, Tsai SY. Postoperative wound infection after posterior spinal instrumentation: analysis of long-term treatment outcomes. Eur Spine J. 2015;24(3):561–70.
46. Hegde V, Meredith DS, Huang RC, Kepler CK. Management of postoperative spinal infections. World J Orthop [Internet]. 2012 Nov 11 [cited 2024 Apr 11];3(11):182. Available from: /pmc/articles/PMC3547112/
47. Abbey DM, Turner DM, Warson JS, Wirt TC, Scalley RD. Treatment of postoperative wound infections following spinal fusion with instrumentation. J Spinal Disord [Internet]. 1995 [cited 2024 Apr 12];8(4):278–83. Available from: https://pubmed.ncbi.nlm.nih.gov/8547767/
48. Picada R, Winter RB, Lonstein JE, Denis F, Pinto MR, Smith MD, et al. Postoperative deep wound infection in adults after posterior lumbosacral spine fusion with instrumentation: incidence and management. J Spinal Disord [Internet]. 2000 [cited 2024 Apr 12];13(1):42–5. Available from: https://pubmed.ncbi.nlm.nih.gov/10710149/
49. Clark CE, Shufflebarger HL. Late-developing infection in instrumented idiopathic scoliosis. Spine (Phila Pa 1976) [Internet]. 1999 Sep 15 [cited 2024 Apr 12];24(18):1909–12. Available from: https://pubmed.ncbi.nlm.nih.gov/10515015/
50. Hahn F, Zbinden R, Min K. Late implant infections caused by Propionibacterium acnes in scoliosis surgery. Eur Spine J [Internet]. 2005 Oct [cited 2024 Apr 12];14(8):783–8. Available from: https://pubmed.ncbi.nlm.nih.gov/15841406/
51. Richards BS, Emara KM. Delayed infections after posterior TSRH spinal instrumentation for idiopathic scoliosis: Revisited. Spine (Phila Pa 1976) [Internet]. 2001 Sep 15 [cited 2024 Apr 12];26(18):1990–6. Available from: https://www.researchgate.net/publication/11800492_Delayed_Infections_After_Posterior_TSRH_Spinal_Instrumentation_for_Idiopathic_Scoliosis
52. Atesok K, Vaccaro A, Stippler M, Striano BM, Carr M, Heffernan M, et al. Fate of hardware in spinal Infections. Surg Infect. 2020;21(5):404–10.

53. Chahoud J, Kanafani Z, Kanj SS. Surgical site infections following spine surgery: eliminating the controversies in the diagnosis. Front Med [Internet]. 2014 [cited 2024 Apr 10];1(MAR):7. Available from: http://www.ncbi.nlm.nih.gov/pubmed/25705620
54. Thavarajasingam SG, Vemulapalli KV, Vishnu KS, Ponniah HS, Vogel ASM, Vardanyan R, et al. Conservative versus early surgical treatment in the management of pyogenic spondylodiscitis: a systematic review and meta-analysis. Sci Rep. 2023;13(1):15647.
55. Gelalis ID, Arnaoutoglou CM, Politis AN, Batzaleksis NA, Katonis PG, Xenakis TA. Bacterial wound contamination during simple and complex spinal procedures. A prospective clinical study. Spine J [Internet]. 2011 [cited 2024 Apr 12];11(11):1042–8. Available from: https://pubmed.ncbi.nlm.nih.gov/22122837/
56. Cruse PJE, Foord R. A five-year prospective study of 23,649 surgical wounds. Arch Surg [Internet]. 1973 [cited 2024 Apr 12];107(2):206–10. Available from: https://pubmed.ncbi.nlm.nih.gov/4719566/
57. Dipaola CP, Saravanja DD, Boriani L, Zhang H, Boyd MC, Kwon BK, et al. Postoperative infection treatment score for the spine (PITSS): construction and validation of a predictive model to define need for single versus multiple irrigation and debridement for spinal surgical site infection. Spine J [Internet]. 2012 [cited 2024 Apr 12];12(3):218–30. Available from: https://pubmed.ncbi.nlm.nih.gov/22386957/

MIX
Papier aus verantwortungsvollen Quellen
Paper from responsible sources
FSC® C105338
FSC
www.fsc.org

If you have any concerns about our products,
you can contact us on
**ProductSafety@springernature.com**

In case Publisher is established outside the EU,
the EU authorized representative is:
**Springer Nature Customer Service Center GmbH**
**Europaplatz 3, 69115 Heidelberg, Germany**

Printed by Libri Plureos GmbH
in Hamburg, Germany